Clinical Pathways in Neuro-Ophthalmology

An Evidence-Based Approach

Third Edition

Stacy V. Smith, MD
Neuro-ophthalmologist
Assistant Professor
Department of Neurology
Houston Methodist Neurological Institute
Blanton Eye Institute
Houston Methodist The Woodlands Hospital
The Woodlands, Texas
Assistant Professor
Weill Cornell Medical College
New York, New York

Andrew G. Lee, MD
Chairman
Department of Ophthalmology
Blanton Eye Institute
Houston Methodist Hospital
Houston, Texas
Professor of Ophthalmology, Neurology, and Neurosurgery
Weill Cornell Medical College
New York, New York
Professor of Ophthalmology, UTMB and UT MD
Anderson Cancer Center and Texas A and M College of Medicine (Adjunct)
Houston, Texas
Adjunct Professor
Baylor College of Medicine and The Center for Space Medicine
Houston, Texas
Adjunct Professor
The University of Iowa Hospitals and Clinics
Iowa City, Iowa
Adjunct Professor
The University of Buffalo
Buffalo, New York

Paul W. Brazis, MD
Neuro-ophthalmologist
Professor Emeritus
Departments of Neurology and Ophthalmology
Mayo Clinic
Jacksonville, Florida

32 illustrations

Thieme
New York • Stuttgart • Delhi • Rio de Janeiro

Executive Editor: William Lamsback
Managing Editor: Elizabeth Palumbo
Director, Editorial Services: Mary Jo Casey
Assistant Managing Editor: Haley Paskalides
Production Editor: Naamah Schwartz
International Production Director: Andreas Schabert
Editorial Director: Sue Hodgson
International Marketing Director: Fiona Henderson
International Sales Director: Louisa Turrell
Director of Institutional Sales: Adam Bernacki
Senior Vice President and Chief Operating Officer: Sarah Vanderbilt
President: Brian D. Scanlan

Library of Congress Cataloging-in-Publication Data

Names: Smith, Stacy, (Stacy V.), author. | Lee, Andrew G. | Brazis, Paul W.
Title: Clinical pathways in neuro-ophthalmology : an evidence-based approach / Stacy Smith, Houston Methodist Academic Medicine Associates, The Woodlands, TX, USA, Andrew G. Lee, Blanton Eye Institute, Houston Methodist Eye Associates, Houston, TX, USA, Paul W. Brazis, Dept. of Neurology (Professor Emeritus), Mayo Clinic, Jacksonville, FL, USA.
Description: 3 [edition]. | New York : Thieme, [2019] | Revision of: Clinical pathways in neuro-ophthalmology / Andrew G. Lee, Paul W. Brazis. c2003. 2nd ed. | Includes bibliographical references and index.
Identifiers: LCCN 2018006221 | ISBN 9781626232853 (print) | ISBN 9781626232860 (e-book)
Subjects: LCSH: Neuroophthalmology. | Medical protocols. | Evidence-based medicine.
Classification: LCC RE725 .L44 2019 | DDC 617.7–dc23 LC record available at https://lccn.loc.gov/2018006221

© 2019 Thieme Medical Publishers, Inc.
Thieme Publishers New York
333 Seventh Avenue, New York, NY 10001 USA
+1 800 782 3488, customerservice@thieme.com

Thieme Publishers Stuttgart
Rüdigerstrasse 14, 70469 Stuttgart, Germany
+49 [0]711 8931 421, customerservice@thieme.de

Thieme Publishers Delhi
A-12, Second Floor, Sector-2, Noida-201301
Uttar Pradesh, India
+91 120 45 566 00, customerservice@thieme.in

Thieme Publishers Rio de Janeiro, Thieme Publicações Ltda.
Edifício Rodolpho de Paoli, 25º andar
Av. Nilo Peçanha, 50 – Sala 2508,
Rio de Janeiro 20020-906 Brasil
+55 21 3172-2297 / +55 21 3172-1896

Cover design: Thieme Publishing Group
Typesetting by Thomson Digital, India

Printed in The United States of America by King Printing Company, Inc.   5 4 3 2 1

ISBN 978-1-62623-285-3

Also available as an e-book:
eISBN 978-1-62623-286-0

Important note: Medicine is an ever-changing science undergoing continual development. Research and clinical experience are continually expanding our knowledge, in particular our knowledge of proper treatment and drug therapy. Insofar as this book mentions any dosage or application, readers may rest assured that the authors, editors, and publishers have made every effort to ensure that such references are in accordance with **the state of knowledge at the time of production of the book.**

Nevertheless, this does not involve, imply, or express any guarantee or responsibility on the part of the publishers in respect to any dosage instructions and forms of applications stated in the book. **Every user is requested to examine carefully** the manufacturers' leaflets accompanying each drug and to check, if necessary in consultation with a physician or specialist, whether the dosage schedules mentioned therein or the contraindications stated by the manufacturers differ from the statements made in the present book. Such examination is particularly important with drugs that are either rarely used or have been newly released on the market. Every dosage schedule or every form of application used is entirely at the user's own risk and responsibility. The authors and publishers request every user to report to the publishers any discrepancies or inaccuracies noticed. If errors in this work are found after publication, errata will be posted at www.thieme.com on the product description page.

Some of the product names, patents, and registered designs referred to in this book are in fact registered trademarks or proprietary names even though specific reference to this fact is not always made in the text. Therefore, the appearance of a name without designation as proprietary is not to be construed as a representation by the publisher that it is in the public domain.

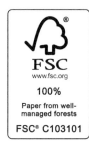

Contents

Contents

Foreword

Never in the history of medicine have physicians had so many ways to both diagnose and treat disease, and never have physicians had so many bureaucratic barriers to performing these activities. This paradox has necessitated a return to the days when clinical judgment was at least as important as diagnostic testing. The challenge to all of us who care for patients is thus to understand the signs and symptoms that distinguish between many different local and systemic disorders so that we can perform the most logical, expeditious, safe, and economic assessment.

Andrew G. Lee is the Chair of the Blanton Eye Institute, Houston Methodist Hospital. He is an ophthalmology-trained neuro-ophthalmologist and holds academic appointments at Weill Cornell Medicine (New York); the University of Texas Medical Branch (UTMB) at Galveston; Baylor College of Medicine (Houston); the University of Texas MD Anderson Cancer Center (UTMDACC) in Houston; Texas A & M College of Medicine; The University of Buffalo (New York); and the University of Iowa Hospitals and Clinics in Iowa City, Iowa.

Paul W. Brazis is a neurology-trained neuro-ophthalmologist and was the head of the neuro-ophthalmology service at the Mayo Clinic in Jacksonville, Florida. He is now Professor Emeritus at Mayo Clinic.

Stacy V. Smith is a neurology-trained neuro-ophthalmologist and headache medicine specialist at Houston Methodist Neurological Institute, Houston Methodist The Woodlands Hospital.

The authors have extensive training and experience in the field of neuro-ophthalmology, and have contributed singly and together to the field of neuro-ophthalmology with numerous articles, chapters, and textbooks. In this book, the authors provide the reader with a triumvirate of information. First, they describe the symptoms and signs of a variety of neuro-ophthalmologic disorders, such as anterior and retrobulbar optic neuropathies, ocular motor nerve pareses, and other disorders of ocular motility and alignment, and anisocoria. Second, they provide algorithms for differentiating, both in the office and using laboratory and neuroimaging studies, between conditions that often have overlapping clinical manifestations. Third, they provide a basic set of references about each subject that the reader can use to expand his or her knowledge.

By providing basic, clinically relevant information regarding various disorders, as well as their diagnoses and treatments, this book teaches the reader how to approach a patient with a known or presumed neuro-ophthalmologic problem in a logical, straightforward, and cost-effective manner. As such, it is a welcome addition to the neuro-ophthalmologic repertoire.

Neil R. Miller, MD
Baltimore, Maryland

Preface

The primary goal of the first edition of this book was to provide the reader with an easy-to-follow, heavily referenced guide to the management of common neuro-ophthalmologic conditions. In this edition, we have specifically chosen to focus on recent references, and we emphasize the best available clinical evidence. To this end, we include letters or case reports if they add significant new information. We include pre-1990 references only if they are of historical significance. We have tried to be inclusive, however, in the construction of our tables and charts, and provide the references as needed. The secondary goal of this book is to discuss and classify the available clinical evidence concerning the evaluation and treatment of various neuro-ophthalmologic processes and grade the strength of any recommendations that are made. Readers will have to judge for themselves which is the best approach for the individual patient; the authors emphasize that these guidelines are not meant to define any particular standard of care for these conditions.

In this edition, we classify the clinical evidence into the following four categories and, where appropriate, summarize the class of evidence for each section.

1. Class I: Well-designed, randomized, power-controlled clinical trials including meta-analyses of such trials.

2. Class II: Well-designed controlled studies without randomization including meta-analyses of such studies.
3. Class III: Retrospective observational studies, cohort, or case–control studies, or multiple time series with or without intervention.
4. Class IV: Expert opinion, case series, case reports.

We grade the strength of the recommendations from each section as follows:

1. Level A: A principle for patient management reflecting a high degree of clinical certainty (usually requires class I evidence that directly addresses the clinical question).
2. Level B: A recommendation reflecting moderate clinical certainty based on either class II evidence or strong consensus of class III evidence with significant and consistent results.
3. Level C: An acceptable practice option with low clinical certainty based on class III or class IV evidence.
4. Level U: Inconclusive or conflicting evidence, or opinion that is insufficient to support an evidence-based recommendation.

Stacy V. Smith, MD
Andrew G. Lee, MD
Paul W. Brazis, MD (Professor Emeritus)

Acknowledgments

We would again like to thank our mentor, colleague, and friend Dr. Neil R. Miller for his encouragement and example. Dr. Brazis would also like to thank the following individuals for their guidance: Drs. James Corbett, Jonathan Trobe, James Bolling, and Frank Rubino. He is appreciative of the encouragement and support of his family, especially Elizabeth, Erica, Paul, and Kelly Brazis.

Dr. Lee acknowledges the support and encouragement of the seven outstanding chairmen of ophthalmology with whom he has had the honor to serve over the years: Drs. Mort Goldberg, Dan B. Jones, Thomas Weingeist, Keith Carter, Tim Stout, Bernard Godley, and Kevin Merkley. He thanks his parents Drs. Alberto C. Lee and Rosalind G. Lee for instilling in a young man the thirst for knowledge and intellectual curiosity. He is particularly thankful to his loving, patient, and tolerant wife, Dr. Hilary A. Beaver, who has been both a source of academic inspiration and a creative muse. Dr. Lee also thanks his two children, Rachael Elizabeth Lee and Virginia Anne Lee, for keeping his priorities straight and his mind and soul humble. He hopes that one day they will join the tradition and long line of Lee family physicians.

Dr. Smith especially thanks her mentors Drs. Deborah I. Friedman and Andrew G. Lee for their support and guidance, as well as all the many dedicated coauthors on this project. Dr. Smith also acknowledges the unwavering support and encouragement of her friends and family, especially her husband, Joseph, mother, Charlene, and father, Thomas.

We appreciate the assistance of our editors at Thieme Medical Publishers. We thank the faculty and residents of the Departments of Ophthalmology, Neurology, and Neurosurgery at the Houston Methodist Hospital, Baylor College of Medicine, and UTMB as well as the faculty and staff in the Departments of Neurology and Ophthalmology at the Mayo Clinic in Jacksonville, Florida, for their academic support and stimulation.

The Editors

Contributors

Alec L. Amram, MD
Resident
Department of Ophthalmology
University of Texas Medical Branch
Galveston, Texas

Shauna Berry, DO
Pediatric Ophthalmology and Adult Strabismus Fellow
University of California, Los Angeles
Los Angeles, California

Paul W. Brazis, MD
Neuro-ophthalmologist
Professor Emeritus
Departments of Neurology and Ophthalmology
Mayo Clinic
Jacksonville, Florida

Paul D. Chamberlain
Medical Student
Baylor College of Medicine
Houston, Texas

Benjamin A. Dake, MD
Resident
Department of Ophthalmology
University of South Florida
Tampa, Florida

Angeline Mariani Derham, MD
Ophthalmology Resident
New York Medical College
Jamaica Hospital Medical Center
Queens, New York

John D. Eatman, MD
Assistant Professor
University of Missouri-Kansas City School of Medicine
Neurologist
Saint Luke's Neurology
Kansas City, Missouri

William J. Hertzing
Medical Student
University of Texas Medical Branch
Department of Ophthalmology and Visual Sciences
Galveston, Texas

Andrew G. Lee, MD
Chairman
Department of Ophthalmology
Blanton Eye Institute
Houston Methodist Hospital
Houston, Texas
Professor of Ophthalmology, Neurology, and Neurosurgery
Weill Cornell Medical College
New York, New York
Professor of Ophthalmology, UTMB and UT MD
Anderson Cancer Center and Texas A & M College of
    Medicine (Adjunct)
Houston, Texas
Adjunct Professor
Baylor College of Medicine and The Center for Space
    Medicine
Houston, Texas
Adjunct Professor
The University of Iowa Hospitals and Clinics
Iowa City, Iowa
Adjunct Professor
The University of Buffalo
Buffalo, New York

Weijie V. Lin
Medical Student
Baylor College of Medicine
Houston, Texas

Leanne M. Little
Medical Student
Baylor College of Medicine
Houston, Texas

Murtaza M. Mandviwala
Medical Student
University of Texas Medical Branch
Galveston, Texas

Austin S. Nakatsuka, MD
Resident
Department of Ophthalmology
University of Texas Medical Branch
Galveston, Texas

Mohammad Obadah Nakawah, MD
Neurologist
Department of Neurology
Houston Methodist Neurological Institute
Weill Cornell Medical College
Houston, Texas

Andres S. Parra, BA
Medical Student
Baylor College of Medicine
Houston, Texas

Grecia Rico, MD
Graduate Research Fellow
Department of Pathology and Genomic Medicine
Houston Methodist Hospital
Houston, Texas

Mohammed Rigi, MD, MS
Resident
Department of Pathology
University of Alabama at Birmingham
Birmingham, Alabama

Elsa Rodarte, MD
Resident
Department of Neurology
The University of Texas Health Science Center
  at Houston
Houston, Texas

Ama Sadaka, MD
Assistant Professor
Ophthalmologist
Lebanese American University Medical Center Rizk Hospital
Beirut, Lebanon

Beena M. Shah, BBA
Medical Student
Baylor College of Medicine
Houston, Texas

Noreen Shaikh, MD
Ophthalmology Resident
MedStar Georgetown University Hospital/
  Washington Hospital Center
Washington, DC

Stacy V. Smith, MD
Neuro-ophthalmologist
Assistant Professor
Department of Neurology
Houston Methodist Neurological Institute
Houston Methodist The Woodlands Hospital
The Woodlands, Texas

Alison K. Yoder
Medical Student
Baylor College of Medicine
Houston, Texas

1 The Diagnosis of Optic Neuropathies

Ama Sadaka, Paul D. Chamberlain, Leanne M. Little, and Shauna Berry

Abstract

Optic neuropathy refers to disease or damage to the optic nerve, typically characterized by decreased visual acuity, decreased color vision, visual field defect, relative afferent pupillary defect, optic disc edema, and/or optic disc atrophy. Possible etiologies include hereditary, inflammatory, infiltrative, ischemic, demyelinating (optic neuritis), toxic, and compressive optic neuropathies. This chapter discusses the clinical pathway for evaluating and diagnosing optic neuropathy, reviewing the literature in detail.

Keywords: optic neuropathy, hereditary optic neuropathy, radiation optic neuropathy, compressive optic neuropathy, toxic/nutritional optic neuropathy

1.1 Introduction

The diagnosis of an optic neuropathy is usually made on clinical grounds alone. Several excellent references discuss in detail the anatomy of the optic nerve as well as examination techniques.[1,2,3] The clinical features of optic neuropathies include decreased visual acuity, decreased color vision, visual field defect, relative afferent pupillary defect (RAPD), optic disc edema, and/or optic disc atrophy. Other more complex (and time-consuming) testing for optic neuropathy, such as visual evoked potentials (VEPs), flicker fusion, formal color vision testing, and contrast sensitivity, can be performed but in general are not required to establish the clinical diagnosis of optic neuropathy and are not discussed here.

Once the diagnosis of optic neuropathy has been made, it is important to consider a wide differential diagnosis of possible etiologies, including hereditary, inflammatory, infiltrative, ischemic, demyelinating (optic neuritis [ON]), toxic, and compressive optic neuropathies. We refer the reader to the specific chapter on each type of optic neuropathy for further details.

1.2 Can the Appearance of the Optic Nerve Differentiate Etiology?

In general, the appearance of the optic nerve (e.g., normal, swollen, or pale) is not specific and cannot differentiate among various possible etiologies for optic neuropathy. Trobe et al[4] reviewed 163 color fundus photographs of several entities resulting in optic atrophy, including glaucoma, central retinal artery occlusion (CRAO), ischemic optic neuropathy (ION), ON, hereditary optic neuropathy (Leber and non-Leber types), compressive optic neuropathy (CON), and traumatic optic neuropathy (TON). These photographs were reviewed by five ophthalmologists as "unknowns." Glaucoma, CRAO, and ION were correctly identified as the etiology by at least one of the five observers with an accuracy above 80%, but the remaining etiologies were correctly identified in less than 50% of cases. Helpful features in differentiating the entities included the following:

1. The presence of retinal arteriolar attenuation and sheathing in ischemic lesions (e.g., CRAO or ION).
2. Temporal pallor in entities selectively involving central vision and central visual field with sparing of peripheral visual field (e.g., ON and toxic optic neuropathies).
3. Superior or inferior (sector) optic disc pallor in ION.

Although optic disc cupping was often identified in glaucoma, it was also seen in 20% of cases not associated with glaucoma. Optic disc cupping in glaucoma cases, however, was more profound than in nonglaucomatous cases and greater neuroretinal rim pallor occurred in the nonglaucomatous cases. In patients with glaucoma, there is often absence of at least part of the neuroretinal rim, and the color of the remaining rim is normal. With nonglaucomatous optic neuropathy, rarely is any area of the rim completely absent and the remaining rim is often pale. Interestingly, only 11% of these cases with a known history of papillitis or ION had sufficient clues to identify previous disc swelling.[4]

Another study suggested that optic disc appearance may help differentiate anterior ischemic optic neuropathy (AION) from ON, although there are overlapping features. Optic disc stereographs were reviewed by masked observers (87 AION and 68 ON).[5] Altitudinal disc swelling was more than three times more common in AION than ON, although most discs were diffusely swollen. Most patients with AION had hemorrhages, whereas most ON cases did not. Almost all discs with ON had normal color or were hyperemic; only 35% of discs with AION had pallid swelling. Pallid swelling was so rare in ON, however, that of discs with pallor, 93% had AION. Arterial attenuation was also much more typical of AION. AION was the clinical diagnosis in 82% of cases with altitudinal edema, 81% of cases with disc hemorrhage, 93% of cases with pallid edema, and 90% of cases with arterial attenuation. A pale optic nerve with hemorrhage, regardless of type of edema, always represented AION (100%). A hyperemic optic nerve with hemorrhage represented AION in 82% of cases, but if altitudinal edema was also present, the incidence of AION increased to 93%. Conversely, a normal color optic nerve without hemorrhage represented ON in 91% of cases.

In addition, numerous authors have stressed the localizing value to the optic chiasm or optic tract of a special type of optic atrophy caused by specific involvement of the nerve fiber layer of the nasal and temporal retina, respectively. A lesion of the optic tract may result in "band" (or "bow tie") atrophy in the eye contralateral to the involved optic tract. Band atrophy correlates clinically with loss of vision in the temporal visual field and is due to atrophy of the nerve fibers from the nasal half of the retina that then enter the optic disc nasally and temporally. Band atrophy may be unilateral or bilateral with lesions of the optic chiasm.

Neither the pattern (e.g., central scotoma, arcuate, altitudinal) of ipsilateral visual field impairment nor the severity of visual loss is pathognomonic for any specific optic neuropathy, and virtually any visual field defect may occur with any optic neuropathy.[6] In their report on 35 eyes in 20 patients with CON and 70 eyes in 54 patients with ON, Trobe and Glaser[6] found central scotomas in 33% of cases of CON (vs. 75% in ON) and felt that a central scotoma could not be used as a differentiating feature between the two entities.

The following sections describe the evaluation of optic neuropathy; this approach is summarized in ▶ Fig. 1.1. We begin with an age-based differential diagnosis of an acute optic neuropathy. Two of the most common causes of acute optic neuropathy are AION and ON. Although there is considerable overlap in their clinical presentation, age can be used as an initial differentiating feature in many cases.[7] In younger patients (< 40 years

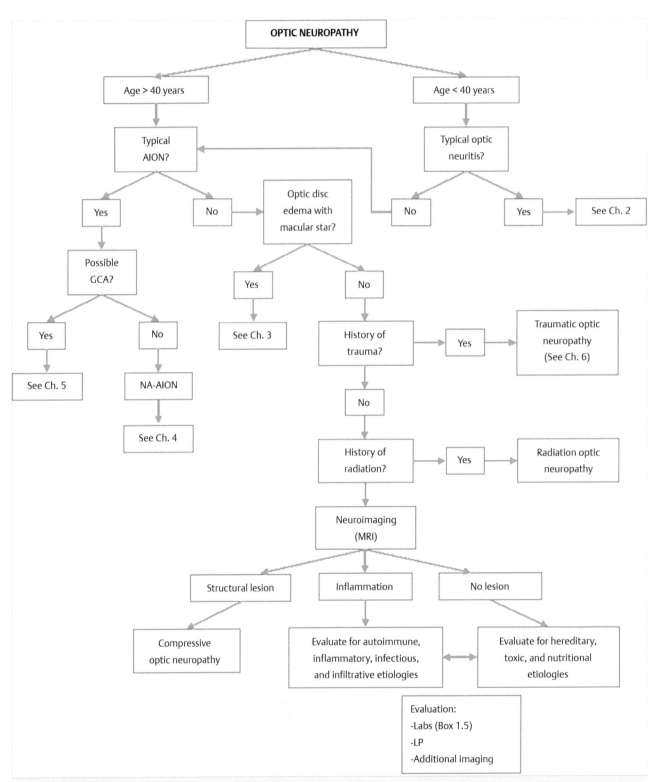

Fig. 1.1 Evaluation of an optic neuropathy. Please refer to the respective chapters on each disorder for additional evaluation and treatment recommendations.

old) with acute unilateral optic disc edema and evidence for an optic neuropathy, ON is more likely than AION. Conversely, in the older patient with acute optic disc edema and visual loss, AION is more common (class III).

1.3 Is the Clinical Presentation Typical for Anterior Ischemic Optic Neuropathy?

The features of typical AION are discussed in Chapter 4. If these features are present, the patient should undergo an evaluation for underlying vasculopathic risk factors and giant cell arteritis (classes III–IV, level B).

1.4 Is the Clinical Presentation Typical for Optic Neuritis?

The features and evaluation of typical ON are described in Chapter 2.

1.5 Is the Clinical Presentation Consistent with Optic Disc Edema with a Macular Star?

The evaluation of optic disc edema with a macular star (ODEMS) is outlined in Chapter 3.

1.6 Is a Compressive Optic Neuropathy Present?

CON usually causes painless, progressive, gradual loss of visual function (visual acuity, visual field, and color vision), a RAPD (in unilateral or asymmetric cases), and optic disc edema or atrophy (but the optic disc may initially appear normal).[1,2,6] Unfortunately, CON may also present acutely or be steroid responsive and may masquerade as an inflammatory or demyelinating optic neuropathy.

CON that is due to orbital or intracanalicular lesions may result in ipsilateral optic disc edema, followed by optic atrophy and may be associated with the development of abnormal blood vessels on the disc head called optociliary shunt vessels. These vessels probably represent collateral circulation between the retinal and choroidal venous circulation that allows venous blood to bypass the compression at the level of the optic nerve. The presence of an unexplained RAPD or unexplained optic atrophy should prompt appropriate neuroimaging studies (usually magnetic resonance imaging [MRI] of the involved optic nerve).[8] Optical coherence tomography (OCT) also may help differentiate compressive and glaucomatous optic neuropathy.[9,10,11] Orbital signs such as proptosis, chemosis, or conjunctival injection should direct the imaging studies to the orbit (classes III–IV, level B). Box 1.1 lists some possible causes of CON. Optic atrophy in the presence of painless and progressive vision loss, hemianopic field loss, and bilateral disease indicate the

increased likelihood of a compressive etiology.[12] Common tumors affecting the anterior visual pathways include meningiomas, optic nerve gliomas, and craniopharyngiomas.[13,14]

Box 1.1 Lesions causing compressive optic neuropathy

- Intracranial or intraorbital benign and malignant tumors[1,15,16,17,18,19]:
  - Meningioma.[20]
  - Meningocele.[21]
  - Glioma.
  - Craniopharyngioma.
  - Pituitary adenoma.[22,23]
  - Germinoma.[24]
  - Lymphoma and leukemia.[25,26,27,28,29]
  - Sinus histiocytosis with massive lymphadenopathy.[30,31,32,33]
  - Langerhans cell histiocytosis.[34]
  - Nasopharyngeal cancer.[35]
  - Metastasis.[36,37,38,39,40,41,42,43,44,45]
  - Sellar/suprasellar arachnoid cyst.[46]
  - Melanocytoma of the optic nerve.[47,48]
- Dermoid cyst.[49]
- Orbital cyst.[50]
- Extramedullary hematopoiesis.[51,52,53,54]
- Orbital fractures.
- Pneumatocele.[55,56]
- Inflammatory or infectious diseases (e.g., mucoceles, sclerosing orbital inflammation, cholesterol granuloma, neurosarcoidosis, acute febrile neutrophilic dermatosis, sphenoidal sinus inflammation, perinuclear antineutrophil cytoplasmic antibody [p-ANCA]/cytoplasmic cytoplasmic antibody [c-ANCA] vasculitis, fungal hypertrophic cranial pachymeningitis, amyloidosis, aspergillosis, and nodular fasciitis).[57,58,59,60,61,62,63,64,65,66,67,68,69,70,71,72,73,74,75,76]
- Idiopathic hypertrophic cranial pachymeningitis.[77,78,79,80,81,82,83,84,85,86,87,88,89,90,91]
- Primary bone diseases (e.g., osteopetrosis, fibrous dysplasia, craniometaphyseal dysplasia, fibrosclerosis, Paget disease, aneurysmal bone cyst, pneumosinus dilatans, etc.).[52,92,93,94,95,96,97,98,99,100,101,102,103,104,105,106,107,108]
- Vascular etiologies:
  - Orbital hemorrhage.[109,110,111,112,113,114,115]
  - Subperiosteal hematoma.[116,117,118]
  - Orbital venous anomalies.[119,120]
  - Arteriovenous malformations (e.g., carotid cavernous sinus fistula).[121]
  - Hemangioma.[122,123]
  - Carotid artery and anterior communicating artery aneurysms.[52,124,125,126,127,128,129,130]
  - Dolichoectasia of the carotid artery.[131,132,133]
  - Compression by supraclinoid carotid artery.[132,134,135]
  - Hypertensive intracranial ophthalmic artery.[136]
- Lymphatic malformation.[137,138,139]
- Thyroid ophthalmopathy (see Chapter 16).
- Hydrocephalus.
- Iatrogenic:
  - Intracranial catheters.[140]
  - Intranasal balloon catheter.

- ○ Intracranial oxidized cellulose hemostat.[141]
- ○ Postoperative (e.g., postoptic canal decompression, sinus surgery, postcraniotomy, following use of oxidized regenerated cellulose).[142,143,144,145]
- ○ Muslinoma.[146,147]
- ○ Maxillary artery embolization.[148]

1.6.1 Meningioma

Meningiomas are more commonly seen in middle-aged (peak in the fifth decade), white females (female:male = 3:1).[149] They can be present anywhere along optic pathway.[14,150] They can be bilateral especially if associated with neurofibromatosis type 2.[151,152,153,154,155] Symptoms can vary from asymptomatic to gradually progressive loss of vision or visual field defects, and may have mental status changes if involving frontal lobe, diplopia if cavernous sinus involved, and anosmia if involving the olfactory groove.[156,157,158] Patients may experience pain with orbital meningiomas, even before noting vision loss.[159] These lesions tend to grow slow but may grow faster during pregnancy, or shrink afterward.[160,161,162,163,164,165,166,167]

Examination findings can include RAPD, optic disc edema, optic atrophy, optociliary shunt vessels (retinochoroidal venous collaterals), proptosis, visual field deficits, and motility deficits.[168,169,170,171,172,173] Indocyanine green videoangiography may show abnormal hemodynamics of choroidal circulation in patients with sheath meningiomas.[174] Different visual field defects can be observed depending on the location of the tumor including generalized depression or constriction (orbital/canal/sphenoid), central/paracentral/cecocentral (orbital/canal), homonymous hemianopia (suprasellar/sphenoid), and bitemporal hemianopia (suprasellar/sphenoid).[175,176,177,178,179] The motility deficits are usually secondary to a restrictive pattern if the tumor is in the orbit or from a paretic pattern if there is compression of any of the cranial nerves, with the most common being the sixth nerve palsy.[180] Exophthalmos can also be visualized in the presence of an orbital or sphenoid meningioma.[181]

The differential diagnosis for an optic nerve sheath meningioma can include sarcoidosis and other granulomatous diseases, meningocele, ON, hypertrophic cranial pachymeningitis, inflammatory pseudotumor, immunoglobulin G4 (IgG4) related disease, sinus histiocytosis with massive lymphadenopathy, and metastasis.[45,168,182,183,184,185,186,187,188,189,190,191,192,193,194,195,196,197,198,199,200]

Treatment of a meningioma affecting the optic pathway depends on the location and whether they are causing compressive damage. If asymptomatic, the lesions are usually observed.[201] Treatment with vascular endothelial growth factor antagonists (VEGF-A; bevacizumab)[202] and hormonal agents have demonstrated some modest success in recurrent meningiomas.[203] More invasive measures include debulking surgery,[196,204,205,206,207,208,209,210,211] gamma knife radiosurgery,[212,213,214] and radiation therapy.[215,216,217,218,219,220,221,222,223,224,225,226,227,228,229,230,231,232,233,234,235] The algorithm for management of meningiomas affecting the optic pathway is delineated in ▶ Fig. 1.2.

1.6.2 Optic Nerve Glioma

Optic pathway gliomas (OPGs) are predominantly classified as pilocytic astrocytomas with 10 to 30% confined to unilateral optic nerve. They can present at any age, but the majority present before the age of 10 years (mean 8.8 years) with no sex predilection. The more anterior their location, the better the prognosis usually.[236] The location of infiltration can be nerve alone (24%), optic disc (1.6%), optic chiasm, or tract (75.7%).[237,238,239,240,241,242,243,244,245,246,247,248,249,250,251,252,253,254,255,256,257,258,259,260,261,262,263,264,265,266,267,268,269,270,271,272,273,274,275,276,277,278] Parenchymal optic nerve enlargement, along with optic nerve sheath meningioma and metastasis, should be considered on the differential diagnosis.[279,280,281,282,283,284] More information about malignant gliomas of the anterior visual pathway in adults is outlined in Box 1.2.

> **Box 1.2 Clinical features of adult malignant gliomas of the anterior visual pathway**
>
> - Epidemiology:
>   - ○ Age at presentation: middle-age; range 6 to 79 years, mean 47.8; 73% were 40 years or older.
>   - ○ Sex: 65% males and 35% females.
>   - ○ No association with NF1 (neurofibromatosis).
> - Clinical signs and symptoms[285,286,287,288,289,290,291,292,293,294,295,296]:
>   - ○ Decreased vision:
>   - – Bilateral or unilateral.
>   - – Visual acuity usually falls to blindness over average of 11.1 weeks (range 1–60 weeks).
>   - – Optic nerve visual field defects.
>   - ○ Normal discs, optic disc swelling, or atrophy.
>   - ○ Proptosis.
>   - ○ Ophthalmoplegia.
>   - ○ Retro-orbital pain common.
>   - ○ Macular edema, cherry-red spot, and flame hemorrhage or hemorrhagic papillopathy may mimic central retinal vein occlusion (CRVO).
> - Location:
>   - ○ Involves chiasm and at least one contiguous optic nerve; often involves hypothalamus, third ventricle, basal ganglia, and temporal lobe.
>   - ○ Primarily affects chiasm and intracranial optic nerves.
> - Treatment[243,245,246,248,249,251,252,255,256,257,264,265,266,267,268,270,271,272,273,275,276,277,297,298,299,300,301,302,303,304,305,306,307,308,309,310,311,312,313,314,315,316,317,318,319]:
>   - ○ Radiation.
>   - ○ Chemotherapy.
>   - ○ Treatment may temporarily improve or rarely stabilize vision.
> - Pathology: malignant astrocytoma.
> - Prognosis[262,269,289,320,321,322,323,324]:
>   - ○ Poor.
>   - ○ Overall mortality 97%.
>   - ○ Mean survival 8.7 months (3–24 months).

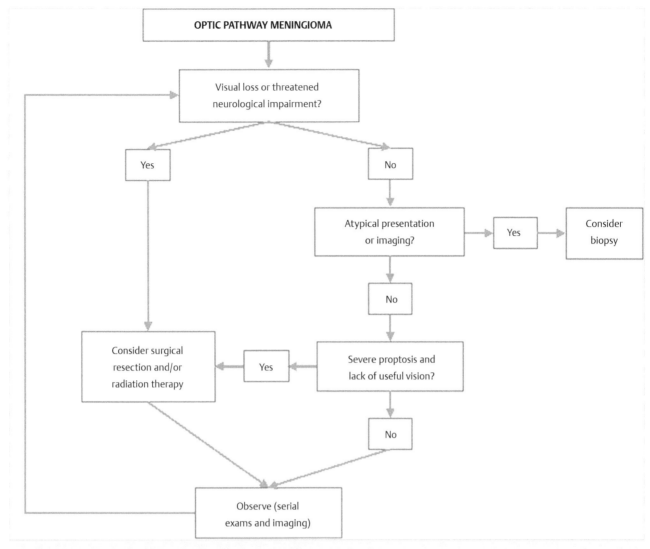

Fig. 1.2 Treatment algorithm for meningiomas affecting optic pathway.

The majority of patients (87.5%) with OPG have vision loss at presentation. Hypothalamic or endocrinologic symptoms such as diabetes insipidus, diencephalic wasting, precocious puberty, somnolence, and growth failure may be present in up to a quarter of the patients. Optic nerve gliomas are commonly associated with NF1 (29%), with 15% of NF1 patients with no visual symptoms having a glioma.[312,325,326]

Treatment recommendations include observation if stable (classes III–IV, level B), chemotherapy (classes III–IV, level C) as first line for progressive tumors, radiation therapy (classes III–IV, level C), and surgery (classes III–IV, level C) if considered resectable.[299,300,301,303,304,305,306,307,309,310,313,314,315,316,317,319,327,328] Magnetic resonance scan with gadolinium, while superior to computed tomography (CT), does not consistently predict visual field defects.[240,253,329,330,331] In a pediatric population and in those patients with NF1, OCT has been used as a clinical tool for detection of tumor.[294,332,333,334,335] Treatment options are outlined in ▶ Fig. 1.3.[297] The prognosis is generally good with 80% maintaining stable vision after an initial period of visual loss.[336] Spontaneous regression may occur.

1.6.3 Craniopharyngioma

Please refer to Box 1.3 for the clinical features of craniopharyngioma.

> **Box 1.3 Clinical features of craniopharyngiomas**[337,338,339,340,341,342,343,344,345]
>
> - Any age:
>   - Bimodal incidence.
>   - Peak age: younger than 20 years and 50 to 70 years.
> - Equal sex distribution.
> - Clinical:
>   - Decreased visual acuity (optic nerve, chiasm, optic tract).
>   - In children—often decreased acuity and papilledema (50%).
>   - In adults—less commonly papilledema.
>   - Signs of increased intracranial pressure (headache, nausea, vomiting).

○ Endocrine:
  – Absent or precocious sexual development.
  – Growth disturbances.
  – Variable hypopituitarism.
  – Diabetes insipidus.
  – Obesity.
  – Impotence.
  – Amenorrhea/galactorrhea.
○ Somnolence, confusion, or dementia (especially in older patients).
○ Ocular findings.
○ Seesaw nystagmus.
○ Visual field defects:
  – Inferior bitemporal field defect (most have field defects).
  – May have incongruous, asymmetric defect.

  – May involve optic tract.
  – May cause ocular motor nerve palsies.
• Neuroimaging:
○ MRI delineates tumor and intracranial anatomy.
○ CT shows calcification better.
○ Occasionally may infiltrate optic nerve, chiasm tract, mimicking primary intrinsic tumor such as optic glioma ("potbelly" appearance of optic nerve).
• Treatment:
○ Surgical: complete versus partial resection.
○ Radiotherapy.
○ Cyst aspiration and P32 instillation.
○ Consider intracystic chemotherapy (bleomycin).
○ Secondary malignant glioma can develop after radiation therapy.

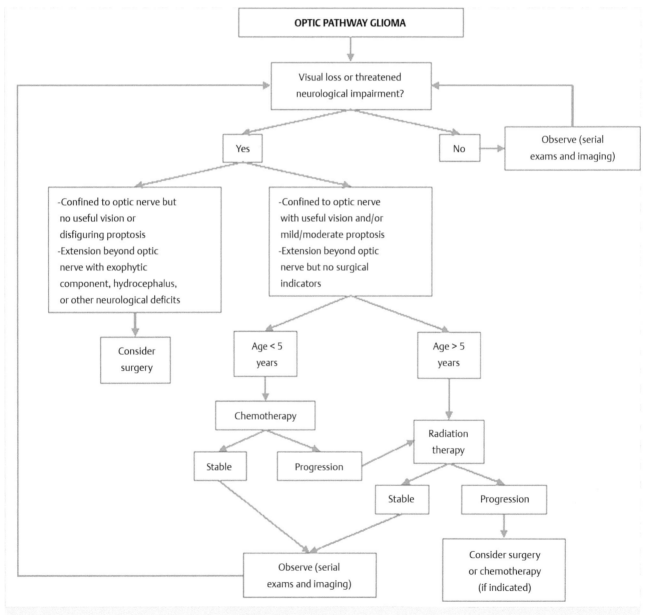

Fig. 1.3 Treatment algorithm for optic pathway gliomas.[218]

1.7 Is There Clinical Evidence for an Infiltrative or Inflammatory Optic Neuropathy?

Infiltrative or inflammatory optic neuropathy may present with the typical features of an optic neuropathy discussed earlier. As described in Chapter 2, the clinical profile of typical ON (e.g., pain with eye movement, typical age of onset, etc.) should be differentiated from atypical ON (e.g., lack of pain, atypical age of onset, anterior or posterior segment inflammation, etc.). Atypical cases should undergo an evaluation for infiltrative or inflammatory etiologies as listed in Box 1.4 (class IV, level C).

Patients with inflammatory autoimmune optic neuropathy often have a progressive or recurrent steroid-responsive or steroid-dependent clinical course. A more detailed discussion of the evaluation of atypical ON and these alternative etiologies is found in Chapter 2. Evaluation should include infectious, inflammatory, neoplastic, toxic, and hereditary etiologies. The appropriate specific laboratory studies should be directed by the pertinent history and examination findings (Box 1.5). In addition to an MRI of the brain and orbits with and without contrast, a lumbar puncture and chest radiograph also may be reasonable first-line tests in this setting.

Box 1.4 Infiltrative or inflammatory optic neuropathies

- Neoplastic:
  - Plasmacytoma and multiple myeloma.[346]
  - Carcinomatous meningitis.[36,347,348,349,350,351]
  - Leukemia.[352,353,354,355,356,357,358,359]
  - Lymphoma.[360,361,362,363,364,365,366,367,368,369,370,371,372,373]
  - Metastases.[374]
  - Infiltrative orbitopathy in POEMS (polyneuropathy, organomegaly, endocrinopathy, monoclonal protein, skin changes) syndrome.
- Paraneoplastic disease.[348,375,376,377,378,379,380,381,382]
- Calciphylaxis.[383]
- Infectious etiologies:
  - Cryptococcal meningitis.[384]
  - Aspergillus.[385,386,387,388]
  - Mucormycosis.[389]
  - Cysticercosis.[390,391,392,393]
  - Lyme disease.[330,394]
  - Tuberculosis.[382]
  - Toxoplasmosis.[395,396]
  - Syphilis.[382,397,398]
  - Cat-scratch disease.[382,399]
  - Human immunodeficiency virus (HIV; acquired immunodeficiency syndrome [AIDS]).[396,400]
  - Human herpes virus 6.[401]
  - Herpes simplex virus.[402]
  - West Nile virus.[382]
- Inflammatory diseases[1,403]:
  - Eosinophilic granulomatosis with polyangiitis (previously Churg–Strauss syndrome).[404]
  - Contiguous sinus disease.
  - Behçet disease.[405,406]
  - Sarcoidosis.[382,407,408,409,410,411,412,413,414,415,416,417]

- Granulomatosis with polyangiitis (previously Wegener granulomatosis).[382,405,418,419]
- Systemic lupus erythematosus.[382,405,420,421,422,423]
- Sjögren syndrome.[382,405,424]
- Relapsing polychondritis.
- Rheumatoid meningitis.[425,426]
- Polyarteritis nodose.[405]
- Inflammatory bowel disease.[427,428]
- Granulomatous hypophysitis.[429]
- Isolated optic nerve pseudotumor.[430]
- Reactive lymphocytosis with pseudolymphoma from phenytoin.[431]
- Immunoglobulin G4-related disease

Box 1.5 Laboratory evaluation of an atypical or unexplained optic neuropathy

- Infectious etiologies:
  - Syphilis serology, interferon gamma release assay (IGRA), *Bartonella* titers for cat-scratch disease, toxoplasmosis titers, toxocara titers, and Lyme titers.
- Inflammatory etiologies:
  - Erythrocyte sedimentation rate, antinuclear antibody, anti-double-stranded deoxyribonucleic acid (DNA), rheumatoid factor, anticyclic citrullinated peptide antibodies, anticyclic complement levels, antineutrophil cytoplasmic antibody, angiotensin-converting enzyme, aquaporin-4 antibody, and myelin oligodendrocyte glycoprotein antibody.
- Neoplastic etiologies:
  - Complete blood count and paraneoplastic antibody profile.
- Toxic etiologies:
  - Serum vitamin B12, methylmalonic acid, folate levels, and heavy metal screen.
- Hereditary etiologies:
  - Leber hereditary optic neuropathy mutation blood test.

1.7.1 Immunoglobulin G4–Related Optic Neuropathy

Patients with IgG4-related disease may harbor destructive tissue fibrosis or sclerosis in numerous organs, as well as the tendency to form tumefactive lesions in more than one site.[186,432,433] The disease may induce lesions involving the orbit, extraocular muscles, lacrimal system, optic nerve, or sclera.[434,435,436,437,438] This may present as orbital myositis, perineuritis of the optic and trigeminal nerves, and orbital inflammation.[433,439,440] Lacrimal involvement is a common orbital manifestation of the disease, with orbital mass/optic nerve lesions being less common.[186,441]

The proposed diagnostic criteria include elevated IgG4+ plasma cells within affected tissue, along with characteristic histological features including a dense lymphoplasmacytic infiltrate, fibrosis typically arranged in a storiform pattern, and obliterative phlebitis.[432] It is notable that up to 40% of patients with biopsy-proven IgG4-related disease have normal serum levels of IG.[432] In the case of suspected optic nerve involvement, MRI may demonstrate infraorbital nerve enlargement.[442] Confirmatory diagnosis can be made with biopsy of affected tissue and immunostaining for IgG and IgG4, with the presence of greater than 30 IgG4 + plasma cells per high-powered field.[432]

Differential diagnosis for intraorbital IgG4-related disease includes idiopathic orbital inflammatory syndrome and the Tolosa–Hunt syndrome, as well as other etiologies of mass lesions including sarcoidosis, Castleman's disease, granulomatosis with polyangiitis (Wegener granulomatosis), lymphoma, pleomorphic adenoma, hemangioma, and carcinoma.[186,432] While low-grade B-cell lymphomas can also produce elevated IgG4, this diagnosis can be excluded with genetic testing and careful histopathologic analysis.[186,432]

Treatment of IgG4-related disease includes systemic corticosteroids, rituximab, azathioprine, and antirheumatic drugs such as methotrexate.[186,434,435,441] Recurrence is unlikely, but has been reported, especially during tapering of pharmacotherapy.[186,433] Prognosis is typically good for patients with IgG4-related disease; however, the incidence of developing cancer within 3 years is increased as compared to the general population.[433]

1.8 Is There Evidence for Traumatic Optic Neuropathy?

The features and evaluation of TON are discussed in Chapter 6.

1.9 Is There Evidence for a Toxic or Nutritional Optic Neuropathy?

Patients with toxic optic neuropathies usually present with painless, bilaterally symmetric, and slowly progressive visual loss. The visual field defect is typically bilateral central or cecocentral scotomas. The optic nerves may appear normal until late in the course of the disease when optic atrophy (often temporal pallor) usually develops. Occasionally, the discs may be swollen and slightly hyperemic. A number of medications and toxins may result in optic neuropathy.[443,444,445,446] These are summarized in Box 1.6. Most of these etiologies can be excluded by a careful and detailed exposure and occupational history.

Box 1.6 Etiologies for toxic optic neuropathy

- Common etiologies:
  - Ethambutol—tuberculosis therapy.[447,448,449,450,451,452,453, 454,455,456,457,458,459,460]
  - Ethanol and tobacco (nutritional optic neuropathy—formerly tobacco-alcohol amblyopia).[444,445,446,455,456,457, 461,462,463]
- Less common etiologies:
  - Amantadine—antiviral, treatment of Parkinson disease.
  - Amiodarone—cardiac disease.[446,455,456,457,458,460,464,465,466, 467,468,469]
  - Amoproxan—vasodilator and antiarrhythmic.
  - Aniline dyes.
  - Antitumor necrosis factor alpha (TNF-alpha) agents—anti-inflammatory.[470,471,472]
  - Arnica-30—homeopathic medication.[473]
  - Aspidium (male fern).
  - Barbiturates—sedative, anticonvulsant.

- Cafergot—headache.
- Carbon disulfide—manufacture of viscose rayon fibers and cellophane films.
- Carbon monoxide.[468,474,475]
- Carbon tetrachloride—manufacturing of refrigerants and aerosols, dry-cleaning fluid, fat solvent, fire extinguishers, insecticides, shampoo.
- Cephaloridine—antibiotic.
- Chloramphenicol—antibiotic.[452,458]
- Chloronitrobenzene and dinitrobenzene—explosives.
- Chloroquine—antimalarial.[458,460]
- Chlorpromazine—antipsychotic.[458]
- Chlorpropamide—diabetes.
- Cimetidine.[476]
- Ciprofloxacin—antibiotic.[455,477,478]
- Cisplatin plus carboplatin—chemotherapy.[479]
- Cisplatin plus carmustine—chemotherapy.[480]
- Clioquinol—antibiotic.[481]
- Cobalt chloride.[456,482]
- Corticosteroids.[458,460,483,484]
- Cyanide intoxication (dietary).[485]
- Cyclosporine—chemotherapy.[460,486]
- Cytosine arabinoside—chemotherapy.[458]
- Dapsone.[455]
- D-penicillamine—rheumatologic.
- Deferoxamine—for removal of excess iron in patients requiring long-term transfusions.[487]
- Dichloromethane—solvent, fuel.[488]
- Dichlorodiphenyltrichloroethane (DDT)—insecticide.
- Digitalis (digoxin)—cardiac disease.[460]
- Diiodohydroxyquin—amebicide.
- Dinitrotoluene—explosive.
- Disulfiram—alcohol addiction.[460]
- Docetaxel—antineoplastic.[458,489]
- Dopamine agonists (e.g., bromocriptine, cabergoline, pergolide).[472]
- Elcatonin—synthetic analogue of calcitonin.[490]
- Emetine—amebicide.
- Ethchlorvynol—hypnotic.
- Ethylene glycol—antifreeze, moistener for tobacco, lacquer softener, solvent.[468]
- Etoposide phosphate and carboplatin (intracarotid)—chemotherapy.[491]
- 5-Fluorouracil—antineoplastic.[458]
- Gallium nitrate—antineoplastic.[492]
- Halogenated hydroxyquinoline (e.g., iodochlorhydroxyquin, boxyquinolone, chlorquinaldol, diiodohydroxyquin)—gastrointestinal disorders.
- Heavy metals (e.g., arsenic, iron, lead, mercury).[488,493]
- Hexachlorophene—detergent cleanser.
- Hymenoptera sting (e.g., wasps, bees).[494,495]
- Hydrogen peroxide—bleaching agent, disinfectant.[496]
- Hydroxychloroquine—antimalarial.[458]
- Indocyanine green—retinal stain.[459]
- Interferon—adjuvant chemotherapeutic agent.[458,460]
- Intravitreal silicone oil—retinal tamponade in retinal detachments.[471]
- Iodoform—disinfectant.
- Iodopyracet—radiologic contrast media.

- Isoniazid (isonicotinylhydrazide)—tuberculosis therapy.[452, 455,456,457,458,460]
- Linezolid—antibiotic.[455,456,458,468,497]
- Lithium—mood stabilizer.[460]
- Lysol—disinfectant.
- Manganese—skin exposure or inhalation of fumes in pottery or electroplating industry.[498]
- Melatonin, sertraline, and a high-protein diet.[499]
- Methamphetamine (intranasal abuse.)[500]
- Methanol—wood alcohol, solvent, combustible, antifreeze, and adulterant of alcohol.[298,455,456,457,468,501,502,503]
- Methotrexate—antineoplastic and rheumatologic.[458,460,504]
- Methyl acetate—solvent for nitrocellulose, resins, and oils, and manufacture of artificial leather.
- Methyl bromide—fumigant, fire extinguishers, refrigerant, and insecticide.
- Nalidixic acid—antibiotic.[460]
- Neem oil (Margosa oil)—accidental ingestion or traditional medicine use.[505]
- Octamoxin—monoamine oxidase inhibitor.
- Organophosphate pesticides.
- Oxymetholone—hematopoietic stimulator.[471]
- Paclitaxel—antineoplastic.[458]
- Pamidronate—treatment of hypercalcemia.[506]
- Penicillamine—treatment of Wilson disease, rheumatologic diseases.
- Phenazone—analgesic and antipyretic.
- Pheniprazine—monoamine oxidase inhibitor for hypertension and depression.
- Phosphodiesterase type 5 (PDE5) inhibitors—treatment of erectile dysfunction.[455,456,458,468]
- Plasmocid—antimalarial.
- Quinine—antimalarial, cramps.
- Snake venom and antisnake venom.[507]
- Sodium fluoride.
- Statins—antihyperlipidemic.[458]
- Streptomycin—tuberculosis therapy.[458]
- Styrene (vinyl benzyl)—synthetic rubber and fiberglass production.
- Sulfonamides—antibiotics.
- Tacrolimus (FK 506)—immunosuppressant.[508,509,510]
- Tamoxifen—chemotherapy.[458]
- Tamsulosin—benign prostatic hypertrophy agent.[458]
- Tetracycline—antibiotic.[460]
- Thioridazine—antipsychotic.[458]
- Thallium—rodenticides and insecticides.
- Tolbutamide—diabetes.
- Toluene—glue sniffing.[468,511]
- Topiramate—antiepileptic.[458,471]
- Trichloroethylene—industrial solvent and degreasing compound used in dry cleaning and in manufacture of rubber.
- Tricresyl phosphate—plasticizer and lubricant.
- Vigabatrin—antiepileptic.[455,458,460,472]
- Vincristine—antineoplastic agent.[458,460]

Ethambutol is a commonly used medication that may cause toxic optic neuropathy. The mechanism of ethambutol toxicity is poorly understood but may be related to zinc depletion.[450] The incidence of toxicity is dose and duration dependent,[447,448,449,450,451,452,453,512] with the incidence of optic neuropathy being as high as 6% at doses of 25 mg/kg/day. Doses less than 15 mg/kg/day are thought to be relatively safe.

Barron et al[513] reported ethambutol optic neuropathy in 3 of 304 (0.99%) patients treated with ethambutol at 25 mg/kg/day for 60 days, followed by 15 mg/kg/day. Leibold[514] described two types of visual loss due to ethambutol toxicity: a central toxicity (e.g., decreased visual acuity, central scotomas, and impaired color perception) and a periaxial toxicity (e.g., normal or almost normal visual acuity, normal color perception, and peripheral quadrantic scotomas or constriction). There was a 20% incidence of central toxicity and an 11% incidence of periaxial toxicity in 35 patients receiving doses higher than 35 mg/kg/day for a minimum of 185 days. A 5.3% incidence of periaxial toxicity occurred in the 38 patients receiving less than 35 mg/kg/day.[514] Although many authors feel that doses of 25 mg/kg/day for less than 2 months, followed by maintenance doses of 15 mg/kg/day are safe, there are cases of visual loss even at "safe" doses.[452,453,515] Brontë-Stewart et al[516] reported five patients with severe visual loss after doses of 25 mg/kg/day for 2 months, followed by 15 mg/kg/day. Three of these five patients had renal disease that may have increased drug levels because 70% of the ethambutol dose is excreted by the kidneys.[517] Tsai and Lee[453] reported 10 patients with ethambutol optic neuropathy from "safe" doses, stressing that there is in fact no risk-free dose of ethambutol. Toxicity in this study was most prominent in individuals older than 60 years, and thus this drug must be used with caution, especially in elderly patients. Isoniazid (isonicotinic acid hydrazide [INH]), especially in combination with ethambutol, has also been reported to cause a toxic optic neuropathy, and isoniazid toxicity should be suspected as the etiology in cases of persistent visual loss despite discontinuation of ethambutol.[518] VEP studies may be useful in evaluating patients with early ethambutol toxicity.[448]

Nutritional deficiencies may result in optic neuropathy.[519,520] Vitamins and nutrient deficiencies causing optic neuropathy include thiamine (B_1) deficiency,[457] B_6 deficiency, B_{12} deficiency, folate deficiency,[457,521] niacin deficiency,[457] riboflavin deficiency,[457] copper deficiency,[522] zinc deficiency,[522] and iatrogenic malabsorption (e.g., postbiliopancreatic bypass procedure).[523]

Pernicious anemia or dietary deficiency (e.g., vegetarian) may result in a vitamin B_{12} deficiency optic neuropathy. The pathophysiology of "alcohol amblyopia," now termed nutritional optic neuropathy, is related to a deficiency of B_{12}, thiamine, and/or folate (rather than a direct toxic effect of alcohol).[463] The ability of tobacco alone to cause a toxic optic neuropathy has been asserted by several authors.[524,525] Samples and Younge,[525] for example, state that central and cecocentral scotomas may occur in association with smoking alone, especially cigar smoking. A toxic effect of cyanide may be the basis for tobacco optic neuropathy.[516] Smoking may also impair intestinal vitamin B_{12} absorption.

Patients suspected of harboring a toxic or nutritional optic neuropathy should be screened for nutritional deficiencies and treated with appropriate supplementation (class IV, level C). These patients should be urged to discontinue alcohol and tobacco use. Both serum and erythrocyte folate levels should be checked because there may be variability in the serum folate level alone (especially related to recent meals).[399,521]

Toxic or nutritional optic neuropathies are painless, subacute in onset, and bilateral, and usually involve central visual acuity and visual fields (e.g., central and cecocentral scotomas), but their clinical presentations may be variable. Neuroimaging is recommended because CON may mimic the clinical presentation of toxic optic neuropathy. The determination of presumed toxic or nutritional optic neuropathy should include a complete evaluation to exclude other etiologies of bilateral, painless, and progressive optic neuropathies (e.g., hereditary optic neuropathy, bilateral CON, etc.).

1.10 Is There a History of Radiation Exposure to the Optic Nerves?

Radiation optic neuropathy (RON) is thought to be an ischemic disorder of the optic nerve that usually results in irreversible severe visual loss months to years (majority within first 3 years) after radiation therapy to the brain or orbit.[63,169,201,262,381,526,527,528,529,530,531,532,533,534,535,536,537,538,539,540,541,542,543,544,545,546,547,548,549,550,551] It is most often a retrobulbar optic neuropathy, and thus the optic nerve may appear normal on initial examination. Approximately three-fourths of patients have bilateral involvement.[551,552] The visual loss is characteristically rapid and progressive, with the disc becoming pale over a period of 4 to 6 weeks.[546,547] Final vision is no light perception (NLP) in 45% and worse than 20/200 in an additional 40% of affected eyes (i.e., 85% of eyes with RON have a final visual acuity of 20/200 or worse).[547] More rarely, RON may present as an anterior optic neuropathy with optic disc swelling.[540] Such cases usually occur in the setting of radiation retinopathy following treatment of orbital or intraocular lesions. Associated findings of radiation retinopathy resemble those of diabetic retinopathy and variably include peripapillary hard exudates, hemorrhages, subretinal fluid, cotton-wool spots, focal arteriolar narrowing, macular edema, capillary nonperfusion, capillary telangiectasia, microaneurysms, neovascularization of the disc and retina, perivascular sheathing, vitreous hemorrhage, neovascular glaucoma, CRAO, and CRVO.[553,554] Loss of vision with anterior cases may be due to macular edema, macular hemorrhages, macular exudates, or perifoveal capillary nonperfusion, as well as from optic nerve involvement.[554,555]

Factors that may increase the risk of RON include concomitant chemotherapy, hormone-secreting pituitary adenoma, increased age, and dosage.[547,556] Radiation doses thought to cause RON are cumulative dose greater than 60 Gy total or greater than 1.8 Gy/fraction.[536,546,557,558,559,560] The risk of RON with stereotactic radiosurgery increases significantly if dosage to the visual apparatus is greater than 12 Gy, though dosages from 8 to 12 Gy also have some increased risk and caution is warranted with these doses.[530,538,546,561,562,563,564] Doses less than 8 Gy are generally not associated with increased risk of RON. Other factors that increase the risk of RON following stereotactic radiosurgery are large tumor volume, prior visual dysfunction, prior radiation exposure, or treatment isocenter within 5 mm of anterior visual pathway.[530,547] The diagnosis of

RON is suspected from the clinical setting and may be confirmed by MRI. In RON, the unenhanced T1- and T2-weighted images show no abnormalities, but there is enhancement of the optic nerves, chiasm, and possibly the optic tracts in some cases.[201,391,397,527,539,543,544,545,547,561,565,566] This enhancement usually resolves over several months. Recurrence of the primary tumor and radiation-induced tumors remain important differential diagnoses.

Patients with RON may rarely improve with corticosteroids.[542] Hyperbaric oxygen therapy may be of benefit if given early in the course (e.g., within 72 hours of onset of symptoms), although some patients show no improvement.[262,527,528,542,545] Anticoagulation therapy was of no help in at least two cases.[531,537,567,568] There have been several case reports and series suggesting improvement after using anti-VEGF antibodies (bevacizumab) with or without pentoxifylline and vitamin E.[569,570,571,572] Mohamed et al[573] reported improved vision following optic nerve sheath fenestration in several patients. However, there is no proven effective therapy for RON (class IV, level U).[551]

1.11 Is There Clinical Evidence for a Hereditary Optic Neuropathy?

Miller et al[125] divided the hereditary optic neuropathies into three groups:
1. Patients without associated neurologic signs and symptoms.
2. Patients with neurologic signs and symptoms.
3. Patients in whom the optic neuropathy is secondary to the underlying systemic disease.

The hereditary optic neuropathies may have an isolated, dominant (e.g., Kjer optic neuropathy), recessive, or mitochondrial (e.g., Leber hereditary optic neuropathy [LHON]) inheritance pattern.

1.11.1 Kjer Autosomal-Dominant Optic Neuropathy

Kjer autosomal-dominant optic neuropathy (ADON) or autosomal-dominant optic atrophy usually appears in the first decade of life (usually 4–6 years). However, due to slow progression of the disease, vision loss may not be noticed by patients until years later.[41,69] Mutations in the OPA1 gene on chromosome 3q are thought to account for a majority of ADON cases.[574,575,576,577,578,579] While ADON is inherited in an autosomal-dominant fashion, nearly 50% of cases have either a sporadic mutation or unknown familial history.[576] The prevalence of OPA1 mutations is approximately 1:50,000 people in most populations, and as high as 1:10,000 in Denmark.[580,581,582]

Patients generally present with bilateral, symmetric, painless, and slowly progressive visual acuity and color vision (often blue–yellow dyschromatopsia) loss.[583,584,585] Visual acuity is usually better than 20/60 in 40% of patients, with only 15% developing vision worse than 20/200.[576] Unlike LHON (discussed below), spontaneous recovery of vision is extremely rare.[584]

Fundus examination may be normal, show mild pseudoedema, or may show subtle temporal optic atrophy. There may be peripapillary atrophy, absent foveal reflex, mild macular pigmentary changes, arterial attenuation, and nonglaucomatous cupping.[581,586] Visual field testing might show central, paracentral, or cecocentral scotomas. Sometimes there is inversion of the peripheral field with the field being more constricted to blue than red isopters.[587,588,589,590] VEP may be reduced in amplitude and delayed.[576,587,588,589] OCT may be normal or later show macular retinal nerve fiber layer thinning in the papillomacular bundle.[576,591,592] MRI findings are nonspecific and include bilateral optic atrophy with prominent optic nerve perineural cerebrospinal fluid. MRI is used to rule out other etiologies.[576] OPA1 mutations may be identified by commercial testing, though the rate of OPA1 mutation detection varies from 5 to 65% depending on whether it is a sporadic or inherited case.[576]

Some patients may have other neurological deficits in addition to the visual symptoms. These are termed ADON-plus (ADON+).[576,578,581,592,593] People with ADON+ may have sensorineural hearing loss, progressive external ophthalmoplegia, myopathy, or ataxia. While onset of visual loss does not differ between ADON and ADON+, ADON+ patients generally have more severe visual symptoms.[576] In addition, the "plus" symptoms generally appear later, in the second to fourth decades of life. There are currently no effective treatments for ADON,[594,595] but patients should be offered genetic counseling.

1.11.2 Leber Hereditary Optic Neuropathy

LHON usually occurs in young males (80–90% of cases in the United States) with onset between 13 and 35 years of age (range 5–80 years), although it may rarely affect females and develop at any age.[594,596,597,598,599,600,601,602,603,604,605,606,607,608] It is a mitochondrial disease, meaning every son and daughter of a female carrier inherit LHON trait, while only women pass the trait.[565,585,593,609] Affected women are more likely to have affected children, especially daughters, than unaffected woman carriers. LHON demonstrates incomplete penetrance, and men with an inherited LHON mutation are at a higher risk of vision loss (20–83%) than females (4–32%).[608] Some authors suggest that secondary mutations affect penetrance and phenotype, as additional mutations further reduce the energy production of the mitochondrial complex.[610,611,612,613] "Primary" mitochondrial DNA mutations include 11778, 3460, and 14484, with better prognosis seen in patients with a mutation at position 14484 patients (37–65% improve spontaneously).[565,601,608,614,615,616,617,618,619] Patients carrying the mutation at position 11778 carry the worst prognosis with only 4% of patients showing spontaneous improvement.[620,621] A number of other less common mutations also have been implicated in the disorder.[141,236,622,623] Some patients with presumed toxic or nutritional deficiency amblyopia may harbor a LHON mutation,[604,624,625] and therefore testing for Leber mutations may be indicated in these patients. If suspected, diagnosis of LHON can be confirmed by serologic testing for the known LHON mutations.

Patients generally present with acute to subacute bilateral, sequential, painless vision loss with the second eye becoming involved in weeks to months after the first.[607,626] Visual prognosis is usually poor, with visual acuity from 20/200 to hand motion. Some patients experience spontaneous improvement, which may occur gradually over 6 months to 1 year, or even up to 10 years after onset with return of a small island of vision within the large central scotoma.[607] Those that improve appear to have a lower mean age of onset.

Visual field loss is usually central or cecocentral involving the central 25 to 30 degrees.[626] Those patients occasionally experience positive Uhthoff's phenomenon. Fundus examination during the acute vision loss event shows telangiectatic microangiopathy, apparent swelling of nerve fiber layer around the optic disc ("pseudoedema") with occasional disc or retinal hemorrhages, and macular edema or exudate.[627] Fluorescein angiogram often shows "pseudoedema," but may rarely show disc leakage. MRI may show increased signal in middle or posterior intraorbital sections of the optic nerves.[602,628] Fundus appearance after the acute event shows attenuated arterioles, nerve fiber layer loss especially affecting the papillomacular bundle, and temporal optic disc pallor that can also progress to nonglaucomatous cupping.

LHON has been associated with other syndromes like Wolff–Parkinson–White syndrome, Lawn–Ganong–Levine syndrome, prolonged QT dystonia (described with 11778 and 3460 mutations), myoclonus (with 11778 mutations),[629] and Charcot–Marie–Tooth disease. Postural tremor occurs with increased frequency in all forms. A multiple sclerosis (MS) like illness has been found in up to 45% of females with 11778 mutations and is termed Harding's disease.[630,631,632]

Although the diagnosis of LHON can be confirmed by serologic testing for the known LHON mutations, little consensus exists regarding the treatment of LHON.[594,633] Historically, treatment (class IV, level U) has included multivitamins, folate, vitamin B_{12}, thiamine, ubiquinate (coenzyme Q10), ibedinone, and other coenzyme Q10 analogs.[594,595,604,634,635,636] More recently, however, there have been great efforts to find an efficacious treatment for LHON. Although it is still in the early stages of clinical trials, gene therapy for two different target genes is currently under investigation as a possible therapeutic approach.[594,607,637] There has also been renewed interest in Idebenone therapy. Some recent studies suggest possible efficacy in select patients with LHON, including patients who begin treatment when only one eye is affected and those with the 11778 mutation.[638,639,640,641] In addition to medical therapy, patients should avoid alcohol, tobacco, and other environmental toxins.[606,635,642,643] Low-vision services should always be offered to these patients early on.

Other forms of hereditary optic neuropathy are outlined in Box 1.7.

Box 1.7 Other hereditary optic neuropathies[2]

- No associated neurologic deficits:
  - Apparent sex-linked optic atrophy.
- Associated with other neurologic or systemic diseases:
  - Autosomal-dominant progressive optic atrophy with congenital deafness.
  - Autosomal-dominant progressive optic atrophy with progressive hearing loss and ataxia.
  - Autosomal-dominant progressive optic atrophy with peripheral neuropathy.[644]

- Autosomal-dominant optic atrophy with ataxia and pes cavus.
- Hereditary optic atrophy with progressive hearing loss and polyneuropathy.
- Familial bulbospinal neuronopathy with optic atrophy.[645]
- Dominant optic atrophy, deafness, ophthalmoplegia, and myopathy.
- Autosomal-recessive optic atrophy with progressive hearing loss, spastic quadriplegia, mental deterioration, and death (opticocochleodentate degeneration).
- Opticoacoustic atrophy with dementia.
- Sex-linked recessive optic atrophy, ataxia, deafness, tetraplegia, and areflexia.
- Progressive encephalopathy with edema, hypsarrhythmia, and optic atrophy (PEHO syndrome).
- Juvenile diabetes insipidus, diabetes mellitus, progressive optic atrophy, and deafness (Wolfram's syndrome or diabetes insipidus, diabetes mellitus, optic atrophy, and deafness [DIDMOAD]).[646,647]
- Complicated hereditary infantile optic atrophy (Behr's syndrome).
- Optic atrophy with hereditary ataxias (Friedreich's ataxia, Marie's ataxia).
- Optic atrophy with Charcot–Marie–Tooth disease (hereditary sensorimotor neuropathy).
- Optic atrophy with myotonic muscular dystrophy.[648]

1.12 Is This an Atypical or Unexplained Optic Neuropathy?

A number of patients with optic neuropathy do not fit into the categories listed in our approach. For patients with unexplained optic neuropathy or atypical optic neuropathy, a suggested evaluation is listed in Box 1.5. In addition to the suggested labs, consider neuroimaging with an MRI of the brain and orbits with and without contrast, a lumbar puncture, and a chest radiograph.

References

[1] Burde REM, Savino PJ, Trobe JD. Clinical Decisions in Neuro-ophthalmology. St. Louis, MO: Mosby-Year Book; 1992:56–57

[2] Miller NR, Newman NJ. Walsh and Hoyt's Clinical Neuro-ophthalmology. 5th ed. Baltimore, MD: Williams & Wilkins; 1998

[3] Trobe JD. The Neurology of Vision. Oxford: Oxford University Press; 2001

[4] Trobe JD, Glaser JS, Cassady JC. Optic atrophy. Differential diagnosis by fundus observation alone. Arch Ophthalmol. 1980; 98(6):1040–1045

[5] Warner JEA, Lessell S, Rizzo JF, III, Newman NJ. Does optic disc appearance distinguish ischemic optic neuropathy from optic neuritis? Arch Ophthalmol. 1997; 115(11):1408–1410

[6] Trobe JD, Glaser JS. Quantitative perimetry in compressive optic neuropathy and optic neuritis. Arch Ophthalmol. 1978; 96(7):1210–1216

[7] Rizzo JF, III, Lessell S. Optic neuritis and ischemic optic neuropathy. Overlapping clinical profiles. Arch Ophthalmol. 1991; 109(12):1668–1672

[8] Guy J, Mancuso A, Quisling RG, Beck R, Moster M. Gadolinium-DTPA-enhanced magnetic resonance imaging in optic neuropathies. Ophthalmology. 1990; 97(5):592–599, discussion 599–600

[9] Danesh-Meyer HV, Yap J, Frampton C, Savino PJ. Differentiation of compressive from glaucomatous optic neuropathy with spectral-domain optical coherence tomography. Ophthalmology. 2014; 121(8):1516–1523

[10] Miki A, Endo T, Morimoto T, Matsushita K, Fujikado T, Nishida K. Retinal nerve fiber layer and ganglion cell complex thicknesses measured with spectral-domain optical coherence tomography in eyes with no light perception due to nonglaucomatous optic neuropathy. Jpn J Ophthalmol. 2015; 59(4):230–235

[11] Hata M, Miyamoto K, Oishi A, et al. Comparison of optic disc morphology of optic nerve atrophy between compressive optic neuropathy and glaucomatous optic neuropathy. PLoS One. 2014; 9(11):e112403

[12] Lee AG, Chau FY, Golnik KC, Kardon RH, Wall M. The diagnostic yield of the evaluation for isolated unexplained optic atrophy. Ophthalmology. 2005; 112(5):757–759

[13] Dutton JJ. Optic nerve gliomas and meningiomas. Neurol Clin. 1991; 9(1):163–177

[14] Fayaz I, Gentili F, Mackenzie IR. Optic nerve sheath meningioma. J Neurol Neurosurg Psychiatry. 1999; 67(3):408

[15] Golnik KC, Hund PW, III, Stroman GA, Stewart WC. Magnetic resonance imaging in patients with unexplained optic neuropathy. Ophthalmology. 1996; 103(3):515–520

[16] Katz B. Disc edema, transient obscurations of vision, and a temporal fossa mass. Surv Ophthalmol. 1991; 36(2):133–139

[17] Kazim M, Kennerdell JS, Rothfus W, Marquardt M. Orbital lymphangioma. Correlation of magnetic resonance images and intraoperative findings. Ophthalmology. 1992; 99(10):1588–1594

[18] Kodsi SR, Younge BR, Leavitt JA, Campbell RJ, Scheithauer BW. Intracranial plasma cell granuloma presenting as an optic neuropathy. Surv Ophthalmol. 1993; 38(1):70–74

[19] Lee AG, Phillips PH, Newman NJ, et al. Neuro-ophthalmologic manifestations of adenoid cystic carcinoma. J Neuroophthalmol. 1997; 17(3):183–188

[20] Yin S, Zhou P, Li Q, Jiang S. Intrasellar clear cell meningioma mimicking invasive pituitary adenoma: a case report and review of the literature. Turk Neurosurg. 2015; 25(6):976–979

[21] Garrity JA, Trautmann JC, Bartley GB, et al. Optic nerve sheath meningoceles. Clinical and radiographic features in 13 cases with a review of the literature. Ophthalmology. 1990; 97(11):1519–1531

[22] Osaguona VB, Okeigbemen VW. Nonglaucomatous optic atrophy in Benin City. Ann Afr Med. 2015; 14(2):109–113

[23] Jayaraman M, Ambika S, Gandhi RA, Bassi SR, Ravi P, Sen P. Multifocal visual evoked potential recordings in compressive optic neuropathy secondary to pituitary adenoma. Doc Ophthalmol. 2010; 121(3):197–204

[24] Nakajima T, Kumabe T, Jokura H, Yoshimoto T. Recurrent germinoma in the optic nerve: report of two cases. Neurosurgery. 2001; 48(1):214–217, discussion 217–218

[25] Brazis PW, Menke DM, McLeish WM, et al. Angiocentric T-cell lymphoma presenting with multiple cranial nerve palsies and retrobulbar optic neuropathy. J Neuroophthalmol. 1995; 15(3):152–157

[26] Nygaard R, Garwicz S, Haldorsen T, et al. The Nordic Society of Pediatric Oncology and Hematology (NOPHO). Second malignant neoplasms in patients treated for childhood leukemia. A population-based cohort study from the Nordic countries. Acta Paediatr Scand. 1991; 80(12):1220–1228

[27] Park KL, Goins KM. Hodgkin's lymphoma of the orbit associated with acquired immunodeficiency syndrome. Am J Ophthalmol. 1993; 116(1):111–112

[28] Roth DB, Siatkowski RM. Bilateral blindness as the initial presentation of lymphoma of the sphenoid sinus. Am J Ophthalmol. 2000; 129(2):256–258

[29] Esmaeli B, Ahmadi MA, Manning J, McLaughlin PW, Ginsberg L. Clinical presentation and treatment of secondary orbital lymphoma. Ophthal Plast Reconstr Surg. 2002; 18(4):247–253

[30] Goldberg S, Mahadevia P, Lipton M, Rosenbaum PS. Sinus histiocytosis with massive lymphadenopathy involving the orbit: reversal of compressive optic neuropathy after chemotherapy. J Neuroophthalmol. 1998; 18(4):270–275

[31] Siu RC, Tan IL, Davidson AS, Robertson A, Fraser CL. Clinical reasoning: compressive optic neuropathy secondary to intracranial Rosai-Dorfman disease. Neurology. 2015; 85(12):e89–e92

[32] Wu SY, Ma L, Tsai YJ. Partial removal of orbital tumor in Rosai-Dorfman disease. Jpn J Ophthalmol. 2004; 48(2):154–157

[33] Pless M, Chang BM. Rosai-Dorfman disease. Extranodal sinus histiocytosis in three co-existing sites. A case report. J Neurooncol. 2003; 61(2):137–141

[34] Bae JW, Kim YH, Kim SK, et al. Langerhans cell histiocytosis causing acute optic neuropathy. Childs Nerv Syst. 2015; 31(4):615–619

[35] Chua CN, Alhady M, Ngo CT, Swethadri GK, Singh A, Tan S. Solitary nasal neurofibroma presenting as compressive optic neuropathy. Eye (Lond). 2006; 20(12):1406–1408

[36] Kattah JC, Chrousos GC, Roberts J, Kolsky M, Zimmerman L, Manz H. Metastatic prostate cancer to the optic canal. Ophthalmology. 1993; 100 (11):1711–1715

[37] Newman NJ, Grossniklaus HE, Wojno TH. Breast carcinoma metastatic to the optic nerve. Arch Ophthalmol. 1996; 114(1):102–103

[38] Newsom RSB, Simcock P, Zambarakji H. Cerebral metastasis presenting with altitudinal field defect. J Neuroophthalmol. 1999; 19(1):10–11

[39] Pengel J, Crevits L, Wynants P, De Poorter MC, Mastenbroek GG, De Reuck J. Optic nerve metastasis simulating optic neuritis. Clin Neurol Neurosurg. 1997; 99(1):46–49

[40] Chiam PJ, Ho VW, Hubbard AD, Weerasinghe S. A case of misconstrue proptosis. BMJ Case Rep. 2013; 2013:bcr2012008410

[41] Tagg NT, Lee AG, Syed NA, Golnik KC. Artery, vein, neither, both? Surv Ophthalmol. 2009; 54(3):408–411

[42] Fang KH, Chen CK, Hao SP. Acute visual loss in a head and neck cancer patient with ocular metastasis and sphenoid pyocele. Auris Nasus Larynx. 2007; 34(4):569–571

[43] Konuk O, Pehlivanli Z, Yirmibesoglu E, Erkal HS, Erekul S, Unal M. Compressive optic neuropathy due to orbital metastasis of a sacral chordoma: case report. Ophthal Plast Reconstr Surg. 2005; 21(3):245–247

[44] Berney C, Borruat FX, de Tribolet N. Spontaneous visual improvement in pituitary metastasis. Eur J Ophthalmol. 2003; 13(1):105–107

[45] Li CZ, Li CC, Lin MC, et al. A clinical pitfall: optimal management of single dural-based metastatic carcinoma of the breast mimicking meningioma. Neurologist. 2015; 20(5):93–95

[46] Dawkins RL, Hackney JR, Riley KO. Penetration of an optic nerve by a sellar/suprasellar arachnoid cyst. World Neurosurg. 2016; 87:662.e7–662.e11

[47] Shields JA, Demirci H, Mashayekhi A, Eagle RC, Jr, Shields CL. Melanocytoma of the optic disk: a review. Surv Ophthalmol. 2006; 51(2):93–104

[48] Besada E, Shechtman D, Barr RD. Melanocytoma inducing compressive optic neuropathy: the ocular morbidity potential of an otherwise invariably benign lesion. Optometry. 2002; 73(1):33–38

[49] Tannan A, Jhaveri M, Moftakhar R, Munich S, Harbhajanka A, Cohen AJ. Compressive optic neuropathy secondary to a lateral rectus muscle dermoid cyst. Ophthal Plast Reconstr Surg. 2015; 31(3):e63–e64

[50] Touitou V, Vignal-Clermont C, Berges O, Morax S, Gaudric A. Orbital cyst associated with ocular pit in an adult without microphthalmos. Orbit. 2009; 28(2–3):98–100

[51] Aarabi B, Haghshenas M, Rakeii V. Visual failure caused by suprasellar extramedullary hematopoiesis in beta thalassemia: case report. Neurosurgery. 1998; 42(4):922–925, discussion 925–926

[52] Sawaya R, El Ayoubi N, Hamam R. Acute neurological visual loss in young adults: causes, diagnosis and management. Postgrad Med J. 2015; 91(1082):698–703

[53] Ittipunkul N, Martin T, Siriwanasan R, Olanratanachai K, Rootman J. Extra-medullary hematopoiesis causing bilateral optic atrophy in beta thalassemia/Hb E disease. J Med Assoc Thai. 2007; 90(4):809–812

[54] Pless M, Rizzo JF, III, Shang J. Orbital apex syndrome: a rare presentation of extramedullary hematopoiesis: case report and review of literature. J Neurooncol. 2002; 57(1):37–40

[55] Wein FB, Gans MS. The perils of a sneeze. J Neuroophthalmol. 1999; 19(2):128–130

[56] Chaudhry IA, Al-Amri A, Shamsi FA, Al-Rashed W. Visual recovery after evacuation of orbital emphysema. Orbit. 2007; 26(4):283–285

[57] Hao SP. Mucocele of the sphenoid sinus with acute bilateral blindness: report of a case. J Formos Med Assoc. 1994; 93(6):519–521

[58] Loehrl TA, Leopold DA. Sphenoethmoidal mucocele presenting with bilateral visual compromise. Ann Otol Rhinol Laryngol. 2000; 109(6):608–610

[59] Thorne JE, Volpe NJ, Wulc AE, Galetta SL. Caught by a masquerade: sclerosing orbital inflammation. Surv Ophthalmol. 2002; 47(1):50–54

[60] Yamaguchi K, Ohnuma I, Takahashi S, et al. Magnetic resonance imaging in acute optic neuropathy by sphenoidal mucocele. Int Ophthalmol. 1997; 21(1):9–11

[61] Lin CC, Chao TK, Chen TH, Wang JK. Compressive optic neuropathy caused by cholesterol granuloma in the posterior ethmoid sinus. Eye Sci. 2015; 30(1):31–33

[62] Lally E, Murchison AP, Moster ML, Bilyk JR. Compressive optic neuropathy from neurosarcoidosis. Ophthal Plast Reconstr Surg. 2015; 31(3):e79

[63] Gupta D, Tailor TD, Keene CD, Rostomily RC, Jian-Amadi A. A case of nodular fasciitis causing compressive optic neuropathy. Ophthal Plast Reconstr Surg. 2014; 30(2):e47–e49

[64] Koay CL, Chew FL, Chong KY, Subrayan V. Compressive optic neuropathy: a unique presentation of Sweet syndrome. Indian J Ophthalmol. 2013; 61(3):140–141

[65] Taflan T, Güngör I, Cengel Kurnaz S, Güngör L. Optic neuropathy secondary to inflammation of sphenoidal sinuses and Onodi cell polyps: a case report. Ocul Immunol Inflamm. 2013; 21(3):247–250

[66] Salvi F, Mascalchi M, Pasini E, et al. p-ANCA pachymeningitis presenting with isolated "optic neuropathy". Neurol Sci. 2010; 31(5):639–641

[67] Hwang DJ, Chung YS, Jun SY, Kim YJ, Lee JY, Park IW. A case of compressive optic neuropathy caused by sphenoid sinus cholesterol granuloma. Jpn J Ophthalmol. 2009; 53(4):441–442

[68] Aakalu VK, Ahmad AZ. Wegener granulomatosis causing compressive optic neuropathy in a child. Ophthal Plast Reconstr Surg. 2009; 25(4):327–328

[69] Liewluck T, Schatz NJ, Potter PF, Romaguera RL. Compressive retrobulbar optic neuropathy due to hypertrophic pachymeningitis. Intern Med. 2008; 47(19):1761–1762

[70] Oono S, Kurimoto T, Fukazawa K, Mimura O. Compressive optic neuropathy caused by a paranasal sinus cyst of Wegener's granulomatosis. Jpn J Ophthalmol. 2007; 51(6):480–481

[71] Toh ST, Lee JC. Onodi cell mucocele: rare cause of optic compressive neuropathy. Arch Otolaryngol Head Neck Surg. 2007; 133(11):1153–1156

[72] Thurtell MJ, Besser M, Halmagyi GM. Anterior clinoid mucocele causing acute monocular blindness. Clin Experiment Ophthalmol. 2007; 35(7):675–676

[73] Ismail AR, Clifford L, Meacock WR. Compressive optic neuropathy in fungal hypertrophic cranial pachymeningitis. Eye (Lond). 2007; 21(4):568–569

[74] Oishi A, Miyamoto K, Yoshimura N. Orbital amyloidosis-induced compressive optic neuropathy accompanied by characteristic eyelid pigmentation. Ophthal Plast Reconstr Surg. 2006; 22(6):485–487

[75] Lee LA, Huang CC, Lee TJ. Prolonged visual disturbance secondary to isolated sphenoid sinus disease. Laryngoscope. 2004; 114(6):986–990

[76] Kitagawa K, Hayasaka S, Shimizu K, Nagaki Y. Optic neuropathy produced by a compressed mucocele in an Onodi cell. Am J Ophthalmol. 2003; 135(2):253–254

[77] Aylward GW, Sullivan TJ, Garner A, Moseley I, Wright JE. Orbital involvement in multifocal fibrosclerosis. Br J Ophthalmol. 1995; 79(3):246–249

[78] Botella C, Orozco M, Navarro J, Riesgo P. Idiopathic chronic hypertrophic craniocervical pachymeningitis: case report. Neurosurgery. 1994; 35(6):1144–1149

[79] Girkin CA, Perry JD, Miller NR, Reich SG. Pachymeningitis with multiple cranial neuropathies and unilateral optic neuropathy secondary to Pseudomonas aeruginosa: case report and review. J Neuroophthalmol. 1998; 18(3):196–200

[80] Hamilton SR, Smith CH, Lessell S. Idiopathic hypertrophic cranial pachymeningitis. J Clin Neuroophthalmol. 1993; 13(2):127–134

[81] Jacobson DM, Anderson DR, Rupp GM, Warner JJ. Idiopathic hypertrophic cranial pachymeningitis: clinical-radiological-pathological correlation of bone involvement. J Neuroophthalmol. 1996; 16(4):264–268

[82] Kawano Y, Kira J. Chronic hypertrophic cranial pachymeningitis associated with HTLV-I infection. J Neurol Neurosurg Psychiatry. 1995; 59(4):435–437

[83] Lam BL, Barrett DA, Glaser JS, Schatz NJ, Brown HH. Visual loss from idiopathic intracranial pachymeningitis. Neurology. 1994; 44(4):694–698

[84] Levine MR, Kaye L, Mair S, Bates J. Multifocal fibrosclerosis. Report of a case of bilateral idiopathic sclerosing pseudotumor and retroperitoneal fibrosis. Arch Ophthalmol. 1993; 111(6):841–843

[85] Mamelak AN, Kelly WM, Davis RL, Rosenblum ML. Idiopathic hypertrophic cranial pachymeningitis. Report of three cases. J Neurosurg. 1993; 79(2):270–276

[86] Nishizaki T, Iwamoto F, Uesugi S, Akimura T, Yamashita K, Ito H. Idiopathic cranial pachymeningoencephalitis focally affecting the parietal dura mater and adjacent brain parenchyma: case report. Neurosurgery. 1997; 40(4):840–843, discussion 843

[87] Olmos PR, Falko JM, Rea GL, Boesel CP, Chakeres DW, McGhee DB. Fibrosing pseudotumor of the sella and parasellar area producing hypopituitarism and multiple cranial nerve palsies. Neurosurgery. 1993; 32(6):1015–1021, discussion 1021

[88] Parney IF, Johnson ES, Allen PBR. "Idiopathic" cranial hypertrophic pachymeningitis responsive to antituberculous therapy: case report. Neurosurgery. 1997; 41(4):965–971

[89] Rootman J, McCarthy M, White V, Harris G, Kennerdell J. Idiopathic sclerosing inflammation of the orbit. A distinct clinicopathologic entity. Ophthalmology. 1994; 101(3):570–584

[90] Tamai H, Tamai K, Yuasa H. Pachymeningitis with pseudo-Foster Kennedy syndrome. Am J Ophthalmol. 2000; 130(4):535–537

[91] Prabhakar S, Bhatia R, Lal V, Singh P. Hypertrophic pachymeningitis: varied manifestations of a single disease entity. Neurol India. 2002; 50(1):45–52

[92] Arroyo JG, Lessell S, Montgomery WW. Steroid-induced visual recovery in fibrous dysplasia. J Clin Neuroophthalmol. 1991; 11(4):259–261

[93] Bland LI, Marchese MJ, McDonald JV. Acute monocular blindness secondary to fibrous dysplasia of the skull: a case report. Ann Ophthalmol. 1992; 24(7):263–266

[94] Bocca G, de Vries J, Cruysberg JR, Boers GH, Monnens LA. Optic neuropathy in McCune-Albright syndrome: an indication for aggressive treatment. Acta Paediatr. 1998; 87(5):599–600

[95] Caldemeyer KS, Smith RR, Edwards-Brown MK. Familial hypophosphatemic rickets causing ocular calcification and optic canal narrowing. AJNR Am J Neuroradiol. 1995; 16(6):1252–1254

[96] Chen YR, Breidahl A, Chang CN. Optic nerve decompression in fibrous dysplasia: indications, efficacy, and safety. Plast Reconstr Surg. 1997; 99(1):22–30, discussion 31–33

[97] Daly BD, Chow CC, Cockram CS. Unusual manifestations of craniofacial fibrous dysplasia: clinical, endocrinological and computed tomographic features. Postgrad Med J. 1994; 70(819):10–16

[98] Grimm MA, Hazelton T, Beck RW, Murtagh FR. Postgadolinium enhancement of a compressive neuropathy of the optic nerve. AJNR Am J Neuroradiol. 1995; 16(4):779–781

[99] Joseph MP. Commentary on Papay FA, Morales L Jr, Flaharty P, et al. Optic nerve decompression in cranial base fibrous dysplasia. J Craniofac Surg. 1995; 6:11–13

[100] Katz BJ, Nerad JA. Ophthalmic manifestations of fibrous dysplasia: a disease of children and adults. Ophthalmology. 1998; 105(12):2207–2215

[101] Michael CB, Lee AG, Patrinely JR, Stal S, Blacklock JB. Visual loss associated with fibrous dysplasia of the anterior skull base. Case report and review of the literature. J Neurosurg. 2000; 92(2):350–354

[102] Saito K, Suzuki Y, Nehashi K, Sugita K. Unilateral extradural approach for bilateral optic canal release in a patient with fibrous dysplasia. Surg Neurol. 1990; 34(2):124–128

[103] Schaffler GJ, Simbrunner J, Lechner H, et al. Idiopathic sclerotic inflammation of the orbit with left optic nerve compression in a patient with multifocal fibrosclerosis. AJNR Am J Neuroradiol. 2000; 21(1):194–197

[104] Skolnick CA, Mafee MF, Goodwin JA. Pneumosinus dilatans of the sphenoid sinus presenting with visual loss. J Neuroophthalmol. 2000; 20(4):259–263

[105] Steel DHW, Potts MJ. Bilateral sudden visual loss in Albright's syndrome. Br J Ophthalmol. 1995; 79(12):1149

[106] Stretch JR, Poole MD. Pneumosinus dilatans as the aetiology of progressive bilateral blindness. Br J Plast Surg. 1992; 45(6):469–473

[107] Weisman JS, Hepler RS, Vinters HV. Reversible visual loss caused by fibrous dysplasia. Am J Ophthalmol. 1990; 110(3):244–249

[108] MacNally SP, Ashida R, Williams TJ, King AT, Leatherbarrow B, Rutherford SA. A case of acute compressive optic neuropathy secondary to aneurysmal bone cyst formation in fibrous dysplasia. Br J Neurosurg. 2010; 24(6):705–707

[109] Amrith S, Baratham G, Khoo CY, Low CH, Sinniah R. Spontaneous hematic cysts of the orbit presenting with acute proptosis. A report of three cases. Ophthal Plast Reconstr Surg. 1990; 6(4):273–277

[110] Buus DR, Tse DT, Farris BK. Ophthalmic complications of sinus surgery. Ophthalmology. 1990; 97(5):612–619

[111] Dolman PJ, Glazer LC, Harris GJ, Beatty RL, Massaro BM. Mechanisms of visual loss in severe proptosis. Ophthal Plast Reconstr Surg. 1991; 7(4):256–260

[112] Moorthy RS, Yung CW, Nunery WR, Sondhi N, Fogle N. Spontaneous orbital subperiosteal hematomas in patients with liver disease. Ophthal Plast Reconstr Surg. 1992; 8(2):150–152

[113] Muthukumar N. Traumatic haemorrhagic optic neuropathy: case report. Br J Neurosurg. 1997; 11(2):166–167

[114] Nemiroff J, Baharestani S, Juthani VV, Klein KS, Zoumalan C. Cirrhosis-related coagulopathy resulting in disseminated intravascular coagulation and spontaneous orbital hemorrhages. Orbit. 2014; 33(5):372–374

[115] Jamal BT, Diecidue RJ, Taub D, Champion A, Bilyk JR. Orbital hemorrhage and compressive optic neuropathy in patients with midfacial fractures receiving low-molecular weight heparin therapy. J Oral Maxillofac Surg. 2009; 67(7):1416–1419

[116] Yazici B, Gönen T. Posttraumatic subperiosteal hematomas of the orbit in children. Ophthal Plast Reconstr Surg. 2011; 27(1):33–37

[117] Sokol JA, Baron E, Lantos G, Kazim M. Orbital compression syndrome in sickle cell disease. Ophthal Plast Reconstr Surg. 2008; 24(3):181–184

[118] Yip CC, McCulley TJ, Kersten RC, Kulwin DR. Proptosis after hair pulling. Ophthal Plast Reconstr Surg. 2003; 19(2):154–155

[119] Wright JE, Sullivan TJ, Garner A, Wulc AE, Moseley IF. Orbital venous anomalies. Ophthalmology. 1997; 104(6):905–913

[120] Hwang CS, Lee S, Yen MT. Optic neuropathy following endovascular coiling of an orbital varix. Orbit. 2012; 31(6):418–419

[121] Tan AC, Farooqui S, Li X, et al. Ocular manifestations and the clinical course of carotid cavernous sinus fistulas in Asian patients. Orbit. 2014; 33(1):45–51

[122] Lee BJ, Schoenfield L, Perry JD. Orbital intramuscular hemangioma enlarging during pregnancy. Ophthal Plast Reconstr Surg. 2009; 25(6):491–493

[123] Wiwatwongwana D, Rootman J. Management of optic neuropathy from an apical orbital-cavernous sinus hemangioma with radiotherapy. Orbit. 2008; 27(3):219–221

[124] Bakker SL, Hasan D, Bijvoet HW. Compression of the visual pathway by anterior cerebral artery aneurysm. Acta Neurol Scand. 1999; 99(3):204–207

[125] Miller NR, Savino PJ, Schneider T. Rapid growth of an intracranial aneurysm causing apparent retrobulbar optic neuritis. J Neuroophthalmol. 1995; 15(4):212–218

[126] Misra M, Mohanty AB, Rath S. Giant aneurysm of internal carotid artery presenting features of retrobulbar neuritis. Indian J Ophthalmol. 1991; 39(1):28–29

[127] Ortiz JR, Newman NJ, Barrow DL. CREST-associated multiple intracranial aneurysms and bilateral optic neuropathies. J Clin Neuroophthalmol. 1991; 11(4):233–240

[128] Shutter LA, Kline LB, Fisher WS. Visual loss and a suprasellar mass complicated by pregnancy. Surv Ophthalmol. 1993; 38(1):63–69

[129] Vargas ME, Kupersmith MJ, Setton A, Nelson K, Berenstein A. Endovascular treatment of giant aneurysms which cause visual loss. Ophthalmology. 1994; 101(6):1091–1098

[130] Koskela E, Setälä K, Kivisaari R, Hernesniemi J, Laakso A. Neuro-ophthalmic presentation and surgical results of unruptured intracranial aneurysms: prospective Helsinki experience of 142 patients. World Neurosurg. 2015; 83(4):614–619

[131] Colapinto EV, Cabeen MA, Johnson LN. Optic nerve compression by a dolichoectatic internal carotid artery: case report. Neurosurgery. 1996; 39(3):604–606

[132] Jacobson DM. Symptomatic compression of the optic nerve by the carotid artery: clinical profile of 18 patients with 24 affected eyes identified by magnetic resonance imaging. Ophthalmology. 1999; 106(10):1994–2004

[133] Savy LE, Moseley IF. Intracranial arterial calcification and ectasia in visual failure. Br J Radiol. 1996; 69(821):394–401

[134] Ishikawa T, Ito T, Shoji E, Inukai K. Compressive optic nerve atrophy resulting from a distorted internal carotid artery. Pediatr Neurol. 2000; 22(4):322–324

[135] Rebolleda G, Corcóstegui J, Arruabarrena C, Martínez San Millán J, Muñoz-Negrete FJ. Optociliary shunt vessels in compressive optic neuropathy by the intracranial internal carotid artery. Eur J Ophthalmol. 2008; 18(2):316–319

[136] Hikage F, Hashimoto M, Ohguro H. Vascular compressive optic neuropathy caused by hypertensive intracranial ophthalmic artery. Jpn J Ophthalmol. 2010; 54(5):511–514

[137] Kiratli H, Tarlan B. Total clinical regression of an orbital macrocystic lymphatic malformation following intralesional sodium tetradecyl sulphate injection. J AAPOS. 2015; 19(1):78–80

[138] Zimmermann AP, Eivazi B, Wiegand S, Werner JA, Teymoortash A. Orbital lymphatic malformation showing the symptoms of orbital complications of acute rhinosinusitis in children: a report of 2 cases. Int J Pediatr Otorhinolaryngol. 2009; 73(10):1480–1483

[139] Gündüz K, Demirel S, Yagmurlu B, Erden E. Correlation of surgical outcome with neuroimaging findings in periocular lymphangiomas. Ophthalmology. 2006; 113(7):1231.e1–1231.e8

[140] Shults WT, Hamby S, Corbett JJ, Kardon R, Winterkorn JS, Odel JG. Neuro-ophthalmic complications of intracranial catheters. Neurosurgery. 1993; 33(1):135–138

[141] Dutton JJ, Tse DT, Anderson RL. Compressive optic neuropathy following use of intracranial oxidized cellulose hemostat. Ophthalmic Surg. 1983; 14(6):487–490

[142] Carter K, Lee AG, Tang RA, et al. Neuro-ophthalmologic complications of sinus surgery. Neuro-ophthalmology. 1998; 19(2):75–82

[143] Edelstein C, Goldberg RA, Rubino G. Unilateral blindness after ipsilateral prophylactic transcranial optic canal decompression for fibrous dysplasia. Am J Ophthalmol. 1998; 126(3):469–471

[144] Yoon MK, Piluek WJ, Ruggiero JP, McDermott MW, McCulley TJ. Orbital cerebrospinal fluid accumulation after complicated pterional-orbitozygomatic craniotomy. J Neuroophthalmol. 2014; 34(4):346–349

[145] Arat YO, Dorotheo EU, Tang RA, Boniuk M, Schiffman JS. Compressive optic neuropathy after use of oxidized regenerated cellulose in orbital surgery: review of complications, prophylaxis, and treatment. Ophthalmology. 2006; 113(2):333–337

[146] Bhatti MT, Holder CA, Newman NJ, Hudgins PA. MR characteristics of muslin-induced optic neuropathy: report of two cases and review of the literature. AJNR Am J Neuroradiol. 2000; 21(2):346–352

[147] Lee AG, Cech DA, Rose JE, et al. Recurrent visual loss due to muslin-induced optochiasmatic arachnoiditis. Neuro-ophthalmology. 1997; 18(4):199–204

[148] Finnerty KN, Mancini R. Vision loss after maxillary artery embolization secondary to compressive optic neuropathy. Ophthal Plast Reconstr Surg. 2013; 29(4):e108–e110

[149] Mafee MF, Goodwin J, Dorodi S. Optic nerve sheath meningiomas. Role of MR imaging. Radiol Clin North Am. 1999; 37(1):37–58, ix

[150] Dutton JJ. Optic nerve sheath meningiomas. Surv Ophthalmol. 1992; 37(3): 167–183

[151] Cunliffe IA, Moffat DA, Hardy DG, Moore AT. Bilateral optic nerve sheath meningiomas in a patient with neurofibromatosis type 2. Br J Ophthalmol. 1992; 76(5):310–312

[152] Misra S, Misra N, Gogri P, Mehta R. A rare case of bilateral optic nerve sheath meningioma. Indian J Ophthalmol. 2014; 62(6):728–730

[153] Nickel M, Löbel U, Holst B, et al. Unexplained loss of vision in a child: consider bilateral primary optic nerve sheath meningioma. Neuropediatrics. 2014; 45(5):321–324

[154] Kothari NA, Kulkarni KM, Lam BL. Untreated bilateral optic nerve sheath meningiomas observed for 27 years. J Neuroophthalmol. 2013; 33(1):45–47

[155] Sawaya RA, Sidani C, Farah N, Hourani-Risk R. Presumed bilateral optic nerve sheath meningiomas presenting as optic neuritis. J Neuroophthalmol. 2008; 28(1):55–57

[156] Kang KB, Lim JI. Blurred vision in a woman who had sphenoid wing meningioma. JAMA Ophthalmol. 2015; 133(9):1081–1082

[157] Zielinski G, Grala B, Koziarski A, Kozlowski W. Skull base secretory meningioma. Value of histological and immunohistochemical findings for peritumoral brain edema formation. Neuroendocrinol Lett. 2013; 34(2): 111–117

[158] Bassiouni H, Asgari S, Stolke D. Olfactory groove meningiomas: functional outcome in a series treated microsurgically. Acta Neurochir (Wien). 2007; 149(2):109–121, discussion 121

[159] Wroe SJ, Thompson AJ, McDonald WI. Painful intraorbital meningiomas. J Neurol Neurosurg Psychiatry. 1991; 54(11):1009–1010

[160] Grunberg SM, Weiss MH, Spitz IM, et al. Treatment of unresectable meningiomas with the antiprogesterone agent mifepristone. J Neurosurg. 1991; 74(6):861–866

[161] Wan WL, Geller JL, Feldon SE, Sadun AA. Visual loss caused by rapidly progressive intracranial meningiomas during pregnancy. Ophthalmology. 1990; 97(1):18–21

[162] Rubinstein AB, Loven D, Geier A, Reichenthal E, Gadoth N. Hormone receptors in initially excised versus recurrent intracranial meningiomas. J Neurosurg. 1994; 81(2):184–187

[163] Kerschbaumer J, Freyschlag CF, Stockhammer G, et al. Hormone-dependent shrinkage of a sphenoid wing meningioma after pregnancy: case report. J Neurosurg. 2016; 124(1):137–140

[164] Moscovici S, Fraifeld S, Cohen JE, et al. Parasellar meningiomas in pregnancy: surgical results and visual outcomes. World Neurosurg. 2014; 82(3–4):e503–e512

[165] Shitara S, Nitta N, Fukami T, Nozaki K. Tuberculum sellae meningioma causing progressive visual impairment during pregnancy. Case report. Neurol Med Chir (Tokyo). 2012; 52(8):607–611

[166] Chacko JG, Miller JL, Angtuaco EJ. Spontaneous postpartum resolution of vision loss caused by a progesterone receptor-positive tuberculum sellae meningioma. J Neuroophthalmol. 2010; 30(2):132–134

[167] Ebner FH, Bornemann A, Wilhelm H, Ernemann U, Honegger J. Tuberculum sellae meningioma symptomatic during pregnancy: pathophysiological considerations. Acta Neurochir (Wien). 2008; 150(2):189–193, discussion 193

[168] Vaphiades MS. Disk edema and cranial MRI optic nerve enhancement: how long is too long? Surv Ophthalmol. 2001; 46(1):56–58

[169] Örnek N, Büyüktortop-Gökçinar N, Dağ E, Örnek K. Compressive optic neuropathy presenting with psychiatric symptoms. J Craniofac Surg. 2014; 25(2):e163–e164

[170] Ling JD, Chao D, Al Zubidi N, Lee AG. Big red flags in neuro-ophthalmology. Can J Ophthalmol. 2013; 48(1):3–7

[171] Semeraro F, Forbice E, Duse S, Costagliola C. Pseudo-Foster Kennedy syndrome in a young woman with meningioma infiltrating the superior sagittal sinus. Clin Neurol Neurosurg. 2012; 114(3):272–274

[172] Kitthaweesin K, Ployprasith C. Ocular manifestations of suprasellar tumors. J Med Assoc Thai. 2008; 91(5):711–715

[173] Saeed P, Rootman J, Nugent RA, White VA, Mackenzie IR, Koornneef L. Optic nerve sheath meningiomas. Ophthalmology. 2003; 110(10):2019–2030

[174] Muci-Mendoza R, Arevalo JF, Ramella M, et al. Optociliary veins in optic nerve sheath meningioma. Indocyanine green videoangiography findings. Ophthalmology. 1999; 106(2):311–318

[175] Kinjo T, al-Mefty O, Ciric I. Diaphragma sellae meningiomas. Neurosurgery. 1995; 36(6):1082–1092

[176] Klink DF, Sampath P, Miller NR, Brem H, Long DM. Long-term visual outcome after nonradical microsurgery patients with parasellar and cavernous sinus meningiomas. Neurosurgery. 2000; 47(1):24–31, discussion 31–32

[177] Maroon JC, Kennerdell JS, Vidovich DV, Abla A, Sternau L. Recurrent spheno-orbital meningioma. J Neurosurg. 1994; 80(2):202–208

[178] Weaver DT, Garrity JA, Meyer FA, Laws ER. Visual prognosis in sphenoid ridge meningioma. Presented at the 19th annual meeting of the North American Neuro-Ophthalmology Society, Big Sky, MT; 1993

[179] Wadud SA, Ahmed S, Choudhury N, Chowdhury D. Evaluation of ophthalmic manifestations in patients with intracranial tumours. Mymensingh Med J. 2014; 23(2):268–271

[180] Larson JJ, van Loveren HR, Balko MG, Tew JM, Jr. Evidence of meningioma infiltration into cranial nerves: clinical implications for cavernous sinus meningiomas. J Neurosurg. 1995; 83(4):596–599

[181] Scarone P, Leclerq D, Héran F, Robert G. Long-term results with exophthalmos in a surgical series of 30 sphenoorbital meningiomas. Clinical article. J Neurosurg. 2009; 111(5):1069–1077

[182] Kudrimoti JK, Gaikwad MJ, Puranik SC, Chugh AP. Primary dural non-hodgkin's lymphoma mimicking meningioma: A case report and review of literature. J Cancer Res Ther. 2015; 11(3):648

[183] Suresh S, Abel AS, Younge BR, Bilyk JR, Lee MS. Masses in the membranes. Surv Ophthalmol. 2016; 61(3):357–362

[184] Lok JY, Yip NK, Chong KK, Li CL, Young AL. Idiopathic hypertrophic pachymeningitis mimicking prolactinoma with recurrent vision loss. Hong Kong Med J. 2015; 21(4):360–362

[185] Nassif S, Boulos F. Extranodal (dural) Rosai-Dorfman disease radiologically and histologically mimicking meningioma: a case report. Anal Quant Cytopathol Histpathol. 2015; 37(2):144–146

[186] Noshiro S, Wanibuchi M, Akiyama Y, et al. IgG4-related disease initially presented as an orbital mass lesion mimicking optic nerve sheath meningioma. Brain Tumor Pathol. 2015; 32(4):286–290

[187] Okano A, Nakatomi H, Shibahara J, Tsuchiya T, Saito N. Intracranial inflammatory pseudotumors associated with immunoglobulin G4-related disease mimicking multiple meningiomas: a case report and review of the literature. World Neurosurg. 2015; 83(6):1181.e1–1181.e4

[188] Malhotra G, Asopa RV, Sridhar E. Unusual case of isolated parasellar metastasis from carcinoma of thyroid. Clin Nucl Med. 2013; 38(2):145–148

[189] Tariq R, Ahmed R. Tuberculous hypertrophic pachymeningitis presenting as visual blurring and headaches. J Pak Med Assoc. 2012; 62(9):966–968

[190] Lim AC, Cerra C, Pal P, Kearney T, Gnanalingham KK. Visual loss from a pituitary mass: collision tumors of prostatic metastasis and suprasellar meningioma. J Neurol Surg A Cent Eur Neurosurg. 2013; 74 Suppl 1:e81–e84

[191] Ali H, Price RF. Cranial meningioma co-localised with Langerhans cell histiocytosis. Br J Neurosurg. 2013; 27(1):122–124

[192] Kulkarni KM, Sternau L, Dubovy SR, Lam BL. Primary dural lymphoma masquerading as a meningioma. J Neuroophthalmol. 2012; 32(3):240–242

[193] Gupta K, Bagdi N, Sunitha P, Ghosal N. Isolated intracranial Rosai-Dorfman disease mimicking meningioma in a child: a case report and review of the literature. Br J Radiol. 2011; 84(1003):e138–e141

[194] Chaturvedi S, Gupta S, Kumari R. Meningioma with metastasis from follicular carcinoma thyroid. Indian J Pathol Microbiol. 2010; 53(2):316–318

[195] Prabhu K, Daniel RT, Chacko G, Chacko AG. Optic nerve haemangioblastoma mimicking a planum sphenoidale meningioma. Br J Neurosurg. 2009; 23(5): 561–563

[196] Arvold ND, Lessell S, Bussiere M, et al. Visual outcome and tumor control after conformal radiotherapy for patients with optic nerve sheath meningioma. Int J Radiat Oncol Biol Phys. 2009; 75(4):1166–1172

[197] George KJ, Price R. Nasoethmoid schwannoma with intracranial extension. Case report and review of literature. Br J Neurosurg. 2009; 23(1):83–85

[198] Kasliwal MK, Suri A, Gupta DK, Suri V, Rishi A, Sharma BS. Sphenoid wing inflammatory pseudotumor mimicking a clinoidal meningioma: case report and review of the literature. Surg Neurol. 2008; 70(5):509–513, discussion 513

[199] Roberti F, Lee HH, Caputy AJ, Katz B. "Shave" biopsy of the optic nerve in isolated neurosarcoidosis. J Neurosurg Sci. 2005; 49(2):59–63, discussion 63

[200] Selva D, Rootman J, Crompton J. Orbital lymphoma mimicking optic nerve meningioma. Orbit. 2004; 23(2):115–120

[201] Zimmerman CF, Schatz NJ, Glaser JS. Magnetic resonance imaging of optic nerve meningiomas. Enhancement with gadolinium-DTPA. Ophthalmology. 1990; 97(5):585–591

[202] Ly KI, Hamilton SR, Rostomily RC, Rockhill JK, Mrugala MM. Improvement in visual fields after treatment of intracranial meningioma with bevacizumab. J Neuroophthalmol. 2015; 35(4):382–386

[203] Sadun AA, Weiss MH. Reversal of visual losses following RU 486 therapy for meningioma. Presented at the 19th annual meeting of the North American Neuro-Ophthalmology Society, Big Sky, MT; 1993

[204] DeMonte F, Smith HK, al-Mefty O. Outcome of aggressive removal of cavernous sinus meningiomas. J Neurosurg. 1994; 81(2):245–251

[205] Hirsch WL, Sekhar LN, Lanzino G, Pomonis S, Sen CN. Meningiomas involving the cavernous sinus: value of imaging for predicting surgical complications. AJR Am J Roentgenol. 1993; 160(5):1083–1088

[206] Stafford SL, Perry A, Leavitt JA, et al. Anterior visual pathway meningiomas primarily resected between 1978 and 1988: the Mayo Clinic Rochester experience. J Neuroophthalmol. 1998; 18(3):206–210

[207] Berhouma M, Jacquesson T, Abouaf L, Vighetto A, Jouanneau E. Endoscopic endonasal optic nerve and orbital apex decompression for nontraumatic optic neuropathy: surgical nuances and review of the literature. Neurosurg Focus. 2014; 37(4):E19

[208] Taha AN, Erkmen K, Dunn IF, Pravdenkova S, Al-Mefty O. Meningiomas involving the optic canal: pattern of involvement and implications for surgical technique. Neurosurg Focus. 2011; 30(5):E12

[209] Yu HJ, Wu YT, Chen HK, Lin JW. Primary orbital meningioma: a study of six cases at a single institution. APMIS. 2011; 119(1):36–43

[210] Saeed P, van Furth WR, Tanck M, et al. Surgical treatment of sphenoorbital meningiomas. Br J Ophthalmol. 2011; 95(7):996–1000

[211] Cannon PS, Rutherford SA, Richardson PL, King A, Leatherbarrow B. The surgical management and outcomes for spheno-orbital meningiomas: a 7-year review of multi-disciplinary practice. Orbit. 2009; 28(6):371–376

[212] Sethi RA, Rush SC, Liu S, et al. Dose-response relationships for meningioma radiosurgery. Am J Clin Oncol. 2015; 38(6):600–604

[213] Zeiler FA, McDonald PJ, Kaufmann AM, et al. Gamma Knife radiosurgery of cavernous sinus meningiomas: an institutional review. Can J Neurol Sci. 2012; 39(6):757–762

[214] Kim MS, Park K, Kim JH, Kim YD, Lee JI. Gamma knife radiosurgery for orbital tumors. Clin Neurol Neurosurg. 2008; 110(10):1003–1007

[215] al-Mefty O, Kersh JE, Routh A, Smith RR. The long-term side effects of radiation therapy for benign brain tumors in adults. J Neurosurg. 1990; 73 (4):502–512

[216] Fineman MS, Augsburger JJ. A new approach to an old problem. Surv Ophthalmol. 1999; 43(6):519–524

[217] Goldsmith BJ, Wara WM, Wilson CB, Larson DA. Postoperative irradiation for subtotally resected meningiomas. A retrospective analysis of 140 patients treated from 1967 to 1990. J Neurosurg. 1994; 80(2):195–201

[218] Lee AG, Woo SY, Miller NR, Safran AB, Grant WH, Butler EB. Improvement in visual function in an eye with a presumed optic nerve sheath meningioma after treatment with three-dimensional conformal radiation therapy. J Neuroophthalmol. 1996; 16(4):247–251

[219] Lunsford LD. Contemporary management of meningiomas: radiation therapy as an adjuvant and radiosurgery as an alternative to surgical removal? J Neurosurg. 1994; 80(2):187–190

[220] Moyer PD, Golnik KC, Breneman J. Treatment of optic nerve sheath meningioma with three-dimensional conformal radiation. Am J Ophthalmol. 2000; 129(5):694–696

[221] Newman SA. Meningiomas: a quest for the optimum therapy. J Neurosurg. 1994; 80(2):191–194

[222] Peele KA, Kennerdell JS, Maroon JC, et al. The role of postoperative irradiation in the management of sphenoid wing meningiomas. A preliminary report. Ophthalmology. 1996; 103(11):1761–1766, discussion 1766–1767

[223] Wilson CB. Meningiomas: genetics, malignancy, and the role of radiation in induction and treatment. The Richard C. Schneider Lecture. J Neurosurg. 1994; 81(5):666–675

[224] Malloy KA, Chigbu DI. Anterior temporal chordoid meningioma causing compressive optic neuropathy. Optom Vis Sci. 2011; 88(5):645–651

[225] Eddleman CS, Liu JK. Optic nerve sheath meningioma: current diagnosis and treatment. Neurosurg Focus. 2007; 23(5):E4

[226] Kim BS, Im YS, Woo KI, Kim YD, Lee JI. Multisession gamma knife radiosurgery for orbital apex tumors. World Neurosurg. 2015; 84(4):1005–1013

[227] Marwaha G, Macklis R, Singh AD. Radiation therapy: orbital tumors. Dev Ophthalmol. 2013; 52:94–101

[228] Adams G, Roos DE, Crompton JL. Radiotherapy for optic nerve sheath meningioma: a case for earlier intervention? Clin Oncol (R Coll Radiol). 2013; 25(6):356–361

[229] Bloch O, Sun M, Kaur G, Barani IJ, Parsa AT. Fractionated radiotherapy for optic nerve sheath meningiomas. J Clin Neurosci. 2012; 19(9):1210–1215

[230] Saeed P, Blank L, Selva D, et al. Primary radiotherapy in progressive optic nerve sheath meningiomas: a long-term follow-up study. Br J Ophthalmol. 2010; 94(5):564–568

[231] Schick U, Jung C, Hassler WE. Primary optic nerve sheath meningiomas: a follow-up study. Cent Eur Neurosurg. 2010; 71(3):126–133

[232] Milker-Zabel S, Huber P, Schlegel W, Debus J, Zabel-du Bois A. Fractionated stereotactic radiation therapy in the management of primary optic nerve sheath meningiomas. J Neurooncol. 2009; 94(3):419–424

[233] Smee RI, Schneider M, Williams JR. Optic nerve sheath meningiomas–non-surgical treatment. Clin Oncol (R Coll Radiol). 2009; 21(1):8–13

[234] Stieber VW. Radiation therapy for visual pathway tumors. J Neuroophthalmol. 2008; 28(3):222–230

[235] Vagefi MR, Larson DA, Horton JC. Optic nerve sheath meningioma: visual improvement during radiation treatment. Am J Ophthalmol. 2006; 142(2):343–344

[236] Alvord EC, Jr, Lofton S. Gliomas of the optic nerve or chiasm. Outcome by patients' age, tumor site, and treatment. J Neurosurg. 1988; 68(1):85–98

[237] Brodovsky S, ten Hove MW, Pinkerton RM, Ludwin SK, Smith RM. An enhancing optic nerve lesion: malignant glioma of adulthood. Can J Ophthalmol. 1997; 32(6):409–413

[238] Chateil JF, Soussotte C, Pédespan JM, Brun M, Le Manh C, Diard F. MRI and clinical differences between optic pathway tumours in children with and without neurofibromatosis. Br J Radiol. 2001; 74(877):24–31

[239] Créange A, Zeller J, Rostaing-Rigattieri S, et al. Neurological complications of neurofibromatosis type 1 in adulthood. Brain. 1999; 122(Pt 3):473–481

[240] Cummings TJ, Provenzale JM, Hunter SB, et al. Gliomas of the optic nerve: histological, immunohistochemical (MIB-1 and p53), and MRI analysis. Acta Neuropathol. 2000; 99(5):563–570

[241] Deliganis AV, Geyer JR, Berger MS. Prognostic significance of type 1 neurofibromatosis (von Recklinghausen Disease) in childhood optic glioma. Neurosurgery. 1996; 38(6):1114–1118, discussion 1118–1119

[242] DiMario FJ, Jr, Ramsby G, Greenstein R, Langshur S, Dunham B. Neurofibromatosis type 1: magnetic resonance imaging findings. J Child Neurol. 1993; 8(1):32–39

[243] Drake JM, Joy M, Goldenberg A, Kreindler D. Computer- and robot-assisted resection of thalamic astrocytomas in children. Neurosurgery. 1991; 29(1):27–33

[244] Dunn DW, Purvin V. Optic pathway gliomas in neurofibromatosis. Dev Med Child Neurol. 1990; 32(9):820–824

[245] Dutton JJ. Gliomas of the anterior visual pathway. Surv Ophthalmol. 1994; 38(5):427–452

[246] Epstein MA, Packer RJ, Rorke LB, et al. Vascular malformation with radiation vasculopathy after treatment of chiasmatic/hypothalamic glioma. Cancer. 1992; 70(4):887–893

[247] Friedman JM, Birch P. An association between optic glioma and other tumours of the central nervous system in neurofibromatosis type 1. Neuropediatrics. 1997; 28(2):131–132

[248] Fuss M, Hug EB, Schaefer RA, et al. Proton radiation therapy (PRT) for pediatric optic pathway gliomas: comparison with 3D planned conventional photons and a standard photon technique. Int J Radiat Oncol Biol Phys. 1999; 45(5):1117–1126

[249] Garvey M, Packer RJ. An integrated approach to the treatment of chiasmatic-hypothalamic gliomas. J Neurooncol. 1996; 28(2–3):167–183

[250] Gayre GS, Scott IU, Feuer W, Saunders TG, Siatkowski RM. Long-term visual outcome in patients with anterior visual pathway gliomas. J Neuroophthalmol. 2001; 21(1):1–7

[251] Grill J, Couanet D, Cappelli C, et al. Radiation-induced cerebral vasculopathy in children with neurofibromatosis and optic pathway glioma. Ann Neurol. 1999; 45(3):393–396

[252] Hoffman HJ, Humphreys RP, Drake JM, et al. Optic pathway/hypothalamic gliomas: a dilemma in management. Pediatr Neurosurg. 1993; 19(4):186–195

[253] Imes RK, Hoyt WF. Magnetic resonance imaging signs of optic nerve gliomas in neurofibromatosis 1. Am J Ophthalmol. 1991; 111(6):729–734

[254] Janss AJ, Grundy R, Cnaan A, et al. Optic pathway and hypothalamic/chiasmatic gliomas in children younger than age 5 years with a 6-year follow-up. Cancer. 1995; 75(4):1051–1059

[255] Jenkin D, Angyalfi S, Becker L, et al. Optic glioma in children: surveillance, resection, or irradiation? Int J Radiat Oncol Biol Phys. 1993; 25(2):215–225

[256] Kestle JRW, Hoffman HJ, Mock AR. Moyamoya phenomenon after radiation for optic glioma. J Neurosurg. 1993; 79(1):32–35

[257] Kovalic JJ, Grigsby PW, Shepard MJ, Fineberg BB, Thomas PR. Radiation therapy for gliomas of the optic nerve and chiasm. Int J Radiat Oncol Biol Phys. 1990; 18(4):927–932

[258] Levin LA, Jakobiec FA. Optic nerve tumors of childhood: a decision-analytical approach to their diagnosis. Int Ophthalmol Clin. 1992; 32(1):223–240

[259] Listernick R, Charrow J, Greenwald M. Emergence of optic pathway gliomas in children with neurofibromatosis type 1 after normal neuroimaging results. J Pediatr. 1992; 121(4):584–587

[260] Listernick R, Charrow J, Greenwald M, Mets M. Natural history of optic pathway tumors in children with neurofibromatosis type 1: a longitudinal study. J Pediatr. 1994; 125(1):63–66

[261] Listernick R, Louis DN, Packer RJ, Gutmann DH. Optic pathway gliomas in children with neurofibromatosis 1: consensus statement from the NF1 Optic Pathway Glioma Task Force. Ann Neurol. 1997; 41(2):143–149

[262] Liu GT, Lessell S. Spontaneous visual improvement in chiasmal gliomas. Am J Ophthalmol. 1992; 114(2):193–201

[263] Liu GT. Visual loss in childhood. Surv Ophthalmol. 2001; 46(1):35–42

[264] Moghrabi A, Friedman HS, Burger PC, Tien R, Oakes WJ. Carboplatin treatment of progressive optic pathway gliomas to delay radiotherapy. J Neurosurg. 1993; 79(2):223–227

[265] Nishio S, Takeshita I, Fujiwara S, Fukui M. Optico-hypothalamic glioma: an analysis of 16 cases. Childs Nerv Syst. 1993; 9(6):334–338

[266] Oaks W. Recent experience with resection of pilocytic astrocytomas of the hypothalamus. Concepts Pediatr Neurosurg. 1990; 10:108–117

[267] Packer RJ, Ater JC, Phillips P, et al. Efficacy of chemotherapy for children with newly diagnosed progressive low-grade glioma. (abstract). Ann Neurol. 1994; 36:496

[268] Packer RJ, Lange B, Ater J, et al. Carboplatin and vincristine for recurrent and newly diagnosed low-grade gliomas of childhood. J Clin Oncol. 1993; 11(5):850–856

[269] Parsa CF, Hoyt CS, Lesser RL, et al. Spontaneous regression of optic gliomas: thirteen cases documented by serial neuroimaging. Arch Ophthalmol. 2001; 119(4):516–529

[270] Petronio J, Edwards MS, Prados M, et al. Management of chiasmal and hypothalamic gliomas of infancy and childhood with chemotherapy. J Neurosurg. 1991; 74(5):701–708

[271] Pierce SM, Barnes PD, Loeffler JS, McGinn C, Tarbell NJ. Definitive radiation therapy in the management of symptomatic patients with optic glioma. Survival and long-term effects. Cancer. 1990; 65(1):45–52

[272] Rodriguez LA, Edwards MSB, Levin VA. Management of hypothalamic gliomas in children: an analysis of 33 cases. Neurosurgery. 1990; 26(2):242–246, discussion 246–247

[273] Shuper A, Horev G, Kornreich L, et al. Visual pathway glioma: an erratic tumour with therapeutic dilemmas. Arch Dis Child. 1997; 76(3):259–263

[274] Sutton LN. Visual pathway gliomas of childhood. Contemporary Neurosurg. 1994; 16(8):1–6

[275] Sutton LN, Molloy PT, Sernyak H, et al. Long-term outcome of hypothalamic/chiasmatic astrocytomas in children treated with conservative surgery. J Neurosurg. 1995; 83(4):583–589

[276] Wisoff JH. Management of optic pathway tumors of childhood. Neurosurg Clin N Am. 1992; 3(4):791–802

[277] Wisoff JH, Abbott R, Epstein F. Surgical management of exophytic chiasmatic-hypothalamic tumors of childhood. J Neurosurg. 1990; 73(5):661–667

[278] Gupta V, Sabri K, Whelan KF, Viscardi V. Rare case of optic pathway glioma with extensive intra-ocular involvement in a child with neurofibromatosis type 1. Middle East Afr J Ophthalmol. 2015; 22(1):117–118

[279] Vassal F, Pommier B, Boutet C, Forest F, Campolmi N, Nuti C. Isolated primary central nervous system lymphoma arising from the optic chiasm. Neurochirurgie. 2014; 60(6):312–315

[280] Tahir MZ, Shaikh F, Siddiqui AA. Primary chiasmal sarcoid granuloma masquerading as glioma of the optic chiasm. J Coll Physicians Surg Pak. 2010; 20(10):695–696

[281] Pollock JM, Greiner FG, Crowder JB, Crowder JW, Quindlen E. Neurosarcoidosis mimicking a malignant optic glioma. J Neuroophthalmol. 2008; 28(3):214–216

[282] Bergmann M, Brück W, Neubauer U, Probst-Cousin S. Diagnostic pitfall: optic neuritis mimicking optic nerve glioma. Neuropathology. 2009; 29(4):450–453

[283] Tumialán LM, Dhall SS, Biousse V, Newman NJ. Optic nerve glioma and optic neuritis mimicking one another: case report. Neurosurgery. 2005; 57(1):E190–, discussion E190

[284] Aversa do Souto A, Fonseca AL, Gadelha M, Donangelo I, Chimelli L, Domingues FS. Optic pathways tuberculoma mimicking glioma: case report. Surg Neurol. 2003; 60(4):349–353

[285] Parness-Yossifon R, Listernick R, Charrow J, Barto H, Zeid JL. Strabismus in patients with neurofibromatosis type 1-associated optic pathway glioma. J AAPOS. 2015; 19(5):422–425

[286] Dansingani KK, Jung JJ, Belinsky I, Marr BP, Freund KB. Ischemic retinopathy in neurofibromatosis type 1. Retin Cases Brief Rep. 2015; 9(4):290–294

[287] Avery RA, Cnaan A, Schuman JS, et al. Longitudinal change of circumpapillary retinal nerve fiber layer thickness in children with optic pathway gliomas. Am J Ophthalmol. 2015; 160(5):944–952.e1

[288] Toledano H, Muhsinoglu O, Luckman J, Goldenberg-Cohen N, Michowiz S. Acquired nystagmus as the initial presenting sign of chiasmal glioma in young children. Eur J Paediatr Neurol. 2015; 19(6):694–700

[289] Brodsky MC, Keating GF. Chiasmal glioma in spasmus nutans: a cautionary note. J Neuroophthalmol. 2014; 34(3):274–275

[290] Della Puppa A, Rustemi O, Gioffre' G. The rare event of optic-chiasmatic hemorrhagic low grade glioma in adulthood. Considerations on treatment strategy. Neurol Sci. 2014; 35(4):623–625

[291] Arrese I, Sarabia R, Zamora T. Chiasmal haemorrhage secondary to glioma with unusual MRI appearance. Neurocirugia (Astur). 2014; 25(3):136–139

[292] Varan A, Batu A, Cila A, et al. Optic glioma in children: a retrospective analysis of 101 cases. Am J Clin Oncol. 2013; 36(3):287–292

[293] Hill JD, Rhee MS, Edwards JR, Hagen MC, Fulkerson DH. Spontaneous intraventricular hemorrhage from low-grade optic glioma: case report and review of the literature. Childs Nerv Syst. 2012; 28(2):327–330

[294] Avery RA, Liu GT, Fisher MJ, et al. Retinal nerve fiber layer thickness in children with optic pathway gliomas. Am J Ophthalmol. 2011; 151(3):542–9.e2

[295] Jacob FD, Ramaswamy V, Goez HR. Acquired monocular nystagmus as the initial presenting sign of a chiasmal glioma. Can J Neurol Sci. 2010; 37(1):96–97

[296] Yokoyama S, Takayama K, Sueda M, Ishikawa Y, Hirano H. Optic nerve glioma manifesting as intratumoral hemorrhage in a pregnant woman: case report. Neurol Med Chir (Tokyo). 2003; 43(11):559–562

[297] Lee AG, Dutton JJ. A practice pathway for the management of gliomas of the anterior visual pathway: an update and evidence-based approach. Neuroophthalmology. 1999; 22(3):139–155

[298] Sullivan-Mee M, Solis K. Methanol-induced vision loss. J Am Optom Assoc. 1998; 69(1):57–65

[299] Dodgshun AJ, Elder JE, Hansford JR, Sullivan MJ. Long-term visual outcome after chemotherapy for optic pathway glioma in children: site and age are strongly predictive. Cancer. 2015; 121(23):4190–4196

[300] Shofty B, Mauda-Havakuk M, Weizman L, et al. The effect of chemotherapy on optic pathway gliomas and their sub-components: a volumetric MR analysis study. Pediatr Blood Cancer. 2015; 62(8):1353–1359

[301] Kaul A, Toonen JA, Cimino PJ, Gianino SM, Gutmann DH. Akt- or MEK-mediated mTOR inhibition suppresses Nf1 optic glioma growth. Neuro-oncol. 2015; 17(6):843–853

[302] Shofty B, Ben-Sira L, Kesler A, Constantini S. Optic pathway gliomas. Adv Tech Stand Neurosurg. 2015; 42:123–146

[303] Cappellano AM, Petrilli AS, da Silva NS, et al. Single agent vinorelbine in pediatric patients with progressive optic pathway glioma. J Neurooncol. 2015; 121(2):405–412

[304] Rodriguez FJ, Raabe EH. mTOR: a new therapeutic target for pediatric low-grade glioma? CNS Oncol. 2014; 3(2):89–91

[305] Nair AG, Pathak RS, Iyer VR, Gandhi RA. Optic nerve glioma: an update. Int Ophthalmol. 2014; 34(4):999–1005

[306] Cardellicchio S, Bacci G, Farina S, et al. Low-dose cisplatin-etoposide regimen for patients with optic pathway glioma: a report of four cases and literature review. Neuropediatrics. 2014; 45(1):42–49

[307] Avery RA, Hwang EI, Jakacki RI, Packer RJ. Marked recovery of vision in children with optic pathway gliomas treated with bevacizumab. JAMA Ophthalmol. 2014; 132(1):111–114

[308] Hütt-Cabezas M, Karajannis MA, Zagzag D, et al. Activation of mTORC1/ mTORC2 signaling in pediatric low-grade glioma and pilocytic astrocytoma reveals mTOR as a therapeutic target. Neuro-oncol. 2013; 15(12):1604–1614

[309] Okada K, Yamasaki K, Tanaka C, Fujisaki H, Osugi Y, Hara J. Phase I study of bevacizumab plus irinotecan in pediatric patients with recurrent/refractory solid tumors. Jpn J Clin Oncol. 2013; 43(11):1073–1079

[310] Liu GT, Katowitz JA, Rorke-Adams LB, Fisher MJ. Optic pathway gliomas: neoplasms, not hamartomas. JAMA Ophthalmol. 2013; 131(5):646–650

[311] Uslu N, Karakaya E, Dizman A, Yegen D, Guney Y. Optic nerve glioma treatment with fractionated stereotactic radiotherapy. J Neurosurg Pediatr. 2013; 11(5):596–599

[312] Fried I, Tabori U, Tihan T, Reginald A, Bouffet E. Optic pathway gliomas: a review. CNS Oncol. 2013; 2(2):143–159

[313] Ashur-Fabian O, Blumenthal DT, Bakon M, Nass D, Davis PJ, Hercbergs A. Long-term response in high-grade optic glioma treated with medically induced hypothyroidism and carboplatin: a case report and review of the literature. Anticancer Drugs. 2013; 24(3):315–323

[314] Chong AL, Pole JD, Scheinemann K, et al. Optic pathway gliomas in adolescence–time to challenge treatment choices? Neuro-oncol. 2013; 15 (3):391–400

[315] Avery RA, Fisher MJ, Liu GT. Optic pathway gliomas. J Neuroophthalmol. 2011; 31(3):269–278

[316] Peyrl A, Azizi A, Czech T, et al. Tumor stabilization under treatment with imatinib in progressive hypothalamic-chiasmatic glioma. Pediatr Blood Cancer. 2009; 52(4):476–480

[317] Diaz RJ, Laughlin S, Nicolin G, Buncic JR, Bouffet E, Bartels U. Assessment of chemotherapeutic response in children with proptosis due to optic nerve glioma. Childs Nerv Syst. 2008; 24(6):707–712

[318] Sharif S, Ferner R, Birch JM, et al. Second primary tumors in neurofibromatosis 1 patients treated for optic glioma: substantial risks after radiotherapy. J Clin Oncol. 2006; 24(16):2570–2575

[319] Mantadakis E, Raissaki M, Danilatou V, Kambourakis A, Stiakaki E, Kalmanti M. Remission of a chiasmatic glioma in a non-NF1 patient after brief chemotherapy with vincristine and carboplatin: case report and literature review. J Neurooncol. 2004; 67(1–2):95–100

[320] Pruzan NL, de Alba Campomanes A, Gorovoy IR, Hoyt C. Spontaneous regression of a massive sporadic chiasmal optic pathway glioma. J Child Neurol. 2015; 30(9):1196–1198

[321] Parsa CF. Why visual function does not correlate with optic glioma size or growth. Arch Ophthalmol. 2012; 130(4):521–522

[322] Mishra MV, Andrews DW, Glass J, et al. Characterization and outcomes of optic nerve gliomas: a population-based analysis. J Neurooncol. 2012; 107 (3):591–597

[323] Hwang JM, Cheon JE, Wang KC. Visual prognosis of optic glioma. Childs Nerv Syst. 2008; 24(6):693–698

[324] Piccirilli M, Lenzi J, Delfinis C, Trasimeni G, Salvati M, Raco A. Spontaneous regression of optic pathways gliomas in three patients with neurofibromatosis type I and critical review of the literature. Childs Nerv Syst. 2006; 22(10):1332–1337

[325] Blanchard G, Lafforgue MP, Lion-François L, et al. NF France network. Systematic MRI in NF1 children under six years of age for the diagnosis of optic pathway gliomas. Study and outcome of a French cohort. Eur J Paediatr Neurol. 2016; 20(2):275–281

[326] Levin MH, Armstrong GT, Broad JH, et al. Risk of optic pathway glioma in children with neurofibromatosis type 1 and optic nerve tortuosity or nerve sheath thickening. Br J Ophthalmol. 2016; 100(4):510–514

[327] Binning MJ, Liu JK, Kestle JR, Brockmeyer DL, Walker ML. Optic pathway gliomas: a review. Neurosurg Focus. 2007; 23(5):E2

[328] Lee AG. Neuroophthalmological management of optic pathway gliomas. Neurosurg Focus. 2007; 23(5):E1

[329] Aquilina K, Daniels DJ, Spoudeas H, Phipps K, Gan HW, Boop FA. Optic pathway glioma in children: does visual deficit correlate with radiology in focal exophytic lesions? Childs Nerv Syst. 2015; 31(11):2041–2049

[330] Prada CE, Hufnagel RB, Hummel TR, et al. The use of magnetic resonance imaging screening for optic pathway gliomas in children with neurofibromatosis type 1. J Pediatr. 2015; 167(4):851–856.e1

[331] Yeom KW, Lober RM, Andre JB, et al. Prognostic role for diffusion-weighted imaging of pediatric optic pathway glioma. J Neurooncol. 2013; 113(3):479–483

[332] Topcu-Yilmaz P, Kasim B, Kiratli H. Investigation of retinal nerve fiber layer thickness in patients with neurofibromatosis-1. Jpn J Ophthalmol. 2014; 58 (2):172–176

[333] Avery RA, Hwang EI, Ishikawa H, et al. Handheld optical coherence tomography during sedation in young children with optic pathway gliomas. JAMA Ophthalmol. 2014; 132(3):265–271

[334] Parrozzani R, Clementi M, Kotsafti O, et al. Optical coherence tomography in the diagnosis of optic pathway gliomas. Invest Ophthalmol Vis Sci. 2013; 54 (13):8112–8118

[335] Chang L, El-Dairi MA, Frempong TA, et al. Optical coherence tomography in the evaluation of neurofibromatosis type-1 subjects with optic pathway gliomas. J AAPOS. 2010; 14(6):511–517

[336] Nicolin G, Parkin P, Mabbott D, et al. Natural history and outcome of optic pathway gliomas in children. Pediatr Blood Cancer. 2009; 53(7):1231–1237

[337] Brummitt ML, Kline LB, Wilson ER. Craniopharyngioma: pitfalls in diagnosis. J Clin Neuroophthalmol. 1992; 12(2):77–81, discussion 82–84

[338] Crotty TB, Scheithauer BW, Young WF, Jr, et al. Papillary craniopharyngioma: a clinicopathological study of 48 cases. J Neurosurg. 1995; 83(2):206–214

[339] el-Mahdy W, Powell M. Transsphenoidal management of 28 symptomatic Rathke's cleft cysts, with special reference to visual and hormonal recovery. Neurosurgery. 1998; 42(1):7–16, discussion 16–17

[340] Fahlbusch R, Honegger J, Paulus W, Huk W, Buchfelder M. Surgical treatment of craniopharyngiomas: experience with 168 patients. J Neurosurg. 1999; 90(2):237–250

[341] Honegger J, Buchfelder M, Fahlbusch R. Surgical treatment of craniopharyngiomas: endocrinological results. J Neurosurg. 1999; 90(2): 251–257

[342] Petito CK. Craniopharyngioma: prognostic importance of histologic features. AJNR Am J Neuroradiol. 1996; 17(8):1441–1442

[343] Rao GP, Blyth CP, Jeffreys RV. Ophthalmic manifestations of Rathke's cleft cysts. Am J Ophthalmol. 1995; 119(1):86–91

[344] Weiner HL, Wisoff JH, Rosenberg ME, et al. Craniopharyngiomas: a clinicopathological analysis of factors predictive of recurrence and functional outcome. Neurosurgery. 1994; 35(6):1001–1010, discussion 1010–1011

[345] Youl BD, Plant GT, Stevens JM, Kendall BE, Symon L, Crockard HA. Three cases of craniopharyngioma showing optic tract hypersignal on MRI. Neurology. 1990; 40(9):1416–1419

[346] Maini R, Macewen CJ. Intracranial plasmacytoma presenting with optic nerve compression. Br J Ophthalmol. 1997; 81(5):417–418

[347] Freilich RJ, Krol G, DeAngelis LM. Neuroimaging and cerebrospinal fluid cytology in the diagnosis of leptomeningeal metastasis. Ann Neurol. 1995; 38(1):51–57

[348] Ing EB, Augsburger JJ, Eagle RC. Lung cancer with visual loss. Surv Ophthalmol. 1996; 40(6):505–510

[349] McFadzean R, Brosnahan D, Doyle D, Going J, Hadley D, Lee W. A diagnostic quartet in leptomeningeal infiltration of the optic nerve sheath. J Neuroophthalmol. 1994; 14(3):175–182

[350] Sung JU, Lam BL, Curtin VT, Tse DT. Metastatic gastric carcinoma to the optic nerve. Arch Ophthalmol. 1998; 116(5):692–693

[351] Teare JP, Whitehead M, Rake MO, Coker RJ. Rapid onset of blindness due to meningeal carcinomatosis from an oesophageal adenocarcinoma. Postgrad Med J. 1991; 67(792):909–911

[352] Brown DM, Kimura AE, Ossoinig KC, Weiner GJ. Acute promyelocytic infiltration of the optic nerve treated by oral trans-retinoic acid. Ophthalmology. 1992; 99(9):1463–1467

[353] Camera A, Piccirillo G, Cennamo G, et al. Optic nerve involvement in acute lymphoblastic leukemia. Leuk Lymphoma. 1993; 11(1–2):153–155

[354] Costagliola C, Rinaldi M, Cotticelli L, Sbordone S, Nastri G. Isolated optic nerve involvement in chronic myeloid leukemia. Leuk Res. 1992; 16(4):411–413

[355] Cramer SC, Glaspy JA, Efird JT, Louis DN. Chronic lymphocytic leukemia and the central nervous system: a clinical and pathological study. Neurology. 1996; 46(1):19–25

[356] Horton JC, Garcia EC, Becker EK. Magnetic resonance imaging of leukemic invasion of the optic nerve. Arch Ophthalmol. 1992; 110(9):1207–1208

[357] Pierro L, Brancato R, Zaganelli E, Guarisco L, Lanzetta P. Ocular involvement in acute lymphoblastic leukemia: an echographic study. Int Ophthalmol. 1992; 16(3):159–162

[358] Shibasaki H, Hayasaka S, Noda S, Masaki Y, Yamamoto D. Radiotherapy resolves leukemic involvement of the optic nerves. Ann Ophthalmol. 1992; 24(10):395–397

[359] Wallace RT, Shields JA, Shields CL, Ehya H, Ewing M. Leukemic infiltration of the optic nerve. Arch Ophthalmol. 1991; 109(7):1027

[360] Dunker S, Reuter U, Rösler A, et al. Optic nerve infiltration in well-differentiated B-cell lymphoma. Ophthalmology. 1996; 93:351–353

[361] Fierz AB, Sartoretti S, Thoelen AM. Optic neuropathy and central retinal artery occlusion in non-Hodgkin lymphoma. J Neuroophthalmol. 2001; 21 (2):103–105

[362] Forman S, Rosenbaum PS. Lymphomatoid granulomatosis presenting as an isolated unilateral optic neuropathy. A clinicopathologic report. J Neuroophthalmol. 1998; 18(2):150–152

[363] Guyer DR, Green WR, Schachat AP, Bastacky S, Miller NR. Bilateral ischemic optic neuropathy and retinal vascular occlusions associated with lymphoma and sepsis. Clinicopathologic correlation. Ophthalmology. 1990; 97(7):882–888

[364] Noda S, Hayasaka S, Setogawa T. Intraocular lymphoma invades the optic nerve and orbit. Ann Ophthalmol. 1993; 25(1):30–34

[365] Siatkowski RM, Lam BL, Schatz NJ, Glaser JS, Byrne SF, Hughes JR. Optic neuropathy in Hodgkin's disease. Am J Ophthalmol. 1992; 114(5):625–629

[366] Strominger MB, Schatz NJ, Glaser JS. Lymphomatous optic neuropathy. Am J Ophthalmol. 1993; 116(6):774–776

[367] Yamamoto N, Kiyosawa M, Kawasaki T, Miki T, Fujino T, Tokoro T. Successfully treated optic nerve infiltration with adult T-cell lymphoma. J Neuroophthalmol. 1994; 14(2):81–83

[368] Zaman AG, Graham EM, Sanders MD. Anterior visual system involvement in non-Hodgkin's lymphoma. Br J Ophthalmol. 1993; 77(3):184–187

[369] Wong D, Danesh-Meyer H, Pon JA. Infiltrative lymphomatous optic neuropathy in non-Hodgkin lymphoma. J Clin Neurosci. 2015; 22(9):1513–1515

[370] Kim JL, Mendoza PR, Rashid A, Hayek B, Grossniklaus HE. Optic nerve lymphoma: report of two cases and review of the literature. Surv Ophthalmol. 2015; 60(2):153–165

[371] Tavallali A, Shields CL, Bianciotto C, Shields JA. Choroidal lymphoma masquerading as anterior ischemic optic neuropathy. Eur J Ophthalmol. 2010; 20(5):959–962

[372] Millar MJ, Tumuluri K, Murali R, Ng T, Beaumont P, Maloof A. Bilateral primary optic nerve lymphoma. Ophthal Plast Reconstr Surg. 2008; 24(1):71–73

[373] Lee LC, Howes EL, Bhisitkul RB. Systemic non-Hodgkin's lymphoma with optic nerve infiltration in a patient with AIDS. Retina. 2002; 22(1):75–79

[374] Cerovski B, Vidović T, Stiglmayer N, Popović Suić S. Prostatic carcinoma metastatic to the optic nerve. Coll Antropol. 2009; 33(4):1421–1422

[375] Cross SA, Salomao D, Lennon VA. A paraneoplastic syndrome of combined optic neuritis and retinitis defined serologically by CRMP-5-IgG. Presented at the 28th annual meeting of the North American Neuro-Ophthalmology Society, Copper Mountain, Colorado, February 9–14, 2002

[376] Lieberman FS, Odel J, Hirsh J, Heinemann M, Michaeli J, Posner J. Bilateral optic neuropathy with IgGkappa multiple myeloma improved after myeloablative chemotherapy. Neurology. 1999; 52(2):414–416

[377] Luiz JE, Lee AG, Keltner JL, Thirkill CE, Lai EC. Paraneoplastic optic neuropathy and autoantibody production in small-cell carcinoma of the lung. J Neuroophthalmol. 1998; 18(3):178–181

[378] Malik S, Furlan AJ, Sweeney PJ, Kosmorsky GS, Wong M. Optic neuropathy: a rare paraneoplastic syndrome. J Clin Neuroophthalmol. 1992; 12(3):137–141

[379] Oohira A, Inoue T, Fukuda N, Uchida K-I. A case with paraneoplastic optic neuropathy presenting bitemporal hemianopsia. Neuro-ophthalmology. 1991; 11(6):325–328

[380] Thambisetty MR, Scherzer CR, Yu Z, Lennon VA, Newman NJ. Paraneoplastic optic neuropathy and cerebellar ataxia with small cell carcinoma of the lung. J Neuroophthalmol. 2001; 21(3):164–167

[381] Yu Z, Kryzer TJ, Griesmann GE, Kim K, Benarroch EE, Lennon VA. CRMP-5 neuronal autoantibody: marker of lung cancer and thymoma-related autoimmunity. Ann Neurol. 2001; 49(2):146–154

[382] Costello F. Inflammatory optic neuropathies. Continuum (Minneap Minn). 2014; 20 4 Neuro-ophthalmology:816–837

[383] Huerva V, Sánchez MC, Ascaso FJ, Craver L, Fernández E. Calciphylaxis and bilateral optic neuropathy. J Fr Ophtalmol. 2011; 34(9):651.e1–651.e4

[384] Cohen DB, Glasgow BJ. Bilateral optic nerve cryptococcosis in sudden blindness in patients with acquired immune deficiency syndrome. Ophthalmology. 1993; 100(11):1689–1694

[385] Brown P, Demaerel P, McNaught A, et al. Neuro-ophthalmological presentation of non-invasive Aspergillus sinus disease in the non-immunocompromised host. J Neurol Neurosurg Psychiatry. 1994; 57(2):234–237

[386] Dinowitz M, Leen JS, Hameed M, Wolansky L, Frohman L. Sudden painless visual loss. Surv Ophthalmol. 2001; 46(2):143–148

[387] Hutnik CML, Nicolle DA, Munoz DG. Orbital aspergillosis. A fatal masquerader. J Neuroophthalmol. 1997; 17(4):257–261

[388] Johnson TE, Casiano RR, Kronish JW, Tse DT, Meldrum M, Chang W. Sino-orbital aspergillosis in acquired immunodeficiency syndrome. Arch Ophthalmol. 1999; 117(1):57–64

[389] Balch K, Phillips PH, Newman NJ. Painless orbital apex syndrome from mucormycosis. J Neuroophthalmol. 1997; 17(3):178–182

[390] Chandra S, Vashisht S, Menon V, Berry M, Mukherji SK. Optic nerve cysticercosis: imaging findings. AJNR Am J Neuroradiol. 2000; 21(1):198–200

[391] Gulliani BP, Dadeya S, Malik KPS, Jain DC. Bilateral cysticercosis of the optic nerve. J Neuroophthalmol. 2001; 21(3):217–218

[392] Gurha N, Sood A, Dhar J, Gupta S. Optic nerve cysticercosis in the optic canal. Acta Ophthalmol Scand. 1999; 77(1):107–109

[393] Sudan R, Muralidhar R, Sharma P. Optic nerve cysticercosis: case report and review of current management. Orbit. 2005; 24(2):159–162

[394] Lesser RL, Kornmehl EW, Pachner AR, et al. Neuro-ophthalmologic manifestations of Lyme disease. Ophthalmology. 1990; 97(6):699–706

[395] Song A, Scott IU, Davis JL, Lam BL. Atypical anterior optic neuropathy caused by toxoplasmosis. Am J Ophthalmol. 2002; 133(1):162–164

[396] Lee MW, Fong KS, Hsu LY, Lim WK. Optic nerve toxoplasmosis and orbital inflammation as initial presentation of AIDS. Graefes Arch Clin Exp Ophthalmol. 2006; 244(11):1542–1544

[397] Danesh-Meyer H, Kubis KC, Sergott RC. Not so slowly progressive visual loss. Surv Ophthalmol. 1999; 44(3):247–252

[398] Li SY, Birnbaum AD, Tessler HH, Goldstein DA. Posterior syphilitic uveitis: clinical characteristics, co-infection with HIV, response to treatment. Jpn J Ophthalmol. 2011; 55(5):486–494

[399] Golnik KC, Marotto ME, Fanous MM, et al. Ophthalmic manifestations of Rochalimaea species. Am J Ophthalmol. 1994; 118(2):145–151

[400] Cacciatori M, Ling CS, Dhillon B. Retrobulbar neuritis in a patient with acquired immune deficiency syndrome. Acta Ophthalmol Scand. 1996; 74 (2):194–196

[401] Khairallah M, Kahloun R. Ocular manifestations of emerging infectious diseases. Curr Opin Ophthalmol. 2013; 24(6):574–580

[402] Francis PJ, Jackson H, Stanford MR, Graham EM. Inflammatory optic neuropathy as the presenting feature of herpes simplex acute retinal necrosis. Br J Ophthalmol. 2003; 87(4):512–514

[403] Peter J, Andrew NH, Smith C, Figueira E, Selva D. Idiopathic inflammatory orbital myositis presenting with vision loss. Orbit. 2014; 33(6):449–452

[404] Acheson JF, Cockerell OC, Bentley CR, Sanders MD. Churg-Strauss vasculitis presenting with severe visual loss due to bilateral sequential optic neuropathy. Br J Ophthalmol. 1993; 77(2):118–119

[405] Vodopivec I, Lobo AM, Prasad S. Ocular inflammation in neurorheumatic disease. Semin Neurol. 2014; 34(4):444–457

[406] Kidd DP. Optic neuropathy in Behçet's syndrome. J Neurol. 2013; 260(12):3065–3070

[407] Achiron L, Strominger M, Witkin N, Primo S. Sarcoid optic neuropathy: a case report. J Am Optom Assoc. 1995; 66(10):646–651

[408] Beck AD, Newman NJ, Grossniklaus HE, Galetta SL, Kramer TR. Optic nerve enlargement and chronic visual loss. Surv Ophthalmol. 1994; 38(6):555–566

[409] Carmody RF, Mafee MF, Goodwin JA, Small K, Haery C. Orbital and optic pathway sarcoidosis: MR findings. AJNR Am J Neuroradiol. 1994; 15(4):775–783

[410] DeBroff BM, Donahue SP. Bilateral optic neuropathy as the initial manifestation of systemic sarcoidosis. Am J Ophthalmol. 1993; 116(1):108–111

[411] Ing EB, Garrity JA, Cross SA, Ebersold MJ. Sarcoid masquerading as optic nerve sheath meningioma. Mayo Clin Proc. 1997; 72(1):38–43

[412] Kosmorsky GS, Prayson R. Primary optic pathway sarcoidosis in a 38-year-old white man. J Neuroophthalmol. 1996; 16(3):188–190

[413] Pelton RW, Lee AG, Orengo-Nania SD, Patrinely JR. Bilateral optic disk edema caused by sarcoidosis mimicking pseudotumor cerebri. Am J Ophthalmol. 1999; 127(2):229–230

[414] Sharma OP, Sharma AM. Sarcoidosis of the nervous system. A clinical approach. Arch Intern Med. 1991; 151(7):1317–1321

[415] Silver MR, Messner LV. Sarcoidosis and its ocular manifestations. J Am Optom Assoc. 1994; 65(5):321–327

[416] Thorne JE, Galetta SL. Disc edema and retinal periphlebitis as the initial manifestation of sarcoidosis. Arch Neurol. 1998; 55(6):862–863

[417] Pasadhika S, Rosenbaum JT. Ocular sarcoidosis. Clin Chest Med. 2015; 36(4):669–683

[418] Belden CJ, Hamed LM, Mancuso AA. Bilateral isolated retrobulbar optic neuropathy in limited Wegener's granulomatosis. J Clin Neuroophthalmol. 1993; 13(2):119–123

[419] Shunmugam M, Morley AM, Graham E, D'Cruz D, O'Sullivan E, Malhotra R. Primary Wegener's granulomatosis of the orbital apex with initial optic nerve infiltration. Orbit. 2011; 30(1):24–26

[420] Ahmadieh H, Roodpeyma S, Azarmina M, Soheilian M, Sajjadi SH. Bilateral simultaneous optic neuritis in childhood systemic lupus erythematosus. A case report. J Neuroophthalmol. 1994; 14(2):84–86

19

[421] Rosenbaum JT, Simpson J, Neuwelt CM. Successful treatment of optic neuropathy in association with systemic lupus erythematosus using intravenous cyclophosphamide. Br J Ophthalmol. 1997; 81(2):130–132

[422] Siatkowski RM, Scott IU, Verm AM, et al. Optic neuropathy and chiasmopathy in the diagnosis of systemic lupus erythematosus. J Neuroophthalmol. 2001; 21(3):193–198

[423] Ohsie LH, Murchison AP, Wojno TH. Lupus erythematosus profundus masquerading as idiopathic orbital inflammatory syndrome. Orbit. 2012; 31 (3):181–183

[424] Béjot Y, Osseby GV, Ben Salem D, et al. Bilateral optic neuropathy revealing Sjögren's syndrome. Rev Neurol (Paris). 2008; 164(12):1044–1047

[425] Ağildere AM, Tutar NU, Yücel E, Coşkun M, Benli S, Aydin P. Pachymeningitis and optic neuritis in rheumatoid arthritis: MRI findings. Br J Radiol. 1999; 72(856):404–407

[426] Weinstein GW, Powell SR, Thrush WP. Chiasmal neuropathy secondary to rheumatoid pachymeningitis. Am J Ophthalmol. 1987; 104(4):439–440

[427] Ferro JM, Oliveira SN, Correia L. Neurologic manifestations of inflammatory bowel diseases. Handb Clin Neurol. 2014; 120:595–605

[428] Calvo P, Pablo L. Managing IBD outside the gut: ocular manifestations. Dig Dis. 2013; 31(2):229–232

[429] Arsava EM, Uluç K, Kansu T, Dogulu CF, Soylemezoglu F, Selekler K. Granulomatous hypophysitis and bilateral optic neuropathy. J Neuroophthalmol. 2001; 21(1):34–36

[430] Patankar T, Prasad S, Krishnan A, Laxminarayan R. Isolated optic nerve pseudotumour. Australas Radiol. 2000; 44(1):101–103

[431] Galetta SL, Stadtmauer EA, Hicks DG, Raps EC, Plock G, Oberholtzer JC. Reactive lymphohistiocytosis with recurrence in the optic chiasm. J Clin Neuroophthalmol. 1991; 11(1):25–30

[432] Deshpande V, Zen Y, Chan JK, et al. Consensus statement on the pathology of IgG4-related disease. Mod Pathol. 2012; 25(9):1181–1192

[433] Yamamoto M, Hashimoto M, Takahashi H, Shinomura Y. IgG4 disease. J Neuroophthalmol. 2014; 34(4):393–399

[434] Chen TS, Figueira E, Lau OC, et al. Successful "medical" orbital decompression with adjunctive rituximab for severe visual loss in IgG4-related orbital inflammatory disease with orbital myositis. Ophthal Plast Reconstr Surg. 2014; 30(5):e122–e125

[435] Behbehani RS, Al-Nomas HS, Al-Herz AA, Katchy KC. Bilateral intracranial optic nerve and chiasmal involvement in IgG4-related disease. J Neuroophthalmol. 2015; 35(2):229–231

[436] Takahashi Y, Kitamura A, Kakizaki H. Bilateral optic nerve involvement in immunoglobulin G4-related ophthalmic disease. J Neuroophthalmol. 2014; 34(1):16–19

[437] Koizumi S, Kamisawa T, Kuruma S, et al. Clinical features of IgG4-related dacryoadenitis. Graefes Arch Clin Exp Ophthalmol. 2014; 252(3):491–497

[438] Sogabe Y, Ohshima K, Azumi A, et al. Location and frequency of lesions in patients with IgG4-related ophthalmic diseases. Graefes Arch Clin Exp Ophthalmol. 2014; 252(3):531–538

[439] Soussan M, Medjoul A, Badelon I, Guyot A, Martin A, Abad S. IgG4-related diffuse perineural disease. Neurology. 2014; 83(20):1877–1878

[440] Tomio R, Ohira T, Wenlin D, Yoshida K. Immunoglobulin G4-related intracranial inflammatory pseudotumours along both the oculomotor nerves. BMJ Case Rep. 2013; 2013:bcr2012007320

[441] Caputo C, Bazargan A, McKelvie PA, Sutherland T, Su CS, Inder WJ. Hypophysitis due to IgG4-related disease responding to treatment with azathioprine: an alternative to corticosteroid therapy. Pituitary. 2014; 17(3): 251–256

[442] Ohshima K, Sogabe Y, Sato Y. The usefulness of infraorbital nerve enlargement on MRI imaging in clinical diagnosis of IgG4-related orbital disease. Jpn J Ophthalmol. 2012; 56(4):380–382

[443] Brazis PW, Lee AG. Neuro-ophthalmic problems caused by medications. Focal Points. 1998; 16:1–13

[444] Danesh-Meyer H, Kubis KC, Wolf MA. Chiasmopathy? Surv Ophthalmol. 2000; 44(4):329–335

[445] Sedwick LA. The perils of Pauline: visual loss in a tippler. Surv Ophthalmol. 1991; 35(6):454–462

[446] Sedwick LA. Getting to the heart of visual loss: when cardiac medication may be dangerous to the optic nerves. Surv Ophthalmol. 1992; 36(5):366–372

[447] Harcombe A, Kinnear W, Britton J, Macfarlane J. Ocular toxicity of ethambutol. Respir Med. 1991; 85(2):151–153

[448] Kumar A, Sandramouli S, Verma L, Tewari HK, Khosla PK. Ocular ethambutol toxicity: is it reversible? J Clin Neuroophthalmol. 1993; 13(1):15–17

[449] Russo PA, Chaglasian MA. Toxic optic neuropathy associated with ethambutol: implications for current therapy. J Am Optom Assoc. 1994; 65(5):332–338

[450] Schild HS, Fox BC. Rapid-onset reversible ocular toxicity from ethambutol therapy. Am J Med. 1991; 90(3):404–406

[451] Seth V, Khosla PK, Semwal OP, D'Monty V. Visual evoked responses in tuberculous children on ethambutol therapy. Indian Pediatr. 1991; 28(7):713–717

[452] Thomas RJ. Neurotoxicity of antibacterial therapy. South Med J. 1994; 87(9): 869–874

[453] Tsai RK, Lee YH. Reversibility of ethambutol optic neuropathy. J Ocul Pharmacol Ther. 1997; 13(5):473–477

[454] Libershteyn Y. Ethambutol/linezolid toxic optic neuropathy. Optom Vis Sci. 2016; 93(2):211–217

[455] Grzybowski A, Zülsdorff M, Wilhelm H, Tonagel F. Toxic optic neuropathies: an updated review. Acta Ophthalmol. 2015; 93(5):402–410

[456] Altiparmak UE. Toxic optic neuropathies. Curr Opin Ophthalmol. 2013; 24 (6):534–539

[457] Sharma P, Sharma R. Toxic optic neuropathy. Indian J Ophthalmol. 2011; 59 (2):137–141

[458] Blomquist PH. Ocular complications of systemic medications. Am J Med Sci. 2011; 342(1):62–69

[459] Gandorfer A, Haritoglou C, Kampik A. Toxicity of indocyanine green in vitreoretinal surgery. Dev Ophthalmol. 2008; 42:69–81

[460] Orssaud C, Roche O, Dufier JL. Nutritional optic neuropathies. J Neurol Sci. 2007; 262(1–2):158–164

[461] Chiotoroiu SM, Noaghi M, Stefaniu GI, Secureanu FA, Purcarea VL, Zemba M. Tobacco-alcohol optic neuropathy: clinical challenges in diagnosis. J Med Life. 2014; 7(4):472–476

[462] Ramkumar HL, Savino PJ. Toxic optic neuropathy: an unusual cause. Indian J Ophthalmol. 2014; 62(10):1036–1039

[463] Syed S, Lioutas V. Tobacco-alcohol amblyopia: a diagnostic dilemma. J Neurol Sci. 2013; 327(1–2):41–45

[464] Macaluso DC, Shults WT, Fraunfelder FT. Features of amiodarone-induced optic neuropathy. Am J Ophthalmol. 1999; 127(5):610–612

[465] Speicher MA, Goldman MH, Chrousos GA. Amiodarone optic neuropathy without disc edema. J Neuroophthalmol. 2000; 20(3):171–172

[466] Sreih AG, Schoenfeld MH, Marieb MA. Optic neuropathy following amiodarone therapy. Pacing Clin Electrophysiol. 1999; 22(7):1108–1110

[467] Kervinen M, Falck A, Hurskainen M, Hautala N. Bilateral optic neuropathy and permanent loss of vision after treatment with amiodarone. J Cardiovasc Pharmacol. 2013; 62(4):394–396

[468] Lloyd MJ, Fraunfelder FW. Drug-induced optic neuropathies. Drugs Today (Barc). 2007; 43(11):827–836

[469] Mindel JS, Anderson J, Hellkamp A, et al. SCD-HeFT Investigators. Absence of bilateral vision loss from amiodarone: a randomized trial. Am Heart J. 2007; 153(5):837–842

[470] Chan JW, Castellanos A. Infliximab and anterior optic neuropathy: case report and review of the literature. Graefes Arch Clin Exp Ophthalmol. 2010; 248(2):283–287

[471] Iuorno JD, Kolostyak KP, Mejico LJ. Therapies with potential toxicity of neuro-ophthalmic interest. Curr Opin Ophthalmol. 2003; 14(6):339–343

[472] ten Tusscher MP, Jacobs PJ, Busch MJ, de Graaf L, Diemont WL. Bilateral anter-ior toxic optic neuropathy and the use of infliximab. BMJ. 2003; 326(7389):579

[473] Venkatramani DV, Goel S, Ratra V, Gandhi RA. Toxic optic neuropathy following ingestion of homeopathic medication Arnica-30. Cutan Ocul Toxicol. 2013; 32(1):95–97

[474] Simmons IG, Good PA. Carbon monoxide poisoning causes optic neuropathy. Eye (Lond). 1998; 12(Pt 5):809–814

[475] Kobayashi A, Ando A, Tagami N, et al. Severe optic neuropathy caused by dichloromethane inhalation. J Ocul Pharmacol Ther. 2008; 24(6):607–612

[476] Sa'adah MA, Al Salem M, Ali AS, Araj G, Zuriqat M. Cimetidine-associated optic neuropathy. Eur Neurol. 1999; 42(1):23–26

[477] Vrabec TR, Sergott RC, Jaeger EA, Savino PJ, Bosley TM. Reversible visual loss in a patient receiving high-dose ciprofloxacin hydrochloride (Cipro). Ophthalmology. 1990; 97(6):707–710

[478] Samarakoon N, Harrisberg B, Ell J. Ciprofloxacin-induced toxic optic neuropathy. Clin Experiment Ophthalmol. 2007; 35(1):102–104

[479] Caraceni A, Martini C, Spatti G, Thomas A, Onofrj M. Recovering optic neuritis during systemic cisplatin and carboplatin chemotherapy. Acta Neurol Scand. 1997; 96(4):260–261

[480] Wang MY, Arnold AC, Vinters HV, Glasgow BJ. Bilateral blindness and lumbosacral myelopathy associated with high-dose carmustine and cisplatin therapy. Am J Ophthalmol. 2000; 130(3):367–368

[481] Nakae K, Yamamoto S, Shigematsu I, Kono R. Relation between subacute myelo-optic neuropathy (S.M.O.N.) and clioquinol: nationwide survey. Lancet. 1973; 1(7796):171–173

[482] Catalani S, Rizzetti MC, Padovani A, Apostoli P. Neurotoxicity of cobalt. Hum Exp Toxicol. 2012; 31(5):421–437

[483] Teus MA, Teruel JL, Pascual J, Martin-Escobar E. Corticosteroid-induced toxic optic neuropathy. Am J Ophthalmol. 1991; 112(5):605–606

[484] Giralt J, Rey A, Villanueva R, Alforja S, Casaroli-Marano RP. Severe visual loss in a breast cancer patient on chemotherapy. Med Oncol. 2012; 29(4):2567–2569

[485] Román GC. Tropical myelopathies. Handb Clin Neurol. 2014; 121:1521–1548

[486] Avery R, Jabs DA, Wingard JR, Vogelsang G, Saral R, Santos G. Optic disc edema after bone marrow transplantation. Possible role of cyclosporine toxicity. Ophthalmology. 1991; 98(8):1294–1301

[487] Pinna A, Corda L, Carta F. Rapid recovery with oral zinc sulphate in deferoxamine-induced presumed optic neuropathy and hearing loss. J Neuroophthalmol. 2001; 21(1):32–33

[488] Loh A, Hadziahmetovic M, Dunaief JL. Iron homeostasis and eye disease. Biochim Biophys Acta. 2009; 1790(7):637–649

[489] Moloney TP, Xu W, Rallah-Baker K, Oliveira N, Woodward N, Farrah JJ. Toxic optic neuropathy in the setting of docetaxel chemotherapy: a case report. BMC Ophthalmol. 2014; 14:18

[490] Kimura H, Masai H, Kashii S. Optic neuropathy following elcatonin therapy. J Neuroophthalmol. 1996; 16(2):134–136

[491] Lauer AK, Wobig JL, Shults WT, Neuwelt EA, Wilson MW. Severe ocular and orbital toxicity after intracarotid etoposide phosphate and carboplatin therapy. Am J Ophthalmol. 1999; 127(2):230–233

[492] Csaky KG, Caruso RC. Gallium nitrate optic neuropathy. Am J Ophthalmol. 1997; 124(4):567–568

[493] Ekinci M, Ceylan E, Cağatay HH, et al. Occupational exposure to lead decreases macular, choroidal, and retinal nerve fiber layer thickness in industrial battery workers. Curr Eye Res. 2014; 39(8):853–858

[494] Lai P, Yang J, Cui H, Xie H. Prognosis of corneal wasp sting: case report and review of the literature. Cutan Ocul Toxicol. 2011; 30(4):325–327

[495] Teoh SC, Lee JJ, Fam HB. Corneal honeybee sting. Can J Ophthalmol. 2005; 40 (4):469–471

[496] Domaç FM, Koçer A, Tanidir R. Optic neuropathy related to hydrogen peroxide inhalation. Clin Neuropharmacol. 2007; 30(1):55–57

[497] Karuppannasamy D, Raghuram A, Sundar D. Linezolid-induced optic neuropathy. Indian J Ophthalmol. 2014; 62(4):497–500

[498] Lewis JR. Bilateral optic neuropathy secondary to manganese toxicity. Presented at the 27th Annual Meeting of the North American Neuro-Ophthalmology Society, Rancho Mirage, California, February 18–22, 2001

[499] Lehman NL, Johnson LN. Toxic optic neuropathy after concomitant use of melatonin, zoloft, and a high-protein diet. J Neuroophthalmol. 1999; 19(4):232–234

[500] Wijaya J, Salu P, Leblanc A, Bervoets S. Acute unilateral visual loss due to a single intranasal methamphetamine abuse. Bull Soc Belge Ophtalmol. 1999; 271:19–25

[501] Khan AH, Rahaman MF, Mollah RI, Alam A, Hassan SN, Chowdhury MA. Methanol induced toxic amblyopia: a case report. Mymensingh Med J. 2016; 25(1):176–178

[502] Zakharov S, Pelclova D, Diblik P, et al. Long-term visual damage after acute methanol poisonings: Longitudinal cross-sectional study in 50 patients. Clin Toxicol (Phila). 2015; 53(9):884–892

[503] Ranjan R, Kushwaha R, Gupta RC, Khan P. An unusual case of bilateral multifocal retinal pigment epithelial detachment with methanol-induced optic neuritis. J Med Toxicol. 2014; 10(1):57–60

[504] Johansson BA. Visual field defects during low-dose methotrexate therapy. Doc Ophthalmol. 1992; 79(1):91–94

[505] Suresha AR, Rajesh P, Anil Raj KS, Torgal R. A rare case of toxic optic neuropathy secondary to consumption of neem oil. Indian J Ophthalmol. 2014; 62(3):337–339

[506] des Grottes JM, Schrooyen M, Dumon JC, Body JJ. Retrobulbar optic neuritis after pamidronate administration in a patient with a history of cutaneous porphyria. Clin Rheumatol. 1997; 16(1):93–95

[507] Kumar PK, Ahuja S, Kumar PS. Bilateral acute anterior uveitis and optic disc edema following a snake bite. Korean J Ophthalmol. 2014; 28(2):186–188

[508] Brazis PW, Spivey JR, Bolling JP, Steers JL. A case of bilateral optic neuropathy in a patient on tacrolimus (FK506) therapy after liver transplantation. Am J Ophthalmol. 2000; 129(4):536–538

[509] Ascaso FJ, Mateo J, Huerva V, Cristóbal JA. Unilateral tacrolimus-associated optic neuropathy after liver transplantation. Cutan Ocul Toxicol. 2012; 31 (2):167–170

[510] Venneti S, Moss HE, Levin MH, et al. Asymmetric bilateral demyelinating optic neuropathy from tacrolimus toxicity. J Neurol Sci. 2011; 301(1–2):112–115

[511] Kiyokawa M, Mizota A, Takasoh M, Adachi-Usami E. Pattern visual evoked cortical potentials in patients with toxic optic neuropathy caused by toluene abuse. Jpn J Ophthalmol. 1999; 43(5):438–442

[512] Choi SY, Hwang JM. Optic neuropathy associated with ethambutol in Koreans. Korean J Ophthalmol. 1997; 11(2):106–110

[513] Barron GJ, Tepper L, Iovine G. Ocular toxicity from ethambutol. Am J Ophthalmol. 1974; 77(2):256–260

[514] Leibold JE. The ocular toxicity of ethambutol and its relation to dose. Ann N Y Acad Sci. 1966; 135(2):904–909

[515] Alvarez KL, Krop LC. Ethambutol-induced ocular toxicity revisited. Ann Pharmacother. 1993; 27(1):102–103

[516] Brontë-Stewart J, Pettigrew AR, Foulds WS. Toxic optic neuropathy and its experimental production. Trans Ophthalmol Soc U K. 1976; 96(3):355–358

[517] Citron KM, Thomas GO. Ocular toxicity from ethambutol. Thorax. 1986; 41 (10):737–739

[518] Jimenez-Lucho VE, del Busto R, Odel J. Isoniazid and ethambutol as a cause of optic neuropathy. Eur J Respir Dis. 1987; 71(1):42–45

[519] Bourne RR, Dolin PJ, Mtanda AT, Plant GT, Mohamed AA. Epidemic optic neuropathy in primary school children in Dar es Salaam, Tanzania. Br J Ophthalmol. 1998; 82(3):232–234

[520] Lessell S. Nutritional amblyopia. J Neuroophthalmol. 1998; 18(2):106–111

[521] Golnik KC, Schaible ER. Folate-responsive optic neuropathy. J Neuroophthalmol. 1994; 14(3):163–169

[522] Ugarte M, Osborne NN, Brown LA, Bishop PN. Iron, zinc, and copper in retinal physiology and disease. Surv Ophthalmol. 2013; 58(6):585–609

[523] Smets RM, Waeben M. Unusual combination of night blindness and optic neuropathy after biliopancreatic bypass. Bull Soc Belge Ophtalmol. 1999; 271:93–96

[524] Rizzo JF, III, Lessell S. Tobacco amblyopia. Am J Ophthalmol. 1993; 116(1):84–87

[525] Samples JR, Younge BR. Tobacco-alcohol amblyopia. J Clin Neuroophthalmol. 1981; 1(3):213–218

[526] Arnold AC. Radiation optic neuropathy. Presented at the North American Neuro-Ophthalmology meeting, Tucson, Arizona; 1995

[527] Borruat F-X, Schatz NJ, Glaser JS, Feun LG, Matos L. Visual recovery from radiation-induced optic neuropathy. The role of hyperbaric oxygen therapy. J Clin Neuroophthalmol. 1993; 13(2):98–101

[528] Borruat F-X, Schatz NJ, Glaser JS, et al. Radiation optic neuropathy: report of cases, role of hyperbaric oxygen therapy, and literature review. Neuro-ophthalmology. 1996; 16(4):255–266

[529] Ebner R, Slamovits TL, Friedland S, Pearlman JL, Fowble B. Visual loss following treatment of sphenoid sinus carcinoma. Surv Ophthalmol. 1995; 40(1):62–68

[530] Girkin CA, Comey CH, Lunsford LD, Goodman ML, Kline LB. Radiation optic neuropathy after stereotactic radiosurgery. Ophthalmology. 1997; 104(10):1634–1643

[531] Glantz MJ, Burger PC, Friedman AH, Radtke RA, Massey EW, Schold SC, Jr. Treatment of radiation-induced nervous system injury with heparin and warfarin. Neurology. 1994; 44(11):2020–2027

[532] Goldsmith BJ, Rosenthal SA, Wara WM, Larson DA. Optic neuropathy after irradiation of meningioma. Radiology. 1992; 185(1):71–76

[533] Guy J, Mancuso A, Beck R, et al. Radiation-induced optic neuropathy: a magnetic resonance imaging study. J Neurosurg. 1991; 74(3):426–432

[534] Guy J, Schatz NJ. Radiation-induced optic neuropathy. In: Tusa RJ, Newman SA, eds. Neuro-ophthalmological Disorders. New York, NY: Marcel Dekker; 1995:437–450

[535] Hudgins PA, Newman NJ, Dillon WP, Hoffman JC, Jr. Radiation-induced optic neuropathy: characteristic appearances on gadolinium-enhanced MR. AJNR Am J Neuroradiol. 1992; 13(1):235–238

[536] Jiang GL, Tucker SL, Guttenberger R, et al. Radiation-induced injury to the visual pathway. Radiother Oncol. 1994; 30(1):17–25

[537] Landau K, Killer HE. Radiation damage. Neurology. 1996; 46(3):889

[538] Leber KA, Berglöff J, Pendl G. Dose-response tolerance of the visual pathways and cranial nerves of the cavernous sinus to stereotactic radiosurgery. J Neurosurg. 1998; 88(1):43–50

[539] McClellan RL, el Gammal T, Kline LB. Early bilateral radiation-induced optic neuropathy with follow-up MRI. Neuroradiology. 1995; 37(2):131–133

[540] Parsons JT, Bova FJ, Fitzgerald CR, Mendenhall WM, Million RR. Radiation optic neuropathy after megavoltage external-beam irradiation: analysis of time-dose factors. Int J Radiat Oncol Biol Phys. 1994; 30(4):755–763

[541] Polak BCP, Wijngaarde R. Radiation neuropathy in patients with both diabetes mellitus and ophthalmic Graves' disease. Orbit. 1995; 14:71–74

[542] Roden D, Bosley TM, Fowble B, et al. Delayed radiation injury to the retrobulbar optic nerves and chiasm. Clinical syndrome and treatment with hyperbaric oxygen and corticosteroids. Ophthalmology. 1990; 97(3):346–351

[543] Tachibana O, Yamaguchi N, Yamashima T, Yamashita J. Radiation necrosis of the optic chiasm, optic tract, hypothalamus, and upper pons after radiotherapy for pituitary adenoma, detected by gadolinium-enhanced, T1-weighted magnetic resonance imaging: case report. Neurosurgery. 1990; 27(4):640–643

[544] Zimmerman CF, Schatz NJ, Glaser JS. Magnetic resonance imaging of radiation optic neuropathy. Am J Ophthalmol. 1990; 110(4):389–394

[545] Li CQ, Gerson S, Snyder B. Case report: hyperbaric oxygen and MRI findings in radiation-induced optic neuropathy. Undersea Hyperb Med. 2014; 41(1):59–63

[546] Mayo C, Martel MK, Marks LB, Flickinger J, Nam J, Kirkpatrick J. Radiation dose-volume effects of optic nerves and chiasm. Int J Radiat Oncol Biol Phys. 2010; 76(3) Suppl:S28–S35

[547] Danesh-Meyer HV. Radiation-induced optic neuropathy. J Clin Neurosci. 2008; 15(2):95–100

[548] Astradsson A, Wiencke AK, Munck af Rosenschold P, et al. Visual outcome after fractionated stereotactic radiation therapy of benign anterior skull base tumors. J Neurooncol. 2014; 118(1):101–108

[549] Thariat J, Grange JD, Mosci C, et al. Visual outcomes of parapapillary uveal melanomas following proton beam therapy. Int J Radiat Oncol Biol Phys. 2016; 95(1):328–335

[550] Mackley HB, Reddy CA, Lee SY, et al. Intensity-modulated radiotherapy for pituitary adenomas: the preliminary report of the Cleveland Clinic experience. Int J Radiat Oncol Biol Phys. 2007; 67(1):232–239

[551] Lee MS, Borruat FX. Should patients with radiation-induced optic neuropathy receive any treatment? J Neuroophthalmol. 2011; 31(1):83–88

[552] Wijers OB, Levendag PC, Luyten GP, et al. Radiation-induced bilateral optic neuropathy in cancer of the nasopharynx. Case failure analysis and a review of the literature. Strahlenther Onkol. 1999; 175(1):21–27

[553] Gupta A, Dhawahir-Scala F, Smith A, Young L, Charles S. Radiation retinopathy: case report and review. BMC Ophthalmol. 2007; 7:6

[554] Zamber RW, Kinyoun JL. Radiation retinopathy. West J Med. 1992; 157(5):530–533

[555] Gragoudas ES, Li W, Lane AM, Munzenrider J, Egan KM. Risk factors for radiation maculopathy and papillopathy after intraocular irradiation. Ophthalmology. 1999; 106(8):1571–1577, discussion 1577–1578

[556] Lessell S. Friendly fire: neurogenic visual loss from radiation therapy. J Neuroophthalmol. 2004; 24(3):243–250

[557] Bhandare N, Monroe AT, Morris CG, Bhatti MT, Mendenhall WM. Does altered fractionation influence the risk of radiation-induced optic neuropathy? Int J Radiat Oncol Biol Phys. 2005; 62(4):1070–1077

[558] Dunavoelgyi R, Georg D, Zehetmayer M, et al. Dose-response of critical structures in the posterior eye segment to hypofractionated stereotactic photon radiotherapy of choroidal melanoma. Radiother Oncol. 2013; 108(2):348–353

[559] Zhao Z, Lan Y, Bai S, et al. Late-onset radiation-induced optic neuropathy after radiotherapy for nasopharyngeal carcinoma. J Clin Neurosci. 2013; 20(5):702–706

[560] Riechardt AI, Cordini D, Willerding GD, et al. Proton beam therapy of parapapillary choroidal melanoma. Am J Ophthalmol. 2014; 157(6):1258–1265

[561] Stafford SL, Pollock BE, Leavitt JA, et al. A study on the radiation tolerance of the optic nerves and chiasm after stereotactic radiosurgery. Int J Radiat Oncol Biol Phys. 2003; 55(5):1177–1181

[562] Leavitt JA, Stafford SL, Link MJ, Pollock BE. Long-term evaluation of radiation-induced optic neuropathy after single-fraction stereotactic radiosurgery. Int J Radiat Oncol Biol Phys. 2013; 87(3):524–527

[563] Carvounis PE, Katz B. Gamma knife radiosurgery in neuro-ophthalmology. Curr Opin Ophthalmol. 2003; 14(6):317–324

[564] Al-Wassia R, Dal Pra A, Shun K, et al. Stereotactic fractionated radiotherapy in the treatment of juxtapapillary choroidal melanoma: the McGill University experience. Int J Radiat Oncol Biol Phys. 2011; 81(4):e455–e462

[565] Howell N. Leber hereditary optic neuropathy: mitochondrial mutations and degeneration of the optic nerve. Vision Res. 1997; 37(24):3495–3507

[566] Young WC, Thornton AF, Gebarski SS, Cornblath WT. Radiation-induced optic neuropathy: correlation of MR imaging and radiation dosimetry. Radiology. 1992; 185(3):904–907

[567] Barbosa AP, Carvalho D, Marques L, et al. Inefficiency of the anticoagulant therapy in the regression of the radiation-induced optic neuropathy in Cushing's disease. J Endocrinol Invest. 1999; 22(4):301–305

[568] Danesh-Meyer HV, Savino PJ, Sergott RC. Visual loss despite anticoagulation in radiation-induced optic neuropathy. Clin Experiment Ophthalmol. 2004; 32(3):333–335

[569] Chahal HS, Lam A, Khaderi SK. Is pentoxifylline plus vitamin E an effective treatment for radiation-induced optic neuropathy? J Neuroophthalmol. 2013; 33(1):91–93

[570] Farooq O, Lincoff NS, Saikali N, Prasad D, Miletich RS, Mechtler LL. Novel treatment for radiation optic neuropathy with intravenous bevacizumab. J Neuroophthalmol. 2012; 32(4):321–324

[571] Finger PT, Chin KJ. Antivascular endothelial growth factor bevacizumab for radiation optic neuropathy: secondary to plaque radiotherapy. Int J Radiat Oncol Biol Phys. 2012; 82(2):789–798

[572] Finger PT. Anti-VEGF bevacizumab (Avastin) for radiation optic neuropathy. Am J Ophthalmol. 2007; 143(2):335–338

[573] Mohamed IG, Roa W, Fulton D, et al. Optic nerve sheath fenestration for a reversible optic neuropathy in radiation oncology. Am J Clin Oncol. 2000; 23(4):401–405

[574] Eiberg H, Kjer B, Kjer P, Rosenberg T. Dominant optic atrophy (OPA1) mapped to chromosome 3q region. I. Linkage analysis. Hum Mol Genet. 1994; 3(6):977–980

[575] Johnston RL, Burdon MA, Spalton DJ, Bryant SP, Behnam JT, Seller MJ. Dominant optic atrophy, Kjer type. Linkage analysis and clinical features in a large British pedigree. Arch Ophthalmol. 1997; 115(1):100–103

[576] Skidd PM, Lessell S, Cestari DM. Autosomal dominant hereditary optic neuropathy (ADOA): a review of the genetics and clinical manifestations of ADOA and ADOA+. Semin Ophthalmol. 2013; 28(5–6):422–426

[577] Almind GJ, Grønskov K, Milea D, Larsen M, Brøndum-Nielsen K, Ek J. Genomic deletions in OPA1 in Danish patients with autosomal dominant optic atrophy. BMC Med Genet. 2011; 12:49

[578] Yu-Wai-Man P, Griffiths PG, Gorman GS, et al. Multi-system neurological disease is common in patients with OPA1 mutations. Brain. 2010; 133(Pt 3):771–786

[579] Newman NJ. Hereditary optic neuropathies: from the mitochondria to the optic nerve. Am J Ophthalmol. 2005; 140(3):517–523

[580] Kjer B, Eiberg H, Kjer P, Rosenberg T. Dominant optic atrophy mapped to chromosome 3q region. II. Clinical and epidemiological aspects. Acta Ophthalmol Scand. 1996; 74(1):3–7

[581] Lenaers G, Hamel C, Delettre C, et al. Dominant optic atrophy. Orphanet J Rare Dis. 2012; 7:46

[582] Yu-Wai-Man P, Griffiths PG, Burke A, et al. The prevalence and natural history of dominant optic atrophy due to OPA1 mutations. Ophthalmology. 2010; 117(8):1538–1546, 1546.e1

[583] Eliott D, Traboulsi EI, Maumenee IH. Visual prognosis in autosomal dominant optic atrophy (Kjer type). Am J Ophthalmol. 1993; 115(3):360–367

[584] Johnston RL, Seller MJ, Behnam JT, Burdon MA, Spalton DJ. Dominant optic atrophy. Refining the clinical diagnostic criteria in light of genetic linkage studies. Ophthalmology. 1999; 106(1):123–128

[585] Yu-Wai-Man P, Griffiths PG, Hudson G, Chinnery PF. Inherited mitochondrial optic neuropathies. J Med Genet. 2009; 46(3):145–158

[586] Barboni P, Carbonelli M, Savini G, et al. OPA1 mutations associated with dominant optic atrophy influence optic nerve head size. Ophthalmology. 2010; 117(8):1547–1553

[587] Berninger TA, Jaeger W, Krastel H. Electrophysiology and colour perimetry in dominant infantile optic atrophy. Br J Ophthalmol. 1991; 75(1):49–52

[588] Del Porto G, Vingolo EM, Steindl K, et al. Clinical heterogeneity of dominant optic atrophy: the contribution of visual function investigations to diagnosis. Graefes Arch Clin Exp Ophthalmol. 1994; 232(12):717–727

[589] Votruba M, Fitzke FW, Holder GE, Carter A, Bhattacharya SS, Moore AT. Clinical features in affected individuals from 21 pedigrees with dominant optic atrophy. Arch Ophthalmol. 1998; 116(3):351–358

[590] Maresca A, la Morgia C, Caporali L, Valentino ML, Carelli V. The optic nerve: a "mito-window" on mitochondrial neurodegeneration. Mol Cell Neurosci. 2013; 55:62–76

[591] Milea D, Sander B, Wegener M, et al. Axonal loss occurs early in dominant optic atrophy. Acta Ophthalmol. 2010; 88(3):342–346

[592] Yu-Wai-Man P, Bailie M, Atawan A, Chinnery PF, Griffiths PG. Pattern of retinal ganglion cell loss in dominant optic atrophy due to OPA1 mutations. Eye (Lond). 2011; 25(5):596–602

[593] Milea D, Amati-Bonneau P, Reynier P, Bonneau D. Genetically determined optic neuropathies. Curr Opin Neurol. 2010; 23(1):24–28

[594] Yu-Wai-Man P, Votruba M, Moore AT, Chinnery PF. Treatment strategies for inherited optic neuropathies: past, present and future. Eye (Lond). 2014; 28(5):521–537

[595] Newman NJ. Treatment of hereditary optic neuropathies. Nat Rev Neurol. 2012; 8(10):545–556

[596] Ajax ET, Kardon R. Late-onset Leber's hereditary optic neuropathy. J Neuroophthalmol. 1998; 18(1):30–31

[597] al-Salem M. Leber's congenital amaurosis in 22 affected members of one family. J Pediatr Ophthalmol Strabismus. 1997; 34(4):254–257

[598] Hackett SE. Leber's hereditary optic neuropathy: a genetic disorder of the eye. Insight. 1997; 22(3):94–96

[599] Kerrison JB, Newman NJ. Clinical spectrum of Leber's hereditary optic neuropathy. Clin Neurosci. 1997; 4(5):295–301

[600] Mackey DA, Buttery RC. Leber hereditary optic neuropathy in Australia. Aust N Z J Ophthalmol. 1992; 20:177–184

[601] Macmillan C, Kirkham T, Fu K, et al. Pedigree analysis of French Canadian families with T14484C Leber's hereditary optic neuropathy. Neurology. 1998; 50(2):417–422

[602] Mashima Y, Oshitari K, Imamura Y, Momoshima S, Shiga H, Oguchi Y. Orbital high resolution magnetic resonance imaging with fast spin echo in the acute stage of Leber's hereditary optic neuropathy. J Neurol Neurosurg Psychiatry. 1998; 64(1):124–127

[603] Newman NJ. Leber's hereditary optic neuropathy. New genetic considerations. Arch Neurol. 1993; 50(5):540–548

[604] Purohit SS, Tomsak RL. Nutritional deficiency amblyopia or Leber's hereditary optic neuropathy? Neuroophthalmology. 1997; 18:111–116

[605] Saadati HG, Hsu HY, Heller KB, Sadun AA. A histopathologic and morphometric differentiation of nerves in optic nerve hypoplasia and Leber hereditary optic neuropathy. Arch Ophthalmol. 1998; 116(7):911–916

[606] Tsao K, Aitken PA, Johns DR. Smoking as an aetiological factor in a pedigree with Leber's hereditary optic neuropathy. Br J Ophthalmol. 1999; 83(5):577–581

[607] Rasool N, Lessell S, Cestari DM. Leber hereditary optic neuropathy: bringing the lab to the clinic. Semin Ophthalmol. 2016; 31(1–2):107–116

[608] Yen MY, Wang AG, Wei YH. Leber's hereditary optic neuropathy: a multifactorial disease. Prog Retin Eye Res. 2006; 25(4):381–396

[609] Huoponen K, Vilkki J, Aula P, Nikoskelainen EK, Savontaus ML. A new mtDNA mutation associated with Leber hereditary optic neuroretinopathy. Am J Hum Genet. 1991; 48(6):1147–1153

[610] Brown MD, Voljavec AS, Lott MT, Torroni A, Yang CC, Wallace DC. Mitochondrial DNA complex I and III mutations associated with Leber's hereditary optic neuropathy. Genetics. 1992; 130(1):163–173

[611] Howell N, Kubacka I, Halvorson S, Mackey D. Leber's hereditary optic neuropathy: the etiological role of a mutation in the mitochondrial cytochrome b gene. Genetics. 1993; 133(1):133–136

[612] Johns DR, Neufeld MJ. Cytochrome c oxidase mutations in Leber hereditary optic neuropathy. Biochem Biophys Res Commun. 1993; 196(2):810–815

[613] Johns DR, Smith KH, Savino PJ, Miller NR. Leber's hereditary optic neuropathy. Clinical manifestations of the 15257 mutation. Ophthalmology. 1993; 100(7):981–986

[614] Cock HR, Tabrizi SJ, Cooper JM, Schapira AHV. The influence of nuclear background on the biochemical expression of 3460 Leber's hereditary optic neuropathy. Ann Neurol. 1998; 44(2):187–193

[615] Hedges TR, III, Sedwick LA, Newman NJ. Two brothers with bilateral optic neuropathy. Surv Ophthalmol. 1995; 39(5):417–424

[616] Johns DR, Heher KL, Miller NR, Smith KH. Leber's hereditary optic neuropathy: clinical manifestations of the 14484 mutation. Arch Ophthalmol. 1993; 111:495–498

[617] Johns DR, Smith KH, Miller NR. Leber's hereditary optic neuropathy. Clinical manifestations of the 3460 mutation. Arch Ophthalmol. 1992; 110(11):1577–1581

[618] Nakamura M, Yamamoto M. Variable pattern of visual recovery of Leber's hereditary optic neuropathy. Br J Ophthalmol. 2000; 84(5):534–535

[619] Tońska K, Kodroń A, Bartnik E. Genotype-phenotype correlations in Leber hereditary optic neuropathy. Biochim Biophys Acta. 2010; 1797(6–7):1119–1123

[620] Newman NJ, Lott MT, Wallace DC. The clinical characteristics of pedigrees of Leber's hereditary optic neuropathy with the 11778 mutation. Am J Ophthalmol. 1991; 111(6):750–762

[621] Stone EM, Newman NJ, Miller NR, Johns DR, Lott MT, Wallace DC. Visual recovery in patients with Leber's hereditary optic neuropathy and the 11778 mutation. J Clin Neuroophthalmol. 1992; 12(1):10–14

[622] Kerrison JB, Howell N, Miller NR, Hirst L, Green WR. Leber hereditary optic neuropathy. Electron microscopy and molecular genetic analysis of a case. Ophthalmology. 1995; 102(10):1509–1516

[623] Shoffner JM, Brown MD, Stugard C, et al. Leber's hereditary optic neuropathy plus dystonia is caused by a mitochondrial DNA point mutation. Ann Neurol. 1995; 38(2):163–169

[624] Cullom ME, Heher KL, Miller NR, Savino PJ, Johns DR. Leber's hereditary optic neuropathy masquerading as tobacco-alcohol amblyopia. Arch Ophthalmol. 1993; 111(11):1482–1485

[625] Shaikh S, Ta C, Basham AA, Mansour S. Leber hereditary optic neuropathy associated with antiretroviral therapy for human immunodeficiency virus infection. Am J Ophthalmol. 2001; 131(1):143–145

[626] Newman NJ, Biousse V, Newman SA, et al. Progression of visual field defects in leber hereditary optic neuropathy: experience of the LHON treatment trial. Am J Ophthalmol. 2006; 141(6):1061–1067

[627] Barboni P, Carbonelli M, Savini G, et al. Natural history of Leber's hereditary optic neuropathy: longitudinal analysis of the retinal nerve fiber layer by optical coherence tomography. Ophthalmology. 2010; 117(3):623–627

[628] Vaphiades MS, Newman NJ. Optic nerve enhancement on orbital magnetic resonance imaging in Leber's hereditary optic neuropathy. J Neuroophthalmol. 1999; 19(4):238–239

[629] Carelli V, Valentino ML, Liguori R, et al. Leber's hereditary optic neuropathy (LHON/11778) with myoclonus: report of two cases. J Neurol Neurosurg Psychiatry. 2001; 71(6):813–816

[630] Bhatti MT, Newman NJ. A multiple sclerosis-like illness in a man harboring the mtDNA 14484 mutation. J Neuroophthalmol. 1999; 19(1):28–33

[631] Pfeffer G, Burke A, Yu-Wai-Man P, Compston DA, Chinnery PF. Clinical features of MS associated with Leber hereditary optic neuropathy mtDNA mutations. Neurology. 2013; 81(24):2073–2081

[632] Palace J. Multiple sclerosis associated with Leber's hereditary optic neuropathy. J Neurol Sci. 2009; 286(1–2):24–27

[633] Peragallo JH, Newman NJ. Is there treatment for Leber hereditary optic neuropathy? Curr Opin Ophthalmol. 2015; 26(6):450–457

[634] Mashima Y, Hiida Y, Oguchi Y. Remission of Leber's hereditary optic neuropathy with idebenone. Lancet. 1992; 340(8815):368–369

[635] Mashima Y, Hiida Y, Oguchi Y. Lack of differences among mitochondrial DNA in family members with Leber's hereditary optic neuropathy and differing visual outcomes. J Neuroophthalmol. 1995; 15(1):15–19

[636] Mashima Y, Kigasawa K, Wakakura M, Oguchi Y. Do idebenone and vitamin therapy shorten the time to achieve visual recovery in Leber hereditary optic neuropathy? J Neuroophthalmol. 2000; 20(3):166–170

[637] Feuer WJ, Schiffman JC, Davis JL, et al. Gene therapy for leber hereditary optic neuropathy: initial results. Ophthalmology. 2016; 123(3):558–570

[638] Carelli V, La Morgia C, Valentino ML, et al. Idebenone treatment in Leber's hereditary optic neuropathy. Brain. 2011; 134(Pt 9):e188

[639] Klopstock T, Metz G, Yu-Wai-Man P, et al. Persistence of the treatment effect of idebenone in Leber's hereditary optic neuropathy. Brain. 2013; 136(Pt 2):e230

[640] Klopstock T, Yu-Wai-Man P, Dimitriadis K, et al. A randomized placebo-controlled trial of idebenone in Leber's hereditary optic neuropathy. Brain. 2011; 134(Pt 9):2677–2686

[641] Rudolph G, Dimitriadis K, Büchner B, et al. Effects of idebenone on color vision in patients with leber hereditary optic neuropathy. J Neuroophthalmol. 2013; 33(1):30–36

[642] Kerrison JB, Miller NR, Hsu F, et al. A case-control study of tobacco and alcohol consumption in Leber hereditary optic neuropathy. Am J Ophthalmol. 2000; 130(6):803–812

[643] Kirkman MA, Yu-Wai-Man P, Korsten A, et al. Gene-environment interactions in Leber hereditary optic neuropathy. Brain. 2009; 132(Pt 9):2317–2326

[644] Chalmers RM, Bird AC, Harding AE. Autosomal dominant optic atrophy with asymptomatic peripheral neuropathy. J Neurol Neurosurg Psychiatry. 1996; 60(2):195–196

[645] Paradiso G, Micheli F, Taratuto AL, Parera IC. Familial bulbospinal neuronopathy with optic atrophy: a distinct entity. J Neurol Neurosurg Psychiatry. 1996; 61(2):196–199

[646] Barrett TG, Bundey SE, Fielder AR, Good PA. Optic atrophy in Wolfram (DIDMOAD) syndrome. Eye (Lond). 1997; 11(Pt 6):882–888

[647] Scolding NJ, Kellar-Wood HF, Shaw C, Shneerson JM, Antoun N. Wolfram syndrome: hereditary diabetes mellitus with brainstem and optic atrophy. Ann Neurol. 1996; 39(3):352–360

[648] Gamez J, Montane D, Martorell L, Minoves T, Cervera C. Bilateral optic nerve atrophy in myotonic dystrophy. Am J Ophthalmol. 2001; 131(3):398–400

2 Optic Neuritis

Leanne M. Little

Abstract

Optic neuritis is an inflammatory optic neuropathy. The etiology may be inflammatory, infectious, demyelinating, or idiopathic. This chapter discusses the clinical pathway for diagnosing and treating optic neuritis, as well as a detailed review of the relevant literature.

Keywords: optic neuritis, multiple sclerosis, neuromyelitis optica, optic neuritis treatment trial, optic neuropathy

2.1 Introduction

Optic neuritis (ON) is a general term for an optic neuropathy resulting from an idiopathic, inflammatory, infectious, or demyelinating etiology. If the optic nerve is swollen on ophthalmoscopy, then the term *papillitis* or *anterior ON* is used. If the optic nerve is normal on ophthalmoscopy, then it is called *retrobulbar ON*. In clinical practice, most ophthalmologists use the term *ON* to describe idiopathic or demyelinating ON.

2.2 What Are the Features of Typical Optic Neuritis?

Patients with idiopathic or demyelinating ON usually present with a "typical" clinical profile as shown in Box 2.1.

Box 2.1 Features of typical optic neuritis[1,2,3,4,5,6, 7,8,9,10,11,12,13,14,15,16,17,18,19,20]

- Acute, usually unilateral loss of vision:
  - Visual acuity (variable visual loss 20/20 to no light perception [NLP]).
  - Visual field (variable optic nerve visual field defects).[21]
- A relative afferent pupillary defect (RAPD) in unilateral or bilateral but asymmetric cases.
- Periocular pain (90%), especially with eye movement.[12]
- Normal (65%) or swollen (35%) optic nerve head.
- A young adult patient (< 40 years), but ON may occur at any age.
- Eventual visual improvement:
  - Improvement over several weeks in most patients (90%) to normal or near-normal visual acuity; 88% improve at least one Snellen line by day 15.
  - 96% improve at least one line by day 30.
  - Visual recovery may continue for months (up to 1 year).

Patients may complain of residual deficits in contrast sensitivity, color vision, stereopsis, light brightness, visual acuity, or visual field.[10,22,23,24]

The clinical characteristics of 455 patients with ON enrolled in the Optic Neuritis Treatment Trial (ONTT), a study sponsored by the National Eye Institute conducted at 15 clinical centers in the United States between the years 1988 and 1991, are outlined in ▶ Table 2.1.

Table 2.1 The clinical profile of the Optic Neuritis Treatment Trial (ONTT) patients[25]

Clinical characteristic	Patients
Demographics	
• Female	77%
• White	85%
• Age (y; mean ± SD)	32±6.7
• Mean days of visual symptoms before entry	5.0±1.6
• Ocular pain present	92%
• Pain worsened by eye movement	87%
Ophthalmoscopic findings	
Optic disc appearance	
• Optic disc swollen	35%
• Optic disc normal (retrobulbar)	65%
Characteristics of swollen optic disc	
• Mild and focal	28.6%
• Mild and diffuse	51%
• Severe and focal	3.1%
• Severe and diffuse	16.8%
Retinal or optic disc hemorrhage	
• None	84.5%
• On disc	6.2%
• On retina	3.7%
• On both disc and retina	5.0%
Vitreous	
• Normal	93.8%
• Trace cells	6.2%
• More than trace cells	0%
Retinal exudates	
• Present on or adjacent to disc	3.1%
• Present in the macula	0%
• Present elsewhere	0.6%
Visual acuity	
• 20/20 or better	11%
• 20/25–20/40	25%
• 20/50–20/190	29%
• 20/200–20/800	20%
• Counting fingers	4%
• Hand motions	6%
• Light perception	3%
• No light perception (NLP)	3%
Visual function deficits in fellow eye	**67%**
• Visual acuity	14%
• Contrast sensitivity	15%
• Color vision	22%
Abnormal MRI (one or more white matter lesion)	**49%**

Abbreviation: MRI, magnetic resonance imaging.
Note: Percentage represents the percentage of patients with the characteristic.

The majority of patients with ON with eye or ophthalmic trigeminal distribution pain or pain with eye movement have involvement of the orbital segment of the optic nerve.[26,27] The absence of pain, particularly with eye movement, suggests the disorder is limited to the canalicular or intracranial portion of the optic nerve.[26,27]

2.3 What Visual Field Defects Are Noted with Optic Neuritis?

Final analysis of the ONTT showed that the most common abnormality in the affected eyes on presentation was a diffuse field defect (66.2%), which dropped to 8.6% prevalence after 15 years. Central/cecocentral losses were seen in 28.8% of affected eyes initially, and 4.7% at 15 years. Altitudinal/arcuate defects were found in 23.6% of affected eyes on presentation and 5.6% at 15 years.[21] Classic teaching (in the Goldmann and tangent perimetry era) indicated that central scotoma was the most common pattern of visual field loss in ON, and the finding of only 28.8% in this category at first seems surprising. However, many early studies involved Goldmann's perimetry in which a central scotoma represented depressed sensitivity within the central 30 degrees. The pattern of diffuse field loss in the ONTT actually may represent this same pattern. If one includes both the diffuse and the central/cecocentral categories of the ONTT, this study actually confirms that central visual field loss is the most common defect in ON.[28] Moreover, the study of Fang et al[29] regarding global field loss involvement in ON suggests that within the central 30 degrees even cases with focal (central scotoma, arcuate) defects usually show an element of superimposed general depression.[29] The report of Keltner et al,[30] which incorporated central and peripheral visual field testing (the latter by Goldmann's perimetry) in the ONTT, supports this concept; although 97.1% of patients initially showed defects within the central 30 degrees, only 69.9% had abnormal peripheral fields.

Although it is not unusual for patients with ON to have central loss without peripheral loss, it is rare for the peripheral field to be abnormal in the presence of normal central 30-degree fields. Keltner et al[30] showed that in most cases peripheral testing does not increase sensitivity, with only 2.9% of eyes in the study having abnormal peripheral fields with normal central fields. When the results obtained through Humphrey automated central static visual fields and Goldmann's peripheral kinetic isopters are compared, the far periphery appears to recover more rapidly than the central field, at least in more severe cases of ON.[30] Thus, in most cases recovery in ON can probably be monitored effectively with automated perimetry of the central visual fields alone. However, in cases of severe loss of central field, a peripheral kinetic visual field obtained with a Goldmann perimeter may provide additional information about the patient's vision in the far periphery.[30] Gerling et al[1] noted that peripheral testing may better define defects that are diffuse in the central 30 degrees but are actually altitudinal when the nasal periphery is tested.

Although it has long been postulated that ON tends to affect the papillomacular bundle with resultant central/cecocentral scotoma, the pattern loss in ON in the ONTT revealed pure papillomacular involvement in only 28%.[21] Fang et al[29] showed that ON affects the entire 30 degrees (global field involvement) even in patients who appear to have localized depression of visual threshold, indicating that ON does not have a true predilection for the papillomacular bundle, or any specific nerve fiber bundle. In another study, Fang et al[31] assessed specific nerve fiber group involvement by analyzing recovery of field within concentric field rings in the central 30 degrees and found that return of field function does not appear to differ between patients with diffuse or localized defects. They postulate that reduced redundancy of axons in the periphery of the field compared with near fixation may be responsible for the greater recovery of threshold near fixation.

The final analysis of the ONTT trial on visual defects in the contralateral eye to the eye with ON revealed that diffuse loss only accounted for 6.2% of the fellow eye at baseline, and 5.1% at 15 years. The contralateral eye was normal in 25.3% of presenting ON cases, and normal in 64.4% of cases after 15 years.[21]

2.4 What Are the Features of Atypical Optic Neuritis?

Patients who meet the criteria listed in Box 2.1 are considered to have typical ON. Conversely, patients with the features listed in Box 2.2 have atypical ON. For example, the fundus features that should lead the examiner to consider an alternate diagnosis to ON include lipid maculopathy, very severe disc edema with marked hemorrhages, cotton-wool spots, vitreous cells, pale optic disc edema, retinal arteriolar narrowing, and retinopathy.

Box 2.2 Features of atypical optic neuritis (ON)[4,5,6,7,15,32,33,34,35,36,37]

- Bilateral simultaneous onset of ON in an adult patient.
- Painless loss of vision to less than 6/60 with no early recovery.
- Severe or persistent pain for more than 2 weeks after onset of symptoms.
- Severe headache (e.g., sphenoid sinusitis).
- Optic atrophy at presentation without previously documented ON or multiple sclerosis (MS).
- Ocular findings suggestive of an inflammatory process:
  ○ Anterior uveitis.
  ○ Posterior chamber inflammation more than trace.
  ○ Macular exudate or star figure.
  ○ Retinal infiltrate or retinal inflammation.
- Severe optic disc edema.
- Marked optic disc hemorrhages.
- Lack of significant improvement of visual function or worsening of visual function after 30 days.
- Lack of at least one line of visual acuity improvement within the first 3 weeks after onset of symptoms.
- Loss of vision to no perception of light with no early recovery.
- Age older than 50 years.
- African or Afro-Caribbean patients with vision less than 6/12 and no early recovery.

- Preexisting diagnosis or evidence of other systemic condition:
  - Neoplasia.
  - Inflammatory (e.g., sarcoidosis, Wegener granulomatosis, systemic lupus erythematosus).
  - Infectious disease (e.g., Lyme disease, tuberculosis, human immunodeficiency virus [HIV] infection).
  - Severe hypertension, diabetes, or other systemic vasculopathy.
- Exquisitely steroid-sensitive or steroid-dependent optic neuropathy.

2.5 What Disorders May Be Associated with Optic Neuritis?

Box 2.3 lists a number of disorders that may be associated with typical or atypical ON. The presence of one of these disorders is usually suggested by the historical or examination findings.

Box 2.3 Disorders associated with optic neuritis

- Polyneuropathies:
  - Guillain–Barré syndrome.[38,39]
  - Miller Fisher syndrome.[40]
  - Chronic inflammatory demyelinating polyradiculoneuropathy (CIDP).[41,42]
- Infections:
  - Bacteria:
    - Syphilis.[43,44,117]
    - Tuberculosis.[45]
    - Lyme disease.[46,47,48,49,50,51]
    - *Bartonella henselae* (cat-scratch disease).[52,53,54,55]
    - Mycoplasma.[38,56,57]
    - Whipple disease.
    - Brucellosis.[58,59,60]
    - ®-hemolytic streptococcus.
    - Meningococcus.[61]
    - *Propionibacterium acnes*.[62]
  - Fungi:
    - Aspergillus.
    - Histoplasmosis.[63,64]
    - Cryptococcus.[65]
  - Rickettsiae (e.g., Q fever, epidemic typhus, ehrlichiosis[66]).
  - Protozoa:
    - Toxoplasmosis.[67,68,69,70,71,72]
  - Parasites:
    - Toxocariasis.[73]
    - Cysticercosis.[74,75]
  - Viruses:
    - Adenovirus.
    - Hepatitis A.[76]
    - Hepatitis B.[77]
    - Cytomegalovirus (CMV).[78,79,80,81,82]
    - Coxsackie B.
    - Chikungunya.[83,84]
    - Dengue fever.[85]
    - Rubella.
    - Chickenpox.[86]
    - Herpes zoster.[86,87,88,89,90,91,92,118 ,119,120,121,122,123]
    - Smallpox.[93]
    - Herpes simplex virus 1.[94]
    - Epstein–Barr (EB) virus (infectious mononucleosis).[95,96,97,98,99]
    - Measles.[100,101]
    - Mumps.[102,103]
    - Influenza.
    - HTLV-1.[104,105,106]
    - West Nile virus.[107,108]
    - Human immunodeficiency virus (HIV)/acquired immunodeficiency syndrome (AIDS).[109,110,111,112,113,114,115,116]
  - Prions (Jakob–Creutzfeldt disease).
- Postvaccination[124,125,126,127,128,129,130,131,132,133,134,135]:*
  - Smallpox.[93]
  - Tetanus.[129]
  - Rabies.
  - Influenza.[125]
  - Hepatitis B.[124,128]
  - Bacille Calmette–Guérin (BCG.)[131]
  - Anthrax.[133,134]
  - Trivalent measles–mumps–rubella vaccine.
  - Mantoux tuberculin skin test.[127]
- Focal infection or inflammation[136]:
  - Paranasal sinusitis.[137]
  - Mucocele.
  - Postinfectious.[138]
  - Malignant otitis externa.[139]
- Systemic inflammations and diseases:
  - Giant cell arteritis.[140]
  - Behçet disease.[141]
  - Inflammatory bowel disease.[142,143]
  - Reiter syndrome.
  - Sarcoidosis.[2,34,144,145,146,147]
  - Systemic lupus erythematosus.[148,149,150,151,152,153,154,155]
  - Sjögren syndrome.[156]
  - Mixed connective tissue disease.
  - Rheumatoid arthritis.[157,158]
  - Anti-tumor necrosis factor (TNF) alpha therapy.[158,159,160,161,162]
- Miscellaneous:
  - Multifocal choroiditis.
  - Birdshot chorioretinopathy.
  - Acute posterior multifocal placoid pigment epitheliopathy (APMPPE).[163]
  - Autoimmune optic neuropathy.[164,165,166,167]
  - Familial Mediterranean fever.[168]
  - Bee or wasp sting.[169,170,171,172]
  - Snake bite.[173]
  - Radiation induced.[174]
  - Postpartum optic neuritis.[175]
  - Retrobulbar optic neuritis with retinitis pigmentosa sine pigmento.[176]

○ Neuromyelitis optica (Devic disease).[167,177,178,179,180,181,182, 183,184,185,186,187,188,189,190,191,192]

○ Recurrent optic neuromyelitis with endocrinopathies.[193]

*Hepatitis B, tetanus, influenza, measles, and rubella vaccination are not associated with an increased risk of optic neuritis.[135]

2.6 Is It Neuromyelitis Optica?

The association of acute or subacute loss of vision in one or both eyes caused by optic neuropathy preceded or followed by a transverse or ascending myelopathy that is associated with aquaporin-4 immunoglobulin G (AQP4-IgG) antibodies is referred to as neuromyelitis optica (Devic disease).[194] It is a neuroinflammatory disease distinct from multiple sclerosis (MS).[194] On presentation, visual loss is usually due to unilateral ON, but bilateral visual impairment can be seen.[195,196] Females are more affected than males (9:1),[194,197] and prevalence can vary between races.[198,199,200,201,202] The loss of vision is notably rapid and severe, with complete blindness not uncommon.[196] Because of limitations to the original clinical definition of NMO, variations are now included as a member of the neuromyelitis optica spectrum disorders (NMOSD).[194] Criteria for NMOSD, as well as the clinical features of NMO (Devic disease), are outlined in Box 2.4.

Box 2.4 Clinical features of neuromyelitis optica spectrum disorders (NMOSD)[194,203,204,205,206, 207,208,209,210]

Neuromyelitis optica (NMO):
- AQP4-IgG seropositive patients with limited, or partial, forms of NMO.[203,211,212]
- Otherwise typical NMO patients with cerebral, diencephalic, and brainstem lesions.[213,214,215,216,217,218,219, 220,221,222,223,224,225]
- Asian opticospinal multiple sclerosis.[226,227]
- AQP4-IgG seropositive optic neuritis or longitudinal spinal cord lesions associated with systemic autoimmune disease.[193,228,229,230,231,232,233,234,235,236,237,238,239,240,241]

Neuromyelitis optica (Devic disease)[178,179,180,181,182,183, 184,185,186,187,188,189,190,191,192,193,199,242,243,244,245,246,247]:
- Age: typically younger patients.
- Gender: 9:1 female:male in adults; 3:1 female:male in children.[194,197]
- Race:
  ○ May be more common in African Americans who develop ON.[199,200]
  ○ May be more common in Asians who develop ON.[198,200]
  ○ May be more common in Caucasians than previously thought.[201,202]
- Familial cases: rare.[244,248]
- Pathology: differs from multiple sclerosis (MS)[249,250]:

○ Activation of the humoral immune system and eosinophil activation exclusively in the cerebrospinal fluid (CSF).[251,252]
○ Possible role of T cells.
○ AQP4-IgG antibodies have pathologic effect.[253,254,255,256, 257,258]
○ Astrocytes are targeted early in the disease process.[255,259,260]
○ More severe axonal damage than MS.[261]
○ Blood–brain barrier breakdown.[262,263]
○ Cerebellum is almost never affected.
○ Excavation of affected tissue with formation of cavities common in Devic disease but rare in MS.
○ Gliosis characteristic of MS absent or minimal with Devic disease.
○ Arcuate fibers in cerebral subcortex relatively unaffected in Devic disease but severely damaged in MS.
○ Similar pathogenesis in children and adults.[194,264,265]
- Clinical features—Note: no single clinical feature is diagnostic for NMOSD in the absence of AQP4-IgG antibodies[194]:
  ○ May have prodrome of fever, sore throat, and headache.
  ○ Visual loss:
    – May precede or follow paraplegia.
    – ON usually unilateral.[195,196]
    – Bilateral visual impairment.[196]
    – Rapid and usually severe (complete blindness not uncommon).[196]
    – Central scotoma most common visual field defect.
- Ophthalmoscopy:
  ○ Typical presentation with unilateral optic neuritis, but can be bilateral simultaneously.[195]
  ○ Majority have mild disc swelling of both discs but may be normal.
  ○ Occasional severe swelling with dilation of veins and extensive peripapillary exudates.
  ○ May have slight narrowing of retinal vessel.
- Neuroimaging:
  ○ Magnetic resonance imaging (MRI)[266,267,268]:
    – Sparing of the cortex.[269,270,271]
    – Longitudinally extensive transverse myelitis (over ≥ 3 segments).[195]
    – Hippocampal volume as a predictor of cognition.[272]
    – Variations for NMOSD.[273,274,275,276]
  ○ Optical coherence tomography (OCT)[277,278,279]:
    – ON with thinner retinal nerve fiber layer (RNFL) compared to MS.[280,281]
    – Superior and inferior quadrants more severely affected than MS.[280]
- Visual prognosis[200]:
  ○ Greater final visual impairment than MS.[243]
  ○ Usually some recovery of vision.
  ○ Often recovers within weeks to months.
  ○ Some cases severe and permanent.[202]
- Paraplegia (transverse myelitis):
  ○ Usually sudden and severe.
  ○ Often recover to some degree but may be permanent complete paralysis.[282]
  ○ Spinal cord MRI often shows abnormality extending over three or more segments.[283]

○ May have Lhermitte symptom, paroxysmal tonic spasms,[284,285] and radicular pain.[286,287]

- Course: typically relapsing, but can be monophasic.[177,195,200,242,288]
- Associations:
  ○ Rarely associated with demyelinating peripheral neuropathy.
  ○ Rarely associated with HIV-1 infection, pulmonary tuberculosis, human papillomavirus (HPV) vaccination, and as a paraneoplastic disorder.[289,290,291,292]
  ○ Course of disease influenced by pregnancy.[293,294,295,296]
  ○ Rarely, opportunistic retinal infections (with immunosuppressive therapy).[297]
  ○ Possibly syndrome of inappropriate antidiuresis (SIAD).[298,299]
  ○ Persistent hiccups and nausea.[219,300,301,302,303]
- Laboratory studies:
  ○ Often AQP4-IgG antibodies.[255,304,305,306,307,308,309,310,311,312,313,314,315,316]
  ○ Myelin oligodendrocyte glycoprotein (MOG) antibodies.[317,318,319,320]
  ○ Often CSF pleocytosis (e.g., > 50 white blood cell [WBC], often polymorphonuclear cells).
  ○ Oligoclonal bands uncommon.[321,322]
  ○ Rare increased intracranial pressure.
- Treatment:
  ○ Immunomodulatory mechanisms (azathioprine, rituximab, tocilizumab, mycophenolate mofetil, methotrexate, and mitoxantrone).[323,324,325,326,327,328,329,330,331,332,333,334,335,336,337,338,339,340,341,342]
  ○ Possible response to intravenous (IV) steroids.
  ○ IV gamma globulin.
  ○ Plasma exchange when associated with optic neuritis.[343]
- Mortality less than 10 to 33%.

The current consensus for NMOSD includes syndromes that may or may not be associated with AQP4-IgG antibodies, and may show findings on imaging with lesions that are not necessarily restricted to the spinal cord.[194] Lesions can also be seen on the optic nerve, spinal cord, area postrema, brainstem, diencephalon, and cerebral areas.[194,213,214,215,216,217,218,219,220,221,222,223,224,225] Patients may only show limited, or partial, forms of NMO.[203,211,212] In addition, the new criteria includes Asian opticospinal MS,[226,227] as well as AQP4-IgG seropositive ON or other spinal cord lesions associated with systemic autoimmune disease.[193,228,229,230,231,232,233,234,235,236,237,238,239,240,241]

AQP4-IgG has been found to contribute to the pathophysiology of NMOSD,[253,254,255,256,257,258] which is different from that of MS.[249,250] There is early astrocyte involvement in the disease process,[255,259,260] as well as blood–brain barrier breakdown[262,263]; typically, there is more severe axonal damage than in MS.[261] Therefore, serologic testing for AQP4-IgG is imperative diagnostically. For many patients with suspected NMOSD with no detection of AQP4-IgG, serum myelin oligodendrocyte glycoprotein (MOG) antibodies have been detected—these patients may also have differing clinical characteristics and some early

evidence suggests that the MOG antibody disease may have a more favorable prognosis than AQP4-IgG + NMO.[194]

For adult patients with NMOSD, the diagnostic criteria depend on whether or not AQP4-IgG is present in the serum. If AQP4-IgG is present, then at least *one* core clinical characteristic must be included along with exclusion of all other alternative diagnoses. Core clinical criteria include ON, acute myelitis, area postrema syndrome (unexplained hiccups or nausea and vomiting), acute brainstem syndrome, symptomatic narcolepsy or acute diencephalic clinical syndrome with NMOSD-diencephalic magnetic resonance imaging (MRI) lesions, and symptomatic cerebral syndrome with NMOSD-typical brain lesions.[194] For diagnosis of NMOSD, patients lacking AQP4-IgG or of unknown serostatus must meet other diagnostic criteria, including at least *two* clinical criteria occurring as a result of attacks (with at least one of the criteria being ON, acute myelitis with longitudinally extensive transverse myelitis [LETM], or area postrema syndrome).[194] Additional MRI requirements for NMOSD without AQP4-IgG are indicated.[194]

The course of disease for NMOSD is typically relapsing, but can also be monophasic.[177,195,200,242,288] Visual prognosis for NMOSD indicates greater impairment than for MS; some recovery of vision usually occurs over weeks to months, but vision loss can be severe and permanent.[202,243] Recovery after LETM is possible, but can also be permanent complete paralysis.[282] Lhermitte symptom, paroxysmal tonic spasms,[284,285] and exquisite radicular pain[286,287] are also associated with LETM.

2.7 What Are the Clinical Features of Optic Neuritis in Children?

The clinical features of ON in children differ from those in adults. It is more likely to be a bilateral disease, and to have papillitis.[344] Children may present with worse vision than adults, but may have similar, if not better, visual outcomes.[344,345,346,347] It is more likely to be associated with a viral/parainfectious etiology, and less likely to be associated with MS.[344] Brady et al[346] concluded that younger patients are more likely to have bilateral disease and a better visual prognosis. A lack of MRI abnormalities at the time of diagnosis of ON indicates a lower chance of developing MS.[348]

Unlike Brady et al, Wan et al[345] did not find a trend toward better visual outcomes in younger patients; however, children with ON were found to have at least as good, and possibly better, visual outcomes as compared to adults. Patients who regained visual acuity took an average of 61 days to recover; this could be separated into a mean of 97 days to recover normal vision for those presenting with vision to counting fingers or worse, and a mean of 35 days for those above that vision threshold at presentation. A poor visual outcome at 1 year (< 20/40) was associated with vision of less than 20/20 at 3 months.

In another study of 47 children with MS, 38 (80.9%) had ON at least once, and 10 (21.3%) had two or more attacks of ON.[349] The presence of tumor necrosis factor α7 (TNF- α7) locus on chromosome 6 was proposed as a possible marker of early MS onset in these patients.

Wilejto et al[350] found that ON in childhood was more likely to be unilateral, MS risk was high (36% at 2 years), and bilateral ON was associated with a greater likelihood for MS.

2.8 What Is the Evaluation of Optic Neuritis?

Formal evaluation of ON requires a thorough history and physical examination, along with various imaging techniques (see section on Neuroimaging) and laboratory workup. The National Eye Institute Visual Function Questionnaire (NEI-VFQ-25) and a 10-item Neuro-Ophthalmic Supplement can be used to assess self-reported visual dysfunction, which may not be elicited by tests for visual acuity, and is especially useful in MS-associated ON.[351,352,353,354,355] The differential diagnosis of acute demyelinating ON should include anterior ischemic optic neuropathy and Leber hereditary optic neuropathy (especially in men with a central scotoma and painless loss of vision), as well as a variety of other inflammatory, compressive, infectious, ischemic, toxic, inherited, and other ophthalmologic conditions; distinction can be made through the history of the illness and clinical findings.[84,85]

In atypical cases, consideration should be given to doing a lumbar puncture and additional laboratory studies; in the ONTT, syphilis serology, antinuclear antibody (ANA), and chest X-ray were performed.[25] The required evaluation depends on the history and examination, with specific attention to infectious or inflammatory etiologies as listed in (Box 2.3 (p. 26)). In addition, patients with inflammatory autoimmune ON often have progressive or recurrent steroid-responsive or steroid-dependent optic neuropathy.[2,164,165]

2.9 What Were the Results of the Optic Neuritis Treatment Trial?

The ONTT was developed to evaluate the efficacy of corticosteroid treatment for acute ON and to investigate the relationship between ON and MS.[3,4,5,6,7,33,356,357] The ONTT was sponsored by the National Eye Institute as a randomized, controlled clinical trial that enrolled 457 patients at 15 clinical centers in the United States between the years 1988 and 1991. The ONTT entry criteria specified that patients be between the ages of 18 and 46 years, that they have a relative afferent pupillary defect as well as a visual field defect in the affected eye, and that they were examined within 8 days of the onset of visual symptoms of a first attack of acute unilateral ON. Patients were excluded if they had previous episodes of ON in the affected eye, previous corticosteroid treatment for ON or MS, or systemic disease other than MS that might be a cause of the ON.[3,4,5,6,7,33,356] The clinical features of the ONTT patients are outlined in ▶ Table 2.1.

In the ONTT, all patients underwent testing for collagen vascular disease (ANA), serologic testing for syphilis (fluorescent treponemal antibody absorption [FTA-ABS]), and a chest radiograph for sarcoidosis. Lumbar puncture was optional. An ANA test was positive in a titer less than 1:320 in 13% of patients, and 1:320 or greater in 3%. Only one patient was eventually diagnosed with a collagen vascular disease. Overall, these additional tests (e.g., ANA, FTA-ABS, chest radiograph, lumbar puncture) were not found to be helpful in identifying alternative causes for ON in the study's patients.[25]

Visual and neurologic outcomes in these patients were no different from those of the other ONTT patients. The FTA-ABS was positive in six patients (1.3%), but none had syphilis. A chest radiograph did not reveal sarcoidosis in any patient. However, in a separate report, Jacobson et al[46] described 4 of 20 patients with isolated ON with a positive serology for Lyme disease. These authors recommended serologic testing for Lyme disease in patients with ON, with or without the typical rash of erythema migrans, who live in or have visited Lyme endemic areas. Cerebrospinal fluid (CSF) analysis was recommended for patients with positive serology and intravenous (IV) antibiotic therapy for unexplained pleocytosis.[46] We do not order Lyme titers for patients with ON from nonendemic regions (class IV, level C).

A controversial outcome of the ONTT was that for patients with abnormal MRI results, IV steroids were found to be temporarily protective against the development of demyelinating lesions consistent with MS.[357] In the ONTT, although 16% of patients who received IV treatment developed MS at 2 years, while 30% of patients treated orally or with placebo developed MS.[25] However, by 5 years, the treatment had no significant effect on the development of MS.[358] At 10 years, patients in the prednisone treatment group had a higher recurrence rate of ON (44%) than those in the IV (29%) or placebo group (31%).

The evaluation recommendations of the ONTT study group for patients with typical acute ON are listed in Box 2.5.

> ### Box 2.5 Modified evaluation recommendations based on the Optic Neuritis Treatment Trial for optic neuritis
>
> - No laboratory studies or lumbar puncture required for typical optic neuritis.[25]
> - Potential testing for atypical optic neuritis:
>   - Chest radiograph.
>   - Syphilis serology.
>   - Collagen vascular disease screen.
>   - Serum chemistries.
>   - Complete blood counts.
>   - Lumbar puncture.
>   - Lyme serology in patients from endemic areas.
>   - Aquaporin-4 and myelin oligodendrocyte glycoprotein antibodies.
> - Neuroimaging:
>   - MRI of the brain for all optic neuritis (classes I–II, level B).
>   - Consider MR orbit with fat suppression views to examine optic nerve course, especially in atypical optic neuritis.

2.10 What Are the Neuroimaging Findings in Optic Neuritis?

Periventricular white matter signal abnormalities on MRI consistent with MS[359,360] have been reported in 40 to 70% of cases of isolated ON.[8,359,361,362,363,364,365] MRI with gadolinium may show enhancing lesions in 26 to 37% of patients with isolated ON[361,366] and may increase the detection of disease activity.[366, 367,368,369] Although computed tomography (CT) scan of the head may also show abnormalities in MS and ON, CT has been relatively insensitive to the detection of MS plaques compared to MRI. MRI is a very sensitive test for detecting lesions consistent with MS.[360,370] Paty[371] reported 19 cases of clinically definite MS (CDMS) out of 200 consecutive patients with suspected MS comparing predictive value of MR scanning with CT scanning, evoked potentials (EPs), and CSF analysis for oligoclonal bands. Eighteen of these 19 (95%) patients had MR scans that were "strongly suggestive of MS" at first evaluation. Fourteen of 19 (74%) patients had positive oligoclonal bands. Ten of 19 (53%) patients had abnormal somatosensory EPs, 9 of 19 (47%) patients had abnormal visual EPs (VEPs), and 9 of 19 (47%) patients had abnormal CT scans. Combining multiple reports, the risk of developing MS within 1 to 4 years is about 30% (range 23–35%) in patients with isolated ON and an abnormal MR scan.[4,372,373,374] Morrisey et al[364] reported 89 patients (44 with ON, 17 with brainstem involvement, and 28 with spinal cord involvement) with an acute clinical demyelinating attack. Of these 89 patients, 57 (64%) had one or more MR scan abnormalities and 32 had no MR scan abnormalities. Only 1 of the 32 patients with normal MR scans developed MS, versus development of MS in 37 of 57 patients (65%) with an abnormal MR scan. Of the three isolated clinical syndromes (optic nerve, brainstem, and spinal cord), ON with an abnormal MR scan had the highest rate of progression to MS—82%. Jacobs et al[359] reported 42 patients with isolated monosymptomatic ON. During 5.6 years of follow-up, 21 patients developed MS. Of these 21 patients, 16 (76%) had abnormal MR scans and 5 had normal MR scans.[359]

Söderström et al[374] performed a prospective study of 147 consecutive patients with acute monosymptomatic ON. Of 116 patients examined with MR scans, 64 (55%) had three or more high-signal lesions, 11 (9%) had one or two high-signal lesions, and 41 (35%) had a normal MRI. Among 146 patients undergoing CSF studies, oligoclonal bands were demonstrated in 103 (71%) patients. During the 6-year study period, 53 patients (36%) developed CDMS. Three or more MS lesions on MR scan or CSF oligoclonal bands were strongly associated with MS. Jacobs et al[373] found that 42 of 74 (57%) patients with isolated monosymptomatic ON had 1 to 20 brain lesions by MR scans. All of the brain lesions were clinically silent and had characteristics consistent with MS. During 5.6 years of follow-up, 21 patients (28%) developed CDMS. Sixteen of the 21 converting patients (76%) had abnormal MR scans; the other 5 (24%) had MR scans that were normal initially (when they had ON only) and normal in 4 of the 5 when repeated after they had developed clinical MS. Of the 53 patients who had not developed CDMS, 26 (49%) had abnormal MR scans and 27 (51%) had normal MR scans. The authors concluded that the findings of an abnormal MR scan at the time of ON was significantly related to the subsequent development of MS. The interpretation of the strength of that relationship must be tempered by the fact that some of the converting patients had normal MR scans and approximately half of the patients who did not develop clinical MS had abnormal MR scans. Thus, it should be emphasized that MS is a clinical diagnosis that cannot be made on the basis of MR scan abnormalities alone,[375,376] and the absence of MR scan abnormalities does not protect against the future development of

MS.[6,359] Magnetization transfer ratio (MTR), a quantitative MRI measure, can be used to detect abnormalities in normal-appearing gray matter on MRI, as well as to monitor symptomatic demyelinating lesions.[377,378,379,380] However, the ONTT found that some patients with monosymptomatic ON showed no clinical signs or MRI evidence of demyelination after 10 years; in addition, MRI abnormalities that had no implication for clinical manifestation of CDMS were observed in some patients.[381]

The ONTT prospectively studied 388 patients who did not have probable or definite MS at study entry and who were followed for the development of CDMS.[358] The 5-year cumulative probability of CDMS was 30% and did not differ by treatment group. Neurologic impairment in patients who developed CDMS was generally mild. Brain MR scans performed at study entry was a strong predictor of CDMS, with the 5-year risk of CDMS ranging from 16% in 202 patients with no MR lesions to 51% in 89 patients with three or more MR lesions. The 5-year risk of CDMS following ON is dependent on the number of lesions present on brain MR scan. Even a normal brain MRI, however, did not preclude the development of CDMS.

MR scans may demonstrate contrast-enhancing lesions within the optic nerve in patients with ON.[26,382,383,384] Less complete visual recovery in ON was associated with longer lesions of the optic nerve and with involvement of the intracanalicular segment in one study.[383] In another study, however, lesions involving the canal or longer segments of the optic nerve had worse starting vision, but the location and length of enhancement were not predictive of recovery.[26] Hickman et al[385] found no evidence for association between mean areas of the optic nerve at baseline, at 1 year, or for the rate of decline and visual outcome.

Optical coherence tomography (OCT) has emerged as an important diagnostic tool for ON. Retinal nerve fiber layer (RNFL) thickness has been found to be a good measure of damage to the afferent visual pathway.[386,387,388,389,390,391,392] Reduced volume of the macula is associated with RNFL axonal loss in MS patients with a history of ON.[390,393] Changes observed via OCT differ between men and women, indicating potential differences in recovery after ON.[394] RNFL atrophy with retinal periphlebitis was found to be associated with MS disease activity.[395] In contrast, Naismith et al[396] found that OCT was less sensitive than VEPs for detecting disability and a worse prognosis for MS. One study showed that OCT did not provide evidence for retinal axonal loss in early clinical stages of MS, and could not predict conversion to MS at 6 months.[397]

Other methods of imaging evaluation for ON include orbital Doppler sonography, which shows increased peak systolic and end diastolic velocities in the ophthalmic artery for patients with acute ON.[398] Near-infrared spectroscopy (NIRS) can be an effective noninvasive measure of visual dysfunction in patients with ON.[399] Positron emission tomography (PET) also shows potential for improvement of the understanding of the pathophysiology of ON.[400] Decreased axial diffusivity shown by diffusion tensor imaging (DTI) predicts worse 6-month visual outcome in acute ON, and increased optic nerve radial diffusivity is correlated with a proportional decline in vision.[401,402,403]

MRI can help determine if optic nerve enhancements are resulting from NMOSD, as the spectrum shows unique characteristics. Enhancement occurs in areas of affected AQP4 receptors.[266,267,268,273,274,275,276,404] NMOSD should be considered in instances where optic nerve segment or optic chiasm enhancement with T1 or T2 gadolinium is longer, and/or bilateral.[194] OCT usually shows ON with a thinner RNFL compared to MS, as well as more severe involvement of the superior and inferior quadrants than MS.[280,281] While these ophthalmologic findings can be unique, the most specific neuroimaging finding of NMOSD is the presence of central and longitudinally extensive transverse myelitis (LETM) on MRI.[194,195,204] While extension of a cervical lesion into the brainstem is usually indicative of NMOSD, MS cord lesions are usually only one vertebral segment in length; however, it has been noted that NMOSD can present with short myelitis lesions.[194] Other neuroimaging characteristics for NMOSD include longitudinally extensive spinal cord atrophy and specific cerebral lesion patterns on T2-weight MRI sequences.[194]

2.11 Should a Lumbar Puncture Be Performed in Patients with Optic Neuritis?

Patients with ON may show abnormalities in CSF analysis consistent with MS. These CSF abnormalities include increased cell count (> 5 cells/mm^3 per cubic millimeter), increased total protein, increased CSF IgG concentration, oligoclonal bands, antibodies to myelin basic protein (MBP) and proteolipid protein (PLP), and increased CSF MBP levels.[372,373,374,405,406,407,408,409,410] Lumbar puncture, however, did not produce any additional unsuspected diagnosis in the 141 patients in the ONTT undergoing CSF analysis. In addition, a normal initial CSF after ON did not preclude the eventual development of MS.[411]

Cole et al[405] investigated the predictive value of CSF oligoclonal banding for MS 5 years after ON in patients enrolled in the ONTT. In 76 patients, the presence of oligoclonal bands was associated with development of CDMS. However, the results suggested that CSF analysis was useful in the risk assessment of ON patients only when the brain MR scan was normal and was not of predictive value when brain MR scan lesions were present at the time of ON. CDMS developed within 5 years in 22 of the 76 patients (29%), in 16 of 38 patients (42%) with oligoclonal bands present and in 6 of 38 patients (16%) without bands. Among the 39 patients with normal MR scans, CDMS developed in 3 of 11 patients (27%) with bands present but in only 1 patient (4%) without bands. In contrast, among 37 patients with abnormal MR scans, CDMS developed in 13 of 27 (48%) with bands and 5 of 10 (50%) without bands. The positive predictive value of bands was 42% and the negative predictive value was 84%. Among the 39 patients with normal MR scans, the positive predictive value was 27% and the negative predictive value was 96%, whereas among the 37 patients with abnormal MR scans the positive predictive value was 48% and the negative predictive value was 50%.

Although several authors have reported that abnormal CSF results may be predictive of eventual MS,[372,373,374,405,411] others have not found CSF abnormalities to have predictive value.[411] Although a lumbar puncture was optional in the ONTT, it should be considered in atypical ON or in cases where the diagnosis of MS might be clarified by CSF analysis (classes I–II, level B). For typical presentations of ON, the ONTT did not find lumbar puncture to be helpful in discerning alternative causes for optic neuropathy in their patients; therefore, the test is not recommended for use in typical ON.[25]

2.12 Should Visual Evoked Potentials Be Performed on Patients with Optic Neuritis?

Increased latencies and reduced amplitudes of waveforms are observed in more than 65% of patients with ON, and encourage a diagnosis of demyelination in the afferent visual pathway.[412,413,414] Although the VEP is often abnormal in patients with ON,[396,415,416,417,418,419,420,421,422,423] an abnormal VEP in the setting of a clinically diagnosed ON does not alter the diagnostic or treatment plan. The VEP does not provide additional prognostic information for visual recovery; however, Fraser et al[414,424] demonstrated that multifocal VEP (MVEP) latency delay can help predict progression to future MS. We do not recommend routine use of VEP in typical ON (classes III–IV, level C). VEP may be useful in identifying a second site of neurologic involvement (previous ON) to strengthen the clinical diagnosis of MS in patients with no history or examination findings of an optic neuropathy.[425]

2.13 What Is the Treatment of Optic Neuritis?

Although corticosteroids have been used for acute ON[32,357,426,427,428] and have been shown to improve symptoms in MS,[429] well-controlled data to support the treatment efficacy of steroids in ON have been lacking until recently.[3] IV methylprednisolone (MP) treatment has been reported to decrease CSF anti-MBP levels, intrathecal IgG synthesis, and CSF oligoclonal bands; to decrease gadolinium enhancement of MS plaques (and presumably blood–brain barrier disruption) on MR scan; and to improve clinical disability. Modulation of the function of inflammatory cells may also contribute to the clinical efficacy or high-dose corticosteroids.[430] The clinical effect of treatment might be due to reduction of inflammation and myelin breakdown.[410,431,432]

Rawson et al[9] reported a more rapid visual recovery, but no difference in visual outcome after 1 year in a double-blind, placebo-controlled, prospective study of 50 patients with ON treated with adrenocorticotropic hormone (ACTH). Rose et al[433] observed similarly more rapid improvement in patients with ON treated with ACTH compared with placebo. Bowden et al,[434] however, reported no benefit from ACTH compared with placebo in 54 patients with ON. Gould et al[435] reported a prospective, single-blind, controlled, randomized clinical trial of 74 patients with ON who experienced more rapid improvement with a retrobulbar injection of triamcinolone, but patients had no difference in outcome after 6 months.

In the ONTT, the patients were randomly assigned to one of three treatment arms in the study:
1. IV MP sodium succinate (250 mg every 6 hours for 3 days), followed by oral prednisone (1 mg/kg daily) for 11 days.
2. Oral prednisone (1 mg/kg daily) for 14 days.
3. Oral placebo for 14 days, followed by a short oral taper.

The major conclusions of the ONTT related to treatment are summarized in Box 2.6. Wakakura et al[436] also performed a randomized trial of IV megadose MP in ON and found that treatment with steroids improved visual recovery at 3 weeks. Visual function at 12 weeks and at 1 year, however, was the same as in control patients. Sellebjerg et al[427] performed a randomized, controlled trial of oral high-dose MP (500 mg daily for 5 days with a 10-day taper) in 30 patients compared to 30 control patients. The visual analog scale but not spatial visual function was better in the steroid group at 3 weeks. After 8 weeks, the visual analog scale and spatial visual function were comparable in both groups. The risk of new demyelinating attacks within 1 year was unaffected by treatment. In another study, 55 patients with acute ON received IV saline or IV MP and were assessed at 6 months.[429] Patients with short lesions of the optic nerve on MR scan presented earlier than those with long lesions (involving three or more 5-mm-thick slices of any part of the optic nerve, as well as its intracanalicular portion). Lesion length was significantly less in patients presenting within a week of onset of symptoms. Treatment did not limit lesion length in either the long or the short lesion subgroups and had no significant effect on final visual outcome. The authors conclude that steroids do not improve visual outcome or lesion length in patients with acute ON.[429]

Box 2.6 Summary of the Optic Neuritis Treatment Trial findings[25,355,357,381,437,438,439]

- Intravenous (IV) methylprednisolone, followed by oral prednisone accelerated visual recovery but provided no long-term visual benefit.[357]
- "Standard dose" oral prednisone alone did not improve the visual outcome and was associated with an increased rate of new attacks of ON.[357]
- IV, followed by oral corticosteroids reduced the rate of development of clinically definite MS (CDMS) during the first 2 years, but by 3 years the effect had subsided.[33,356,357]
- MR findings have the highest prognostic significance for MS.
- Treatment was well tolerated with few major side effects.
- A low-risk profile for ON includes men with normal MRI results, poor vision, severe disc swelling, and no pain.

Based on the ONTT results, it is recommended that treatment with oral prednisone in standard doses be avoided in ON (class I, level A).[440] Treatment with IV MP should be considered in patients with abnormal MR scans of the brain or a particular need (e.g., monocular patient or occupational requirement) to recover visual function more rapidly (class I, level B). Beck et al[3, 4,5,6,7,33,441] thought that although brain MR scan may not be necessary for the diagnosis of ON, imaging was valuable for prognostic purposes. In the ONTT, patients with multiple signal abnormalities on MR scans most clearly benefited from IV corticosteroid therapy in terms of development of MS.[357] The rate of development of MS was too low in the patients with normal MR scans to assess treatment benefit in this group. ON patients in the ONTT had MR scans within 9 days of the onset of visual loss. Some authors have suggested that patients presenting later than this interval with an abnormal MR scan may still benefit from treatment with IV MP within a treatment window of

about 2 months.[375] The results of the ONTT have led to a reduction in the use of oral corticosteroids in the treatment of ON.[442]

Even though the ONTT was a large, well-designed study, several criticisms have been raised:
1. The lack of an intravenous control group.
2. Incomplete masking of all patients (i.e., in-hospital IV-treated patients knew they had received IV MP).
3. Data regarding treatment effect of IV MP on the development of MS were obtained from a retrospective analysis that was primarily designed for a different purpose (to evaluate the treatment effect).
4. The role of retrobulbar steroids was not assessed.
5. The role of higher doses of MP, such as 30 mg/kg dose suggested for the treatment of acute spinal cord injury, was not determined.
6. The efficacy of oral prednisone at higher doses was not assessed.
7. The need or lack of need for oral tapering doses of corticosteroids following IV MP was not addressed.

Despite these concerns, the ONTT is the best well-controlled prospective clinical trial (class I) available in the literature to date on the treatment and evaluation of ON. We follow the evaluation and the treatment recommendations of the ONTT (class I, level B). There are many other new MS therapies that could be considered in addition to interferon, but long-term data is not available, especially for treatment of ON.[323,324,325,326,327,328,329, 330,331,332,333,334,335,336,337,338,339,340,341,343] However, in patients with longitudinally extensive optic nerve enhancement on MRI or ON without typical demyelinating white matter lesions, IV steroids might be useful for covering patients until NMO can be excluded. If NMO is suspected, the disease-modifying MS therapies should be avoided as these have actually precipitated worsening disease in NMO patients.

In a patient with NMOSD-induced ON, treatment involves immunosuppression. Recommendations from the Neuromyelitis Optica Study Group (NEMOS) suggest first-line therapy as azathioprine and rituximab, second-line therapy as mycophenolate mofetil and methotrexate, and third-line therapy as combination therapy or tocilizumab.[342] The use of interferon therapy is contraindicated if NMOSD is suspected.[253,342,443,444]

2.14 Should Interferon Therapy Be Instituted in Patients with Optic Neuritis?

In the double-blind, randomized controlled high-risk Avonex multiple sclerosis (CHAMPS) study, 383 patients who had a first acute demyelinating event (ON, incomplete transverse myelitis, or a brainstem or cerebellar syndrome) were studied. All had evidence of prior subclinical demyelination on MRI of the brain (two or more silent lesions of at least 3 mm in diameter thought characteristic of MS). Patients received either weekly intramuscular injections of 30 mg of interferon-β-1a (193 patients) or placebo (190 patients).[445,446] The patients had received initial treatment with corticosteroids. During 3 years of follow-up, the cumulative probability of the development of CDMS was significantly lower in the interferon-β-1a group than in the placebo group (rate ratio, 0.56). At 3 years, the cumulative probability was 35% in the interferon-β-1a group and 50% in the placebo group. As compared with the patients in the placebo group, patients in the interferon-β-1a group had a relative reduction in the volume of brain lesions, fewer new lesions or enlarging lesions, and fewer gadolinium-enhancing lesions at 18 months.

In Early Treatment of Multiple Sclerosis (ETOMS) trial, 308 patients were enrolled in this double-blind, randomized controlled study, which required four asymptomatic white matter lesions on MRI for entry (including ON). Patients were provided subcutaneous interferon-β-1a or placebo weekly for 2 years. Less patients developed CDMS from the interferon-β-1a treatment group than in the placebo group (34 vs. 45%, respectively). The time for 30% of patients receiving interferon-β-1a to be converted to CDMS was 10 to 11 months longer than for placebo (569 vs. 252 days). Relapse rates were also significantly lower for the interferon-β-1a group than placebo (0.33 and 0.43), as well as the number of new lesions detected by MRI.[447]

The authors concluded that initiating treatment with interferon-β-1a at the time of a first demyelinating event is beneficial for patients with brain lesions on MRI that indicate high risk of CDMS.[445,446,447] Other MS therapies have been developed in recent years and could be considered in addition to interferon, but long-term data is not yet available for treatment of ON.[323,324,325,326,327,328,329,330,331,332,333,334,335,336,337,338,339,340,341,343] Again, interferon treatment is contraindicated if NMOSD is suspected.[443,444]

2.15 Are There Treatments Other than Steroids for Optic Neuritis?

Intravenous immunoglobulin (IVIg) had been initially reported to improve visual acuity in an uncontrolled study of five patients with definite MS and unilateral or bilateral but stable demyelinating ON.[448] However, in a randomized trial in 55 patients, this agent did not reverse persistent visual loss from ON to a degree that merits general use.[449] Another randomized trial showed that in 34 patients receiving IVIg, there was no effect of IVIg on visual function at 6 months, or on preservation of optic nerve axonal function detected via VEP.[450] While it is effective for many other autoimmune neurologic diseases, IVIg has not been shown to be effective in patients with MS who have ON or weakness.[451]

Plasma exchange as an add-on therapy for severe acute ON has been associated with improvement of visual acuity in patients for whom previous high-dose IV corticosteroids were ineffective.[452] A retrospective review showed plasma exchange was associated with clinical improvement in one of four patients presenting with acute ON at discharge, and three of four patients at 6 months; overall, an improvement was seen at 6 months in 63% of 41 patients with severe central nervous system (CNS) demyelination.[453]

2.16 What Is the Long-Term Vision Prognosis of Patients with Optic Neuritis?

In patients with ON, visual recovery generally begins within the first 2 weeks, with much of the recovery occurring by the end of 1 month. If recovery is incomplete at 6 months, some further improvement may continue for up to 1 year.

In the ONTT, there was no significant difference in visual acuity comparing the three treatment groups at 6 months. After 12 months, visual acuity was 20/40 or greater in 93% of patients, greater than 20/20 in 69%, and 20/200 or lower in 3%. Results were similar in each treatment group. The only predictor of poor visual outcome was poor visual acuity at the time of study entry; even so, of 160 patients starting with a visual acuity of 20/200 or worse, all had at least some improvement and only 8 (5%) had visual acuities that were still 20/200 or worse at 6 months. Of 30 patients whose initial visual acuity was light perception (LP) or no light perception (NLP), 20 (67%) recovered to 20/40 or better. One-month visual acuity was the best predictor of 6-month visual acuity outcome[454]; older age was statistically associated with a slightly worse outcome, but this appeared to be of no clinical importance.

Thus, in most patients with ON, visual recovery is rapid. The only factor of value in predicting the visual outcome is initial severity of visual loss. However, even when initial loss is severe, visual recovery is still good in most patients. Patients not following the usual course of visual recovery should be considered atypical and further investigation in regard to etiology of the visual loss is appropriate.

At the 5-year follow-up for 397 (87%) of 454 patients in the ONTT, the affected eyes had normal or only slightly abnormal visual acuities in most patients, and results did not significantly differ by treatment group.[455] Visual acuity in affected eyes was 20/25 or better in 87%, 20/25 to 20/40 in 7%, 20/50 to 20/190 in 3%, and 20/200 or worse in 3%. Recurrence of ON in either eye occurred in 28% of patients and was more frequent in patients with MS and in patients without MS who were in the prednisone treatment group. Most eyes with a recurrence retained normal or almost normal visual function. In conclusion, most patients with ON retain good or excellent vision 5 years following an attack of ON, even if the ON recurs. Recurrences are more frequent in patients with MS and in those treated with oral prednisone alone. Recurrence of ON in either eye occurs in 28% of patients and are twofold more frequent in patients who had or developed CDMS (46%) compared with patients without CDMS (22%).

In the 10-year follow-up for the ONTT of 319 of the original 454 patients with ON, most patients had normal or only slightly abnormal visual function tests in the eyes originally affected by ON. Visual acuity was greater than 20/25 or better in 86% of the affected eyes, and 91% were greater than 20/40 or better. Patients who had MS had worse visual function than those without. Recurrence rate for ON in either eye was 35%, and was much more frequent in patients with CDMS or who later developed CDMS (48%) than those without CDMS (24%). Patients in the prednisone treatment group had a higher recurrence rate (44%) than those in the IV (29%) or placebo group (31%). Ultimately, the 10-year follow-up showed very good regain of vision after an ON attack.[355]

A prospective controlled study found that in 21 patients with unilateral first-time ON, affected eyes had returned to normal via routine visual testing after 4 months. In contrast, motion perception remained impaired over 1 year, and was correlated with functional MRI (fMRI) studies.[456]

In a retrospective study of 253 adult and 38 pediatric patients with CDMS whose first symptom was acute ON, worse recovery was seen in men and people with severe attacks. Pediatric cases had better recovery than adult patients. The level of vitamin D (season adjusted) was associated with the severity of the initial attack, but had no correlation with recovery.[347]

NMOSD patients have a worse long-term visual prognosis than for patients with ON and MS-associated ON.[243] In addition, NMOSD patients are more likely to have a relapsing disease course than monophasic.[177,195,200,242,288] There is usually some recovery of vision over weeks to months, but some cases are severe and permanent.[202]

2.17 What Is the Risk of Developing Multiple Sclerosis following Optic Neuritis?

The risk for the development of MS following ON is quite variable in the literature, with reports ranging from 8 to 85%.[358,373,374,405,457,458,459,460] Most studies of MS and ON indicate a 25 to 35% risk of patients with ON developing MS. This variability is probably related to numerous factors including the following:

- Differences in patient populations (e.g., clinic or hospital vs. population based), sample sizes, study design (retrospective vs. prospective).
- Duration of follow-up (longer interval studies tend to report higher incidence rates).
- Differences in selection criteria and diagnostic evaluation of ON cases.
- Different study diagnostic criteria for both ON and MS.

Rodriguez et al[458] found a cumulative probability of developing CDMS of 24% after 5 years and 39% after 10 years and noted no difference in the risk of developing MS between men and women. Rizzo and Lessell[461] studied 60 patients with ON, with a mean follow-up of 14.9 years. Life table analysis indicated that 74% of the women and 34% of the men developed MS 15 years after their attack of ON, and 91.3% of the women and 44.8% of the men would develop MS after 20 years. MR scan abnormalities are the best predictor for the eventual development of MS after ON.[460] Sørensen et al[459] concluded that ON as the first manifestation of MS (vs. another or unknown onset manifestation of MS) indicates a more favorable prognosis of survival of MS in women. ON was the presenting manifestation of MS in 10% of MS cases.

As noted earlier, in the ONTT prospective study of 388 patients who did not have probable or definite MS at study entry, the 5-year cumulative probability of CDMS was 30%,[358] the 10-year risk was 38%, and the 15-year risk was 50%.[437] Brain MR scans performed at study entry were a strong predictor of CDMS, with the 5-year risk of CDMS ranging from 16% in 202 patients with no MR lesions to 51% in 89 patients with three or more MR lesions. At 10 years, 191 patients with no MR lesions showed a low but not zero (22%) progression rate to CDMS. In contrast, 44 patients with 2 to 4 MR lesions showed 50% progression rate, 37 patients with 5 to 8 MR lesions showed 70% progression, and 28 patients with 9 or more lesions on MR had 57% progression to CDMS.[437] At 15 years, 25% of 191 patients with no MRI lesions at baseline developed MS, while 72% of 161 patients with 1 or more lesions developed MS.[438] The risk of CDMS following ON is highly dependent on the number of lesions present on brain MR scan at the time of attack.[437,438]

Brex et al[462] performed high-resolution, multisequence brain and spinal cord MRI in 60 patients after their first demyelinating event, including 38 patients with ON. At baseline, 73% of patients had lesions on T2-weighted fast spin-echo (FSE) brain images and 42% had asymptomatic spinal cord lesions. Of the 38 patients with ON, 29 had lesions in the brain on FSE images and 16 had spinal cord lesions. Repeat MRI demonstrated new FSE lesions in 43% of the patients overall. After 1 year, 26% of the patients developed MS. The MRI features that provided the best combination of sensitivity and specificity for the development of MS were new FSE lesions at follow-up and enhancing lesions at baseline. The authors concluded that the combination of baseline MR abnormalities on multisequence MRI and new lesions at follow-up, indicating dissemination in space and time, are associated with a high sensitivity and specificity for the early development of clinical MS.

Ghezzi et al[463,464] evaluated the risk of SDMS after acute isolated ON in 102 patients with follow-up duration 6.3 years (10 patients were lost to follow-up). The risk of developing SDMS was 13% after 2 years, 30% after 4 years, 37% after 6 years, and 42% after 8 and 10 years. Gender, age, and season of ON onset did not affect the risk. CDMS occurred in 37 of 71 patients (52.1%) with one MRI lesion or more; no patient with a normal MRI developed CDMS. CDMS developed more frequently in patients with intrathecal IgG synthesis than in those without (43 vs. 28%), but the difference was not statistically significant.[463,464]

Increased risk of MS has been reported in patients with human leukocyte antigen HLA-DR2 and HLA-B7 tissue types, but we do not recommend routine HLA screening for ON.[364,465] Risk factors for developing MS following ON are outlined in ▶ Table 2.2.

Table 2.2 Risk factors for developing multiple sclerosis following optic neuritis

Factor	References
Increased risk	
• Abnormal MR scan (three or more lesions)	Jacobs[373]; ONTT[358,437,438]; Söderström[374]; Mikaeloff[466]; Beck[370]; Tintore[467]
• Prior nonspecific neurologic symptoms	ONTT[358,437,438]
• Increased CSF oligoclonal bands	Cole[405]; Tintore[467]
• Increased CSF IgG	Jacobs[373]; Söderström[374]
• Previous optic neuritis	ONTT[358,437,438]
• HLA-DR2 and HLA-B7	Morrissey[364]
• Increased permeability of blood brain barrier	Cramer[468]
• Each younger decade at onset	Tintore[467]
Decreased risk	
• Normal MR scan	ONTT[437,438]; Brex[370]
• Mental status change	Mikaeloff[466]
• Absence of pain[a]	ONTT[358,437,438]
• Marked disc edema[a]	ONTT[358,437,438]
• Retinal exudates or macular star[a]	ONTT[358,437,438]
• Bilateral simultaneous onset[a]	Frederiksen[469]
• Onset in childhood[a]	Lucchinetti[470]; Mikaeloff[466]

Abbreviation: CSF, cerebrospinal fluid; IgG, immunoglobulin G; MR, magnetic resonance; ONTT, Optic Neuritis Treatment Trial.
[a]We consider these findings in a patient with ON to be atypical and thus likely require further evaluation.

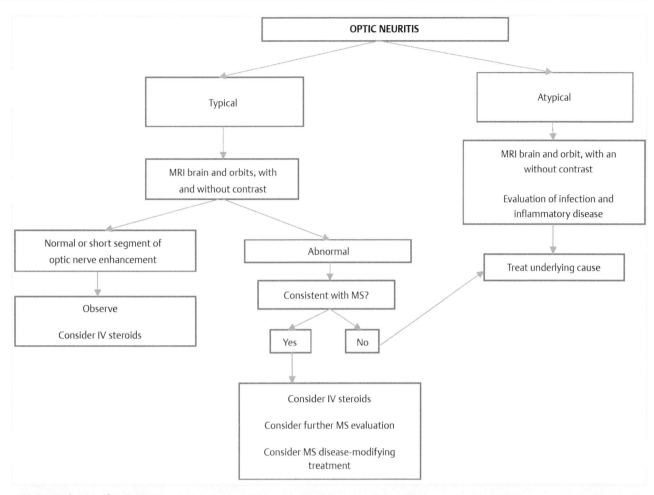

Fig. 2.1 Evaluation of optic neuritis.

Our approach to ON is summarized in ▶ Fig. 2.1.

References

[1] Gerling J, Meyer JH, Kommerell G. Visual field defects in optic neuritis and anterior ischemic optic neuropathy: distinctive features. Graefes Arch Clin Exp Ophthalmol. 1998; 236(3):188–192

[2] Beck AD, Newman NJ, Grossniklaus HE, Galetta SL, Kramer TR. Optic nerve enlargement and chronic visual loss. Surv Ophthalmol. 1994; 38(6): 555–566

[3] Beck RW, The Optic Neuritis Study Group. Corticosteroid treatment of optic neuritis: a need to change treatment practices. Neurology. 1992; 42(6): 1133–1135

[4] Beck RW, Arrington J, Murtagh FR, Cleary PA, Kaufman DI, Experience of the Optic Neuritis Study Group. Brain magnetic resonance imaging in acute optic neuritis. Arch Neurol. 1993; 50(8):841–846

[5] Beck RW, Cleary PA. Optic neuritis treatment trial. One-year follow-up results. Arch Ophthalmol. 1993; 111(6):773–775

[6] Beck RW, Cleary PA, Trobe JD, et al. The Optic Neuritis Study Group. The effect of corticosteroids for acute optic neuritis on the subsequent development of multiple sclerosis. N Engl J Med. 1993; 329(24):1764–1769

[7] Beck RW, Kupersmith MJ, Cleary PA, Katz B. Fellow eye abnormalities in acute unilateral optic neuritis. Experience of the optic neuritis treatment trial. Ophthalmology. 1993; 100(5):691–697, discussion 697–698

[8] Frederiksen JL, Larsson HB, Olesen J, Stigsby B. MRI, VEP, SEP and biothesiometry suggest monosymptomatic acute optic neuritis to be a first manifestation of multiple sclerosis. Acta Neurol Scand. 1991; 83(5):343–350

[9] Jin YP, de Pedro-Cuesta J, Söderström M, Link H. Incidence of optic neuritis in Stockholm, Sweden, 1990–1995: II. Time and space patterns. Arch Neurol. 1999; 56(8):975–980

[10] Cleary PA, Beck RW, Anderson MM, Jr, Kenny DJ, Backlund JY, Gilbert PR. Design, methods, and conduct of the Optic Neuritis Treatment Trial. Control Clin Trials. 1993; 14(2):123–142

[11] Frederiksen JL, Larsson HB, Ottovay E, Stigsby B, Olesen J. Acute optic neuritis with normal visual acuity. Comparison of symptoms and signs with psychophysiological, electrophysiological and magnetic resonance imaging data. Acta Ophthalmol (Copenh). 1991; 69(3):357–366

[12] Gerling J, Janknecht P, Kommerell G. Orbital pain in optic neuritis and anterior ischemic optic neuropathy. Neuro-ophthalmology. 1998; 19(2):93–99

[13] Keltner JL, Johnson CA, Beck RW, Cleary PA, Spurr JO. Quality control functions of the Visual Field Reading Center (VFRC) for the Optic Neuritis Treatment Trial (ONTT). Control Clin Trials. 1993; 14(2):143–159

[14] Keltner JL, Johnson CA, Spurr JO, Beck RW, Optic Neuritis Study Group. Baseline visual field profile of optic neuritis. The experience of the optic neuritis treatment trial. Arch Ophthalmol (Chicago, Ill 1960). 1993; 111(2):231–234

[15] Optic Neuritis Study Group. The clinical profile of optic neuritis. Experience of the Optic Neuritis Treatment Trial. Arch Ophthalmol. 1991; 109(12): 1673–1678

[16] Schneck ME, Haegerstrom-Portnoy G. Color vision defect type and spatial vision in the optic neuritis treatment trial. Invest Ophthalmol Vis Sci. 1997; 38(11):2278–2289

[17] Slamovits TL, Macklin R, Beck RW, Frenkel M, Lim JI, Hillman DS. What to tell the patient with optic neuritis about multiple sclerosis. Surv Ophthalmol. 1991; 36(1):47–50

[18] Wakakura M, Minei-Higa R, Oono S, et al. Optic Neuritis Treatment Trial Multicenter Cooperative Research Group (ONMRG). Baseline features of idiopathic optic neuritis as determined by a multicenter treatment trial in Japan. Jpn J Ophthalmol. 1999; 43(2):127–132

[19] Wall M, Johnson CA, Kutzko KE, Nguyen R, Brito C, Keltner JL. Long- and short-term variability of automated perimetry results in patients with optic neuritis and healthy subjects. Arch Ophthalmol. 1998; 116(1):53–61

[20] Dworak DP, Nichols J. A review of optic neuropathies. Dis Mon. 2014; 60(6): 276–281

[21] Keltner JL, Johnson CA, Cello KE, Dontchev M, Gal RL, Beck RW, Optic Neuritis Study Group. Visual field profile of optic neuritis: a final follow-up report from the optic neuritis treatment trial from baseline through 15 years. Arch Ophthalmol. 2010; 128(3):330–337

[22] Cleary PA, Beck RW, Bourque LB, Backlund JC, Miskala PH. Visual symptoms after optic neuritis. Results from the Optic Neuritis Treatment Trial. J Neuroophthalmol. 1997; 17(1):18–23, quiz 24–28

[23] Frederiksen JL, Sørensen TL, Sellebjerg FT. Residual symptoms and signs after untreated acute optic neuritis. A one-year follow-up. Acta Ophthalmol Scand. 1997; 75(5):544–547

[24] Steel DH, Waldock A. Measurement of the retinal nerve fibre layer with scanning laser polarimetry in patients with previous demyelinating optic neuritis. J Neurol Neurosurg Psychiatry. 1998; 64(4):505–509

[25] December 1991 The Clinical Profile of Optic Neuritis Experience of the Optic Neuritis Treatment Trial Arch Ophthalmol. 1991;109(12):1673-1678. doi:10.1001/archopht.1991.01080120057025

[26] Kupersmith MJ, Alban T, Zeiffer B, Lefton D. Contrast-enhanced MRI in acute optic neuritis: relationship to visual performance. Brain. 2002; 125(Pt 4): 812–822

[27] Kupersmith MJ, Fazzone H, Lefton D. Localization of the pain with optic neuritis. Presented at the 28th Annual Meeting of the North American Neuro-Ophthalmology Society, Copper Mountain, Colorado, February 9–14, 2002

[28] Arnold AC. Visual field defects in the optic neuritis treatment trial: central vs peripheral, focal vs global. Am J Ophthalmol. 1999; 128(5):632–634

[29] Fang JP, Donahue SP, Lin RH. Global visual field involvement in acute unilateral optic neuritis. Am J Ophthalmol. 1999; 128(5):554–565

[30] Keltner JL, Johnson CA, Spurr JO, Beck RW. Comparison of central and peripheral visual field properties in the optic neuritis treatment trial. Am J Ophthalmol. 1999; 128(5):543–553

[31] Fang JP, Lin RH, Donahue SP. Recovery of visual field function in the optic neuritis treatment trial. Am J Ophthalmol. 1999; 128(5):566–572

[32] Hickman SJ, Dalton CM, Miller DH, Plant GT. Management of acute optic neuritis. Lancet. 2002; 360(9349):1953–1962

[33] Beck RW, Cleary PA. Recovery from severe visual loss in optic neuritis. Arch Ophthalmol (Chicago, Ill 1960). 1993; 111(3):300

[34] Beck RW, Cleary PA, Backlund JC. The course of visual recovery after optic neuritis. Experience of the Optic Neuritis Treatment Trial. Ophthalmology. 1994; 101(11):1771–1778

[35] Biousse V, Trichet C, Bloch-Michel E, Roullet E. Multiple sclerosis associated with uveitis in two large clinic-based series. Neurology. 1999; 52(1): 179–181

[36] Lee AG, Brazis PW. The 5-year risk of MS after optic neuritis. Neurology. 1998; 51(4):1236–, author reply 1237–1238

[37] Moschos M. Acute bilateral optic neuritis. Doc Ophthalmol. 1989; 73(3): 225–230

[38] Nadkarni N, Lisak RP. Guillain-Barré syndrome (GBS) with bilateral optic neuritis and central white matter disease. Neurology. 1993; 43(4):842–843

[39] Ropper A, Wijdicks E, Truax B. (1991). Guillain-Barré Syndrome. Philadelphia. PA: FA Davis; 1991

[40] Chan JW. Optic neuritis in anti-GQ1b positive recurrent Miller Fisher syndrome. Br J Ophthalmol. 2003; 87(9):1185–1186

[41] Kaufman D. Peripheral demyelinating and axonal disorders. In: Miller N, Newman N, eds. Walsh and Hoyt's Clinical Neuro-Ophthalmology. 5th ed. Baltimore, MD: Williams and Wilkins; 1998:5677–5719

[42] Lee AG, Galetta SL, Lepore FE, Appel SH. Optic atrophy and chronic acquired polyneuropathy. J Neuroophthalmol. 1999; 19(1):67–69

[43] Frohman L, Wolansky L. Magnetic resonance imaging of syphilitic optic neuritis/perineuritis. J Neuroophthalmol. 1997; 17(1):57–59

[44] Pless ML, Kroshinsky D, LaRocque RC, Buchbinder BR, Duncan LM. Case records of the Massachusetts General Hospital. Case 26-2010. A 54-year-old man with loss of vision and a rash. N Engl J Med. 2010; 363(9):865–874

[45] Mansour AM. Optic disk tubercle. J Neuroophthalmol. 1998; 18(3):201–203

[46] Jacobson DM, Marx JJ, Dlesk A. Frequency and clinical significance of Lyme seropositivity in patients with isolated optic neuritis. Neurology. 1991; 41 (5):706–711

[47] Arnold RW, Schriever G. Lyme amaurosis in a child. J Pediatr Ophthalmol Strabismus. 1993; 30(4):268–270

[48] Karma A, Seppälä I, Mikkilä H, Kaakkola S, Viljanen M, Tarkkanen A. Diagnosis and clinical characteristics of ocular Lyme borreliosis. Am J Ophthalmol. 1995; 119(2):127–135

[49] Lesser RL, Kornmehl EW, Pachner AR, et al. Neuro-ophthalmologic manifestations of Lyme disease. Ophthalmology. 1990; 97(6):699–706

[50] Winterkorn JM. Lyme disease: neurologic and ophthalmic manifestations. Surv Ophthalmol. 1990; 35(3):191–204

[51] Jacobson DM. Lyme disease and optic neuritis: long-term follow-up of seropositive patients. Neurology. 2003; 60(5):881–882

[52] Schwartzman WA, Patnaik M, Angulo FJ, Visscher BR, Miller EN, Peter JB. Bartonella (Rochalimaea) antibodies, dementia, and cat ownership among men infected with human immunodeficiency virus. Clin Infect Dis. 1995; 21(4):954–959

[53] Schwartzman WA, Patnaik M, Barka NE, Peter JB. Rochalimaea antibodies in HIV-associated neurologic disease. Neurology. 1994; 44(7):1312–1316

[54] Brazis PW, Stokes HR, Ervin FR. Optic neuritis in cat scratch disease. J Clin Neuroophthalmol. 1986; 6(3):172–174

[55] Herz AM, Lahey JM. Images in clinical medicine. Optic neuritis due to Bartonella henselae infection. N Engl J Med. 2004; 350(2):e1

[56] Salzman MB, Sood SK, Slavin ML, Rubin LG. Ocular manifestations of Mycoplasma pneumoniae infection. Clin Infect Dis. 1992; 14(5):1137–1139

[57] Sheth RD, Goulden KJ, Pryse-Phillips WE. The focal encephalopathies associated with mycoplasma pneumoniae. Can J Neurol Sci. 1993; 20(4): 319–323

[58] McLean DR, Russell N, Khan MY. Neurobrucellosis: clinical and therapeutic features. Clin Infect Dis. 1992; 15(4):582–590

[59] Abd Elrazak M. Brucella optic neuritis. Arch Intern Med. 1991; 151(4): 776–778

[60] Sahin E, Yilmaz A, Ersöz G, Uğuz M, Kaya A. Multiple cranial nerve involvement caused by Brucella melitensis. South Med J. 2009; 102(8):855–857

[61] Miller N. Walsh and Hoyt's Clinical Neuro-Ophthalmology. 4th ed., Baltimore, MD: Williams and Wilkins; 1998

[62] Kouyoumdjian GA, Larkin TP, Blackburn PJ, Mandava N. Optic disk edema as a presentation of propionibacterium acnes endophthalmitis. Am J Ophthalmol. 2001; 132(2):259–261

[63] Perry JD, Girkin CA, Miller NR, Mann RB. Disseminated histoplasmosis causing reversible gaze palsy and optic neuropathy. J Neuroophthalmol. 1999; 19(2):140–143

[64] Yau TH, Rivera-Velazquez PM, Mark AS, et al. Unilateral optic neuritis caused by Histoplasma capsulatum in a patient with the acquired immunodeficiency syndrome. Am J Ophthalmol. 1996; 121(3):324–326

[65] Golnik KC, Newman SA, Wispelway B. Cryptococcal optic neuropathy in the acquired immune deficiency syndrome. J Clin Neuroophthalmol. 1991; 11 (2):96–103

[66] Lee MS, Goslee TE. Ehrlichiosis optic neuritis. 2003:412–413

[67] Banta J, Lam B. Toxoplasmic anterior optic neuropathy. Presented at the 28th Annual Meeting of the North American Neuro-Ophthalmology Society, Copper Mountain, CO, Febryary 9–14, 2002

[68] Falcone PM, Notis C, Merhige K. Toxoplasmic papillitis as the initial manifestation of acquired immunodeficiency syndrome. Ann Ophthalmol. 1993; 25(2):56–57

[69] Grossniklaus HE, Specht CS, Allaire G, Leavitt JA. Toxoplasma gondii retinochoroiditis and optic neuritis in acquired immune deficiency syndrome. Report of a case. Ophthalmology. 1990; 97(10):1342–1346

[70] Pierce E, D'Amico D. Ocular toxoplasmosis: pathogenesis, diagnosis, and management. Semin Ophthalmol. 1993; 8:40–52

[71] Rose GE. Papillitis, retinal neovascularisation and recurrent retinal vein occlusion in Toxoplasma retinochoroiditis: a case report with uncommon clinical signs. Aust N Z J Ophthalmol. 1991; 19(2):155–157

[72] Song A, Scott IU, Davis JL, Lam BL. Atypical anterior optic neuropathy caused by toxoplasmosis. Am J Ophthalmol. 2002; 133(1):162–164

[73] Komiyama A, Hasegawa O, Nakamura S, Ohno S, Kondo K. Optic neuritis in cerebral toxocariasis. J Neurol Neurosurg Psychiatry. 1995; 59(2):197–198

[74] Chang GY, Keane JR. Visual loss in cysticercosis: analysis of 23 patients. Neurology. 2001; 57(3):545–548

[75] Menon V, Tandon R, Khanna S, et al. Cysticercosis of the optic nerve. J Neuroophthalmol. 2000; 20(1):59–60

[76] McKibbin M, Cleland PG, Morgan SJ. Bilateral optic neuritis after hepatitis A. J Neurol Neurosurg Psychiatry. 1995; 58(4):508

[77] Achiron LR. Postinfectious hepatitis B optic neuritis. Optom Vis Sci. 1994; 71 (1):53–56

[78] Harkins T, Maino JH. Cytomegalovirus retinitis complicated by optic neuropathy: a longitudinal study. J Am Optom Assoc. 1992; 63(1):21–27

[79] Ho M. Cytomegalovirus. In: Mandell G, Bennett J, Dolin R, eds. Principles and Practice of Infectious Disease. 4th ed. New York, NY: Churchill Livingstone; 1995:1351–1364

[80] Mansour AM. Cytomegalovirus optic neuritis. Curr Opin Ophthalmol. 1997; 8(3):55–58

[81] Patel SS, Rutzen AR, Marx JL, Thach AB, Chong LP, Rao NA. Cytomegalovirus papillitis in patients with acquired immune deficiency syndrome. Visual prognosis of patients treated with ganciclovir and/or foscarnet. Ophthalmology. 1996; 103(9):1476–1482

[82] Roarty JD, Fisher EJ, Nussbaum JJ. Long-term visual morbidity of cytomegalovirus retinitis in patients with acquired immune deficiency syndrome. Ophthalmology. 1993; 100(11):1685–1688

[83] Lalitha P, Rathinam S, Banushree K, Maheshkumar S, Vijayakumar R, Sathe P. Ocular involvement associated with an epidemic outbreak of chikungunya virus infection. Am J Ophthalmol. 2007; 144(4):552–556

[84] Mittal A, Mittal S, Bharati MJ, Ramakrishnan R, Saravanan S, Sathe PS. Optic neuritis associated with chikungunya virus infection in South India. Arch Ophthalmol. 2007; 125(10):1381–1386

[85] Haritoglou C, Dotse SD, Rudolph G, Stephan CM, Thurau SR, Klauss V. A tourist with dengue fever and visual loss. Lancet. 2002; 360(9339):1070

[86] Lee CC, Venketasubramanian N, Lam MS. Optic neuritis: a rare complication of primary varicella infection. Clin Infect Dis. 1997; 24(3):515–516

[87] Deane JS, Bibby K. Bilateral optic neuritis following herpes zoster ophthalmicus. Arch Ophthalmol. 1995; 113(8):972–973

[88] Greven CM, Singh T, Stanton CA, Martin TJ. Optic chiasm, optic nerve, and retinal involvement secondary to varicella-zoster virus. Arch Ophthalmol. 2001; 119(4):608–610

[89] Gündüz K, Ozdemir O. Bilateral retrobulbar neuritis following unilateral herpes zoster ophthalmicus. Ophthalmologica. 1994; 208(2):61–64

[90] Miyashita K, Kigasawa K, Mashima Y, Fujino T. Superior altitudinal hemianopia and herpes zoster. Ann Ophthalmol. 1993; 25(1):20–23

[91] Mori T, Terai T, Hatano M, Oda Y, Asada A, Moriwaki M. Stellate ganglion block improved loss of visual acuity caused by retrobulbar optic neuritis after herpes zoster. Anesth Analg. 1997; 85(4):870–871

[92] Nakazawa N, Abe T, Ohmura M. Varicella zoster-associated optic neuropathy with choroidal involvement. Neuroophthalmology. 1999; 21:39–45

[93] Semba RD. The ocular complications of smallpox and smallpox immunization. Arch Ophthalmol. 2003; 121(5):715–719

[94] Tornerup NR, Fomsgaard A, Nielsen NV. HSV-1–induced acute retinal necrosis syndrome presenting with severe inflammatory orbitopathy, proptosis, and optic nerve involvement. Ophthalmology. 2000; 107(2):397–401

[95] Straussberg R, Amir J, Cohen HA, Savir H, Varsano I. Epstein-Barr virus infection associated with encephalitis and optic neuritis. J Pediatr Ophthalmol Strabismus. 1993; 30(4):262–263

[96] Anderson MD, Kennedy CA, Lewis AW, Christensen GR. Retrobulbar neuritis complicating acute Epstein-Barr virus infection. Clin Infect Dis. 1994; 18(5):799–801

[97] Corssmit EP, Leverstein-van Hall MA, Portegies P, Bakker P. Severe neurological complications in association with Epstein-Barr virus infection. J Neurovirol. 1997; 3(6):460–464

[98] Beiran I, Krasnitz I, Zimhoni-Eibsitz M, Gelfand YA, Miller B. Paediatric chiasmal neuritis: typical of post-Epstein-Barr virus infection? Acta Ophthalmol Scand. 2000; 78(2):226–227

[99] Majid A, Galetta SL, Sweeney CJ, et al. Epstein-Barr virus myeloradiculitis and encephalomyeloradiculitis. Brain. 2002; 125(Pt 1):159–165

[100] Totan Y, Cekiç O. Bilateral retrobulbar neuritis following measles in an adult. Eye (Lond). 1999; 13 Pt 3a:383–384

[101] Azuma M, Morimura Y, Kawahara S, Okada AA. Bilateral anterior optic neuritis in adult measles infection without encephalomyelitis. Am J Ophthalmol. 2002; 134(5):768–769

[102] Sugita K, Ando M, Minamitani K, Miyamoto H, Niimi H. Magnetic resonance imaging in a case of mumps postinfectious encephalitis with asymptomatic optic neuritis. Eur J Pediatr. 1991; 150(11):773–775

[103] Khubchandani R, Rane T, Agarwal P, Nabi F, Patel P, Shetty AK. Bilateral neuroretinitis associated with mumps. Arch Neurol. 2002; 59(10):1633–1636

[104] Lehky TJ, Flerlage N, Katz D, et al. Human T-cell lymphotropic virus type II-associated myelopathy: clinical and immunologic profiles. Ann Neurol. 1996; 40(5):714–723

[105] Merle D, Smadja D, Bera O, et al. Uveitis and papillitis in association with HTLV-I associated myelopathy. Ann Ophthalmol. 1997; 29:2895–2896

[106] Yoshida Y, Saiga T, Takahashi H, Hara A. Optic neuritis and human T-lymphotropic virus type 1-associated myelopathy: a case report. Ophthalmologica. 1998; 212(1):73–76

[107] Anninger WV, Lomeo MD, Dingle J, Epstein AD, Lubow M. West Nile virus-associated optic neuritis and chorioretinitis. Am J Ophthalmol. 2003; 136 (6):1183–1185

[108] Vaispapir V, Blum A, Soboh S, Ashkenazi H. West Nile virus meningo-encephalitis with optic neuritis. Arch Intern Med. 2002; 162(5):606–607

[109] Friedman DI. Neuro-ophthalmic manifestations of human immuno-deficiency virus infection. Neurol Clin. 1991; 9(1):55–72

[110] Nichols JW, Goodwin JA. Neuro-ophthalmologic complications of AIDS. Semin Ophthalmol. 1992; 7:24–29

[111] Burton BJ, Leff AP, Plant GT. Steroid-responsive HIV optic neuropathy. J Neuroophthalmol. 1998; 18(1):25–29

[112] Malessa R, Agelink MW, Diener HC. Dysfunction of visual pathways in HIV-1 infection. J Neurol Sci. 1995; 130(1):82–87

[113] Newman NJ, Lessell S. Bilateral optic neuropathies with remission in two HIV-positive men. J Clin Neuroophthalmol. 1992; 12(1):1–5

[114] Quiceno JI, Capparelli E, Sadun AA, et al. Visual dysfunction without retinitis in patients with acquired immunodeficiency syndrome. Am J Ophthalmol. 1992; 113(1):8–13

[115] Sadun AA, Pepose JS, Madigan MC, Laycock KA, Tenhula WN, Freeman WR. AIDS-related optic neuropathy: a histological, virological and ultrastructural study. Graefes Arch Clin Exp Ophthalmol. 1995; 233(7):387–398

[116] Sweeney BJ, Manji H, Gilson RJ, Harrison MJ. Optic neuritis and HIV-1 infection. J Neurol Neurosurg Psychiatry. 1993; 56(6):705–707

[117] McLeish WM, Pulido JS, Holland S, Culbertson WW, Winward K. The ocular manifestations of syphilis in the human immunodeficiency virus type 1-infected host. Ophthalmology. 1990; 97(2):196–203

[118] Friedlander SM, Rahhal FM, Ericson L, et al. Optic neuropathy preceding acute retinal necrosis in acquired immunodeficiency syndrome. Arch Ophthalmol. 1996; 114(12):1481–1485

[119] Lee MS, Cooney EL, Stoessel KM, Gariano RF. Varicella zoster virus retrobulbar optic neuritis preceding retinitis in patients with acquired immune deficiency syndrome. Ophthalmology. 1998; 105(3):467–471

[120] Litoff D, Catalano RA. Herpes zoster optic neuritis in human immunodeficiency virus infection. Arch Ophthalmol. 1990; 108(6):782–783

[121] Margolis TP, Milner MS, Shama A, Hodge W, Seiff S. Herpes zoster ophthalmicus in patients with human immunodeficiency virus infection. Am J Ophthalmol. 1998; 125(3):285–291

[122] Meenken C, van den Horn GJ, de Smet MD, van der Meer JT. Optic neuritis heralding varicella zoster virus retinitis in a patient with acquired immunodeficiency syndrome. Ann Neurol. 1998; 43(4):534–536

[123] Shayegani A, Odel JG, Kazim M, Hall LS, Bamford N, Schubert H. Varicella-zoster virus retrobulbar optic neuritis in a patient with human immunodeficiency virus. Am J Ophthalmol. 1996; 122(4):586–588

[124] Albitar S, Bourgeon B, Genin R, et al. Bilateral retrobulbar optic neuritis with hepatitis B vaccination. Nephrol Dial Transplant. 1997; 12(10):2169–2170

[125] Hull TP, Bates JH. Optic neuritis after influenza vaccination. Am J Ophthalmol. 1997; 124(5):703–704

[126] Kerrison J, Lounsbury D, Lane G, et al. Optic neuritis following anthrax vaccination. Presented at the 27th annual meeting of the North American Neuro-Ophthalmology Society, Rancho Mirage, CA, February 18–22, 2001

[127] Linssen WH, Kruisdijk JJ, Barkhof F, Smit LM. Severe irreversible optic neuritis following Mantoux tuberculin skin test in a child with multiple sclerosis: a case report. Neuropediatrics. 1997; 28(6):338–340

[128] Stewart O, Chang B, Bradbury J. Simultaneous administration of hepatitis B and polio vaccines associated with bilateral optic neuritis. Br J Ophthalmol. 1999; 83(10):1200–1201

[129] Topaloglu H, Berker M, Kansu T, Saatci U, Renda Y. Optic neuritis and myelitis after booster tetanus toxoid vaccination. Lancet. 1992; 339(8786):178–179

[130] van de Geijn EJ, Tukkie R, van Philips LA, Punt H. Bilateral optic neuritis with branch retinal artery occlusion associated with vaccination. Doc Ophthalmol. 1994; 86(4):403–408

[131] Yen MY, Liu JH. Bilateral optic neuritis following bacille Calmette-Guérin (BCG) vaccination. J Clin Neuroophthalmol. 1991; 11(4):246–249

[132] Black S, Eskola J, Siegrist CA, et al. Importance of background rates of disease in assessment of vaccine safety during mass immunisation with pandemic H1N1 influenza vaccines. Lancet. 2009; 374(9707):2115–2122

[133] Payne DC, Rose CE, Jr, Kerrison J, Aranas A, Duderstadt S, McNeil MM. Anthrax vaccination and risk of optic neuritis in the United States military, 1998–2003. Arch Neurol. 2006; 63(6):871–875

[134] Kerrison JB, Lounsbury D, Thirkill CE, Lane RG, Schatz MP, Engler RM. Optic neuritis after anthrax vaccination. Ophthalmology. 2002; 109(1):99–104

[135] DeStefano F, Verstraeten T, Jackson LA, et al. Vaccine Safety Datalink Research Group, National Immunization Program, Centers for Disease Control and Prevention. Vaccinations and risk of central nervous system demyelinating diseases in adults. Arch Neurol. 2003; 60(4):504–509

[136] Moorman CM, Anslow P, Elston JS. Is sphenoid sinus opacity significant in patients with optic neuritis? Eye (Lond). 1999; 13(Pt 1):76–82

[137] Fujimoto N, Adachi-Usami E, Saito E, Nagata H. Optic nerve blindness due to paranasal sinus disease. Ophthalmologica. 1999; 213(4):262–264

[138] Farris BK, Pickard DJ. Bilateral postinfectious optic neuritis and intravenous steroid therapy in children. Ophthalmology. 1990; 97(3):339–345

[139] Bath AP, Rowe JR, Innes AJ. Malignant otitis externa with optic neuritis. J Laryngol Otol. 1998; 112(3):274–277

[140] Garcia-Porrua C, Santamarina R, Armesto V, Gonzalez-Gay MA. Magnetic resonance imaging in optic neuritis due to giant cell arteritis. Arthritis Rheum. 2005; 53(2):313–314

[141] Vaphiades MS, Lee AG, Kansu T. A bad eye and a sore lip. Surv Ophthalmol. 1999; 44(2):148–152

[142] Hutnik CM, Nicolle DA, Canny CL. Papillitis: a rare initial presentation of Crohn's disease. Can J Ophthalmol. 1996; 31(7):373–376

[143] Gupta G, Gelfand JM, Lewis JD. Increased risk for demyelinating diseases in patients with inflammatory bowel disease. Gastroenterology. 2005; 129(3):819–826

[144] Case records of the Massachusetts General Hospital. Weekly clinicopathological exercises. Case 37-1996. A 51-year-old man with visual problems and an intracranial mass. N Engl J Med. 1996; 335(22):1668–1674

[145] DeBroff BM, Donahue SP. Bilateral optic neuropathy as the initial manifestation of systemic sarcoidosis. Am J Ophthalmol. 1993; 116(1):108–111

[146] Haupert CL, Newman NJ. Prolonged Uhthoff phenomenon in sarcoidosis. Am J Ophthalmol. 1997; 124(4):564–566

[147] Kosmorsky GS, Prayson R. Primary optic pathway sarcoidosis in a 38-year-old white man. J Neuroophthalmol. 1996; 16(3):188–190

[148] Ahmadieh H, Roodpeyma S, Azarmina M, Soheilian M, Sajjadi SH. Bilateral simultaneous optic neuritis in childhood systemic lupus erythematosus. A case report. J Neuroophthalmol. 1994; 14(2):84–86

[149] Galindo-Rodríguez G, Aviña-Zubieta JA, Pizarro S, et al. Cyclophosphamide pulse therapy in optic neuritis due to systemic lupus erythematosus: an open trial. Am J Med. 1999; 106(1):65–69

[150] Giorgi D, Balacco Gabrieli C. Optic neuropathy in systemic lupus erythematosus and antiphospholipid syndrome (APS): clinical features, pathogenesis, review of the literature and proposed ophthalmological criteria for APS diagnosis. Clin Rheumatol. 1999; 18(2):124–131

[151] Giorgi D, Balacco Gabrieli C, Bonomo L. The association of optic neuropathy with transverse myelitis in systemic lupus erythematosus. Rheumatology (Oxford). 1999; 38(2):191–192

[152] Ninomiya M, Ohashi K, Sasaki N, et al. A case of optic neuritis accompanying systemic lupus erythematosus several years after onset. Nippon Ganka Kiyo. 1990; 41:636

[153] Ohnuma I, Yamaguchi K, Takahashi S. Retrobulbar neuritis in a patient with mixed connective tissue disease. Nippon Ganka Kiyo. 1996; 47:828–831

[154] Rosenbaum JT, Simpson J, Neuwelt CM. Successful treatment of optic neuropathy in association with systemic lupus erythematosus using intravenous cyclophosphamide. Br J Ophthalmol. 1997; 81(2):130–132

[155] Sivaraj RR, Durrani OM, Denniston AK, Murray PI, Gordon C. Ocular manifestations of systemic lupus erythematosus. Rheumatology (Oxford). 2007; 46(12):1757–1762

[156] Massara A, Bonazza S, Castellino G, et al. Central nervous system involvement in Sjögren's syndrome: unusual, but not unremarkable—clinical, serological characteristics and outcomes in a large cohort of Italian patients. Rheumatology (Oxford). 2010; 49(8):1540–1549

[157] Ağildere AM, Tutar NU, Yücel E, Coşkun M, Benli S, Aydin P. Pachymeningitis and optic neuritis in rheumatoid arthritis: MRI findings. Br J Radiol. 1999; 72(856):404–407

[158] Tauber T, Daniel D, Barash J, Turetz J, Morad Y. Optic neuritis associated with etanercept therapy in two patients with extended oligoarticular juvenile idiopathic arthritis. Rheumatology (Oxford). 2005; 44(3):405

[159] Seror R, Richez C, Sordet C, et al. Club Rhumatismes et Inflammation Section of the SFR. Pattern of demyelination occurring during anti-TNF-α therapy: a French national survey. Rheumatology (Oxford). 2013; 52(5):868–874

[160] Ouakaa-Kchaou A, Gargouri D, Trojet S, et al. Retrobulbar optic neuritis associated with infliximab in a patient with Crohn's disease. J Crohn's Colitis. 2009; 3(2):131–133

[161] Winthrop KL, Chen L, Fraunfelder FW, et al. Initiation of anti-TNF therapy and the risk of optic neuritis: from the safety assessment of biologic ThERapy (SABER) Study. Am J Ophthalmol. 2013; 155(1):183–189.e1

[162] Foroozan R, Buono LM, Sergott RC, Savino PJ. Retrobulbar optic neuritis associated with infliximab. Arch Ophthalmol. 2002; 120(7):985–987

[163] Wolf MD, Folk JC, Goeken NE. Acute posterior multifocal pigment epitheliopathy and optic neuritis in a family. Am J Ophthalmol. 1990; 110(1):89–90

[164] Bielory L, Kupersmith M, Warren F, Bystryn J, Frohman L. Skin biopsies in the evaluation of atypical optic neuropathies. Ocul Immunol Inflamm. 1993; 1(3):231–242

[165] Riedel P, Wall M, Grey A, Cannon T, Folberg R, Thompson HS. Autoimmune optic neuropathy. Arch Ophthalmol. 1998; 116(8):1121–1124

[166] Frohman L, Turbin R, Bielory L, Wolansky L, Lambert WC, Cook S. Autoimmune optic neuropathy with anticardiolipin antibody mimicking multiple sclerosis in a child. Am J Ophthalmol. 2003; 136(2):358–360

[167] Martinez-Hernandez E, Sepulveda M, Rostásy K, et al. Antibodies to aquaporin 4, myelin-oligodendrocyte glycoprotein, and the glycine receptor α1 subunit in patients with isolated optic neuritis. JAMA Neurol. 2015; 72(2):187–193

[168] Lossos A, Eliashiv S, Ben-Chetrit E, Reches A. Optic neuritis associated with familial Mediterranean fever. J Clin Neuroophthalmol. 1993; 13(2):141–143

[169] Berríos RR, Serrano LA. Bilateral optic neuritis after a bee sting. Am J Ophthalmol. 1994; 117(5):677–678

[170] Choi MY, Cho SH. Optic neuritis after bee sting. Korean J Ophthalmol. 2000; 14(1):49–52

[171] Maltzman JS, Lee AG, Miller NR. Optic neuropathy occurring after bee and wasp sting. Ophthalmology. 2000; 107(1):193–195

[172] Song HS, Wray SH. Bee sting optic neuritis. A case report with visual evoked potentials. J Clin Neuroophthalmol. 1991; 11(1):45–49

[173] Menon V, Tandon R, Sharma T, Gupta A. Optic neuritis following snake bite. Indian J Ophthalmol. 1997; 45(4):236–237

[174] Sanda N, Heran F, Daly-Schveitzer N, Sahel JA, Safran AB. Increased optic nerve radiosensitivity following optic neuritis. Neurology. 2014; 82(16):1474–1475

[175] Leiba H, Glaser JS, Schatz NJ, Siatkowski RM. Postpartum optic neuritis: etiologic and pathophysiologic considerations. J Neuroophthalmol. 2000; 20(2):85–88

[176] Hatta M, Hayasaka S, Kato T, Kadoi C. Retrobulbar optic neuritis and rhegmatogenous retinal detachment in a fourteen-year-old girl with retinitis pigmentosa sine pigmento. Ophthalmologica. 2000; 214(2):153–155

[177] Matiello M, Lennon VA, Jacob A, et al. NMO-IgG predicts the outcome of recurrent optic neuritis. Neurology. 2008; 70(23):2197–2200

[178] Ahasan HA, Rafiqueuddin AK, Chowdhury MA, Azhar MA, Kabir F. Neuromyelitis optica (Devic disease) following chicken pox. Trop Doct. 1994; 24(2):75–76

[179] al-Deeb SM, Yaqub BA, Khoja WO. Devic's neuromyelitis optica and varicella. J Neurol. 1993; 240(7):450–451

[180] Barkhof F, Scheltens P, Valk J, Waalewijn C, Uitdehaag BM, Polman CH. Serial quantitative MR assessment of optic neuritis in a case of neuromyelitis optica, using Gadolinium-"enhanced" STIR imaging. Neuroradiology. 1991; 33(1):70–71

[181] Hainfellner JA, Schmidbauer M, Schmutzhard E, Maier H, Budka H. Devic's neuromyelitis optica and Schilder's myelinoclastic diffuse sclerosis. J Neurol Neurosurg Psychiatry. 1992; 55(12):1194–1196

[182] Hershewe G, Corbett J, Thompson H. The NANOS Devic's Study Group. Presented at the North American Neuro-Ophthalmology Society Meeting, Steamboat Springs, Co, February 4–8, 1990

[183] Igarashi Y, Oyachi H, Nakamura Y, Hashimoto M, Ohwada Y, Mito Y. Neuromyelitis optica. Ophthalmologica. 1994; 208(4):226–229

[184] Jain S, Hiran S, Sarma PS. Devic's disease. J Assoc Physicians India. 1994; 42(2):166

[185] Jeffery AR, Buncic JR. Pediatric Devic's neuromyelitis optica. J Pediatr Ophthalmol Strabismus. 1996; 33(5):223–229

[186] Khan MA, Mahar PS, Raghuraman VU. Neuromyelitis optica (Devic's disease). Br J Clin Pract. 1990; 44(12):667–668

[187] Mandler RN, Davis LE, Jeffery DR, Kornfeld M. Devic's neuromyelitis optica: a clinicopathological study of 8 patients. Ann Neurol. 1993; 34(2):162–168

[188] Mandler RN, Ahmed W, Dencoff JE. Devic's neuromyelitis optica: a prospective study of seven patients treated with prednisone and azathioprine. Neurology. 1998; 51(4):1219–1220

[189] O'Riordan JI, Gallagher HL, Thompson AJ, et al. Clinical, CSF, and MRI findings in Devic's neuromyelitis optica. J Neurol Neurosurg Psychiatry. 1996; 60(4):382–387

[190] Piccolo G, Franciotta DM, Camana C, et al. Devic's neuromyelitis optica: long-term follow-up and serial CSF findings in two cases. J Neurol. 1990; 237(4):262–264

[191] Ramelli GP, Deonna T, Roulet E, Zwingli M. Transverse myelitis and optic neuromyelitis in children. Apropos of 3 case reports. Schweiz Rundsch Med Prax. 1992; 81(20):661–663

[192] Silber MH, Willcox PA, Bowen RM, Unger A. Neuromyelitis optica (Devic's syndrome) and pulmonary tuberculosis. Neurology. 1990; 40(6):934–938

[193] Vernant JC, Cabre P, Smadja D, et al. Recurrent optic neuromyelitis with endocrinopathies: a new syndrome. Neurology. 1997; 48(1):58–64

[194] Wingerchuk DM, Banwell B, Bennett JL, et al. International Panel for NMO Diagnosis. International consensus diagnostic criteria for neuromyelitis optica spectrum disorders. Neurology. 2015; 85(2):177–189

[195] Mealy MA, Wingerchuk DM, Greenberg BM, Levy M. Epidemiology of neuromyelitis optica in the United States: a multicenter analysis. Arch Neurol. 2012; 69(9):1176–1180

[196] Papais-Alvarenga RM, Carellos SC, Alvarenga MP, Holander C, Bichara RP, Thuler LC. Clinical course of optic neuritis in patients with relapsing neuromyelitis optica. Arch Ophthalmol (Chicago, Ill 1960). 2008; 126(1):12–16

[197] Collongues N, Marignier R, Zéphir H, et al. Long-term follow-up of neuromyelitis optica with a pediatric onset. Neurology. 2010; 75(12):1084–1088

[198] Sakuma R, Fujihara K, Sato N, Mochizuki H, Itoyama Y. Optic-spinal form of multiple sclerosis and anti-thyroid autoantibodies. J Neurol. 1999; 246(6):449–453

[199] Phillips PH, Newman NJ, Lynn MJ. Optic neuritis in African Americans. Arch Neurol. 1998; 55(2):186–192

[200] Kitley J, Leite MI, Nakashima I, et al. Prognostic factors and disease course in aquaporin-4 antibody-positive patients with neuromyelitis optica spectrum disorder from the United Kingdom and Japan. Brain. 2012; 135(Pt 6):1834–1849

[201] Asgari N, Lillevang ST, Skejoe HPB, Falah M, Stenager E, Kyvik KO. A population-based study of neuromyelitis optica in Caucasians. Neurology. 2011; 76(18):1589–1595

[202] Collongues N, Marignier R, Zéphir H, et al. Neuromyelitis optica in France: a multicenter study of 125 patients. Neurology. 2010; 74(9):736–742

[203] Flanagan EP, Weinshenker BG, Krecke KN, et al. Short myelitis lesions in aquaporin-4-IgG-positive neuromyelitis optica spectrum disorders. JAMA Neurol. 2015; 72(1):81–87

[204] Wingerchuk DM, Lennon VA, Pittock SJ, Lucchinetti CF, Weinshenker BG. Revised diagnostic criteria for neuromyelitis optica. Neurology. 2006; 66(10):1485–1489

[205] Sellner J, Boggild M, Clanet M, et al. EFNS guidelines on diagnosis and management of neuromyelitis optica. Eur J Neurol. 2010; 17(8):1019–1032

[206] Kim SH, Kim W, Li XF, Jung IJ, Kim HJ. Clinical spectrum of CNS aquaporin-4 autoimmunity. Neurology. 2012; 78(15):1179–1185

[207] Jacob A, McKeon A, Nakashima I, et al. Current concept of neuromyelitis optica (NMO) and NMO spectrum disorders. J Neurol Neurosurg Psychiatry. 2013; 84(8):922–930

[208] Sato DK, Nakashima I, Takahashi T, et al. Aquaporin-4 antibody-positive cases beyond current diagnostic criteria for NMO spectrum disorders. Neurology. 2013; 80(24):2210–2216

[209] Pittock SJ, Lucchinetti CF. Neuromyelitis optica and the evolving spectrum of autoimmune aquaporin-4 channelopathies: a decade later. Ann N Y Acad Sci. 2016; 1366(1):20–39

[210] Marignier R, Bernard-Valnet R, Giraudon P, et al. NOMADMUS Study Group. Aquaporin-4 antibody-negative neuromyelitis optica: distinct assay sensitivity-dependent entity. Neurology. 2013; 80(24):2194–2200

[211] Dinkin MJ, Cestari DM, Stein MC, Brass SD, Lessell S. NMO antibody-positive recurrent optic neuritis without clear evidence of transverse myelitis. Arch Ophthalmol. 2008; 126(4):566–570

[212] Collongues N, Cabre P, Marignier R, et al. Group Members for NOMADMUS and CF-SEP. A benign form of neuromyelitis optica: does it exist? Arch Neurol. 2011; 68(7):918–924

[213] Blanc F, Zéphir H, Lebrun C, et al. Cognitive functions in neuromyelitis optica. Arch Neurol. 2008; 65(1):84–88

[214] Chalumeau-Lemoine L, Chretien F, Gaëlle Si Larbi A, et al. Devic disease with brainstem lesions. Arch Neurol. 2006; 63(4):591–593

[215] Eichel R, Meiner Z, Abramsky O, Gotkine M. Acute disseminating encephalomyelitis in neuromyelitis optica: closing the floodgates. Arch Neurol. 2008; 65(2):267–271

[216] Graber JJ, Kister I, Geyer H, Khaund M, Herbert J. Neuromyelitis optica and concentric rings of Baló in the brainstem. Arch Neurol. 2009; 66(2):274–275

[217] Gratton S, Amjad F, Ghavami F, Osborne B, Tornatore C, Mora C. Bilateral hearing loss as a manifestation of neuromyelitis optica. Neurology. 2014; 82(23):2145–2146

[218] Kanbayashi T, Shimohata T, Nakashima I, et al. Symptomatic narcolepsy in patients with neuromyelitis optica and multiple sclerosis: new neurochemical and immunological implications. Arch Neurol. 2009; 66(12):1563–1566

[219] Misu T, Fujihara K, Nakashima I, Sato S, Itoyama Y. Intractable hiccup and nausea with periaqueductal lesions in neuromyelitis optica. Neurology. 2005; 65(9):1479–1482

[220] Newey CR, Bermel RA. Fulminant cerebral demyelination in neuromyelitis optica. Neurology. 2011; 77(2):193

[221] Park KY, Ahn JY, Cho JH, Choi YC, Lee KS. Neuromyelitis optica with brainstem lesion mistaken for brainstem glioma. Case report. J Neurosurg. 2007; 107(3) Suppl:251–254

[222] Pittock SJ, Lennon VA, Krecke K, Wingerchuk DM, Lucchinetti CF, Weinshenker BG. Brain abnormalities in neuromyelitis optica. Arch Neurol. 2006; 63(3):390–396

[223] Pittock SJ, Weinshenker BG, Lucchinetti CF, Wingerchuk DM, Corboy JR, Lennon VA. Neuromyelitis optica brain lesions localized at sites of high aquaporin 4 expression. Arch Neurol. 2006; 63(7):964–968

[224] Roemer SF, Parisi JE, Lennon VA, et al. Pattern-specific loss of aquaporin-4 immunoreactivity distinguishes neuromyelitis optica from multiple sclerosis. Brain. 2007; 130(Pt 5):1194–1205

[225] Rueda Lopes FC, Doring T, Martins C, et al. The role of demyelination in neuromyelitis optica damage: diffusion-tensor MR imaging study. Radiology. 2012; 263(1):235–242

[226] Misu T, Fujihara K, Nakashima I, et al. Pure optic-spinal form of multiple sclerosis in Japan. Brain. 2002; 125(Pt 11):2460–2468

[227] Shimizu J, Hatanaka Y, Hasegawa M, et al. IFNβ-1b may severely exacerbate Japanese optic-spinal MS in neuromyelitis optica spectrum. Neurology. 2010; 75(16):1423–1427

[228] Birnbaum J, Kerr D. Devic's syndrome in a woman with systemic lupus erythematosus: diagnostic and therapeutic implications of testing for the neuromyelitis optica IgG autoantibody. Arthritis Rheum. 2007; 57(2):347–351

[229] Ferreira S, Marques P, Carneiro E, D'Cruz D, Gama G. Devic's syndrome in systemic lupus erythematosus and probable antiphospholipid syndrome. Rheumatology (Oxford). 2005; 44(5):693–695

[230] Gibbs AN, Moroney J, Foley-Nolan D, O'Connell PG. Neuromyelitis optica (Devic's syndrome) in systemic lupus erythematosus: a case report. Rheumatology (Oxford). 2002; 41(4):470–471

[231] Guo Y, Lennon VA, Popescu BFG, et al. Autoimmune aquaporin-4 myopathy in neuromyelitis optica spectrum. JAMA Neurol. 2014; 71(8):1025–1029

[232] Hacohen Y, Zuberi S, Vincent A, Crow YJ, Cordeiro N. Neuromyelitis optica in a child with Aicardi-Goutières syndrome. Neurology. 2015; 85(4):381–383

[233] Iyer A, Rathnasabapathi D, Elsone L, et al. Transverse myelitis associated with an itchy rash and hyperckemia: neuromyelitis optica associated with dermatitis herpetiformis. JAMA Neurol. 2014; 71(5):630–633

[234] Karim S, Majithia V. Devic's syndrome as initial presentation of systemic lupus erythematosus. Am J Med Sci. 2009; 338(3):245–247

[235] Kister I, Gulati S, Boz C, et al. Neuromyelitis optica in patients with myasthenia gravis who underwent thymectomy. Arch Neurol. 2006; 63(6):851–856

[236] Leite MI, Coutinho E, Lana-Peixoto M, et al. Myasthenia gravis and neuromyelitis optica spectrum disorder: a multicenter study of 16 patients. Neurology. 2012; 78(20):1601–1607

[237] McKeon A, Lennon VA, Lotze T, et al. CNS aquaporin-4 autoimmunity in children. Neurology. 2008; 71(2):93–100

[238] Nasir S, Kerr DA, Birnbaum J. Nineteen episodes of recurrent myelitis in a woman with neuromyelitis optica and systemic lupus erythematosus. Arch Neurol. 2009; 66(9):1160–1163

[239] Okada K, Matsushita T, Kira J, Tsuji S. B-cell activating factor of the TNF family is upregulated in neuromyelitis optica. Neurology. 2010; 74(2):177–178

[240] Pittock SJ, Lennon VA, de Seze J, et al. Neuromyelitis optica and non organ-specific autoimmunity. Arch Neurol. 2008; 65(1):78–83

[241] Qiao L, Wang Q, Fei Y, et al. The clinical characteristics of primary Sjogren's syndrome with neuromyelitis optica spectrum disorder in China: a STROBE-compliant article. Medicine (Baltimore). 2015; 94(28):e1145

[242] Wingerchuk DM, Pittock SJ, Lucchinetti CF, Lennon VA, Weinshenker BG. A secondary progressive clinical course is uncommon in neuromyelitis optica. Neurology. 2007; 68(8):603–605

[243] Pirko I, Blauwet LA, Lesnick TG, Weinshenker BG. The natural history of recurrent optic neuritis. Arch Neurol. 2004; 61(9):1401–1405

[244] Yamakawa K, Kuroda H, Fujihara K, et al. Familial neuromyelitis optica (Devic's syndrome) with late onset in Japan. Neurology. 2000; 55(2):318–320

[245] Blanche P, Diaz E, Gombert B, Sicard D, Rivoal O, Brezin A. Devic's neuromyelitis optica and HIV-1 infection. J Neurol Neurosurg Psychiatry. 2000; 68(6):795–796

[246] Filippi M, Rocca MA, Moiola L, et al. MRI and magnetization transfer imaging changes in the brain and cervical cord of patients with Devic's neuromyelitis optica. Neurology. 1999; 53(8):1705–1710

[247] Wingerchuk DM, Hogancamp WF, O'Brien PC, Weinshenker BG. The clinical course of neuromyelitis optica (Devic's syndrome). Neurology. 1999; 53(5): 1107–1114

[248] Matiello M, Kim HJ, Kim W, et al. Familial neuromyelitis optica. Neurology. 2010; 75(4):310–315

[249] Weinshenker BG. Neuromyelitis optica is distinct from multiple sclerosis. Arch Neurol. 2007; 64(6):899–901

[250] Weinshenker BG. Neuromyelitis optica: what it is and what it might be. Lancet. 2003; 361(9361):889–890

[251] Correale J, Fiol M. Activation of humoral immunity and eosinophils in neuromyelitis optica. Neurology. 2004; 63(12):2363–2370

[252] Lucchinetti CF, Mandler RN, McGavern D, et al. A role for humoral mechanisms in the pathogenesis of Devic's neuromyelitis optica. Brain. 2002; 125(Pt 7):1450–1461

[253] Jarius S, Aboul-Enein F, Waters P, et al. Antibody to aquaporin-4 in the long-term course of neuromyelitis optica. Brain. 2008; 131(Pt 11):3072–3080

[254] Jiao Y, Fryer JP, Lennon VA, et al. Aquaporin 4 IgG serostatus and outcome in recurrent longitudinally extensive transverse myelitis. JAMA Neurol. 2014; 71(1):48–54

[255] Misu T, Fujihara K, Kakita A, et al. Loss of aquaporin 4 in lesions of neuromyelitis optica: distinction from multiple sclerosis. Brain. 2007; 130 (Pt 5):1224–1234

[256] Popescu BFG, Guo Y, Jentoft ME, et al. Diagnostic utility of aquaporin-4 in the analysis of active demyelinating lesions. Neurology. 2015; 84(2): 148–158

[257] Takahashi T, Fujihara K, Nakashima I, et al. Anti-aquaporin-4 antibody is involved in the pathogenesis of NMO: a study on antibody titre. Brain. 2007; 130(Pt 5):1235–1243

[258] Yanagawa K, Kawachi I, Toyoshima Y, et al. Pathologic and immunologic profiles of a limited form of neuromyelitis optica with myelitis. Neurology. 2009; 73(20):1628–1637

[259] Almekhlafi MA, Clark AW, Lucchinetti CF, Zhang Y, Power C, Bell RB. Neuromyelitis optica with extensive active brain involvement: an autopsy study. Arch Neurol. 2011; 68(4):508–512

[260] Takano R, Misu T, Takahashi T, Sato S, Fujihara K, Itoyama Y. Astrocytic damage is far more severe than demyelination in NMO: a clinical CSF biomarker study. Neurology. 2010; 75(3):208–216

[261] Miyazawa I, Nakashima I, Petzold A, Fujihara K, Sato S, Itoyama Y. High CSF neurofilament heavy chain levels in neuromyelitis optica. Neurology. 2007; 68(11):865–867

[262] Uzawa A, Mori M, Masuda S, Kuwabara S. Markedly elevated soluble intercellular adhesion molecule 1, soluble vascular cell adhesion molecule 1 levels, and blood-brain barrier breakdown in neuromyelitis optica. Arch Neurol. 2011; 68(7):913–917

[263] Vincent T, Saikali P, Cayrol R, et al. Functional consequences of neuromyelitis optica-IgG astrocyte interactions on blood-brain barrier permeability and granulocyte recruitment. J Immunol. 2008; 181(8):5730–5737

[264] Graves J, Grandhe S, Weinfurtner K, et al. US Network of Pediatric Multiple Sclerosis Centers. Protective environmental factors for neuromyelitis optica. Neurology. 2014; 83(21):1923–1929

[265] Lotze TE, Northrop JL, Hutton GJ, Ross B, Schiffman JS, Hunter JV. Spectrum of pediatric neuromyelitis optica. Pediatrics. 2008; 122(5):e1039–e1047

[266] Rocca MA, Agosta F, Mezzapesa DM, et al. Magnetization transfer and diffusion tensor MRI show gray matter damage in neuromyelitis optica. Neurology. 2004; 62(3):476–478

[267] Yu C, Lin F, Li K, et al. Pathogenesis of normal-appearing white matter damage in neuromyelitis optica: diffusion-tensor MR imaging. Radiology. 2008; 246(1):222–228

[268] Yu CS, Zhu CZ, Li KC, et al. Relapsing neuromyelitis optica and relapsing-remitting multiple sclerosis: differentiation at diffusion-tensor MR imaging of corpus callosum. Radiology. 2007; 244(1):249–256

[269] Calabrese M, Oh MS, Favaretto A, et al. No MRI evidence of cortical lesions in neuromyelitis optica. Neurology. 2012; 79(16):1671–1676

[270] Liu Y, Wang J, Daams M, et al. Differential patterns of spinal cord and brain atrophy in NMO and MS. Neurology. 2015; 84(14):1465–1472

[271] Popescu BFG, Parisi JE, Cabrera-Gómez JA, et al. Absence of cortical demyelination in neuromyelitis optica. Neurology. 2010; 75(23):2103–2109

[272] Liu Y, Fu Y, Schoonheim MM, et al. Structural MRI substrates of cognitive impairment in neuromyelitis optica. Neurology. 2015; 85(17):1491–1499

[273] Kim HJ, Paul F, Lana-Peixoto MA, et al. Guthy-Jackson Charitable Foundation NMO International Clinical Consortium & Biorepository. MRI characteristics of neuromyelitis optica spectrum disorder: an international update. Neurology. 2015; 84(11):1165–1173

[274] Kremer S, Renard F, Achard S, et al. Guthy-Jackson Charitable Foundation (GJCF) Neuromyelitis Optica (NMO) International Clinical Consortium and Biorepository. Use of advanced magnetic resonance imaging techniques in neuromyelitis optica spectrum disorder. JAMA Neurol. 2015; 72(7):815–822

[275] Matthews L, Marasco R, Jenkinson M, et al. Distinction of seropositive NMO spectrum disorder and MS brain lesion distribution. Neurology. 2013; 80 (14):1330–1337

[276] Sinnecker T, Dörr J, Pfueller CF, et al. Distinct lesion morphology at 7-T MRI differentiates neuromyelitis optica from multiple sclerosis. Neurology. 2012; 79(7):708–714

[277] de Seze J, Blanc F, Jeanjean L, et al. Optical coherence tomography in neuromyelitis optica. Arch Neurol. 2008; 65(7):920–923

[278] Gelfand JM, Cree BA, Nolan R, Arnow S, Green AJ. Microcystic inner nuclear layer abnormalities and neuromyelitis optica. JAMA Neurol. 2013; 70(5): 629–633

[279] Sotirchos ES, Saidha S, Byraiah G, et al. In vivo identification of morphologic retinal abnormalities in neuromyelitis optica. Neurology. 2013; 80(15): 1406–1414

[280] Naismith RT, Tutlam NT, Xu J, et al. Optical coherence tomography differs in neuromyelitis optica compared with multiple sclerosis. Neurology. 2009; 72 (12):1077–1082

[281] Ratchford JN, Quigg ME, Conger A, et al. Optical coherence tomography helps differentiate neuromyelitis optica and MS optic neuropathies. Neurology. 2009; 73(4):302–308

[282] Schreiber AL, Fried GW, Formal CS, DeSouza BX. Rehabilitation of neuromyelitis optica (Devic syndrome): three case reports. Am J Phys Med Rehabil. 2008; 87(2):144–148

[283] Scott TF, Kassab SL, Pittock SJ. Neuromyelitis optica IgG status in acute partial transverse myelitis. Arch Neurol. 2006; 63(10):1398–1400

[284] Kim SM, Go MJ, Sung JJ, Park KS, Lee KW. Painful tonic spasm in neuromyelitis optica: incidence, diagnostic utility, and clinical characteristics. Arch Neurol. 2012; 69(8):1026–1031

[285] Usmani N, Bedi G, Lam BL, Sheremata WA. Association between paroxysmal tonic spasms and neuromyelitis optica. Arch Neurol. 2012; 69(1):121–124

[286] Kanamori Y, Nakashima I, Takai Y, et al. Pain in neuromyelitis optica and its effect on quality of life: a cross-sectional study. Neurology. 2011; 77(7):652–658

[287] Qian P, Lancia S, Alvarez E, Klawiter EC, Cross AH, Naismith RT. Association of neuromyelitis optica with severe and intractable pain. Arch Neurol. 2012; 69(11):1482–1487

[288] Wingerchuk DM, Weinshenker BG. Neuromyelitis optica: clinical predictors of a relapsing course and survival. Neurology. 2003; 60(5):848–853

[289] Antoine JC, Camdessanché JP, Absi L, Lassablière F, Féasson L. Devic disease and thymoma with anti-central nervous system and antithymus antibodies. Neurology. 2004; 62(6):978–980

[290] Figueroa M, Guo Y, Tselis A, et al. Paraneoplastic neuromyelitis optica spectrum disorder associated with metastatic carcinoid expressing aquaporin-4. JAMA Neurol. 2014; 71(4):495–498

[291] Menge T, Cree B, Saleh A, et al. Neuromyelitis optica following human papillomavirus vaccination. Neurology. 2012; 79(3):285–287

[292] Pittock SJ, Lennon VA. Aquaporin-4 autoantibodies in a paraneoplastic context. Arch Neurol. 2008; 65(5):629–632

[293] Asgari N, Henriksen TB, Petersen T, Lillevang ST, Weinshenker BG. Pregnancy outcomes in a woman with neuromyelitis optica. Neurology. 2014; 83(17): 1576–1577

[294] Bourre B, Marignier R, Zéphir H, et al. NOMADMUS Study Group. Neuromyelitis optica and pregnancy. Neurology. 2012; 78(12):875–879

[295] Kim W, Kim SH, Nakashima I, et al. Influence of pregnancy on neuromyelitis optica spectrum disorder. Neurology. 2012; 78(16):1264–1267

[296] Saadoun S, Waters P, Leite MI, Bennett JL, Vincent A, Papadopoulos MC. Neuromyelitis optica IgG causes placental inflammation and fetal death. J Immunol. 2013; 191(6):2999–3005

[297] George JS, Leite MI, Kitley JL, et al. Opportunistic infections of the retina in patients with aquaporin-4 antibody disease. JAMA Neurol. 2014; 71(11): 1429–1432 h

[298] Iorio R, Lucchinetti C, Lennon V, et al. Syndrome of inappropriate antidiuresis may herald or accompany neuromyelitis optica (P07.064). Neurology. 2011; 77(17):1644–1646

[299] Suzuki N, Takahashi T, Aoki M, et al. Neuromyelitis optica preceded by hyperCKemia episode. Neurology. 2010; 74(19):1543–1545

[300] Okada S, Takarabe S, Nogawa S, et al. Persistent hiccups followed by cardiorespiratory arrest. Lancet. 2012; 380(9851):1444

[301] Riphagen J, Modderman P, Verrips A. Hiccups, nausea, and vomiting: water channels under attack! Lancet. 2010; 375(9718):954

[302] Popescu BFG, Lennon VA, Parisi JE, et al. Neuromyelitis optica unique area postrema lesions: nausea, vomiting, and pathogenic implications. Neurology. 2011; 76(14):1229–1237

[303] Rison RA, Berkovich R. Teaching NeuroImages: hiccoughs and vomiting in neuromyelitis optica. Neurology. 2010; 75(17):e70

[304] Costa C, Arrambide G, Tintore M, et al. Value of NMO-IgG determination at the time of presentation as CIS. Neurology. 2012; 78(20):1608–1611

[305] Jarius S, Franciotta D, Bergamaschi R, et al. NMO-IgG in the diagnosis of neuromyelitis optica. Neurology. 2007; 68(13):1076–1077

[306] Jiao Y, Fryer JP, Lennon VA, et al. Updated estimate of AQP4-IgG serostatus and disability outcome in neuromyelitis optica. Neurology. 2013; 81(14):1197–1204

[307] Klawiter EC, Alvarez E, III, Xu J, et al. NMO-IgG detected in CSF in seronegative neuromyelitis optica. Neurology. 2009; 72(12):1101–1103

[308] Lennon VA, Wingerchuk DM, Kryzer TJ, et al. A serum autoantibody marker of neuromyelitis optica: distinction from multiple sclerosis. Lancet. 2004; 364(9451):2106–2112

[309] Magaña SM, Pittock SJ, Lennon VA, Keegan BM, Weinshenker BG, Lucchinetti CF. Neuromyelitis optica IgG serostatus in fulminant central nervous system inflammatory demyelinating disease. Arch Neurol. 2009; 66(8):964–966

[310] Matiello M, Schaefer-Klein J, Sun D, Weinshenker BG. Aquaporin 4 expression and tissue susceptibility to neuromyelitis optica. JAMA Neurol. 2013; 70(9):1118–1125

[311] Matiello M, Schaefer-Klein JL, Hebrink DD, Kingsbury DJ, Atkinson EJ, Weinshenker BG, NMO, Genetics Collaborators. Genetic analysis of aquaporin-4 in neuromyelitis optica. Neurology. 2011; 77(12):1149–1155

[312] McKeon A, Fryer JP, Apiwattanakul M, et al. Diagnosis of neuromyelitis spectrum disorders: comparative sensitivities and specificities of immunohistochemical and immunoprecipitation assays. Arch Neurol. 2009; 66(9):1134–1138

[313] Nishiyama S, Ito T, Misu T, et al. A case of NMO seropositive for aquaporin-4 antibody more than 10 years before onset. Neurology. 2009; 72(22):1960–1961

[314] Pittock SJ, Lennon VA, Bakshi N, et al. Seroprevalence of aquaporin-4-IgG in a northern California population representative cohort of multiple sclerosis. JAMA Neurol. 2014; 71(11):1433–1436

[315] Siritho S, Nakashima I, Takahashi T, Fujihara K, Prayoonwiwat N. AQP4 antibody-positive Thai cases: clinical features and diagnostic problems. Neurology. 2011; 77(9):827–834

[316] Waters P, Jarius S, Littleton E, et al. Aquaporin-4 antibodies in neuromyelitis optica and longitudinally extensive transverse myelitis. Arch Neurol. 2008; 65(7):913–919

[317] Kitley J, Waters P, Woodhall M, et al. Neuromyelitis optica spectrum disorders with aquaporin-4 and myelin-oligodendrocyte glycoprotein antibodies: a comparative study. JAMA Neurol. 2014; 71(3):276–283

[318] Kitley J, Woodhall M, Waters P, et al. Myelin-oligodendrocyte glycoprotein antibodies in adults with a neuromyelitis optica phenotype. Neurology. 2012; 79(12):1273–1277

[319] Sato DK, Callegaro D, Lana-Peixoto MA, et al. Distinction between MOG antibody-positive and AQP4 antibody-positive NMO spectrum disorders. Neurology. 2014; 82(6):474–481

[320] Rostasy K, Mader S, Schanda K, et al. Anti-myelin oligodendrocyte glycoprotein antibodies in pediatric patients with optic neuritis. Arch Neurol. 2012; 69(6):752–756

[321] Franciotta D, Jarius S, Aloisi F. More on multiple sclerosis and neuromyelitis optica. Arch Neurol. 2007; 64(12):1802–, author reply 1802–1803

[322] Nakashima I, Fujihara K, Fujimori J, Narikawa K, Misu T, Itoyama Y. Absence of IgG1 response in the cerebrospinal fluid of relapsing neuromyelitis optica. Neurology. 2004; 62(1):144–146

[323] Cree BAC, Lamb S, Morgan K, Chen A, Waubant E, Genain C. An open label study of the effects of rituximab in neuromyelitis optica. Neurology. 2005; 64(7):1270–1272

[324] Jacob A, Weinshenker BG, Violich I, et al. Treatment of neuromyelitis optica with rituximab: retrospective analysis of 25 patients. Arch Neurol. 2008; 65(11):1443–1448

[325] Falcini F, Trapani S, Ricci L, Resti M, Simonini G, de Martino M. Sustained improvement of a girl affected with Devic's disease over 2 years of

mycophenolate mofetil treatment. Rheumatology (Oxford). 2006; 45(7):913–915

[326] Huh S-Y, Kim S-H, Hyun J-W, et al. Mycophenolate mofetil in the treatment of neuromyelitis optica spectrum disorder. JAMA Neurol. 2014; 71(11):1372–1378

[327] Jacob A, Matiello M, Weinshenker BG, et al. Treatment of neuromyelitis optica with mycophenolate mofetil: retrospective analysis of 24 patients. Arch Neurol. 2009; 66(9):1128–1133

[328] Ayzenberg I, Kleiter I, Schröder A, et al. Interleukin 6 receptor blockade in patients with neuromyelitis optica nonresponsive to anti-CD20 therapy. JAMA Neurol. 2013; 70(3):394–397

[329] Araki M, Matsuoka T, Miyamoto K, et al. Efficacy of the anti-IL-6 receptor antibody tocilizumab in neuromyelitis optica: a pilot study. Neurology. 2014; 82(15):1302–1306

[330] Bichuetti DB, Lobato de Oliveira EM, Oliveira DM, Amorin de Souza N, Gabbai AA. Neuromyelitis optica treatment: analysis of 36 patients. Arch Neurol 2010;67:1131–1136

[331] Costanzi C, Matiello M, Lucchinetti CF, et al. Azathioprine: tolerability, efficacy, and predictors of benefit in neuromyelitis optica. Neurology. 2011; 77:659–666

[332] Kieseier BC, Stüve O, Dehmel T, et al. Disease amelioration with tocilizumab in a treatment-resistant patient with neuromyelitis optica: implication for cellular immune responses. JAMA Neurol. 2013; 70(3):390–393

[333] Kim SH, Jeong IH, Hyun JW, et al. Treatment outcomes with rituximab in 100 patients with neuromyelitis optica: influence of FCGR3A polymorphisms on the therapeutic response to rituximab. JAMA Neurol. 2015; 72(9):989–995

[334] Kim SH, Huh SY, Lee SJ, Joung A, Kim HJ. A 5-year follow-up of rituximab treatment in patients with neuromyelitis optica spectrum disorder. JAMA Neurol. 2013; 70(9):1110–1117

[335] Kim SH, Kim W, Li XF, Jung IJ, Kim HJ. Repeated treatment with rituximab based on the assessment of peripheral circulating memory B cells in patients with relapsing neuromyelitis optica over 2 years. Arch Neurol. 2011; 68(11):1412–1420

[336] Kim SH, Kim W, Park MS, Sohn EH, Li XF, Kim HJ. Efficacy and safety of mitoxantrone in patients with highly relapsing neuromyelitis optica. Arch Neurol. 2011; 68(4):473–479

[337] McKeon A, Pittock S. Individualized rituximab treatment for neuromyelitis Optica spectrum disorders. JAMA Neurol. 2013; 70(9):1103–1104

[338] Mealy MA, Wingerchuk DM, Palace J, Greenberg BM, Levy M. Comparison of relapse and treatment failure rates among patients with neuromyelitis optica: multicenter study of treatment efficacy. JAMA Neurol. 2014; 71(3):324–330

[339] Pellkofer HL, Krumbholz M, Berthele A, et al. Long-term follow-up of patients with neuromyelitis optica after repeated therapy with rituximab. Neurology. 2011; 76(15):1310–1315

[340] Ringelstein M, Ayzenberg I, Harmel J, et al. Long-term therapy with interleukin 6 receptor blockade in highly active neuromyelitis optica spectrum disorder. JAMA Neurol. 2015; 72(7):756–763

[341] Yang CS, Yang L, Li T, et al. Responsiveness to reduced dosage of rituximab in Chinese patients with neuromyelitis optica. Neurology. 2013; 81(8):710–713

[342] Trebst C, Jarius S, Berthele A, et al. Neuromyelitis Optica Study Group (NEMOS). Update on the diagnosis and treatment of neuromyelitis optica: recommendations of the Neuromyelitis Optica Study Group (NEMOS). J Neurol. 2014; 261(1):1–16

[343] Merle H, Olindo S, Jeannin S, et al. Treatment of optic neuritis by plasma exchange (add-on) in neuromyelitis optica. Arch Ophthalmol. 2012; 130(7):858–862

[344] Absoud M, Cummins C, Desai N, et al. Childhood optic neuritis clinical features and outcome. Arch Dis Child. 2011; 96(9):860–862

[345] Wan MJ, Adebona O, Benson LA, Gorman MP, Heidary G. Visual outcomes in pediatric optic neuritis. Am J Ophthalmol. 2014; 158(3):503–7.e2

[346] Brady KM, Brar AS, Lee AG, Coats DK, Paysse EA, Steinkuller PG. Optic neuritis in children: clinical features and visual outcome. J AAPOS. 1999; 3(2):98–103

[347] Malik MT, Healy BC, Benson LA, et al. Factors associated with recovery from acute optic neuritis in patients with multiple sclerosis. Neurology. 2014; 82(24):2173–2179

[348] Bonhomme GR, Waldman AT, Balcer LJ, et al. Pediatric optic neuritis: brain MRI abnormalities and risk of multiple sclerosis. Neurology. 2009; 72(10):881–885

[349] Boiko AN, Guseva ME, Guseva MR, et al. Clinico-immunogenetic characteristics of multiple sclerosis with optic neuritis in children. J Neurovirol. 2000; 6 Suppl 2:S152–S155

[350] Wilejto M, Shroff M, Buncic JR, et al. The clinical features, MRI findings, and outcome of optic neuritis in children–Figure E1. Neurology. 2006; 67:8–12

[351] Ma SL, Shea JA, Galetta SL, et al. Self-reported visual dysfunction in multiple sclerosis: new data from the VFQ-25 and development of an MS-specific vision questionnaire. Am J Ophthalmol. 2002; 133(5):686–692

[352] Noble J, Forooghian F, Sproule M, Westall C, O'Connor P. Utility of the National Eye Institute VFQ-25 questionnaire in a heterogeneous group of multiple sclerosis patients. Am J Ophthalmol. 2006; 142(3):464–468

[353] Raphael BA, Galetta KM, Jacobs DA, et al. Validation and test characteristics of a 10-item neuro-ophthalmic supplement to the NEI-VFQ-25. Am J Ophthalmol. 2006; 142(6):1026–1035

[354] Balcer LJ, Miller DH, Reingold SC, Cohen JA. Vision and vision-related outcome measures in multiple sclerosis. Brain. 2015; 138(Pt 1):11–27

[355] Beck RW, Gal RL, Bhatti MT, et al. Optic Neuritis Study Group. Visual function more than 10 years after optic neuritis: experience of the optic neuritis treatment trial. Am J Ophthalmol. 2004; 137(1):77–83

[356] Beck RW. The optic neuritis treatment trial: three-year follow-up results. Arch Ophthalmol. 1995; 113(2):136–137

[357] Beck RW, Gal RL. Treatment of acute optic neuritis: a summary of findings from the optic neuritis treatment trial. Arch Ophthalmol. 2008; 126(7):994–995

[358] Optic Neuritis Study Group. The 5-year risk of MS after optic neuritis. Experience of the optic neuritis treatment trial. Neurology. 1997; 49(5):1404–1413

[359] Jacobs L, Munschauer FE, Kaba SE. Clinical and magnetic resonance in optic neuritis. Neurology. 1991; 41(1):15–19

[360] Baumhefner RW, Tourtellotte WW, Syndulko K, et al. Quantitative multiple sclerosis plaque assessment with magnetic resonance imaging. Its correlation with clinical parameters, evoked potentials, and intra-blood-brain barrier IgG synthesis. Arch Neurol. 1990; 47(1):19–26

[361] Christiansen P, Frederiksen JL, Henriksen O, Larsson HB. Gd-DTPA-enhanced lesions in the brain of patients with acute optic neuritis. Acta Neurol Scand. 1992; 85(2):141–146

[362] Feinstein A, Youl B, Ron M. Acute optic neuritis. A cognitive and magnetic resonance imaging study. Brain. 1992; 115(Pt 5):1403–1415

[363] Francis GS, Evans AC, Arnold DL. Neuroimaging in multiple sclerosis. Neurol Clin. 1995; 13(1):147–171

[364] Morrissey SP, Miller DH, Kendall BE, et al. The significance of brain magnetic resonance imaging abnormalities at presentation with clinically isolated syndromes suggestive of multiple sclerosis. A 5-year follow-up study. Brain. 1993; 116(Pt 1):135–146

[365] Mullins ME. Emergent neuroimaging of intracranial infection/inflammation. Radiol Clin North Am. 2011; 49(1):47–62

[366] Merandi SF, Kudryk BT, Murtagh FR, Arrington JA. Contrast-enhanced MR imaging of optic nerve lesions in patients with acute optic neuritis. AJNR Am J Neuroradiol. 1991; 12(5):923–926

[367] Guy J, Mancuso A, Quisling RG, Beck R, Moster M. Gadolinium-DTPA-enhanced magnetic resonance imaging in optic neuropathies. Ophthalmology. 1990; 97(5):592–599, discussion 599–600

[368] Thompson AJ, Kermode AG, MacManus DG, et al. Patterns of disease activity in multiple sclerosis: clinical and magnetic resonance imaging study. BMJ. 1990; 300(6725):631–634

[369] Swanton JK, Fernando KT, Dalton CM, et al. Early MRI in optic neuritis: the risk for disability. Neurology. 2009; 72(6):542–550

[370] Brex PA, Ciccarelli O, O'Riordan JI, Sailer M, Thompson AJ, Miller DH. A longitudinal study of abnormalities on MRI and disability from multiple sclerosis. N Engl J Med. 2002; 346(3):158–164

[371] Paty DW, Oger JJ, Kastrukoff LF, et al. MRI in the diagnosis of MS: a prospective study with comparison of clinical evaluation, evoked potentials, oligoclonal banding, and CT. Neurology. 1988; 38(2):180–185

[372] Frederiksen JL, Larsson HB, Olesen J. Correlation of magnetic resonance imaging and CSF findings in patients with acute monosymptomatic optic neuritis. Acta Neurol Scand. 1992; 86(3):317–322

[373] Jacobs LD, Kaba SE, Miller CM, Priore RL, Brownscheidle CM. Correlation of clinical, magnetic resonance imaging, and cerebrospinal fluid findings in optic neuritis. Ann Neurol. 1997; 41(3):392–398

[374] Söderström M, Ya-Ping J, Hillert J, Link H. Optic neuritis: prognosis for multiple sclerosis from MRI, CSF, and HLA findings. Neurology. 1998; 50(3):708–714

[375] Guy J, Mancuso A, Quisling R. The role of magnetic resonance imaging in optic neuritis. Ophthalmol Clin North Am. 1994; 7:449–458

[376] Paty DW, Li DK, UBC MS/MRI Study Group and the IFNB Multiple Sclerosis Study Group. Interferon beta-1b is effective in relapsing-remitting multiple sclerosis. II. MRI analysis results of a multicenter, randomized, double-blind, placebo-controlled trial. Neurology. 1993; 43(4):662–667

[377] Audoin B, Fernando KTM, Swanton JK, Thompson AJ, Plant GT, Miller DH. Selective magnetization transfer ratio decrease in the visual cortex following optic neuritis. Brain. 2006; 129(Pt 4):1031–1039

[378] Hickman SJ, Toosy AT, Jones SJ, et al. Serial magnetization transfer imaging in acute optic neuritis. Brain. 2004; 127(Pt 3):692–700

[379] Inglese M, Ghezzi A, Bianchi S, et al. Irreversible disability and tissue loss in multiple sclerosis: a conventional and magnetization transfer magnetic resonance imaging study of the optic nerves. Arch Neurol. 2002; 59(2):250–255

[380] Rovaris M, Gallo A, Riva R, et al. An MT MRI study of the cervical cord in clinically isolated syndromes suggestive of MS. Neurology. 2004; 63(3):584–585

[381] Optic Neuritis Study Group. Long-term brain magnetic resonance imaging changes after optic neuritis in patients without clinically definite multiple sclerosis. Arch Neurol. 2004; 61(10):1538–1541

[382] Cornblath WT, Quint DJ. MRI of optic nerve enlargement in optic neuritis. Neurology. 1997; 48(4):821–825

[383] Dunker S, Wiegand W. Prognostic value of magnetic resonance imaging in monosymptomatic optic neuritis. Ophthalmology. 1996; 103(11):1768–1773

[384] Li M, Li J, He H, et al. Directional diffusivity changes in the optic nerve and optic radiation in optic neuritis. Br J Radiol. 2011; 84(1000):304–314

[385] Hickman SJ, Toosy AT, Jones SJ, et al. A serial MRI study following optic nerve mean area in acute optic neuritis. Brain. 2004; 127(Pt 11):2498–2505

[386] Yeh EA, Marrie RA, Reginald YA, et al. Canadian Pediatric Demyelinating Disease Network. Functional-structural correlations in the afferent visual pathway in pediatric demyelination. Neurology. 2014; 83(23):2147–2152

[387] Fuglø D, Kallenbach K, Tsakiri A, et al. Retinal atrophy correlates with fMRI response in patients with recovered optic neuritis. Neurology. 2011; 77(7):645–651

[388] Gallo A, Esposito F, Sacco R, et al. Visual resting-state network in relapsing-remitting MS with and without previous optic neuritis. Neurology. 2012; 79(14):1458–1465

[389] Kallenbach K, Simonsen H, Sander B, et al. Retinal nerve fiber layer thickness is associated with lesion length in acute optic neuritis. Neurology. 2010; 74(3):252–258

[390] Pulicken M, Gordon-Lipkin E, Balcer LJ, Frohman E, Cutter G, Calabresi PA. Optical coherence tomography and disease subtype in multiple sclerosis. Neurology. 2007; 69(22):2085–2092

[391] Syc SB, Saidha S, Newsome SD, et al. Optical coherence tomography segmentation reveals ganglion cell layer pathology after optic neuritis. Brain. 2012; 135(Pt 2):521–533

[392] Zaveri MS, Conger A, Salter A, et al. Retinal imaging by laser polarimetry and optical coherence tomography evidence of axonal degeneration in multiple sclerosis. Arch Neurol. 2008; 65(7):924–928

[393] Burkholder BM, Osborne B, Loguidice MJ, et al. Macular volume determined by optical coherence tomography as a measure of neuronal loss in multiple sclerosis. Arch Neurol. 2009; 66(11):1366–1372

[394] Costello F, Hodge W, Pan YI, et al. Sex-specific differences in retinal nerve fiber layer thinning after acute optic neuritis. Neurology. 2012; 79(18):1866–1872

[395] Sepulcre J, Murie-Fernandez M, Salinas-Alaman A, García-Layana A, Bejarano B, Villoslada P. Diagnostic accuracy of retinal abnormalities in predicting disease activity in MS. Neurology. 2007; 68(18):1488–1494

[396] Naismith RT, Tutlam NT, Xu J, et al. Optical coherence tomography is less sensitive than visual evoked potentials in optic neuritis. Neurology. 2009; 73(1):46–52

[397] Outteryck O, Zephir H, Defoort S, et al. Optical coherence tomography in clinically isolated syndrome: no evidence of subclinical retinal axonal loss. Arch Neurol. 2009; 66(11):1373–1377

[398] Karaali K, Senol U, Aydin H, Cevikol C, Apaydin A, Lüleci E. Optic neuritis: evaluation with orbital Doppler sonography. Radiology. 2003; 226(2):355–358

[399] Miki A, Nakajima T, Takagi M, et al. Near-infrared spectroscopy of the visual cortex in unilateral optic neuritis. Am J Ophthalmol. 2005; 139(2):353–356

[400] Miller DH, Altmann DR, Chard DT. Advances in imaging to support the development of novel therapies for multiple sclerosis. Clin Pharmacol Ther. 2012; 91(4):621–634

[401] Naismith RT, Xu J, Tutlam NT, et al. Diffusion tensor imaging in acute optic neuropathies: predictor of clinical outcomes. Arch Neurol. 2012; 69(1):65–71

[402] Naismith RT, Xu J, Tutlam NT, Trinkaus K, Cross AH, Song SK. Radial diffusivity in remote optic neuritis discriminates visual outcomes. Neurology. 2010; 74(21):1702–1710

[403] Naismith RT, Xu J, Tutlam NT, et al. Disability in optic neuritis correlates with diffusion tensor-derived directional diffusivities. Neurology. 2009; 72 (7):589–594

[404] Long Y, Chen M, Zhang B, et al. Brain gadolinium enhancement along the ventricular and leptomeningeal regions in patients with aquaporin-4 antibodies in cerebral spinal fluid. J Neuroimmunol. 2014; 269(1–2):62–67

[405] Cole SR, Beck RW, Moke PS, Kaufman DI, Tourtellotte WW, Optic Neuritis Study Group. The predictive value of CSF oligoclonal banding for MS 5 years after optic neuritis. Neurology. 1998; 51(3):885–887

[406] Sellebjerg FT, Frederiksen JL, Olsson T. Anti-myelin basic protein and anti-proteolipid protein antibody-secreting cells in the cerebrospinal fluid of patients with acute optic neuritis. Arch Neurol. 1994; 51(10):1032–1036

[407] Sellebjerg F, Madsen HO, Frederiksen JL, Ryder LP, Svejgaard A. Acute optic neuritis: myelin basic protein and proteolipid protein antibodies, affinity, and the HLA system. Ann Neurol. 1995; 38(6):943–950

[408] Simon JH, McDonald WI. Assessment of optic nerve damage in multiple sclerosis using magnetic resonance imaging. J Neurol Sci. 2000; 172 Suppl 1: S23–S26

[409] Söderström M, Link H, Xu Z, Fredriksson S. Optic neuritis and multiple sclerosis: anti-MBP and anti-MBP peptide antibody-secreting cells are accumulated in CSF. Neurology. 1993; 43(6):1215–1222

[410] Warren KG, Catz I, Johnson E, Mielke B. Anti-myelin basic protein and anti-proteolipid protein specific forms of multiple sclerosis. Ann Neurol. 1994; 35(3):280–289

[411] Sandberg-Wollheim M. Optic neuritis: studies on the cerebrospinal fluid in relation to clinical course in 61 patients. Acta Neurol Scand. 1975; 52(3): 167–178

[412] Balcer LJ. Clinical practice. Optic neuritis. N Engl J Med. 2006; 354(12): 1273–1280

[413] Sisto D, Trojano M, Vetrugno M, Trabucco T, Iliceto G, Sborgia C. Subclinical visual involvement in multiple sclerosis: a study by MRI, VEPs, frequency-doubling perimetry, standard perimetry, and contrast sensitivity. Invest Ophthalmol Vis Sci. 2005; 46(4):1264–1268

[414] Fraser C, Klistorner A, Graham S, Garrick R, Billson F, Grigg J. Multifocal visual evoked potential latency analysis: predicting progression to multiple sclerosis. Arch Neurol. 2006; 63(6):847–850

[415] Rinalduzzi S, Brusa A, Jones SJ. Variation of visual evoked potential delay to stimulation of central, nasal, and temporal regions of the macula in optic neuritis. J Neurol Neurosurg Psychiatry. 2001; 70(1):28–35

[416] Ashworth B, Aspinall PA, Mitchell JD. Visual function in multiple sclerosis. Doc Ophthalmol. 1989; 73(3):209–224

[417] Brusa A, Jones SJ, Kapoor R, Miller DH, Plant GT. Long-term recovery and fellow eye deterioration after optic neuritis, determined by serial visual evoked potentials. J Neurol. 1999; 246(9):776–782

[418] Fotiou F, Koutlas E, Tsorlinis I, et al. The value of neurophysiological and MRI assessment in demyelinating optic neuritis (DON). Electromyogr Clin Neurophysiol. 1999; 39(7):397–404

[419] Frederiksen JL, Petrera J. Serial visual evoked potentials in 90 untreated patients with acute optic neuritis. Surv Ophthalmol. 1999; 44 Suppl 1:S54–S62

[420] Fuhr P, Borggrefe-Chappuis A, Schindler C, Kappos L. Visual and motor evoked potentials in the course of multiple sclerosis. Brain. 2001; 124(Pt 11):2162–2168

[421] Honan WP, Heron JR, Foster DH, Edgar GK, Scase MO, Collins MF. Visual loss in multiple sclerosis and its relation to previous optic neuritis, disease duration and clinical classification. Brain. 1990; 113(Pt 4):975–987

[422] Frohman AR, Schnurman Z, Conger A, et al. Multifocal visual evoked potentials are influenced by variable contrast stimulation in MS. Neurology. 2012; 79(8):797–801

[423] Raz N, Chokron S, Ben-Hur T, Levin N. Temporal reorganization to overcome monocular demyelination. Neurology. 2013; 81(8):702–709

[424] Frohman EM, Costello F, Stüve O, et al. Modeling axonal degeneration within the anterior visual system: implications for demonstrating neuroprotection in multiple sclerosis. Arch Neurol. 2008; 65(1):26–35

[425] Celesia GG, Kaufman DI, Brigell M, et al. Optic neuritis: a prospective study. Neurology. 1990; 40(6):919–923

[426] Lessell S. Corticosteroid treatment of acute optic neuritis. N Engl J Med. 1992; 326(9):634–635

[427] Sellebjerg F, Nielsen HS, Frederiksen JL, Olesen J. A randomized, controlled trial of oral high-dose methylprednisolone in acute optic neuritis. Neurology. 1999; 52(7):1479–1484

[428] Silberberg DH. Corticosteroids and optic neuritis. N Engl J Med. 1993; 329 (24):1808–1810

[429] Kapoor R, Miller DH, Jones SJ, et al. Effects of intravenous methylprednisolone on outcome in MRI-based prognostic subgroups in acute optic neuritis. Neurology. 1998; 50(1):230–237

[430] Sellebjerg F, Christiansen M, Jensen J, Frederiksen JL. Immunological effects of oral high-dose methylprednisolone in acute optic neuritis and multiple sclerosis. Eur J Neurol. 2000; 7(3):281–289

[431] Barkhof F, Frequin ST, Hommes OR, et al. A correlative triad of gadolinium-DTPA MRI, EDSS, and CSF-MBP in relapsing multiple sclerosis patients treated with high-dose intravenous methylprednisolone. Neurology. 1992; 42(1):63–67

[432] Barkhof F, Hommes OR, Scheltens P, Valk J. Quantitative MRI changes in gadolinium-DTPA enhancement after high-dose intravenous methyl-prednisolone in multiple sclerosis. Neurology. 1991; 41(8):1219–1222

[433] Rose AS, Kuzma JW, Kurtzke JF, Namerow NS, Sibley WA, Tourtellotte WW. Cooperative study in the evaluation of therapy in multiple sclerosis. ACTH vs. placebo: final report. Neurology. 1970; 20(5):1–59

[434] Bowden AN, Bowden PM, Friedmann AI, Perkin GD, Rose FC. A trial of corticotrophin gelatin injection in acute optic neuritis. J Neurol Neurosurg Psychiatry. 1974; 37(8):869–873

[435] Gould ES, Bird AC, Leaver PK, McDonald WI. Treatment of optic neuritis by retrobulbar injection of triamcinolone. BMJ. 1977; 1(6075):1495–1497

[436] Wakakura M, Mashimo K, Oono S, et al. Optic Neuritis Treatment Trial Multicenter Cooperative Research Group (ONMRG). Multicenter clinical trial for evaluating methylprednisolone pulse treatment of idiopathic optic neuritis in Japan. Jpn J Ophthalmol. 1999; 43(2):133–138

[437] Beck RW, Trobe JD, Moke PS, et al. Optic Neuritis Study Group. High- and low-risk profiles for the development of multiple sclerosis within 10 years after optic neuritis: experience of the optic neuritis treatment trial. Arch Ophthalmol. 2003; 121(7):944–949

[438] Optic Neuritis Study Group. Multiple sclerosis risk after optic neuritis: final optic neuritis treatment trial follow-up. Arch Neurol. 2008; 65(6):727–732

[439] Moss HE, Gao W, Balcer LJ, Joslin CE. Association of race/ethnicity with visual outcomes following acute optic neuritis: an analysis of the Optic Neuritis Treatment Trial. JAMA Ophthalmol. 2014; 132(4):421–427

[440] Kaufman DI, Trobe JD, Eggenberger ER, Whitaker JN. Practice parameter: the role of corticosteroids in the management of acute monosymptomatic optic neuritis. Report of the Quality Standards Subcommittee of the American Academy of Neurology. Neurology. 2000; 54(11):2039–2044

[441] Beck RW, Cleary PA, Anderson MM, Jr, et al. The Optic Neuritis Study Group. A randomized, controlled trial of corticosteroids in the treatment of acute optic neuritis. N Engl J Med. 1992; 326(9):581–588

[442] Trobe JD. High-dose corticosteroid regimen retards development of multiple sclerosis in optic neuritis treatment trial. Arch Ophthalmol. 1994; 112(1):35–36

[443] Braksick SA, Cutsforth-Gregory JK, Black DF, Weinshenker BG, Pittock SJ, Kantarci OH. Teaching neuroimages: MRI in advanced neuromyelitis optica. Neurology. 2014; 82(12):e101–e102

[444] Palace J, Leite MI, Nairne A, Vincent A. Interferon Beta treatment in neuromyelitis optica: increase in relapses and aquaporin 4 antibody titers. Arch Neurol. 2010; 67(8):1016–1017

[445] CHAMPS Study Group. Interferon beta-1a for optic neuritis patients at high risk for multiple sclerosis. Am J Ophthalmol. 2001; 132(4):463–471

[446] Jacobs LD, Beck RW, Simon JH, et al. CHAMPS Study Group. Intramuscular interferon beta-1a therapy initiated during a first demyelinating event in multiple sclerosis. N Engl J Med. 2000; 343(13):898–904

[447] Comi G, Filippi M, Barkhof F, et al. Early Treatment of Multiple Sclerosis Study Group. Effect of early interferon treatment on conversion to definite multiple sclerosis: a randomised study. Lancet. 2001; 357(9268):1576–1582

[448] van Engelen BG, Hommes OR, Pinckers A, Cruysberg JR, Barkhof F, Rodriguez M. Improved vision after intravenous immunoglobulin in stable demyelinating optic neuritis. Ann Neurol. 1992; 32(6):834–835

[449] Noseworthy JH, O'Brien PC, Petterson TM, et al. A randomized trial of intravenous immunoglobulin in inflammatory demyelinating optic neuritis. Neurology. 2001; 56(11):1514–1522

[450] Roed HG, Langkilde A, Sellebjerg F, et al. A double-blind, randomized trial of IV immunoglobulin treatment in acute optic neuritis. Neurology. 2005; 64 (5):804–810

[451] Dalakas MC. Intravenous immunoglobulin in autoimmune neuromuscular diseases. JAMA. 2004; 291(19):2367–2375

[452] Ruprecht K, Klinker E, Dintelmann T, Rieckmann P, Gold R. Plasma exchange for severe optic neuritis: treatment of 10 patients. Neurology. 2004; 63(6): 1081–1083

[453] Llufriu S, Castillo J, Blanco Y, et al. Plasma exchange for acute attacks of CNS demyelination: predictors of improvement at 6 months. Neurology. 2009; 73(12):949–953

[454] Kupersmith MJ, Gal RL, Beck RW, Xing D, Miller N, Optic Neuritis Study Group. Visual function at baseline and 1 month in acute optic neuritis: predictors of visual outcome. Neurology. 2007; 69(6):508–514

[455] The Optic Neuritis Study Group. Visual function 5 years after optic neuritis: experience of the Optic Neuritis Treatment Trial. Arch Ophthalmol. 1997; 115(12):1545–1552

[456] Raz N, Dotan S, Benoliel T, Chokron S, Ben-Hur T, Levin N. Sustained motion perception deficit following optic neuritis: behavioral and cortical evidence. Neurology. 2011; 76(24):2103–2111

[457] Frith JA, McLeod JG, Hely M. Acute optic neuritis in Australia: a 13 year prospective study. J Neurol Neurosurg Psychiatry. 2000; 68(2):246

[458] Rodriguez M, Siva A, Cross SA, O'Brien PC, Kurland LT. Optic neuritis: a population-based study in Olmsted County, Minnesota. Neurology. 1995; 45 (2):244–250

[459] Sørensen TL, Frederiksen JL, Brønnum-Hansen H, Petersen HC. Optic neuritis as onset manifestation of multiple sclerosis: a nationwide, long-term survey. Neurology. 1999; 53(3):473–478

[460] Fisniku LK, Brex PA, Altmann DR, et al. Disability and T2 MRI lesions: a 20-year follow-up of patients with relapse onset of multiple sclerosis. Brain. 2008; 131(Pt 3):808–817

[461] Rizzo JF, III, Lessell S. Risk of developing multiple sclerosis after uncomplicated optic neuritis: a long-term prospective study. Neurology. 1988; 38(2):185–190

[462] Brex PA, O'Riordan JI, Miszkiel KA, et al. Multisequence MRI in clinically isolated syndromes and the early development of MS. Neurology. 1999; 53 (6):1184–1190

[463] Ghezzi A, Martinelli V, Rodegher M, Zaffaroni M, Comi G. The prognosis of idiopathic optic neuritis. Neurol Sci. 2000; 21(4) Suppl 2:S865–S869

[464] Ghezzi A, Martinelli V, Torri V, et al. Long-term follow-up of isolated optic neuritis: the risk of developing multiple sclerosis, its outcome, and the prognostic role of paraclinical tests. J Neurol. 1999; 246(9): 770–775

[465] Hauser SL, Oksenberg JR, Lincoln R, et al. Optic Neuritis Study Group. Interaction between HLA-DR2 and abnormal brain MRI in optic neuritis and early MS. Neurology. 2000; 54(9):1859–1861

[466] Mikaeloff Y, Suissa S, Vallée L, et al. KIDMUS Study Group. First episode of acute CNS inflammatory demyelination in childhood: prognostic factors for multiple sclerosis and disability. J Pediatr. 2004; 144(2):246–252

[467] Tintore M, Rovira À, Río J, et al. Defining high, medium and low impact prognostic factors for developing multiple sclerosis. Brain. 2015; 138(Pt 7): 1863–1874

[468] Cramer SP, Modvig S, Simonsen HJ, Frederiksen JL, Larsson HB. Permeability of the blood-brain barrier predicts conversion from optic neuritis to multiple sclerosis. Brain. 2015; 138(Pt 9):2571–2583

[469] Frederiksen J. Bilateral acute optic neuritis: prospective clinical, MRI, CSF, neurophysiological and HLA findings. Neuroophthalmology. 1997; 17: 175–183

[470] Lucchinetti CF, Kiers L, O'Duffy A, et al. Risk factors for developing multiple sclerosis after childhood optic neuritis. Neurology. 1997; 49(5):1413–1418

3 Optic Disc Edema with a Macular Star and Neuroretinitis

Stacy V. Smith

Abstract

Optic disc edema associated with macular exudates in a star pattern occurs with a variety of conditions. When optic disc edema with a macular star occurs in the setting of retinitis, particularly due to an infectious etiology, it is termed neuroretinitis. This chapter discusses the clinical pathway for evaluating and diagnosing patients with optic disc edema with a macular star, and includes a detailed review of the literature and reported cases.

Keywords: optic disc edema, macular star, neuroretinitis, Bartonella henselae, optic neuropathy

3.1 Introduction

Optic disc edema with a macular star (ODEMS) is a descriptive term encompassing a heterogeneous group of disorders. In 1916, Leber described patients with idiopathic unilateral visual loss, optic disc edema, and macular exudate.[1] He incorrectly theorized that the pathologic process was primarily retinal and called the condition "stellate retinopathy." The condition subsequently has been called Leber stellate maculopathy, Leber idiopathic stellate neuroretinitis, or simply neuroretinitis. In 1977, Gass suggested that this syndrome was caused by a prelaminar disc vasculitis that results in leakage of disc capillaries and concluded that this entity was not a retinal vasculopathy but a primary optic neuropathy.[2]

This syndrome is characterized by swelling of the optic disc, peripapillary and macular hard exudates that often occur in a star pattern, and (often) vitreous cells. Because the macular exudate likely results from primary optic nerve disease and not a true retinitis, we prefer the term idiopathic ODEMS for idiopathic cases, and use the term neuroretinitis when optic disc swelling and a macular star are associated with retinitis, especially if an infectious cause is documented.[3]

3.2 What Are the Clinical Features of ODEMS and Neuroretinitis?

The clinical features of ODEMS have been described by a number of authors (Brazis and Lee[3]; Hamard et al[4]; King et al[5]) and are summarized in ▶ Table 3.1. Patients are usually children or young adults, with the average age of onset being 20 to 40 years. Men and women are affected equally. Most cases are unilateral, but bilateral involvement has been noted to occur in up to a third of the cases. Most patients present with acute unilateral loss of vision. The condition is often painless, but retrobulbar pain, pain on eye movement, or associated headache may occur. A nonspecific viral illness precedes or accompanies the visual loss in approximately half of the cases.

Visual acuity with ODEMS may range from 20/20 to light perception, but most cases are in the 20/40 to 20/200 range. Dyschromatopsia is often present. Perimetry most often reveals a

Table 3.1 Clinical characteristics of optic disc edema with macular star (ODEMS)

Age at onset	Childhood to young adult (6–50 y)
Gender	Men and women affected equally
Bilateral involvement	5–33%
Pain	Occasional
Antecedent viral illness	Approximately 50%
Initial visual acuity	Variable (20/20—light perception)
Dyschromatopsia	Often prominent
Visual field testing	Central, cecocentral, arcuate, or altitudinal defects; possible generalized constriction
Relative afferent pupil defect	Present, but may be absent if bilateral involvement
Optic disc	Swelling present with subsequent optic atrophy
Macular star	Present, but may take 1 or 2 wk to develop
Vitreous cells	Common (90%)

central or cecocentral scotoma, but other "optic nerve–type" field abnormalities may occur, including arcuate and altitudinal defects or generalized constriction. Depending on the degree of disc edema, there may also be enlargement of the blind spot. Most patients have a relative afferent papillary defect unless involvement is bilateral and relatively symmetric.

Optic disc edema is the earliest sign of ODEMS and may be severe. The disc edema tends to resolve over 2 weeks to 2 months, but in some patients optic atrophy ensues. Optic disc edema is associated with leakage of disc capillaries with the fluid spreading from the disc through the outer plexiform layer of the retina. The serous component of the fluid accumulation in Henle's layer is reabsorbed, and the lipid precipitate forms a macular star. The macular star may be present at the onset of visual loss or may be noted only after 1 to 2 weeks following development of the disc edema. The macular star may even be observed only after the disc swelling is starting to resolve. Patients with acute disc swelling with a normal macula should thus be reexamined within 2 weeks to search for the presence of a macular star, especially because it is of prognostic importance for the patient's subsequent risk of developing multiple sclerosis (see below). Optical coherence tomography (OCT) of the optic nerve and macula can confirm the degree of disc edema as well as the extension of subretinal fluid into the macula.[6] Fluorescein angiography typically shows leakage from the optic disc in the middle to late phases, with abnormal permeability of the deep capillaries in the optic nerve head but no perifoveal leakage.[7]

ODEMS is often associated with cells in the vitreous. Other occasional findings include cells in the anterior chamber, chorioretinitis, inflammatory sheathing of the peripapillary veins, scleritis and uveitis, and (rarely) central or branch retinal artery occlusions.[8] The association of ODEMS with these latter findings suggests a more diffuse vasculitis or an infectious cause.

3.3 What Is the Etiology and Differential of ODEMS and Neuroretinitis?

Most cases of ODEMS are idiopathic and thought to be the result of nonspecific viral infection or some immune-mediated process. In general, ODEMS is usually a benign, self-limited inflammatory process. A number of infectious agents and inflammatory diseases, however, have been reported to cause ODEMS and neuroretinitis. Infectious and other etiologies are summarized in Box 3.1. Some of these infectious agents have been implicated in single case reports, but it appears that syphilis, cat-scratch disease, Lyme disease, and perhaps toxoplasmosis are the most common causes of ODEMS and neuroretinitis in cases where an etiologic agent can be identified. Infectious agents should be aggressively sought in cases of ODEMS and neuroretinitis because appropriate antimicrobial treatment might be indicated. Ray and Gragoudas recommended special emphasis on recent patient travel history (Lyme endemic areas), consumption of unpasteurized or uncooked foods (toxoplasmosis), sexually transmitted disease exposure (syphilis), and animal contacts (cat scratch).[7]

Box 3.1 Etiologies of optic disc edema with macular star or neuroretinitis

- Viruses:
  - Hepatitis B.
  - Herpes simplex.[9]
  - Herpes zoster.[10]
  - Epstein–Barr virus.
  - Influenza A.[11,12]
  - Mumps.[13]
  - Coxsackie B.
  - West Nile virus.[11,14]
  - Chikungunya fever.[9,11,15,16,17]
  - Dengue fever.[11,18]
- Bacteria:
  - Cat-scratch disease (*Bartonella henselae*),[5,8,19,20,21,22,23,24,25,26,27,28,29,30,31,32,33,34,35,36,37,38,39,40,41,42,43,44,45,46,47,48,49,50,51,52,53,54,55] *Bartonella elizabethae*,[56] *Bartonella grahamii*.[57]
  - Tuberculosis.[58]
  - Mycoplasma pneumoniae meningitis.[59]
  - Salmonella.
  - Lyme disease.[60,61,62,63,64,65]
  - Syphilis.[66,67,68]
  - Leptospirosis.
  - Mediterranean spotted fever (*Rickettsia conorii*).[69]
  - Rocky Mountain Spotted Fever (*Rickettsia rickettsii*)[70]
- Fungi:
  - Histoplasmosis.
  - Cryptococcal meningitis (*Cryptococcus neoformans*).[71]
- Parasites and protozoa:
  - Toxoplasmosis.[72,73,74,75]
  - Toxocara.
- Other (Inflammatory, noninfectious*):*
  - Inflammatory:
    - Sarcoidosis.[76,77]
    - Ulcerative colitis.[78]
    - Behçet disease.[79]
    - Vogt–Koyanagi–Harada disease.[80]
    - Primary angiitis of the central nervous system.[81]
    - Polyarteritis nodose.[82]
  - Malignant hypertension.[83,84,85,86,87]
  - Elevated intracranial pressure:
    - Pseudotumor cerebri.[88,89]
    - Meningitis-associated (e.g., *Cryptococcus neoformans, Mycoplasma pneumoniae*).[59,71]
  - Melanocytoma.[90]
  - Parry–Romberg syndrome with progressive hemifacial atrophy.

ODEMS or neuroretinitis may occur as part of syphilitic meningitis (usually bilateral), or may occur as an isolated entity in patients with secondary syphilis, in which case it may be associated with unilateral or bilateral uveitis.[66,67,68] ODEMS or neuroretinitis is common manifestation of cat-scratch disease.[5,8,19,20,21,22,23,24,25,26,27,28,29,30,31,32,33,34,35,36,37,38,39,40,41,42,43,44,45,46,47,48,49,50,51,52,53,54,55] In fact, optic neuritis (papillitis) without a macular star has only rarely been reported with this disease.[27,91]

Cat-scratch disease due to *Bartonella henselae* may cause ODEMS or may cause a neuroretinitis with chorioretinitis at times associated with uveitis, cells in the anterior chamber, and even branch or central retinal artery occlusions.[8,25,27,40,42] This disease may also cause a multifocal retinitis with optic disc edema (without macular star), branch retinal artery occlusion, and vitreitis.[43,92] Optic disc edema associated with peripapillary serous retinal detachment, even without macular star formation, may be an early sign of cat-scratch disease.[93] Solley et al studied 24 patients (35 eyes) with choroidal, retinal, or optic disc manifestations of cat-scratch disease and found that discrete white retinal or choroidal lesions were the most common posterior segment finding (46% of eyes, 63% of patients), followed by macular star (43% of eyes, 63% of patients).[37] Vascular-occlusive events were also seen (14% of eyes, 21% of patients) and the site of occlusion was found to be intimately associated with the aforementioned retinal lesions. Final visual acuity was 20/25 or better in 26 (74%) of 35 eyes and was similar in both treated and untreated patients. Chi et al reviewed 53 patients and 62 eyes (9 cases of bilateral involvement) with serologically confirmed cat-scratch optic neuropath.[43] Only 35 (67%) of patients endorsed a history of cat or kitten contact. Neuroretinitis with a swollen optic disc and macular start was the most common presentation (45% of eyes, 49% of patients, 2 patients with bilateral disease). Additional ocular findings included vitreitis, retinal lesions, branch retinal vascular occlusion, macular hole, and corneal decompensation. A final follow-up visual acuity of 20/40 or better was considered favorable, and achieved by 36 (68%) of 53 eyes. Good visual acuity at presentation was associated with favorable final visual acuity (odds ratio: 0.19; 95% confidence interval: 0.08–0.43; $p < 0.001$). Treatment with antibiotics, corticosteroids, or both was not associated with improvement in vision, similar to Solley et al. In the three patients treated with intravenous corticosteroids, there was an association with poorer visual outcome ($p = 0.028$). However, patients treated with corticosteroids also had a worse initial visual acuity.[43] Cat-scratch disease should be considered in any patient who presents with ODEMS or neuro-retinitis, especially if there is associated lymphadenopathy or retinal artery occlusion (class III, level B). A retrospective case review by Schmalfuss et al noted that when optic nerve enhancement on orbital magnetic resonance imaging (MRI) was present, enhancement was confined to the junction of the nerve to the globe. This finding on MRI may prompt serologic testing for *B. henselae* (class III, level C).[94,95] Visual evoked potentials may show mild abnormalities in patients with optic nerve involvement.[96] The treatment[97] of cat-scratch disease is quite variable in the literature and has included various antibiotic regimens including penicillins, cephalosporins, aminoglycosides, tetracyclines, macrolides, quinolones, trimethoprim-sulfamethoxazole, and rifampin (class III, level C). Reed et al reported seven cases, and concluded that, compared to historic controls, doxycycline and rifampin shortened the course of the disease and improved visual recovery (class III, level C).[33] The ophthalmologic manifestations of cat-scratch disease are outlined in Box 3.2.

ODEMS may also occur with stage II Lyme disease.[60,61,62,63,64,65] Toxoplasmosis may also cause ODEMS or neuroretinitis.[72,73]

Two features that often occur with toxoplasmosis neuroretinitis, but that are uncommon with idiopathic ODEMS, are a prominent anterior chamber inflammation and the presence of toxoplasmosis chorioretinal scars. Toxoplasmosis neuroretinitis is perhaps more likely to cause recurrent episodes of ODEMS or neuroretinitis, compared to the usual monophasic course of idiopathic ODEMS.

ODEMS and neuroretinitis must be differentiated from other entities in which optic disc swelling occurs with or without macular star formation, including vascular causes (e.g., anterior ischemic optic neuropathy, posterior hyaloid detachment, branch or central retinal artery occlusion, hypertension, diabetes, polyarteritis nodosa, inflammatory bowel disease, and Eales' disease), papilledema from increased intracranial pressure, optic nerve tumors or infiltrative processes, diffuse unilateral subacute neuroretinitis (DUSN), optic neuritis, and the acute neuroretinopathy that may occur associated with progressive facial hemiatrophy (Parry–Romberg syndrome).[82,83,107,108,109,110,111,112,113] With many of these etiologies, macular stars are rarely seen and usually the differential diagnosis is not difficult on clinical grounds. However, if a macular star figure is present, further evaluation can aid in the diagnosis. For example, a lumbar puncture can confirm the diagnosis of elevated intracranial pressure and/or meningitis if ODEMS is secondary to central nervous system infection or idiopathic intracranial hypertension. In a patient with otherwise negative infectious and inflammatory workup, an elevated blood pressure should suggest consideration for malignant hypertension as the underlying etiology. In cases of ODEMS due to elevated intracranial and systemic hypertension, vitreous cells would not be expected.[59,71,83,84,85,86,87,88,89] A suggested workup for patients with optic disc edema with macular star is outlined in ▶ Fig. 3.1.

3.4 What Is the Prognosis in Cases of ODEMS?

ODEMS is usually a benign condition that resolves spontaneously without treatment.[34] The disc edema and peripapillary retinal detachment tend to resolve over a period of 2 to 3 months, while the macular star usually begins to disappear after 1 month. The macular star, however, may persist for up to 1 year. Optic atrophy and macular retinal pigment epithelial changes may be residuals of previous ODEMS. The prognosis for visual recovery in ODEMS is usually good, but significant residual visual disability may occasionally occur.[114] Recurrences of ODEMS or neuroretinitis in the same or fellow eye have been described in idiopathic as well as infectious cases, especially in patients with toxoplasmosis.[72,115] Also, Purvin and Chioran described an apparently distinct type of recurrent ODEMS in patients who experienced from two to seven attacks of ODEMS at intervals ranging from 1 to 10 years.[115] The attacks often affected both eyes but never simultaneously. Visual field defects were of the nerve fiber bundle type instead of the central or cecocentral scotomas that are most often noted in benign ODEMS. Patients with the recurrent form of the disease may not experience significant improvement in optic nerve function, and each episode may result in further visual acuity and visual field loss.[116]

Although optic neuritis is a risk factor for the development of multiple sclerosis (see chapter 2), ODEMS or neuroretinitis is

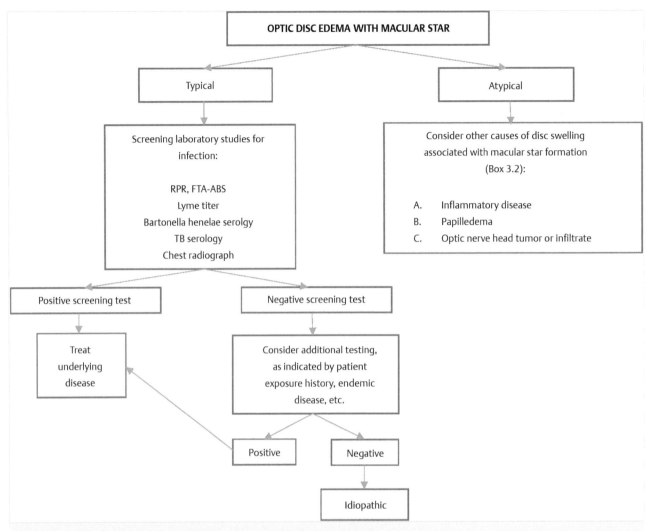

Fig. 3.1 Evaluation of optic disc edema with a macular star (ODEMS) or neuroretinitis.

not.[117] For example, in the Optic Neuritis Treatment Trial (see chapter 2), among patients with swollen discs, clinically definite multiple sclerosis did not develop in any patient who had macular exudates.[117] Because a macular exudate may not develop in cases of ODEMS until 2 weeks after presentation, patients who demonstrate acute papillitis with a normal macula should be reevaluated within 2 weeks for the development of a macular star. Its presence makes the subsequent development of multiple sclerosis extremely unlikely.

In summary, there is no class I or class II evidence for the diagnosis and treatment of ODEMS. Individual history and examination should guide the evaluation focusing on exposure history (e.g., high-risk sexual practices, recent travel, exposure to cats or ticks), systemic findings (e.g., signs and symptoms of viral illness, tuberculosis, increased intracranial pressure, or uncontrolled systemic hypertension), or typical ophthalmoscopic features (e.g., adjacent chorioretinal scar in toxoplasmosis). In typical ODEMS, however, most of the cases remain idiopathic. Cat-scratch disease is emerging as a common etiology in cases with a proven cause and performing a *B. henselae* titer is a reasonable practice option in ODEMS (class III, level C). In the absence of risk factors or clinical suspicion, the yield for

testing for other infectious etiologies is low (class III, level U). Routine testing even for treatable disorders such as syphilis (serology), Lyme disease, or tuberculosis (chest radiography, purified protein derivative skin test, and/or serum interferon gamma release assay (IGRA) are practice options of uncertain yield (class III, level U).

There is no proven treatment for idiopathic ODEMS (class III, level C). Steroids (high-dose oral or intravenous) have been used in some cases with unclear effect (class III, level U). Aggressive immunosuppressive agents such as azathioprine may be considered in the rare recurrent cases (class IV).[115,116,118] Çakir et al report a case of idiopathic neuroretinitis that responded well to intravitreal bevacizumab and triamcinolone acetonide injection after a negative infectious workup. The macular edema resolved within 1 week, but disc edema did not resolve until a 1-month follow-up. The vision improved from 3/10 at presentation to 10/10 1 week postinjection. The only reported complication was intraocular hypertension.[119] However, there is no prospective, randomized data on intravitreal therapy for idiopathic ODEMS. If a specific infectious agent is discovered, then appropriate antimicrobials should be considered, but the data are limited (class III, level B). Specific attention, however, should focus on treatable (e.g., cat-scratch disease, Lyme disease, syphilis, and tuberculosis) infectious etiologies (class III, level B). Atypical cases (e.g., bilateral) might require further evaluation (e.g., neuroimaging or lumbar puncture) to exclude other causes of ODEMS (class III).

References

[1] Leber T. Die pseudonephritischen Netzhauterkrankungen, die Retinitis stellata: die Purtschersche Netzhautaffektion nach schwere Schädelverletzung. In: Graefe AC, Saemisch T, eds. Graefe-Saemisch Handbuch der Gesamten Augenheilkunde. 2nd ed. Vol. 7, Pt. 2. Leipzig: Engelmann; 1916

[2] Gass JDM. Diseases of the optic nerve that may simulate macular disease. Trans Sect Ophthalmol Am Acad Ophthalmol Otolaryngol. 1977; 83(5):763–770

[3] Brazis PW, Lee AG. Optic disk edema with a macular star. Mayo Clin Proc. 1996; 71(12):1162–1166

[4] Hamard P, Hamard H, Ngohou S. La neurorétinite stellaire idiopathique de Leber. A propos de neuf cas. J Fr Ophtalmol. 1994; 17(2):116–123

[5] King MH, Cartwright MJ, Carney MD. Leber's idiopathic stellate neuroretinitis. Ann Ophthalmol. 1991; 23(2):58–60

[6] Stewart MW, Brazis PW, Barrett KM, Eidelman BH, Mendez JC. Optical coherence tomography in a case of bilateral neuroretinitis. J Neuroophthalmol. 2005; 25(2):131–133

[7] Ray S, Gragoudas E. Neuroretinitis. Int Ophthalmol Clin. 2001; 41(1):83–102

[8] May EF, Levi L, Ng JD, Truxal AR. Rochalimaea neuroretinitis and retinal vasculitis. Presented at the meeting of the North American Neuro-Ophthalmology Society, Tucson, AZ, 1995

[9] Murthy KR, Venkataraman N, Satish V, Babu K. Bilateral retinitis following chikungunya fever. Indian J Ophthalmol. 2008; 56(4):329–331

[10] Dhar MY, Goel JL, Sota LD. Optic neuroretinitis, a rare manifestation of herpes zoster ophthalmicus: a case report. J Commun Dis. 1997; 29(1):57–61

[11] Khairallah M, Kahloun R. Ocular manifestations of emerging infectious diseases. Curr Opin Ophthalmol. 2013; 24(6):574–580

[12] Lai CC, Chang YS, Li ML, Chang CM, Huang FC, Tseng SH. Acute anterior uveitis and optic neuritis as ocular complications of influenza A infection in an 11-year-old boy. J Pediatr Ophthalmol Strabismus. 2011; 48 Online: e30–e33

[13] Foster RE, Lowder CY, Meisler DM, Kosmorsky GS, Baetz-Greenwalt B. Mumps neuroretinitis in an adolescent. Am J Ophthalmol. 1990; 110(1):91–93

[14] Sivakumar RR, Prajna L, Arya LK, et al. Molecular diagnosis and ocular imaging of West Nile virus retinitis and neuroretinitis. Ophthalmology. 2013; 120(9):1820–1826

[15] Nair AG, Biswas J, Bhende MP. A case of bilateral chikungunya neuroretinitis. J Ophthalmic Inflamm Infect. 2012; 2(1):39–40

[16] Mahesh G, Giridhar A, Shedbele A, Kumar R, Saikumar SJ. A case of bilateral presumed chikungunya neuroretinitis. Indian J Ophthalmol. 2009; 57(2):148–150

[17] Mittal A, Mittal S, Bharati MJ, Ramakrishnan R, Saravanan S, Sathe PS. Optic neuritis associated with chikungunya virus infection in South India. Arch Ophthalmol. 2007; 125(10):1381–1386

[18] de Amorim Garcia CA, Gomes AH, de Oliveira AG. Bilateral stellar neuroretinitis in a patient with dengue fever. Eye (Lond). 2006; 20(12):1382–1383

[19] Bar S, Segal M, Shapira R, Savir H. Neuroretinitis associated with cat scratch disease. Am J Ophthalmol. 1990; 110(6):703–705

[20] Bhatti MT, Asif R, Bhatti LB. Macular star in neuroretinitis. Arch Neurol. 2001; 58(6):1008–1009

[21] Carithers HA, Margileth AM. Cat-scratch disease. Acute encephalopathy and other neurologic manifestations. Am J Dis Child. 1991; 145(1):98–101

[22] Chrousos GA, Drack AV, Young M, Kattah J, Sirdofsky M. Neuroretinitis in cat scratch disease. J Clin Neuroophthalmol. 1990; 10(2):92–94

[23] Cunningham ET, Koehler JE. Ocular bartonellosis. Am J Ophthalmol. 2000; 130(3):340–349

[24] Earhart KC, Power MH. Images in clinical medicine. Bartonella neuroretinitis. N Engl J Med. 2000; 343(20):1459

[25] Fish RH, Hogan RN, Nightingale SD, Anand R. Peripapillary angiomatosis associated with cat-scratch neuroretinitis. Arch Ophthalmol. 1992; 110(3):323

[26] Ghauri RR, Lee AG, Purvin V. Optic disk edema with a macular star. Surv Ophthalmol. 1998; 43(3):270–274

[27] Golnik KC, Marotto ME, Fanous MM, et al. Ophthalmic manifestations of Rochalimaea species. Am J Ophthalmol. 1994; 118(2):145–151

[28] Gray AV, Reed JB, Wendel RT, Morse LS. Bartonella henselae infection associated with peripapillary angioma, branch retinal artery occlusion, and severe vision loss. Am J Ophthalmol. 1999; 127(2):223–224

[29] Labalette P, Bermond D, Dedes V, Savage C. Cat-scratch disease neuroretinitis diagnosed by a polymerase chain reaction approach. Am J Ophthalmol. 2001; 132(4):575–576

[30] McCrary B, Cockerham W, Pierce P. Neuroretinitis in cat-scratch disease associated with the macular star. Pediatr Infect Dis J. 1994; 13(9):838–839

[31] McCrary B, Cockerham W, Pierce P. Neuroretinitis in cat scratch disease associated with macular star. J Miss State Med Assoc. 1997; 38(5):158–159

[32] Ormerod LD, Skolnick KA, Menosky MM, Pavan PR, Pon DM. Retinal and choroidal manifestations of cat-scratch disease. Ophthalmology. 1998; 105(6):1024–1031

[33] Reed JB, Scales DK, Wong MT, Lattuada CP, Jr, Dolan MJ, Schwab IR. Bartonella henselae neuroretinitis in cat scratch disease. Diagnosis, management, and sequelae. Ophthalmology. 1998; 105(3):459–466

[34] Rosen BS, Barry CJ, Nicoll AM, Constable IJ. Conservative management of documented neuroretinitis in cat scratch disease associated with Bartonella henselae infection. Aust N Z J Ophthalmol. 1999; 27(2):153–156

[35] Schwartzman WA, Patnaik M, Barka NE, Peter JB. Rochalimaea antibodies in HIV-associated neurologic disease. Neurology. 1994; 44(7):1312–1316

[36] Schwartzman WA, Patnaik M, Angulo FJ, Visscher BR, Miller EN, Peter JB. Bartonella (Rochalimaea) antibodies, dementia, and cat ownership among men infected with human immunodeficiency virus. Clin Infect Dis. 1995; 21(4):954–959

[37] Solley WA, Martin DF, Newman NJ, et al. Cat scratch disease: posterior segment manifestations. Ophthalmology. 1999; 106(8):1546–1553

[38] Suhler EB, Lauer AK, Rosenbaum JT. Prevalence of serologic evidence of cat scratch disease in patients with neuroretinitis. Ophthalmology. 2000; 107(5):871–876

[39] Thompson PK, Vaphiades MS, Saccente M. Cat-scratch disease presenting as neuroretinitis and peripheral facial palsy. J Neuroophthalmol. 1999; 19(4):240–241

[40] Ulrich GG, Waecker NJ, Jr, Meister SJ, Peterson TJ, Hooper DG. Cat scratch disease associated with neuroretinitis in a 6-year-old girl. Ophthalmology. 1992; 99(2):246–249

[41] Wade NK, Po S, Wong IG, Cunningham ET, Jr. Bilateral Bartonella-associated neuroretinitis. Retina. 1999; 19(4):355–356

[42] Zhao X, Ge B. Treatment of papillo-retinitis and uveitis associated with cat-scratch disease by combination of TCM and modern drugs. J Tradit Chin Med. 1991; 11(3):184–186

[43] Chi SL, Stinnett S, Eggenberger E, et al. Clinical characteristics in 53 patients with cat scratch optic neuropathy. Ophthalmology. 2012; 119(1):183–187

[44] De Schryver I, Stevens AM, Vereecke G, Kestelyn P. Cat scratch disease (CSD) in patients with stellate neuroretinitis: 3 cases. Bull Soc Belge Ophtalmol. 2002; 286(286):41–46

[45] Ullrich K, Saha N, Lake S. Neuroretinitis following bull ant sting. BMJ Case Rep. 2012; 2012:bcr2012006338

[46] Kalogeropoulos C, Koumpoulis I, Mentis A, Pappa C, Zafeiropoulos P, Aspiotis M. Bartonella and intraocular inflammation: a series of cases and review of literature. Clin Ophthalmol. 2011; 5:817–829

[47] Durá-Travé T, Yoldi-Petri ME, Gallinas-Victoriano F, Lavilla-Oiz A, Bove-Guri M. Neuroretinitis caused by Bartonella henselae (cat-scratch disease) in a 13-year-old girl. Int J Pediatr. 2010; 2010:763105

[48] Hernandez-Da-Mota S, Escalante-Razo F. Bartonellosis causing bilateral Leber neuroretinitis: a case report. Eur J Ophthalmol. 2009; 19(2):307–309

[49] Raihan AR, Zunaina E, Wan-Hazabbah WH, Adil H, Lakana-Kumar T. Neuroretinitis in ocular bartonellosis: a case series. Clin Ophthalmol. 2014; 8:1459–1466

[50] Irshad FA, Gordon RA. Bartonella henselae neuroretinitis in a 15-year-old girl with chronic myelogenous leukemia. J AAPOS. 2009; 13(6):602–604

[51] Ak R, Doganay F, Akoglu EU, Ozturk TC. A challenging differential diagnosis of optic neuropathy in ED: CSD. BMJ Case Rep. 2015; 2015:bcr2015201252

[52] Alterman MA, Young BK, Eggenberger ER, Kaufman DI. Macular hole: a rare complication of ocular bartonellosis. J Neuroophthalmol. 2013; 33(2):153–154

[53] Gajula V, Kamepalli R, Kalavakunta JK. A star in the eye: cat scratch neuroretinitis. Clin Case Rep. 2014; 2(1):17

[54] Gan JJ, Mandell AM, Otis JA, Holmuhamedova M, Perloff MD. Suspecting optic neuritis, diagnosing Bartonella cat scratch disease. Arch Neurol. 2011; 68(1):122–126

[55] Aragão RE, Ramos RM, Bezerra AF, Cavalcanti Júnior RB, Albuquerque TL. Optic neuropathy secondary to cat scratch disease: case report. Arq Bras Oftalmol. 2010; 73(6):537–538

[56] O'Halloran HS, Draud K, Minix M, Rivard AK, Pearson PA. Leber's neuroretinitis in a patient with serologic evidence of Bartonella Elizabethae. Retina. 1998; 18(3):276–278

[57] Kerkhoff FT, Bergmans AM, van Der Zee A, Rothova A. Demonstration of Bartonella grahamii DNA in ocular fluids of a patient with neuroretinitis. J Clin Microbiol. 1999; 37(12):4034–4038

[58] Stechschulte SU, Kim RY, Cunningham ET, Jr. Tuberculous neuroretinitis. J Neuroophthalmol. 1999; 19(3):201–204

[59] Karampsatsas K, Patel H, Basheer SN, Prendergast AJ. Chronic meningitis with intracranial hypertension and bilateral neuroretinitis following Mycoplasma pneumoniae infection. BMJ Case Rep. 2014; 2014:bcr2014207041

[60] Bialasiewicz AA. Augenbefunde bei Lyme-Borreliose. Ophthalmologe. 1992; 89(5):W47–W59

[61] Karma A, Seppälä I, Mikkilä H, Kaakkola S, Viljanen M, Tarkkanen A. Diagnosis and clinical characteristics of ocular Lyme borreliosis. Am J Ophthalmol. 1995; 119(2):127–135

[62] Lesser RL, Kornmehl EW, Pachner AR, et al. Neuro-ophthalmologic manifestations of Lyme disease. Ophthalmology. 1990; 97(6):699–706

[63] Miller NR. In: Miller NR, ed. Walsh and Hoyt's Clinical Neuro-ophthalmology. Baltimore, MD: Williams & Wilkins; 1995:3657–3658

[64] Schönherr U, Lang GE, Meythaler FH. Bilaterale Lebersche neuroretinitis stellata bei Borrelia burgdorferi-Serokonversion. Klin Monatsbl Augenheilkd. 1991; 198(1):44–47

[65] Schönherr U, Wilk CM, Lang GE, Naumann GOH. Intraocular manifestations of Lyme borreliosis. Presented at the Fourth International Conference on Borreliosis, Stockholm, Sweden, June 18–21, 1990

[66] Halperin LS. Neuroretinitis due to seronegative syphilis associated with human immunodeficiency virus. J Clin Neuroophthalmol. 1992; 12(3):171–172

[67] McLeish WM, Pulido JS, Holland S, Culbertson WW, Winward K. The ocular manifestations of syphilis in the human immunodeficiency virus type 1-infected host. Ophthalmology. 1990; 97(2):196–203

[68] Ninomiya H, Hamada T, Akiya S, Kazama H. Three cases of acute syphilitic neuroretinitis. Nippon Ganka Kiyo. 1990; 41:2088–2094

[69] Khairallah M, Ladjimi A, Chakroun M, et al. Posterior segment manifestations of Rickettsia conorii infection. Ophthalmology. 2004; 111(3):529–534

[70] Vaphiades MS. Rocky Mountain spotted fever as a cause of macular star figure. J Neuroophthalmol. 2003; 23(4):276–278

[71] Espino Barros Palau A, Morgan ML, Foroozan R, Lee AG. Neuro-ophthalmic presentations and treatment of Cryptococcal meningitis-related increased intracranial pressure. Can J Ophthalmol. 2014; 49(5):473–477

[72] Fish RH, Hoskins JC, Kline LB. Toxoplasmosis neuroretinitis. Ophthalmology. 1993; 100(8):1177–1182

[73] Moreno RJ, Weisman J, Waller S. Neuroretinitis: an unusual presentation of ocular toxoplasmosis. Ann Ophthalmol. 1992; 24(2):68–70

[74] Wong R, dell'Omo R, Marino M, Hussein B, Okhravi N, Pavesio CE. Toxoplasma gondii: an atypical presentation of toxoplasma as optic disc swelling and hemispherical retinal vein occlusion treated with intravitreal clindamycin. Int Ophthalmol. 2009; 29(3):195–198

[75] Miserocchi E, Modorati G, Rama P. Atypical toxoplasmosis masquerading late occurrence of typical findings. Eur J Ophthalmol. 2009; 19(6):1091–1093

[76] Kosmorsky GS, Prayson R. Primary optic pathway sarcoidosis in a 38-year-old white man. J Neuroophthalmol. 1996; 16(3):188–190

[77] Miller NR. In: Miller NR, ed. Walsh and Hoyt's Clinical Neuro-ophthalmology. Baltimore, MD: Williams & Wilkins; 1995:4487–4489

[78] Shoari M, Katz BJ. Recurrent neuroretinitis in an adolescent with ulcerative colitis. J Neuroophthalmol. 2005; 25(4):286–288

[79] Chan RV, Lee TC, Chaganti RK, Cestari DM, Kim MT, Lee S. Macular star associated with Behçet disease. Retina. 2006; 26(4):468–470

[80] Vaphiades MS, Read RW. Magnetic resonance imaging of choroidal inflammation in Vogt-Koyanagi-Harada disease. J Neuroophthalmol. 2004; 24(4):295–296

[81] Rao NM, Prasad PS, Flippen CC, II, et al. Primary angiitis of the central nervous system presenting as unilateral optic neuritis. J Neuroophthalmol. 2014; 34(4):380–385

[82] Matsuda A, Chin S, Ohashi T. A case of neuroretinitis associated with long-standing polyarteritis nodosa. Ophthalmologica. 1994; 208(3):168–171

[83] Lee AG, Beaver HA, Monsul NT, Miller NR. Acute bilateral optic disk edema with a macular star figure in a 12-year-old girl. Surv Ophthalmol. 2002; 47(1):42–49

[84] Yıldırım A, Mehmet Türkcü F, Yüksel H, Sahin A, Cınar Y, Caça I. Diagnosis of malignant hypertension with ocular examination: a child case. Semin Ophthalmol. 2014; 29(1):32–35

[85] I-Linn ZL, Long QB. An unusual cause of acute bilateral optic disk swelling with macular star in a 9-year-old girl. J Pediatr Ophthalmol Strabismus. 2007; 44(4):245–247

[86] Scott IU, Flynn HW, Jr, Al-Attar L, Ganser GL, V Aragon A, Lam BL. Bilateral optic disc edema in patients with severe systemic arterial hypertension: clinical features and visual acuity outcomes. Ophthalmic Surg Lasers Imaging. 2005; 36(5):374–380

[87] Kasundra GM, Sood I, Prakash S, Mehta DP. Neuroretinitis with abnormal brain imaging in Ask-Upmark kidney: a novel case report. J Pediatr Neurosci. 2014; 9(2):172–174

[88] Nguyen C, Borruat FX. Bilateral peripapillary subretinal neovessel membrane associated with chronic papilledema: report of two cases. Klin Monatsbl Augenheilkd. 2005; 222(3):275–278

[89] Benzimra JD, Simon S, Sinclair AJ, Mollan SP. Sight-threatening pseudotumour cerebri associated with excess vitamin A supplementation. Pract Neurol. 2015; 15(1):72–73

[90] Al-Rashaed S, Abboud EB, Nowilaty SR. Characteristics of optic disc melanocytomas presenting with visual dysfunction. Middle East Afr J Ophthalmol. 2010; 17(3):242–245

[91] Brazis PW, Stokes HR, Ervin FR. Optic neuritis in cat scratch disease. J Clin Neuroophthalmol. 1986; 6(3):172–174

[92] Cohen SM, Davis JL, Gass DM. Branch retinal arterial occlusions in multifocal retinitis with optic nerve edema. Arch Ophthalmol. 1995; 113(10):1271–1276

[93] Wade NK, Levi L, Jones MR, Bhisitkul R, Fine L, Cunningham ET, Jr. Optic disk edema associated with peripapillary serous retinal detachment: an early sign of systemic Bartonella henselae infection. Am J Ophthalmol. 2000; 130(3):327–334

[94] Schmalfuss IM, Dean CW, Sistrom C, Bhatti MT. Optic neuropathy secondary to cat scratch disease: distinguishing MR imaging features from other types of optic neuropathies. AJNR Am J Neuroradiol. 2005; 26(6):1310–1316

[95] Reddy AK, Morriss MC, Ostrow GI, Stass-Isern M, Olitsky SE, Lowe LH. Utility of MR imaging in cat-scratch neuroretinitis. Pediatr Radiol. 2007; 37(8):840–843

[96] Chai Y, Yamamoto S, Hirayama A, Yotsukura J, Yamazaki H. Pattern visual evoked potentials in eyes with disc swelling due to cat scratch disease-associated neuroretinitis. Doc Ophthalmol. 2005; 110(2–3):271–275

[97] Conrad DA. Treatment of cat-scratch disease. Curr Opin Pediatr. 2001; 13(1):56–59

[98] Bafna S, Lee AG. Bilateral optic disc edema and multifocal retinal lesions without loss of vision in cat scratch disease. Arch Ophthalmol. 1996; 114(8):1016–1017

[99] Cunningham ET, Jr, Schatz H, McDonald HR, Johnson RN. Acute multifocal retinitis. Am J Ophthalmol. 1997; 123(3):347–357

[100] Cunningham ET, Jr, McDonald HR, Schatz H, Johnson RN, Ai E, Grand MG. Inflammatory mass of the optic nerve head associated with systemic Bartonella henselae infection. Arch Ophthalmol. 1997; 115(12):1596–1597

[101] Lee WR, Chawla JC, Reid R. Bacillary angiomatosis of the conjunctiva. Am J Ophthalmol. 1994; 118(2):152–157

[102] Ormerod LD, Dailey JP. Ocular manifestations of cat-scratch disease. Curr Opin Ophthalmol. 1999; 10(3):209–216

[103] Soheilian M, Markomichelakis N, Foster CS. Intermediate uveitis and retinal vasculitis as manifestations of cat scratch disease. Am J Ophthalmol. 1996; 122(4):582–584

[104] Zacchei AC, Newman NJ, Sternberg P. Serous retinal detachment of the macula associated with cat scratch disease. Am J Ophthalmol. 1995; 120(6):796–797

[105] Latanza L, Viscogliosi F, Solimeo A, Calabrò F, De Angelis V, De Rosa P. Choroidal neovascularisation as an unusual ophthalmic manifestation of cat-scratch disease in an 8-year-old girl. Int Ophthalmol. 2015; 35(5):709–716

[106] Waisbourd M, Goldstein M, Giladi M, Shulman S, Loewenstein A. Cat-scratch disease associated with branch retinal artery occlusion. Retin Cases Brief Rep. 2010; 4(1):28–30

[107] Akura J, Ikeda T, Sato K, Ikeda N. Macular star associated with posterior hyaloid detachment. Acta Ophthalmol Scand. 2001; 79(3):317–318

[108] Friedrich Y, Feiner M, Gawi H, Friedman Z. Diabetic papillopathy with macular star mimicking clinically significant diabetic macular edema. Retina. 2001; 21(1):80–82

[109] García-Arumí J, Salvador F, Corcostegui B, Mateo C. Neuroretinitis associated with melanocytoma of the optic disk. Retina. 1994; 14(2):173–176

[110] Gass JDM, Harbin TS, Jr, Del Piero EJ. Exudative stellate neuroretinopathy and Coats' syndrome in patients with progressive hemifacial atrophy. Eur J Ophthalmol. 1991; 1(1):2–10

[111] Leavitt JA, Pruthi S, Morgenstern BZ. Hypertensive retinopathy mimicking neuroretinitis in a twelve-year-old girl. Surv Ophthalmol. 1997; 41(6):477–480

[112] Verm A, Lee AG. Bilateral optic disk edema with macular exudates as the manifesting sign of a cerebral arteriovenous malformation. Am J Ophthalmol. 1997; 123(3):422–424

[113] Galvez-Ruiz A. Macular star formation in diabetic patients with non-arteritic anterior ischemic optic neuropathy (NA-AION). Saudi J Ophthalmol. 2015; 29(1):71–75

[114] Lee AG, Brazis PW. Poor visual outcome following optic disc edema with a macular star (neuroretinitis). J Neuro-ophthalmology. 1998; 19:57–61

[115] Purvin VA, Chioran G. Recurrent neuroretinitis. Arch Ophthalmol. 1994; 112 (3):365–371

[116] Sundaram SV, Purvin VA, Kawasaki A. Recurrent idiopathic neuroretinitis: natural history and effect of treatment. Clin Experiment Ophthalmol. 2010; 38(6):591–596

[117] Optic Neuritis Study Group. The 5-year risk of MS after optic neuritis. Experience of the optic neuritis treatment trial. Neurology. 1997; 49(5): 1404–1413

[118] Purvin V, Sundaram S, Kawasaki A. Neuroretinitis: review of the literature and new observations. J Neuroophthalmol. 2011; 31(1):58–68

[119] Çakir M, Cekiç O, Bozkurt E, Pekel G, Yazici AT, Yilmaz OF. Combined intravitreal bevacizumab and triamcinolone acetonide injection for idiopathic neuroretinitis. Ocul Immunol Inflamm. 2009; 17(3):221–223

4 Nonarteritic Ischemic Optic Neuropathy

Murtaza M. Mandviwala, Shauna Berry, Weijie V. Lin, and Ama Sadaka

Abstract

Nonarteritic ischemic optic neuropathy is a common cause of acute painless vision loss. The most common form is anterior ischemic optic neuropathy, identified by the presence of optic disc edema acutely following the onset of symptoms. Posterior ischemic optic neuropathy is less common, and will lack the feature of acute optic disc edema. This chapter discusses the clinical pathway for diagnosing, evaluating, and treating nonarteritic anterior ischemic optic neuropathy, and includes a detailed review of the literature.

Keywords: nonarteritic ischemic optic neuropathy, anterior ischemic optic neuropathy, posterior ischemic optic neuropathy, diabetic papillopathy, optic atrophy

4.1 What Are the Clinical Features for Typical Nonarteritic AION?

Anterior ischemic optic neuropathy (AION) is characterized clinically by the acute onset of usually unilateral visual loss. Although pain may occur in approximately 10% (range 8–30% in various series) of patients, the visual loss is typically painless.[1] Middle-aged to older patients (usually older than 50 years) are the predominant populations at risk for AION. The ocular examination in these patients reveals the following: (1) ipsilateral visual acuity and visual field loss, (2) a relative afferent pupillary defect, and (3) edema of the optic nerve head with or without peripapillary hemorrhages.[2,3,4,5,6,7,8,9,10,11,12,13,14,15,16,17,18,19,20,21,22,23] The presence of optic disc edema (anterior optic neuropathy) in the acute phase is essential for the diagnosis of AION to be made. Rarely, AION may present with asymptomatic disc edema without visual loss or field defect[24] or be associated with macular edema.[25] After resolution of the disc edema, the optic disc develops sector or diffuse pallor. The typical clinical features of nonarteritic (NA-AION) are outlined in Box 4.1.

> ### Box 4.1 Typical clinical features of nonarteritic anterior ischemic optic neuropathy (NA-AION)
>
> - Age usually over 40 years.
> - Unilateral variable loss of visual acuity and/or visual field.
> - Visual field defects consistent with an optic neuropathy (e.g., central, cecocentral, arcuate, or altitudinal).
> - Optic disc edema in the acute phase, followed by optic atrophy that may be sector or diffuse.
> - Small cup and cup-to-disc ratio (< 0.2) in the fellow eye.[3,26,27,28]
> - Often associated with underlying vasculopathic risk factors (e.g., hypertension, diabetes, smoking, ischemic heart disease, hypercholesterolemia).[3,28,29,30,31]
> - Lack of premonitory symptoms (e.g., transient visual loss).

> - Usually visual loss remains static but may improve slightly or progress.
> - End-stage optic disc appearance is segmental or diffuse pallor without significant cupping (unlike arteritic AION).[32]

The optic disc appearance may help differentiate AION from optic neuritis (ON), although there are overlapping features. Optic disc stereo photos were reviewed by masked observers (87 AION and 68 ON).[33] Altitudinal disc swelling was more than three times more common in AION than in ON, although most discs were diffusely swollen. Most patients with AION had hemorrhages, whereas most ON cases did not. Almost all discs with ON had normal color or were hyperemic, and only 35% of discs with AION had pallid swelling. Pallid swelling was so rare in ON, however, that of discs with pallor, 93% had AION. Arterial attenuation was also much more typical of AION. AION was the clinical diagnosis in 82% of cases with altitudinal edema, 81% of the cases with disc hemorrhage, 93% of the cases with pallid edema, and 90% of the cases with arterial attenuation. A pale nerve with hemorrhage, regardless of type of edema, always represented AION (100%). A normal color nerve without hemorrhage reflected ON in 91% of the cases, increased from only 76% if hemorrhage was not considered. A hyperemic nerve with hemorrhage represented AION in 82% of cases, but if altitudinal edema was also present, AION incidence increased to 93%. B-scan ultrasonography has showed that ON may result in a much larger optic nerve diameter than AION and can be useful in differentiating between the two conditions.[34] Similarly, diffusion tensor imaging (DTI) measurement may serve as a biomarker of axonal and myelin damage in AION.[35] Jonas et al examined optic disc photographs of 157 patients with unilateral or bilateral NA-AION and concluded that cup-to-disc ratios were not affected by the disease process and the optic disc size was not related to the final visual acuity outcome.[36] Similarly, another study concluded that eyes with NA-AION have no difference in optic disc size when compared to controls; however, patients with NA-AION may have lower cup-to-disc ratios than the normal population.[37]

Some recent studies have demonstrated the use of optical coherence tomography (OCT) in assessment, diagnosis, and management of NA-AION.[38,39] Findings include increased peripapillary choroid thickness associated with optic disc edema and subretinal fluid on spectral domain OCT (SD-OCT) and macular ganglion cell inner plexiform layer thinning associated with visual field defect in Fourier domain OCT (FD-OCT).[40,41] Ganglion cell layer plus inner plexiform layer (GCL + IPL) thinning has been shown to be better than retinal nerve fiber layer (RNFL) thinning in indicating early structural loss in NA-AION.[42] In addition to GCL + IPL, ganglion cell complex thinning with Bruch's membrane opening enlargement and prelaminar tissue thickening have also been reported in the acute phase of patients presenting with NA-AION.[40,43,44,45,46,47,48,49,50] When comparing the amount of retinal ganglion cell (RGC) loss measured by OCT in patients with AION and patients with open-angle glaucoma (OAG), Danesh-Meyer et al found that AION patients have significantly different disc topography at a given level of RGC loss.[51] The authors describe that patients with AION have smaller cups, larger rims, less cup volume, and more rim volume when compared with OAG patients. Normal lamina cribrosa, anterior lamina cribrosa depth thickness, and choroidal thickness were observed in NA-AION eyes when compared to healthy controls.[52,53] In a prospective, observational case series, Hata et al performed OCT angiography (OCTA) of eyes with NA-AION, which showed that vessels in the peripapillary retina and optic disc were reduced.[54] The thickness abnormalities in RNFLs have been correlated with corresponding visual field abnormalities and may be used as adjunct evidence in diagnosing NA-AION.[55,56] Fluorescein angiography also typically shows delayed filling over the disc in ischemic optic disc edema, whereas optic disc edema from other causes does not demonstrate this filling delay.[57,58,59]

Ischemic optic neuropathy (ION) without acute disc edema is referred to as posterior ischemic optic neuropathy (PION). PION is an atypical presentation of ION, but it may occur in several conditions as listed in Box 4.2.

> ### Box 4.2 Conditions associated with posterior ischemic optic neuropathy
>
> - Atherosclerosis and arteriosclerosis.[60]
> - Severe hypotension or blood loss.
> - Diabetes.[61]
> - Collagen vascular disorders (e.g., systemic lupus erythematosus).
> - Giant cell (temporal) arteritis.[60]
> - Hematologic disorders.
> - Infection (e.g., *Aspergillus*, herpes zoster).
> - Internal carotid artery occlusion or dissection.[62,63]
> - Hypertensive urgency or emergency ("malignant hypertension").
> - Migraine.[64]
> - After surgical procedures, including cataract surgery (hypotension, anemia).[60,65]
> - Severe anemia.
> - Radiation therapy.
> - Thromboembolism (e.g., internal carotid artery disease).

Younger patients (younger than 40 years) with diabetes,[61,66] migraines, severe hypertension including preeclampsia, or oral contraceptive use may also develop ION. We consider the development of ION in patients younger than 40 years to be an atypical presentation.[67] A clinical presentation of AION may occur in young patients without any known vasculopathic risk factors and has been termed AION of the young (AIONY).

AIONY differs from typical AION in that recurrent attacks are more common than with typical NA-AION.

Bilateral simultaneous involvement may occur in NA-AION (up to 15% of cases), but we consider this also an atypical finding. Giant cell arteritis (GCA) and other causes of a bilateral optic neuropathy should be excluded in these cases.[68]

Diabetic papillopathy is probably an atypical form of AION described in diabetics who present with minimal visual symptoms. This entity usually resolves in weeks to months. The clinical features of diabetic papillopathy are outlined in Box 4.3.

> ### Box 4.3 Clinical features of diabetic papillopathy [26,69,70,71,72,73]
>
> - May be unilateral or bilateral (simultaneous or sequential).
> - May have relative afferent pupillary defect if unilateral or bilateral but asymmetric.
> - May be associated with type I or type II diabetes.
> - Disc swelling is mild to moderate and the disc is consistently hyperemic.
> - Disc edema usually resolves within 1 to 10 months.
> - Macular edema and capillary nonperfusion are frequent associated findings.
> - Small cup-to-disc ratio in uninvolved fellow eyes (the "disc at risk").
> - Significant (≥ 5 seconds) delay in fluorescein filling of all or a portion of the optic disc may occur.
> - Minimal if any visual symptoms.
> - May have enlarged blind spot or arcuate defect.
> - Residual visual loss due to associated macular edema and retinopathy.
> - Occasionally residual mild optic atrophy.

4.2 What Other Conditions Are Associated with Ischemic Optic Neuropathy?

ION has been reported in association with a number of systemic conditions listed in Box 4.4.

> ### Box 4.4 Conditions associated with anterior (and posterior) ischemic optic neuropathy
>
> **Systemic vasculopathy:**
> - Common:
>   - Hypertension.[3,31,74,75]
>   - Hypotension.
>   - Diabetes mellitus.[3,31,61,75]
>   - Arteriosclerosis, atherosclerosis, and ischemic heart disease.[31,60,75]
>   - Hypercholesterolemia.[75]
> - Uncommon:
>   - Female carrier of Fabry disease.[76]
>   - Takayasu arteritis.[77,78]
>   - Carotid occlusion and dissection.[62,63,79,80,81,82,83]
>   - Carotid artery hypoplasia.[84]
>   - Thromboangiitis obliterans.
>   - Giant cell arteritis.[85,86,87]
>   - Vasospasm[11,88]:
>   - Migraine.
>   - Raynaud disease.

Acute blood loss or hypotension[89,90,91,92,93,94,95,96]:
- Systemic inflammatory response syndrome (survivors of severe injuries).[92]
- Postsurgical[60,97]:
  - Cardiopulmonary bypass procedures.[98,99,100,101,102,103]
  - Lumbar spine surgery.[89,94,104,105,106,107,108,109,110,111,112,113]
  - Abdominal surgery.[114]
  - Radical neck dissection.[115,116,117,118,119,120,121]
  - Leg vein bypass surgery.[122]
  - Mitral valve surgery.
  - Nasal surgery (intranasal anesthetic).[123]
  - Cholecystectomy.
  - Parathyroidectomy.
  - Radical prostatectomy.[124]
  - Liver transplant.[125]
  - Coronary angiography.
- After treatment for malignant hypertension.[91]
- Hemodialysis.[91,126,127]
- Peritoneal dialysis.[128,129,130]
- Nocturnal hypotension.[31,93,131,132]
- Therapeutic phlebotomy.
- Cardiac arrest.

Surgical (nonhypotensive or nonanemic):
- Cataract surgery.[133,134,135]
- Laser in situ keratomileusis (LASIK).[136,137,138]
- Secondary intraocular lens implantation.
- After lower lid blepharoplasty.[139]
- Pars plana vitrectomy.[140]
- After general surgery without significant blood loss.
- Retinal surgery.

Infectious:
- Aspergillus.
- Herpes zoster.[141,142,143,144]
- Lyme disease.
- Recurrent herpes labialis.[17]
- Staphylococcal cavernous sinus thrombosis.
- Syphilis.
- Acquired immunodeficiency syndrome (AIDS).
- Elevated titers of immunoglobulin G (IgG) antibodies to Chlamydia pneumoniae.[145]

Inflammatory disorders[146]:
- Allergic vasculitis.
- Behçet disease.[147]
- Buerger disease.
- Eosinophilic granulomatosis with polyangiitis (Churg–Strauss syndrome).[148,149,150,151,152]
- Crohn disease.
- Mixed connective tissue disease.
- Myeloperoxidase antineutrophil cytoplasmic antibody (C-ANCA).[153]
- Polyarteritis nodosa.
- Polymyalgia rheumatic.[154]
- Postviral vasculitis.
- Relapsing polychondritis.[155]
- Rheumatoid arthritis.
- Sjögren syndrome.[156,157]
- Systemic lupus erythematosus.[158]
- Vogt–Koyanagi–Harada disease.[159]
- HLA-B27 associated anterior uveitis and ankylosing spondylitis.[160]

Ocular:
- Hyperopia.[161]
- Optic disc drusen.[162,163,164,165,166]
- Papilledema.
- Elevated intraocular pressure.[167,168,169]
- Acute angle-closure glaucoma.[170,171]
- Neovascular glaucoma.[172]
- Birdshot retinochoroidopathy.
- Uveitis.[173]
- Optic glioma.[174]
- Posterior vitreous detachment.[175]
- After intravitreal injection (reported with bevacizumab).[176]

Hematologic abnormalities:
- Anemia (e.g., iron deficiency anemia).[177,178]
- Hyperhomocysteinemia.[179,180,181]
- Antiphospholipid antibodies.[157,182,183,184,185]
- Antiphospholipid antibodies with factor V Leiden mutation.[186]
- Activated protein C resistance.[187]
- Decreased concentrations of protein C, protein S, or antithrombin III.[188]
- Factor V Leiden[189] and prothrombin gene heterozygosity.[190]
- Glucose-6-phosphate dehydrogenase (G-6-PD) deficiency syndrome.
- Hemolysis, Elevated Liver enzymes, and Low Platelet count (HELLP) syndrome.[191]
- Hereditary spherocytosis.[192]
- Leukemia.
- Lipid abnormalities.[193,194]
- Lupus anticoagulant.[195]
- Pernicious anemia.
- Polycythemia vera.[196,197]
- Sickle cell trait and disease.[198]
- Thrombocytopenic purpura.[199]
- Waldenström macroglobulinemia.

Embolic.[200]

Miscellaneous:
- Acute intermittent porphyria.
- Allergic disorders:
  - Serum sickness.
  - Bacille Calmette–Guérin (BCG) vaccination.
  - Urticaria.
  - Quincke edema.
- Cardiac valvular disease.[30]
- Cavernous sinus thrombosis.[201]
- Cervical discopathies and vasospasm.
- Favism.
- Gastrointestinal ulcers.[30]
- Graves disease.[202]
- Human lymphocyte antigen-A29.[18]
- Medications:

- ○ Interferon-alfa.[203,204,205,206,207,208]
- ○ Intracarotid carmustine.
- ○ Sumatriptan.[209]
- ○ Omeprazole.[210]
- ○ Amiodarone.[211]
- ○ Bevacizumab.[51]
- ○ Oxymetazoline nasal spray (nasal decongestant).[212]
- ○ Sildenafil.[213,214,215,216]
- Mitochondrial abnormalities.[217,218,219]
- Lymphoma and sepsis.[220]
- Light-chain amyloidosis.[221]
- Migraine.[209]
- Postimmunization.
- Radiation necrosis.[222,223]
- Renal failure and uremia.[224,225,226]
- Smoking.[15,29,194]
- Trauma.[227]
- After trans-Atlantic airplane journey.[228]
- Familial AION.[229,230,231]

4.3 What Clinical Features Are Atypical for Anterior Ischemic Optic Neuropathy?

There may be overlap in the clinical presentation of AION and other optic neuropathies, including ON.[22,232] Patients with any atypical AION features should undergo a complete evaluation to exclude other causes of an optic neuropathy (e.g., inflammatory, infiltrative, and compressive optic neuropathies; Box 4.5).

Box 4.5 Clinical features atypical for nonarteritic anterior ischemic optic neuropathy

- Age younger than 40 years.
- Bilateral simultaneous onset.
- Visual field defect not consistent with an optic neuropathy (e.g., bitemporal hemianopsia, homonymous hemianopsia).
- Lack of optic disc edema in the acute phase.
- Lack of relative afferent pupillary defect.
- Large cup-to-disc ratio.[233]
- Optic disc appearance of cupped disc after event (present in 2% of patients with NA-AION vs. 92% of patients with arteritic AION).[32]
- Lack of vasculopathic risk factors.
- Presence of premonitory symptoms of transient visual loss (amaurosis fugax).
- Progression of visual loss beyond 2 to 4 weeks.
- Recurrent episodes in the same eye.
- Anterior or posterior segment inflammation (e.g., vitreous cells).

Recurrence of NA-AION in the same eye is uncommon. Hayreh et al studied 594 consecutive patients with a diagnosis of NA-AION and found that recurrence occurred in the same eye in 45

patients (7.6%) with a median follow-up of 3.1 years.[234] Although it is uncommon for NA-AION to recur in the same eye, it may involve the fellow eye in 10 to 73% of cases.[235] Beri et al evaluated 438 patients with AION[236]; 388 had NA-AION and 50 had arteritic AION. The risk of bilateral involvement for the arteritic form was 1.9 times the risk for NA-AION. At 3 years, Beri et al calculated an incidence of bilateral NA-AION of 26%.[236] In patients with bilateral disease, some authors have noted that the final outcome between eyes is similar for acuity, color vision, and visual fields.[235] In another study, visual function in the second eye in patients with bilateral NA-AION correlated poorly with the first eye.[237] In this study, older patients (older than 50 years) with bilateral NA-AION retained better visual function in the second eye, whereas in younger patients the extent of visual loss in the second eye could not be predicted based on the visual loss in the first eye. Kupersmith et al also reported poor correlation of visual acuity and field defects in the second eye compared to the first involved eye.[238] Hayreh et al conducted another study where they also found large differences between the visual acuity and visual field findings of paired eyes at the initial and the final visit in patients with bilateral sequential NA-AION.[239] They concluded that it may not be possible to predict the visual acuity and visual field grade in the second eye based solely on the first.[239]

The visual loss in NA-AION is usually acute and remains relatively static, but may spontaneously improve in up to 42.7% of patients.[12,22,240,241,242] In up to 25% of patients, visual loss may be progressive over several weeks. In our opinion, gradual and progressive visual loss should prompt further evaluation, including neuroimaging, to exclude other causes of a continuing optic neuropathy (e.g., optic nerve sheath meningioma).

4.4 What Is the Evaluation and Treatment for AION?

Patients with typical features of AION (e.g., acute onset, unilateral visual loss, ipsilateral optic disc edema, older/aged patient) do not require neuroimaging (classes II–III, level B). The major entity that must be excluded in AION is GCA (see Chapter 5). An erythrocyte sedimentation rate, C-reactive protein, and other appropriate evaluation for GCA should be considered in cases of AION in patients older than 50 years (class II, level B). Patients with atypical features should be evaluated for other etiologies of an optic neuropathy (see Chapter 1, Box 1.5).

A retrospective cohort study showed that patients with NA-AION have a 3.35 times higher risk of developing a stroke than patients without NA-AION. Thus, the authors concluded a systemic survey for vasculopathies and control of modifiable risk factors should be performed to prevent future neurological consequences.[243] Another study used endothelium-dependent, flow-mediated vasodilation in patients with NA-AION and concluded there may be systemic vascular endothelial dysfunction in patients with NA-AION.[244] Further laboratory studies to investigate the presence of a hypercoagulable state could be considered in patients with NA-AION who do not have the typical risk factors, such as older age, diabetes, hypertension, or tobacco use, or in young patients with bilateral or recurrent attacks of NA-AION, but the data are conflicting (class III, level C). Some authors have recommended laboratory tests for a hypercoagulable state in the following patients: (1) young (younger than 45 years) patients with NA-AION, (2) NA-AION without a small cup-to-disc ratio ("disc at risk") in the fellow eye, (3) bilateral simultaneous NA-AION, (4) recurrent NA-AION in the same eye, (5) NA-AION in a patient with a previous history or family history of recurrent thrombotic events (class III, level U).[245,246] Hyperhomocysteinemia was discovered in two of 12 nondiabetic patients with NA-AION before the age of 50 years.[179] Both of these two patients had experienced NA-AION in both eyes with recurrent episodes (class III).

Unfortunately, although corticosteroids (systemic, retrobulbar, sub-Tenons), anticoagulation, dipyridamole, acetazolamide, hemodilution, vasodilators, vasopressors, atropine, norepinephrine, diphenylhydantoin, and hyperbaric oxygen have been tried in the past, there is no proven therapy for NA-AION.[247,248] The natural history of NA-AION in the past has been difficult to define. In the Ischemic Optic Neuropathy Decompression Trial (IONDT), there was an unexpectedly high rate of spontaneous (three or more lines from baseline at 6 months) improvement of 42.7% (class I, level A). This rate is higher than that noted in the literature on AION before 1989 (< 10%). In the literature since then, visual improvement rates as high as 33% have been reported.[2,22,249]

We believe that any future treatments for NA-AION will have to prove better than the natural history data of the IONDT. Most previously published reports on treatment for NA-AION are limited by retrospective design, nonstandardized methods of data collection or measurement, small sample sizes, and variable (usually relatively short) lengths of follow-up.

Medical control of underlying hypertension, diabetes, and other presumed etiologic vasculopathic risk factors (such as smoking cessation) has been recommended,[29,31] but no well-controlled data on the efficacy of such measures in reducing fellow-eye involvement exist (class III, level C). Despite these recommendations, Hayreh et al found there may be no direct association between NA-AION and tobacco smoking.[250] In addition, overaggressive control of arterial hypertension may be potentially dangerous in patients in whom acute and/or nocturnal hypotension is an underlying etiology for NA-AION (class III, level U).[31] Patients with malignant hypertension in whom the blood pressure is lowered too rapidly may also be at risk for the precipitation of NA-AION in the fellow eye. The occurrence of NA-ION cannot be easily explained by the presence of prothrombotic or atherosclerotic risk factors shift focus to the possibility that mitochondrial abnormalities may be important in the development of NA-ION. Based on these observations, testing for mitochondrial abnormalities may be warranted in NA-ION patients, especially the ones without a medical or family history of a thrombotic or vascular event.[217,251]

A component of a routine complete blood count, neutrophil-to-lymphocyte ratio (NLR) has also been shown to be negatively correlated with visual acuity in NA-AION, with the optimum NLR being 1.94.[252] There is potential use in monitoring this value to indicate the extent of inflammation in NA-AION.

In a small study, plasma endothelin-1, a potent vasoconstrictor, was noted to be significantly elevated (defined as > 2.3 pg/mL) in NA-AION patients compared to controls.[253] These levels may be a risk factor for NA-AION and may warrant further study.

4.5 Are Additional Studies (e.g., Noninvasive Carotid Doppler Studies, Cardiac Studies, Neuroimaging) Warranted in Patients with NA-AION?

Although Guyer et al reported a significantly higher incidence of cerebrovascular and cardiovascular disease in 200 patients with idiopathic AION.[254,255] Hayreh et al found no increased risk for subsequent cerebrovascular or cardiovascular disease.[31] Another study found no increased incidence of cerebrovascular or cardiovascular incidents in patients with NA-AION taking aspirin.[256] Some authors have found no increased incidence of generalized cerebral vascular disease on magnetic resonance imaging (MRI) of the head in nine patients with NA-AION, but Arnold et al reported an increased number of central nervous system white matter lesions on brain MRI in patients with NA-AION.[257] Fry et al found no significant difference in carotid stenosis in 15 patients with AION versus controls.[183] Several authors have reported no significant association between AION and extracranial carotid artery occlusive disease. AION has rarely been attributed to embolic disease.[200] A small study of transcranial Doppler did not identify microemboli in any of the 11 subjects with a recent history of NA-AION.[258] We do not perform additional noninvasive evaluation of the carotid or cardiac systems in patients with NA-AION unless there are other signs of carotid disease, such as ocular ischemic syndrome or retinal emboli, or a history of transient or persistent focal neurologic deficits (class III, level U).[200] We also consider MR angiography in patients with NA-AION with associated ipsilateral head or neck pain to evaluate for carotid artery dissection.[62,79] Neuroimaging studies of the head are not indicated in patients with typical unilateral NA-AION (classes II–III, level B).[257]

In recent years, an interesting link has been studied between obstructive sleep apnea and NA-AION.[259,260] Consider referring NA-AION patients for further sleep evaluation if they are high risk for this disorder.

4.6 Should the Patient with NA-AION Be Placed on Aspirin Therapy?

Aspirin is often given to patients following the development of NA-AION, but there does not seem to be any beneficial effect of treatment on eventual visual outcome.[261] Some authors, however, have suggested that aspirin therapy may reduce the risk of NA-AION in the fellow eye.[262,263] Sanderson et al performed a retrospective review of 101 patients with AION for over 3 years.[263] Fellow-eye involvement occurred in 33 patients, of whom 23 did not take aspirin (compared with 47 patients on aspirin out of 68 patients without fellow-eye involvement). These authors estimated a threefold reduction of second eye involvement ($p = 0.0005$) in the aspirin-treated group and concluded that aspirin therapy significantly reduces the relative risk of NA-AION in the fellow eye. Beck reported on the results of a survey (270 of 350 neuro-ophthalmologist respondents) that among 5,188 ophthalmologists, 60% usually or always prescribed aspirin (usually 325 mg/day), 6% prescribed aspirin about half the time, and 34% occasionally or never prescribed aspirin. Among 582 neurologists, the percentages were 71, 10, and 19%, respectively.[262] In a retrospective study of 431 patients, Beck et al found that the cumulative probability of NA-AION in the fellow eye was 7% in an aspirin group and 15% in a nonaspirin group and the 5-year cumulative probabilities were 17 and 20%, respectively.[262] This study thus suggests a possible short-term benefit of aspirin in reducing the risk of NA-AION in the fellow eye. Kupersmith et al found that aspirin taken two or more times per week decreased the incidence (17.5 vs. 53.5%) of the second-eye involvement in patients with unilateral NA-AION regardless of risk factors.[238] Salomon et al retrospectively evaluated 52 patients.[75] Second-eye involvement was noted in 8 of 16 patients (50%) who did not receive aspirin, in 3 of 8 patients (38%) who received 100 mg/day aspirin, and in only 5 of 28 patients (18%) who received aspirin 325 mg/day. Moreover, the mean time to second-eye involvement was 63 months in patients who did not receive aspirin, versus 156 months in patients who received aspirin 325 mg/day. The authors concluded that aspirin 325 mg/day may be effective in reducing the frequency of second-eye involvement in NA-AION.[75] In light of the possible association between NA-AION and cerebrovascular and cardiac vasculopathic risk factors (e.g., hypertension, diabetes), as well as the recognized reduction in morbidity and mortality for patients with cerebrovascular disease and cardiac disease (e.g., myocardial infarction)[264] treated with aspirin, our current practice (until a prospective trial is performed) is to offer oral aspirin therapy to patients (who have no contraindications to aspirin) with NA-AION (classes II–III, level U).[265] However, other studies and reviews have been mixed in their recommendations regarding aspirin.[266,267]

4.7 Are There Other Treatments for NA-AION?

A pilot clinical trial on the efficacy of levodopa in NA-AION was published with interesting results. Johnson et al reported a prospective, randomized, double-masked, placebo-controlled, clinical trial of 20 subjects with NA-AION of 30 months' mean duration.[16] Subjects were randomized to low-dose levodopa and carbidopa or placebo for 3 weeks. At 12 weeks, the levodopa group was provided a higher, conventional dose of levodopa and carbidopa for an additional 3 weeks. At 12 weeks, the levodopa group experienced a significant ($p = 0.16$) mean difference in improvement of visual acuity of 5.9 letters from the placebo group, and at 24 weeks the treatment effect remained ($p = 0.36$). There was a mean gain of 7.5 letters in the levodopa group compared to the placebo group, and three subjects experienced a doubling of the visual angle, as denoted by a gain of at least 15 letters. No significant improvement was noted for color vision or visual field (classes II–III, level U).

In a follow-up study, Johnson et al further studied the effect of levodopa on visual function in patients treated within 45 days of onset of NA-AION.[268] In a nonrandomized, retrospective study involving 37 patients, 18 were treated with 100-mg levodopa/25-mg carbidopa, whereas 19 patients served as controls.

The proportions of patients with worsened, unchanged, and improved visual acuity at 6 months were compared in the two groups. A higher proportion of the patients in the levodopa group had improved visual acuity with a corresponding lower proportion having worsened acuity as compared to control patients. Ten of the 13 patients (76.9%) in the levodopa group with 20/40 visual acuity or worse at baseline had improved visual acuity at 6 months, and none of the 18 patients had worsened acuity. In contrast, 3 of 10 control patients (30%) with 20/40 visual acuity or worse at baseline had improved visual acuity at 6 months, and 3 of 19 control patients (15.8%) had worsened visual acuity. The proportion of patients with worsened, unchanged, and improved visual fields at 6 months was compared for the two groups and there was no significant difference. The authors concluded that patients treated with levodopa within 45 days of onset of NA-AION were more likely to experience improvement and less likely to have worsened visual acuity than untreated patients.[268]

Unfortunately, there are many flaws in this latter study, and the conclusions are controversial and may well be erroneous for the following reasons (classes II–III, level U).[269] Cox[269] summarized the controversial points:

1. The study was retrospective, unplanned, nonrandomized, and based on a small sample size.
2. The treatment and control groups were very different, mainly in baseline visual functions. The control group actually had better mean acuities and mean field scores at baseline and the imbalance between the groups at baseline makes any results essentially uninterpretable.
3. The study was not randomized, and selection and measurement bias may have been present.
4. The patients placed on the drug may have expected a better visual outcome and, thus, "tested better" than the nontreated group.
5. The statistical analysis used was flawed.

Simsek et al conducted a randomized placebo-controlled trial with $n = 24$ patients to assess the effectiveness of levodopa/carbidopa in treating NA-AION. They found no improvement in visual acuity, color vision, or visual fields.[270] A later study by Lyttle et al performed a retrospective study on 59 patients, and found that the patients administered levodopa/carbidopa had improved visual acuity but not visual fields.[271] However, the retrospective nature of the study and the unequal grouping of patients limits the results of this study as well. Upon a review of these studies, a review by Razeghinejad et al concluded that for a recommendation to treat NA-AION with levodopa to be put into place, larger, randomized, placebo-controlled, double-masked studies need to be performed.[272] It is not the practice of the authors to recommend levodopa for NA-AION based on the available evidence (classes II–III, level U).

Corticosteroids may also have a role in treatment of NA-ION, although the evidence is conflicted. Hayreh et al conducted a study to determine the effect of systemic corticosteroid therapy on NA-AION.[273] The authors found that NA-AION eyes treated with corticosteroids during the acute phase resulted in a significantly higher probability of improvement in visual acuity (VA, hereafter) and visual field (VF) than in the untreated group. When Rebolleda et al examined VA and VFs of 10 eyes with NA-ION treated in the acute phase with systemic corticosteroids, they found conflicting results where the treatment group did not show any beneficial effect when compared to the control group.[274] Similarly, another study examined VA and VF defects of 24 eyes affected by NA-ION treated with intravenous (IV) corticosteroids compared with a control group of 24 eyes at 1, 3, and 6 months. The authors found again that VA and VF defects did not improve in the treatment group when compared to the control group.[275] A recent randomized clinical trial performed by Pakravan et al evaluated 90 eyes diagnosed with NA-AION treated with either normobaric oxygen, corticosteroid, or placebo for VA, VF, and peripapillary RNFL thickness. The results showed no statistical difference in structural and functional outcomes between the three groups.[276]

A retrospective study performed by Radoi et al may show evidence for intravitreal triamcinolone acetonide (IVTA) injections for treatment of NA-AION. Thirty-six patient charts were evaluated for NA-AION where 21 patients had received 4-mg IVTA and 15 patients were not treated. VA significantly improved at the 6-month follow-up in the treated group.[277] Kaderli et al[278] performed a small study comparing four eyes affected by NA-AION treated with IVTA to an untreated control group of six eyes affected by NA-AION. They found that the treated group had improved VA and rapid resolution of optic disc edema when compared to the control group at the 1st and 3rd week follow-ups and 9-month follow-up.[278] Case reports have also been described where patients have marked improvement in VA and VFs after IVTA treatment.[279,280] Despite these results, other case reports show minimal and even decreased VA in patients with NA-AION treated with IVTA.[281]

Erythropoietin injections have also been utilized for treatment of NA-AION. Modarres et al performed a prospective interventional study where 31 eyes with NA-AION received 2,000 units of intravitreal erythropoietin injection within 1 month of onset of the disease. VA improved in 27 eyes (87%), and 17 eyes (54.8%) had three or more lines of visual improvement 6 months after the injection. The authors also report that patients did not have any decline in VA. Despite these results, more studies need to be performed to delineate the effects of erythropoietin.[282]

Even intravitreal antivascular endothelial growth factor (anti-VEGF) injections have been utilized for treatment of NA-AION. One case report noted that bevacizumab was used in a patient, with improvement in vision from count fingers to 20/70.[283] Rootman et al performed a nonrandomized controlled clinical trial where 1.25 mg of intravitreal bevacizumab was injected in 17 new-onset NA-AION eyes. These patients were compared with 8 control eyes undergoing no intervention at 1, 3, and 6 months.[284] The authors found no statistically significant difference between the groups in VF, VA, or optic nerve thickness assessed by OCT. In another study, intravitreal ranibizumab was injected in 17 NA-AION eyes, which resulted in visual gain in 14 eyes. However, all 17 eyes still showed a mean RNFL thickness decrease at follow-up.[285] Furthermore, in a rat model, Huang et al reported that anti-VEGF did not have a neuroprotective effect in NA-AION.[286] Because of conflicting evidence and lack of well-controlled, randomized trials, further studies are required to establish the efficacy of anti-VEGF agents.

Low-density lipoprotein (LDL) apheresis in patients with NA-AION may help accelerate vision recovery.[287,288,289] Eleven patients with NA-AION underwent three sessions of LDL apheresis with steroid treatment, which showed significant vision increase from a mean of 3.7/10 to 7.9/10 after the third session.[288] Furthermore, scotoma caused by NA-AION regressed in all patients at the first session and continued to regress in five more patients after the third session. A prospective study of 20 patients comparing LDL apheresis plus conventional therapy to conventional therapy alone found that mean deviation improved significantly at discharge in the apheresis group, but this difference was no longer present at 6 months.[290]

Dabigatran has also been associated with recovery in visual function in one patient with NA-AION.[291] After failure of standard corticosteroid treatment, two doses of 110 mg of dabigatran etexilate were administered to a female with NA-AION, which led to prompt improvement in VA.[291]

Enhanced extracorporeal counterpulsation (EECP) therapy, a process that increases circulatory flow in the ophthalmic and central retinal arteries, may also be a noninvasive and safe method to improve VA and fields in patients with NA-AION.[292] Zhu et al performed EECP on 16 patients with unilateral NA-AION and found a statistically significant improvement in VA and VF after 12 1-hour treatments.[292] In another study, Yang et al retrospectively analyzed the effect of EECP therapy in a mix of ocular ischemic diseases accompanied by carotid artery stenosis. They found significantly improved VA, VFs, and optical hemodynamics in the patients who received EECP.[293] However, since this study was not focused on a mix of patients and not NA-AION specifically, the implications of these results are not clear.

After reports of vision improvement with diphenylhydantoin in patients with NA-AION, Ellenberger et al conducted a double-blinded, placebo-controlled trial treating 15 patients with diphenylhydantoin.[294] Their results showed no benefit from the drug in VA and fields.

Hyperbaric oxygen has been proposed to reduce the damage of the injured axons in NA-AION by increasing tissue oxygen. Arnold et al found no significant difference in the outcome of patients treated with hyperbaric oxygen versus the untreated control patients. This study was a nonrandomized trial with a small sample size.[247] In a single masked randomized clinical trial, Pakravan et al compared the effects of high-dose steroids against normobaric oxygen therapy against placebo in 90 patients with recent-onset NA-AION, finding no significant improvement from either of these two treatment options compared with the placebo group.[295]

A radial optic neurotomy may reduce the presumed "compartment syndrome" in NA-AION. This technique, previously reported in the treatment of central retinal vein occlusion (CRVO), involves making a transvitreal stab incision at the nasal margin of the optic disc, which opens the scleral canal and relieves the pressure being exerted on the optic nerve.[296] Radial optic neurotomy was described in the case of an 82-year-old male with disc drusen bilateral vision loss and severe VF defects from NA-AION. The neurotomy was performed in the more severely affected eye and there was significant postoperative improvement in VF and acuity.[297] There is debate if this was actually just the natural course of improvement in NA-AION. A study by Soheilian et al showed improvement in six of seven study eyes; however, one patient developed peripapillary choroidal neovascularization.[298] These results should be taken with caution due to the small sample size and the noncontrolled and nonrandomized nature of the study.[270]

Modarres et al studied 16 patients that exhibited partial posterior vitreous detachment (PVD) and underwent pars plana vitrectomy.[299] They conclude that vitreous traction from partial PVD may by a precipitating factor in NA-AION in small discs, and vitrectomy may be indicated. However, replies to this study commented that partial PVD was not seen in many other cases of NA-AION with small discs, that there are significant risks to vitrectomy, and that the pathophysiological explanation is not sound.[300,301,302]

There has been an interest in investigating neuroprotective agents for the treatment of NA-AION. Brimonidine has been hypothesized to assist in treatment of NA-AION due to its neuroprotective effects found in rodents.[303,304] Wilhelm et al conducted a 3-month, double-masked, randomized, placebo-controlled clinical trial on 36 patients older than 40 years with NA-AION.[305] The treatment group received 0.2% brimonidine tartrate and had no statistically significant improvement or worsening in VA at 12 weeks after initial visit compared to the placebo group. In an earlier study, Fazzone et al examined 14 patients with NA-AION and also determined that brimonidine provides no beneficial result.[306]

Citicoline, another neuroprotective agent, was studied in 26 patients with 14 receiving 1,600 mg/day for 60 days.[307] Improvement was seen in pattern electroretinogram, visual evoked potentials, and VA measurements. Another small study with 13 patients administered intravitreal injections of a Rho-kinase inhibitor, fasudil.[308] This agent is believed to be neuroprotective by increasing optic nerve blood flow via suppressing vasoconstriction. Patients showed an average improvement of six lines over a 1-month period. Other neuroprotective agents, N-methyl-D-aspartate receptor antagonist (memantine) and minocycline, have also been proposed for ION treatment for its neuroprotective effects. However, there have not yet been substantial studies regarding their effects on NA-AION.

Additional studies for neuroprotective agents in NA-AION are ongoing. The Neuro-Ophthalmology Research Disease Investigator Consortium (ClinicalTrials.gov: NCT02341560) is actively recruiting patients for a phase III double-masked, randomized, and sham-controlled multicenter trial using QPI-1007 (Quark Pharmaceuticals, Fremont, CA). This agent, administered as a single intravitreal injection, is a small interfering ribonucleic acid (siRNA) that temporarily inhibits the expression caspase-2-preventing apoptosis.[309,310]

Further research on rodent models has shown some promise in the evaluation of new neuroprotective techniques. Optic disc edema and RGC death were decreased when L-arginine was administered during the acute stages of an induced NA-AION. In the future, this may decrease the severity of the anatomical changes and recurrence in the fellow eye. An inflammatory modulator, 15-deoxy 12,14-delta prostaglandin J_2 (PGJ_2), binds and activates the peroxisome proliferator-activated receptor gamma (PPAR-γ) and downregulates nuclear factor kappa B (NF-κB).[311, 312,313] A single intravitreal injection has shown to decrease edema and increase RGC preservation in rodent models[312,313]

4.8 Does Optic Nerve Sheath Fenestration Improve Visual Outcomes in NA-AION?

Initial reports of visual improvement following optic nerve sheath fenestration (ONSF) for NA-AION were encouraging, but anecdotal.[101,314,315,316] Other reports followed with mixed results.[9,101,249,314,316,317,318,319,320,321,322,323,324,325,326] Subsequently, a

well-designed, masked, prospective, randomized IONDT at 25 clinical centers was initiated with the support of the National Eye Institute.[12] The study inclusion criteria were as follows: clinical syndrome consistent with NA-AION (e.g., acute, unilateral visual loss, relative afferent pupillary defect, swollen optic nerve, etc.); age greater than 50 years; visual symptoms for less than 14 days from onset; and VA of 20/64 or worse. Patients were randomly assigned to either ONSF (119 patients) or a control group (125 patients). Experienced protocol-certified study surgeons performed all the surgeries. The primary outcome measure was a three or more line improvement of VA after 6 months, and VF mean deviation on the Humphrey Field Analyzer (Program 24–2) was a secondary outcome measure. Recruitment was halted in September 1994 on the recommendation of the Data and Safety Monitoring Committee. The clinical characteristics of the patients recruited are summarized in ▶ Table 4.1. After 6 months, 32.6% of the ONSF (surgery) group had improved three or more lines of

Table 4.1 Characteristics of patients with nonarteritic anterior ischemic optic neuropathy eligible for the ischemic Optic Neuropathy Decompression Trial

Earliest symptoms	
• Intermittent blurring	5.0%
• Blurred vision	36.1%
• Scotoma	45.4%
• Complete loss of vision	3.8%
Optic disc of affected eye	
• Swollen	100.0%
• Diffuse	75.4%
• Focal	24.6%
• Disc or retinal hemorrhage	71.8%
• Exudates	6.5%
• Abnormal retinal vasculature	19.1%
Optic disc nonstudy eye	
• Pallor	22.5%
• Swollen	0.5%

Note: All percentages = randomized + nonrandomized patients.
• Four hundred twenty patients (258 randomized; 162 not randomized).
• Sixty-two percent men; 95% white.
• Mean age at onset 66.0 (peak age range 60–69).
• Hypertension 47%; diabetes 24%.
• Forty-two percent recalled onset of visual symptoms within 2 hours of awakening.
• Initial visual acuity (VA) 20/20 to light perception (LP), with 49% patients better than 20/64, and 34% 20/200 or worse.
• Mean Westergren erythrocyte sedimentation rate (ESR) 18.4 with 9% greater than 40.
• Nonrandomized patients were younger; 72% were male, and had lower prevalence of hypertension and diabetes.
• Forty-five percent of patients reported worsening (subjective) of vision between onset and baseline examination.
• Twenty-nine percent of eligible patients with baseline VA greater than 20/64 had documented progression to 20/64 or worse during a 30-day period.
• Fifteen percent of randomized patients smoked or discontinued smoking less than 1 year before onset.

Based on The Ischemic Optic Neuropathy Decompression Trial Research Group. Optic nerve decompression surgery for nonarteritic anterior ischemic optic neuropathy (NAION) is not effective and may be harmful. JAMA. 1995; 273(8):625–632

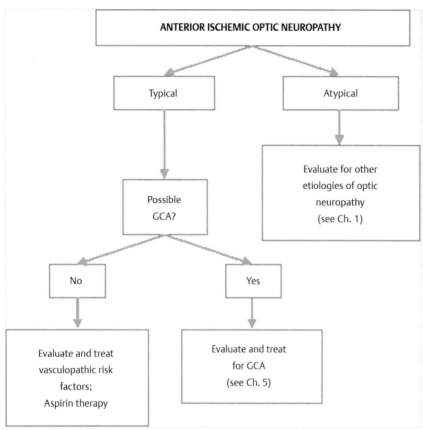

Fig. 4.1 Evaluation of anterior ischemic optic neuropathy.

VA compared with 42.7% of the control group, but 23.9% of the ONSF group had lost three or more lines of VA compared with only 12.4% of the control group. Likewise, VF data confirmed a lack of benefit for surgery. The 3-, 12-, and 24-month data confirmed the findings of the 6-month data.[327] In addition, there was no indication of benefit from ONSF in the subgroup of patients with progressive visual loss. The authors concluded that "ONSF is not effective and may be harmful in NA-AION,"[12] but were careful to state that they could "offer no recommendation regarding the safety and efficacy of this surgery for other conditions."[12] We agree that ONSF should not be performed for NA-AION (class I, level A).[12,328,329,330] The VFs at the 12-month follow-up in the IONDT-enrolled patients did not change significantly from baseline. The authors also concluded that "a VF defect in the non-study eye at baseline was not associated with development of NA-AION during follow-up compared with eyes with normal fields."[218]

Our approach to NA-AION is outlined in ▶ Fig. 4.1.

References

[1] Swartz NG, Beck RW, Savino PJ, et al. Pain in anterior ischemic optic neuropathy. J Neuroophthalmol. 1995; 15(1):9–10

[2] Arnold AC, Hepler RS. Natural history of nonarteritic anterior ischemic optic neuropathy. J Neuroophthalmol. 1994; 14(2):66–69

[3] Feldon SE. Anterior ischemic optic neuropathy: trouble waiting to happen. Ophthalmology. 1999; 106(4):651–652

[4] Friedland S, Winterkorn JM, Burde RM. Luxury perfusion following anterior ischemic optic neuropathy. J Neuroophthalmol. 1996; 16(3):163–171

[5] Gerling J, Jancknecht P, Kommerell G. Orbital pain in optic neuritis and anterior ischemic optic neuropathy. Neuroophthalmology. 1998; 19:93–99

[6] Gerling J, Meyer JH, Kommerell G. Visual field defects in optic neuritis and anterior ischemic optic neuropathy: distinctive features. Graefes Arch Clin Exp Ophthalmol. 1998; 236(3):188–192

[7] Grosvenor T, Malinovsky V, Gelvin J, Tonekaboni K. Diagnosis and management of temporal arteritis: a review and case report. Optom Vis Sci. 1993; 70(9):771–777

[8] Hattenhauer MG, Leavitt JA, Hodge DO, Grill R, Gray DT. Incidence of nonarteritic anterior ischemic optic neuropathy. Am J Ophthalmol. 1997; 123(1):103–107

[9] Hayreh SS. The role of optic nerve sheath fenestration in management of anterior ischemic optic neuropathy. Arch Ophthalmol. 1990; 108(8):1063–1065

[10] Hayreh SS. Acute ischemic disorders of the optic nerve: pathogenesis, clinical manifestations, and management. Ophthalmol Clin North Am. 1996; 9:407–442

[11] Hayreh SS. Anterior ischemic optic neuropathy. Clin Neurosci. 1997; 4(5):251–263

[12] The Ischemic Optic Neuropathy Decompression Trial Research Group. Optic nerve decompression surgery for nonarteritic anterior ischemic optic neuropathy (NAION) is not effective and may be harmful. JAMA. 1995; 273(8):625–632

[13] Ischemic Optic Neuropathy Decompression Trial Research Group. Characteristics of patients with nonarteritic anterior ischemic optic neuropathy eligible for the Ischemic Optic Neuropathy Decompression Trial. Arch Ophthalmol. 1996; 114(11):1366–1374

[14] Johnson LN, Arnold AC. Incidence of nonarteritic and arteritic anterior ischemic optic neuropathy. Population-based study in the state of Missouri and Los Angeles County, California. J Neuroophthalmol. 1994; 14(1):38–44

[15] Johnson LN, Botelho PJ, Kuo HC. Is smoking a risk factor for NAAION? Ophthalmology. 1994; 101(8):1322–1324

[16] Johnson LN, Gould TJ, Krohel GB. Effect of levodopa and carbidopa on recovery of visual function in patients with nonarteritic anterior ischemic optic neuropathy of longer than six months' duration. Am J Ophthalmol. 1996; 121(1):77–83

[17] Johnson LN, Krohel GB, Allen SD, Mozayeni R. Recurrent herpes labialis as a potential risk factor for nonarteritic anterior ischemic optic neuropathy. J Natl Med Assoc. 1996; 88(6):369–373

[18] Johnson LN, Kuo HC, Arnold AC. HLA-A29 as a potential risk factor for nonarteritic anterior ischemic optic neuropathy. Am J Ophthalmol. 1993; 115(4):540–542 (letter)

[19] Kay MC. Ischemic optic neuropathy. Neurol Clin. 1991; 9(1):115–129

[20] Lessell S. Nonarteritic anterior ischemic optic neuropathy: enigma variations. Arch Ophthalmol. 1999; 117(3):386–388

[21] Moro F, Doro D, Mantovani E, Sala M. Ischemic optic neuropathies. Metab Pediatr Syst Ophthalmol (1985). 1990; 13(2–4):75–78

[22] Rizzo JF, III, Lessell S. Optic neuritis and ischemic optic neuropathy. Overlapping clinical profiles. Arch Ophthalmol. 1991; 109(12):1668–1672

[23] Sawle GV, James CB, Russell RW. The natural history of non-arteritic anterior ischaemic optic neuropathy. J Neurol Neurosurg Psychiatry. 1990; 53(10): 830–833

[24] Gordon RN, Burde RM, Slamovits T. Asymptomatic optic disc edema. J Neuroophthalmol. 1997; 17(1):29–32

[25] Tomsak RL, Zakov ZN. Nonarteritic anterior ischemic optic neuropathy with macular edema: visual improvement and fluorescein angiographic characteristics. J Neuroophthalmol. 1998; 18(3):166–168

[26] Burde RM. Optic disk risk factors for nonarteritic anterior ischemic optic neuropathy. Am J Ophthalmol. 1993; 116(6):759–764

[27] Lavin PJ. Optic disk risk factors for nonarteritic anterior ischemic optic neuropathy. Am J Ophthalmol. 1994; 117(6):822

[28] Salomon O, Huna-Baron R, Kurtz S, et al. Analysis of prothrombotic and vascular risk factors in patients with nonarteritic anterior ischemic optic neuropathy. Ophthalmology. 1999; 106(4):739–742

[29] Chung SM, Gay CA, McCrary JA, III. Nonarteritic ischemic optic neuropathy. The impact of tobacco use. Ophthalmology. 1994; 101(4):779–782

[30] Hayreh SS, Joos KM, Podhajsky PA, Long CR. Systemic diseases associated with nonarteritic anterior ischemic optic neuropathy. Am J Ophthalmol. 1994; 118(6):766–780

[31] Hayreh SS, Zimmerman MB, Podhajsky P, Alward WLM. Nocturnal arterial hypotension and its role in optic nerve head and ocular ischemic disorders. Am J Ophthalmol. 1994; 117(5):603–624

[32] Danesh-Meyer HV, Savino PJ, Sergott RC. The prevalence of cupping in end-stage arteritic and nonarteritic anterior ischemic optic neuropathy. Ophthalmology. 2001; 108(3):593–598

[33] Warner JEA, Lessell S, Rizzo JF, III, Newman NJ. Does optic disc appearance distinguish ischemic optic neuropathy from optic neuritis? Arch Ophthalmol. 1997; 115(11):1408–1410

[34] Dehghani A, Giti M, Akhlaghi MR, Karami M, Salehi F. Ultrasonography in distinguishing optic neuritis from nonarteritic anterior ischemic optic neuropathy. Adv Biomed Res. 2012; 1:3

[35] Wang MY, Qi PH, Shi DP. Diffusion tensor imaging of the optic nerve in subacute anterior ischemic optic neuropathy at 3 T. AJNR Am J Neuroradiol. 2011; 32(7):1188–1194

[36] Jonas JB, Hayreh SS, Tao Y, Papastathopoulos KI, Rensch F. Optic nerve head change in non-arteritic anterior ischemic optic neuropathy and its influence on visual outcome. PLoS One. 2012; 7(5):e37499

[37] Contreras I, Rebolleda G, Noval S, Muñoz-Negrete FJ. Optic disc evaluation by optical coherence tomography in nonarteritic anterior ischemic optic neuropathy. Invest Ophthalmol Vis Sci. 2007; 48(9):4087–4092

[38] Han S, Jung JJ, Kim US. Differences between non-arteritic anterior ischemic optic neuropathy and open angle glaucoma with altitudinal visual field defect. Korean J Ophthalmol. 2015; 29(6):418–423

[39] Balogh Z, Kasza M, Várdai J, et al. Analysis of optic disc damage by optical coherence tomography in terms of therapy in non-arteritic anterior ischemic optic neuropathy. Int J Ophthalmol. 2016; 9(9):1352–1354

[40] Han M, Zhao C, Han QH, Xie S, Li Y. Change of retinal nerve layer thickness in non-arteritic anterior ischemic optic neuropathy revealed by Fourier domain optical coherence tomography. Curr Eye Res. 2016; 41(8):1076–1081

[41] Yu C, Ho JK, Liao YJ. Subretinal fluid is common in experimental non-arteritic anterior ischemic optic neuropathy. Eye (Lond). 2014; 28(12): 1494–1501

[42] Kupersmith MJ, Garvin MK, Wang JK, Durbin M, Kardon R. Retinal ganglion cell layer thinning within one month of presentation for non-arteritic anterior ischemic optic neuropathy. Invest Ophthalmol Vis Sci. 2016; 57(8): 3588–3593

[43] De Dompablo E, García-Montesinos J, Muñoz-Negrete FJ, Rebolleda G. Ganglion cell analysis at acute episode of nonarteritic anterior ischemic optic neuropathy to predict irreversible damage. A prospective study. Graefes Arch Clin Exp Ophthalmol. 2016; 254(9):1793–1800

[44] Erlich-Malona N, Mendoza-Santiesteban CE, Hedges TR, III, Patel N, Monaco C, Cole E. Distinguishing ischaemic optic neuropathy from optic neuritis by ganglion cell analysis. Acta Ophthalmol. 2016; 94(8):e721–e726

[45] Rebolleda G, García-Montesinos J, De Dompablo E, Oblanca N, Muñoz-Negrete FJ, González-López JJ. Bruch's membrane opening changes and lamina cribrosa displacement in non-arteritic anterior ischaemic optic neuropathy. Br J Ophthalmol. 2017; 101(2):143–149

[46] Fard MA, Afzali M, Abdi P, Yasseri M, Ebrahimi KB, Moghimi S. Comparison of the pattern of macular ganglion cell-inner plexiform layer defect between ischemic optic neuropathy and open-angle glaucoma. Invest Ophthalmol Vis Sci. 2016; 57(3):1011–1016

[47] Akbari M, Abdi P, Fard MA, et al. Retinal ganglion cell loss precedes retinal nerve fiber thinning in nonarteritic anterior ischemic optic neuropathy. J Neuroophthalmol. 2016; 36(2):141–146

[48] Park SW, Ji YS, Heo H. Early macular ganglion cell-inner plexiform layer analysis in non-arteritic anterior ischemic optic neuropathy. Graefes Arch Clin Exp Ophthalmol. 2016; 254(5):983–989

[49] Larrea BA, Iztueta MG, Indart LM, Alday NM. Early axonal damage detection by ganglion cell complex analysis with optical coherence tomography in nonarteritic anterior ischaemic optic neuropathy. Graefes Arch Clin Exp Ophthalmol. 2014; 252(11):1839–1846

[50] Aggarwal D, Tan O, Huang D, Sadun AA. Patterns of ganglion cell complex and nerve fiber layer loss in nonarteritic ischemic optic neuropathy by Fourier-domain optical coherence tomography. Invest Ophthalmol Vis Sci. 2012; 53(8):4539–4545

[51] Danesh-Meyer HV, Boland MV, Savino PJ, et al. Optic disc morphology in open-angle glaucoma compared with anterior ischemic optic neuropathies. Invest Ophthalmol Vis Sci. 2010; 51(4):2003–2010

[52] Fard MA, Afzali M, Abdi P, et al. Optic nerve head morphology in nonarteritic anterior ischemic optic neuropathy compared to open-angle glaucoma. Invest Ophthalmol Vis Sci. 2016; 57(11):4632–4640

[53] Gonul S, Gedik S, Koktekir BE, Yavuzer K, Okudan S. Evaluation of choroidal thickness in non-arteritic anterior ischaemic optic neuropathy at the acute and chronic stages. Neuroophthalmology. 2016; 40(4):181–187

[54] Hata M, Oishi A, Muraoka Y, et al. Structural and functional analyses in nonarteritic anterior ischemic optic neuropathy: optical coherence tomography angiography study. J Neuroophthalmol. 2017; 37(2):140–148

[55] Deleón-Ortega J, Carroll KE, Arthur SN, Girkin CA. Correlations between retinal nerve fiber layer and visual field in eyes with nonarteritic anterior ischemic optic neuropathy. Am J Ophthalmol. 2007; 143(2):288–294

[56] Contreras I, Noval S, Rebolleda G, Muñoz-Negrete FJ. Follow-up of nonarteritic anterior ischemic optic neuropathy with optical coherence tomography. Ophthalmology. 2007; 114(12):2338–2344

[57] Arnold AC, Badr MA, Hepler RS. Fluorescein angiography in nonischemic optic disc edema. Arch Ophthalmol. 1996; 114(3):293–298

[58] Arnold AC, Hepler RS. Fluorescein angiography in acute nonarteritic anterior ischemic optic neuropathy. Am J Ophthalmol. 1994; 117(2):222–230

[59] Segato T, Piermarocchi S, Midena E. The role of fluorescein angiography in the interpretation of optic nerve head diseases. Metab Pediatr Syst Ophthalmol (1985). 1990; 13(2–4):111–114

[60] Sadda SR, Nee M, Miller NR, Biousse V, Newman NJ, Kouzis A. Clinical spectrum of posterior ischemic optic neuropathy. Am J Ophthalmol. 2001; 132(5):743–750

[61] Inoue M, Tsukahara Y. Vascular optic neuropathy in diabetes mellitus. Jpn J Ophthalmol. 1997; 41(5):328–331

[62] Biousse V, Touboul P-J, D'Anglejan-Chatillon J, Lévy C, Schaison M, Bousser MG. Ophthalmologic manifestations of internal carotid artery dissection. Am J Ophthalmol. 1998; 126(4):565–577

[63] Kerty E. The ophthalmology of internal carotid artery dissection. Acta Ophthalmol Scand. 1999; 77(4):418–421

[64] Lee AG, Brazis PW, Miller NR. Posterior ischemic optic neuropathy associated with migraine. Headache. 1996; 36(8):506–510

[65] Luscavage LE, Volpe NJ, Liss R. Posterior ischemic optic neuropathy after uncomplicated cataract extraction. Am J Ophthalmol. 2001; 132(3):408–409

[66] Jacobson DM, Vierkant RA, Belongia EA. Nonarteritic anterior ischemic optic neuropathy. A case-control study of potential risk factors. Arch Ophthalmol. 1997; 115(11):1403–1407

[67] Rinaldi G, Pastori G, Ammirati M, Bellavitis A. Considerations upon a non-typical anterior ischemic optic neuropathy. Metab Pediatr Syst Ophthalmol (1985). 1990; 13(2–4):92–95

[68] Hayreh SS, Podhajsky PA, Zimmerman B. Occult giant cell arteritis: ocular manifestations. Am J Ophthalmol. 1998; 125(4):521–526

[69] Arnold AC, Petrovich M. Diabetic papillopathy: clinical features and fluorescein angiographic evidence of optic disc ischemia. Presented at the 23rd annual meeting of the North American Neuro-Ophthalmology Society, Keystone, CO, February 9–13, 1997

[70] Katz B. Disc swelling in an adult diabetic patient. Surv Ophthalmol. 1990; 35(2):158–163

[71] Keely KA, Yip B. Diabetic papillopathy: two case reports in individuals with adult onset diabetes mellitus. J Am Optom Assoc. 1997; 68(9):595–603

[72] Regillo CD, Brown GC, Savino PJ, et al. Diabetic papillopathy. Patient characteristics and fundus findings. Arch Ophthalmol. 1995; 113(7):889–895

[73] Vaphiades MS, Regillo CD, Arnold AC. The disk edema dilemma. Surv Ophthalmol. 2002; 47(2):183–188

[74] Hayreh SS. Anterior ischaemic optic neuropathy. Differentiation of arteritic from non-arteritic type and its management. Eye (Lond). 1990; 4(Pt 1):25–41

[75] Salomon O, Huna-Baron R, Steinberg DM, Kurtz S, Seligsohn U. Role of aspirin in reducing the frequency of second eye involvement in patients with non-arteritic anterior ischaemic optic neuropathy. Eye (Lond). 1999; 13 Pt 3a:357–359

[76] Abe H, Sakai T, Sawaguchi S, et al. Ischemic optic neuropathy in a female carrier with Fabry disease. Ophthalmologica. 1992; 205(2):83–88

[77] Schmidt MH, Fox AJ, Nicolle DA. Bilateral anterior ischemic optic neuropathy as a presentation of Takayasu's disease. J Neuroophthalmol. 1997; 17(3):156–161

[78] Malik KP, Kapoor K, Mehta A, et al. Bilateral anterior ischaemic optic neuropathy in Takayasu arteritis. Indian J Ophthalmol. 2002; 50(1):52–54

[79] Biousse V, Schaison M, Touboul P-J, D'Anglejan-Chatillon J, Bousser MG. Ischemic optic neuropathy associated with internal carotid artery dissection. Arch Neurol. 1998; 55(5):715–719

[80] Götte K, Riedel F, Knorz MC, Hörmann K. Delayed anterior ischemic optic neuropathy after neck dissection. Arch Otolaryngol Head Neck Surg. 2000; 126(2):220–223

[81] Mokri B, Silbert PL, Schievink WI, Piepgras DG. Cranial nerve palsy in spontaneous dissection of the extracranial internal carotid artery. Neurology. 1996; 46(2):356–359

[82] Rivkin MJ, Hedges TR, III, Logigian EL. Carotid dissection presenting as posterior ischemic optic neuropathy. Neurology. 1990; 40(9):1469

[83] Strome SE, Hill JS, Burnstine MA, Beck J, Chepeha DB, Esclamado RM. Anterior ischemic optic neuropathy following neck dissection. Head Neck. 1997; 19(2):148–152

[84] Horowitz J, Melamud A, Sela L, Hod Y, Geyer O. Internal carotid artery hypoplasia presenting as anterior ischemic optic neuropathy. Am J Ophthalmol. 2001; 131(5):673–674

[85] Liu TY, Miller NR. Giant cell arteritis presenting as unilateral anterior ischemic optic neuropathy associated with bilateral optic nerve sheath enhancement on magnetic resonance imaging. J Neuroophthalmol. 2015; 35(4):360–363

[86] Yoeruek E, Szurman P, Tatar O, Weckerle P, Wilhelm H. Anterior ischemic optic neuropathy due to giant cell arteritis with normal inflammatory markers. Graefes Arch Clin Exp Ophthalmol. 2008; 246(6):913–915

[87] Kim N, Trobe JD, Flint A, Keoleian G. Late ipsilateral recurrence of ischemic optic neuropathy in giant cell arteritis. J Neuroophthalmol. 2003; 23(2):122–126

[88] Kaiser HJ, Flammer J, Messerli J. Vasospasm: a risk factor for non-arteritic anterior ischemic optic neuropathy? Neuro-ophthalmology. 1996; 16(1):5–10

[89] Brown RH, Schauble JF, Miller NR. Anemia and hypotension as contributors to perioperative loss of vision. Anesthesiology. 1994; 80(1):222–226

[90] Chun DM, Levin DK. Ischemic optic neuropathy after hemorrhage from a cornual ectopic gestation. Am J Obstet Gynecol. 1997; 177(6):1550–1552

[91] Connolly SE, Gordon KB, Horton JC. Salvage of vision after hypotension-induced ischemic optic neuropathy. Am J Ophthalmol. 1994; 117(2):235–242

[92] Cullinane DC, Jenkins JM, Reddy S, et al. Anterior ischemic optic neuropathy: a complication after systemic inflammatory response syndrome. J Trauma. 2000; 48(3):381–386, discussion 386–387

[93] Hayreh SS, Podhajsky P, Zimmerman MB. Role of nocturnal arterial hypotension in optic nerve head ischemic disorders. Ophthalmologica. 1999; 213(2):76–96

[94] Lee AG. Ischemic optic neuropathy following lumbar spine surgery. Case report. J Neurosurg. 1995; 83(2):348–349

[95] Shaked G, Gavriel A, Roy-Shapira A. Anterior ischemic optic neuropathy after hemorrhagic shock. J Trauma. 1998; 44(5):923–925

[96] Teshome T, Alemayehu W. Loss of vision from distant haemorrhage: report of four cases. East Afr Med J. 1999; 76(12):706–708

[97] Williams EL, Hart WM, Jr, Tempelhoff R. Postoperative ischemic optic neuropathy. Anesth Analg. 1995; 80(5):1018–1029

[98] Lund PE, Madsen K. Bilateral blindness after cardiopulmonary bypass. J Cardiothorac Vasc Anesth. 1994; 8(4):448–450

[99] Moster ML, Katz JB, Sedwick LA. Visual loss after coronary artery bypass surgery. Surv Ophthalmol. 1998; 42(5):453–457

[100] Shapira OM, Kimmel WA, Lindsey PS, Shahian DM. Anterior ischemic optic neuropathy after open heart operations. Ann Thorac Surg. 1996; 61(2):660–666

[101] Spoor TC, Wilkinson MJ, Ramocki JM. Optic nerve sheath decompression for the treatment of progressive nonarteritic ischemic optic neuropathy. Am J Ophthalmol. 1991; 111(6):724–728

[102] Dorecka M, Miniewicz-Kurkowska J, Romaniuk D, Gajdzik-Gajdecka U, Wójcik-Niklewska B. Anterior ischemic optic neuropathy after conventional coronary artery bypass graft surgery. Med Sci Monit. 2011; 17(6):CS70–CS74

[103] Tidow-Kebritchi S, Jay WM. Anterior ischemic optic neuropathy following off-pump cardiac bypass surgery. Semin Ophthalmol. 2003; 18(4):166–168

[104] Alexandrakis G, Lam BL. Bilateral posterior ischemic optic neuropathy after spinal surgery. Am J Ophthalmol. 1999; 127(3):354–355

[105] Cheng MA, Sigurdson W, Tempelhoff R, Lauryssen C. Visual loss after spine surgery: a survey. Neurosurgery. 2000; 46(3):625–630, discussion 630–631

[106] Dilger JA, Tetzlaff JE, Bell GR, Kosmorsky GS, Agnor RC, O'Hara JF, Jr. Ischaemic optic neuropathy after spinal fusion. Can J Anaesth. 1998; 45(1):63–66

[107] Katz DM, Trobe JD, Cornblath WT, Kline LB. Ischemic optic neuropathy after lumbar spine surgery. Arch Ophthalmol. 1994; 112(7):925–931

[108] Loftman BA, Shapiro J. Ischemic optic neuropathy. J Neurosurg. 1996; 84(2):306 (letter)

[109] Myers MA, Hamilton SR, Bogosian AJ, Smith CH, Wagner TA. Visual loss as a complication of spine surgery. A review of 37 cases. Spine. 1997; 22(12):1325–1329

[110] Roth S, Nunez R, Schreider BD. Unexplained visual loss after lumbar spinal fusion. J Neurosurg Anesthesiol. 1997; 9(4):346–348

[111] Smith FP. Ischemic optic neuropathy. J Neurosurg. 1996; 84(1):149–150 (letter)

[112] Stevens WR, Glazer PA, Kelley SD, Lietman TM, Bradford DS. Ophthalmic complications after spinal surgery. Spine. 1997; 22(12):1319–1324

[113] Ho VT, Newman NJ, Song S, Ksiazek S, Roth S. Ischemic optic neuropathy following spine surgery. J Neurosurg Anesthesiol. 2005; 17(1):38–44

[114] Stoffelns BM. Anterior ischemic optic neuropathy due to abdominal hemorrhage after laparotomy for uterine myoma. Arch Gynecol Obstet. 2010; 281(1):157–160

[115] Fenton S, Fenton JE, Browne M, Hughes JP, Connor MO, Timon CI. Ischaemic optic neuropathy following bilateral neck dissection. J Laryngol Otol. 2001; 115(2):158–160

[116] Kirkali P, Kansu T. A case of unilateral posterior ischemic optic neuropathy after radical neck dissection. Ann Ophthalmol. 1990; 22(8):297–298

[117] Marks SC, Jaques DA, Hirata RM, Saunders JR, Jr. Blindness following bilateral radical neck dissection. Head Neck. 1990; 12(4):342–345

[118] Nawa Y, Jaques JD, Miller NR, Palermo RA, Green WR. Bilateral posterior optic neuropathy after bilateral radical neck dissection and hypotension. Graefes Arch Clin Exp Ophthalmol. 1992; 230(4):301–308

[119] Schobel GA, Schmidbauer M, Millesi W, Undt G. Posterior ischemic optic neuropathy following bilateral radical neck dissection. Int J Oral Maxillofac Surg. 1995; 24(4):283–287

[120] Wilson JF, Freeman SB, Breene DP. Anterior ischemic optic neuropathy causing blindness in the head and neck surgery patient. Arch Otolaryngol Head Neck Surg. 1991; 117(11):1304–1306

[121] Aydin O, Memisoglu I, Ozturk M, Altintas O. Anterior ischemic optic neuropathy after unilateral radical neck dissection: case report and review. Auris Nasus Larynx. 2008; 35(2):308–312

[122] Remigio D, Wertenbaker C, Katz DM. Post-operative bilateral vision loss. Surv Ophthalmol. 2000; 44(5):426–432

[123] Savino PJ, Burde RM, Mills RP. Visual loss following intranasal anesthetic injection. J Clin Neuroophthalmol. 1990; 10(2):140–144

[124] Williams GC, Lee AG, Adler HL, et al. Bilateral anterior ischemic optic neuropathy and branch retinal artery occlusion after radical prostatectomy. J Urol. 1999; 162(4):1384–1385

[125] Janicki PK, Pai R, Kelly Wright J, Chapman WC, Wright Pinson C. Ischemic optic neuropathy after liver transplantation. Anesthesiology. 2001; 94(2): 361–363

[126] Bartlett S, Cai A, Cairns H. Non-arteritic ischaemic optic neuropathy after first return to haemodialysis. BMJ Case Rep. 2011; 2011:bcr0420114072

[127] Nieto J, Zapata MA. Bilateral anterior ischemic optic neuropathy in patients on dialysis: a report of two cases. Indian J Nephrol. 2010; 20(1):48–50

[128] Jackson TL, Farmer CKT, Kingswood C, Vickers S. Hypotensive ischemic optic neuropathy and peritoneal dialysis. Am J Ophthalmol. 1999; 128(1): 109–111

[129] Di Zazzo G, Guzzo I, De Galasso L, et al. Anterior ischemic optical neuropathy in children on chronic peritoneal dialysis: report of 7 cases. Perit Dial Int. 2015; 35(2):135–139

[130] Dufek S, Feldkoetter M, Vidal E, et al. Anterior ischemic optic neuropathy in pediatric peritoneal dialysis: risk factors and therapy. Pediatr Nephrol. 2014; 29(7):1249–1257

[131] Hayreh SS, Podhajsky PA, Zimmerman B. Nonarteritic anterior ischemic optic neuropathy: time of onset of visual loss. Am J Ophthalmol. 1997; 124 (5):641–647

[132] Landau K, Winterkorn JMS, Mailloux LU, Vetter W, Napolitano B. 24-hour blood pressure monitoring in patients with anterior ischemic optic neuropathy. Arch Ophthalmol. 1996; 114(5):570–575

[133] McCulley TJ, Lam BL, Feuer WJ. Incidence of nonarteritic anterior ischemic optic neuropathy associated with cataract extraction. Ophthalmology. 2001; 108(7):1275–1278

[134] Pérez-Santonja JJ, Bueno JL, Meza J, García-Sandoval B, Serrano JM, Zato MA. Ischemic optic neuropathy after intraocular lens implantation to correct high myopia in a phakic patient. J Cataract Refract Surg. 1993; 19(5):651–654

[135] Lee H, Kim CY, Seong GJ, Ma KT. A case of decreased visual field after uneventful cataract surgery: nonarteritic anterior ischemic optic neuropathy. Korean J Ophthalmol. 2010; 24(1):57–61

[136] Cameron BD, Saffra NA, Strominger MB. Laser in situ keratomileusis-induced optic neuropathy. Ophthalmology. 2001; 108(4):660–665

[137] Cornblath WT, Warren F, Tang R. Optic neuropathy after LASIK. Presented at the 28th annual meeting of the North American Neuro-Ophthalmology Society, Copper Mountain, CO, February 9–14, 2002

[138] Lee AG, Kohnen T, Ebner R, et al. Optic neuropathy associated with laser in situ keratomileusis. J Cataract Refract Surg. 2000; 26(11):1581–1584

[139] Good CD, Cassidy LM, Moseley IF, Sanders MD. Posterior optic nerve infarction after lower lid blepharoplasty. J Neuroophthalmol. 1999; 19(3): 176–179

[140] Cunha LP, Cunha LV, Costa CF, Monteiro ML. Nonarteritic anterior ischemic optic neuropathy following pars plana vitrectomy for macular hole treatment: case report. Arq Bras Oftalmol. 2016; 79(5):342–345

[141] Atmaca LS, Ozmert E. Optic neuropathy and central retinal artery occlusion in a patient with herpes zoster ophthalmicus. Ann Ophthalmol. 1992; 24(2): 50–53

[142] Borruat FX, Herbort CP. Herpes zoster ophthalmicus. Anterior ischemic optic neuropathy and acyclovir. J Clin Neuroophthalmol. 1992; 12(1):37–40

[143] Kothe AC, Flanagan J, Trevino RC. True posterior ischemic optic neuropathy associated with herpes zoster ophthalmicus. Optom Vis Sci. 1990; 67(11): 845–849

[144] Lexa FJ, Galetta SL, Yousem DM, Farber M, Oberholtzer JC, Atlas SW. Herpes zoster ophthalmicus with orbital pseudotumor syndrome complicated by optic nerve infarction and cerebral granulomatous angiitis: MR-pathologic correlation. AJNR Am J Neuroradiol. 1993; 14(1):185–190

[145] Weger M, Haas A, Stanger O, et al. Chlamydia pneumoniae seropositivity and the risk of nonarteritic ischemic optic neuropathy. Ophthalmology. 2002; 109(4):749–752

[146] Coppeto JR, Greco TP. Autoimmune ischemic optic neuropathy associated with positive rheumatoid factor and transient nephrosis. Ann Ophthalmol. 1992; 24(11):434–438

[147] Yamauchi Y, Cruz JM, Kaplan HJ, Goto H, Sakai J, Usui M. Suspected simultaneous bilateral anterior ischemic optic neuropathy in a patient with Behçet's disease. Ocul Immunol Inflamm. 2005; 13(4):317–325

[148] Acheson JF, Cockerell OC, Bentley CR, Sanders MD. Churg-Strauss vasculitis presenting with severe visual loss due to bilateral sequential optic neuropathy. Br J Ophthalmol. 1993; 77(2):118–119

[149] Kattah JC, Chrousos GA, Katz PA, McCasland B, Kolsky MP. Anterior ischemic optic neuropathy in Churg-Strauss syndrome. Neurology. 1994; 44(11): 2200–2202

[150] Sehgal M, Swanson JW, DeRemee RA, Colby TV. Neurologic manifestations of Churg-Strauss syndrome. Mayo Clin Proc. 1995; 70(4):337–341

[151] Vitali C, Genovesi-Ebert F, Romani A, Jeracitano G, Nardi M. Ophthalmological and neuro-ophthalmological involvement in Churg-Strauss syndrome: a case report. Graefes Arch Clin Exp Ophthalmol. 1996; 234(6):404–408

[152] Padovano I, Pazzola G, Pipitone N, Cimino L, Salvarani C. Anterior ischaemic optic neuropathy in eosinophilic granulomatosis with polyangiitis (Churg-Strauss syndrome): a case report and review of the literature. Clin Exp Rheumatol. 2014; 32(3) Suppl 82:S62–S65

[153] Shichinohe N, Shinmei Y, Nitta T, Chin S, Yamada Y, Kase M. Arteritic anterior ischemic optic neuropathy with positive myeloperoxidase antineutrophil cytoplasmic antibody. Jpn J Ophthalmol. 2010; 54(4):344–348

[154] Rodriguez ME, Burris CK, Potter HD. Nonarteritic anterior ischemic optic neuropathy (NAION) in polymyalgia rheumatic. Ophthalmology. 2016; 123 (7):1413

[155] Massry GG, Chung SM, Selhorst JB. Optic neuropathy, headache, and diplopia with MRI suggestive of cerebral arteritis in relapsing polychondritis. J Neuroophthalmol. 1995; 15(3):171–175

[156] Mochizuki A, Hayashi A, Hisahara S, Shoji S. Steroid-responsive Devic's variant in Sjögren's syndrome. Neurology. 2000; 54(6):1391–1392

[157] Rosler DH, Conway MD, Anaya JM, et al. Ischemic optic neuropathy and high-level anticardiolipin antibodies in primary Sjögren's syndrome. Lupus. 1995; 4(2):155–157

[158] Siatkowski RM, Scott IU, Verm AM, et al. Optic neuropathy and chiasmopathy in the diagnosis of systemic lupus erythematosus. J Neuroophthalmol. 2001; 21(3):193–198

[159] Nakao K, Mizushima Y, Abematsu N, Goh N, Sakamoto T. Anterior ischemic optic neuropathy associated with Vogt-Koyanagi-Harada disease. Graefes Arch Clin Exp Ophthalmol. 2009; 247(10):1417–1425

[160] Tham VM, Cunningham E, Jr. Anterior ischaemic optic neuropathy in a patient with HLA-B27 associated anterior uveitis and ankylosing spondylitis. Br J Ophthalmol. 2001; 85(6):756

[161] Katz B, Spencer WH. Hyperopia as a risk factor for nonarteritic anterior ischemic optic neuropathy. Am J Ophthalmol. 1993; 116(6):754–758

[162] Beck RW, Corbett JJ, Thompson HS, Sergott RC. Decreased visual acuity from optic disc drusen. Arch Ophthalmol. 1985; 103(8):1155–1159

[163] Lee AG, Lyle C, Tang R, et al. Optic nerve head drusen and ischemic optic neuropathy. Presented at the 28th annual meeting of the North American Neuro-Ophthalmology Society. Copper Mountain, CO, February 9–14, 2002

[164] Liew SC, Mitchell P. Anterior ischaemic optic neuropathy in a patient with optic disc drusen. Aust N Z J Ophthalmol. 1999; 27(2):157–160

[165] Purvin V, King R, Kawasaki A, Yee R. Anterior ischemic optic neuropathy in eyes with optic disc drusen. Arch Ophthalmol. 2004; 122(1):48–53

[166] Ayhan Z, Yaman A, Söylev Bajin M, Saatci AO. Unilateral acute anterior ischemic optic neuropathy in a patient with an already established diagnosis of bilateral optic disc drusen. Case Rep Ophthalmol Med. 2015; 2015: 730606

[167] Kalenak JW, Kosmorsky GS, Rockwood EJ. Nonarteritic anterior ischemic optic neuropathy and intraocular pressure. Arch Ophthalmol. 1991; 109(5): 660–661

[168] Katz B. Anterior ischemic optic neuropathy and intraocular pressure. Arch Ophthalmol. 1992; 110(5):596–597 (letter)

[169] Katz B, Weinreb RN, Wheeler DT, Klauber MR. Anterior ischaemic optic neuropathy and intraocular pressure. Br J Ophthalmol. 1990; 74(2):99–102

[170] Slavin ML, Margulis M. Anterior ischemic optic neuropathy following acute angle-closure glaucoma. Arch Ophthalmol. 2001; 119(8):1215

[171] Kuriyan AE, Lam BL. Non-arteritic anterior ischemic optic neuropathy secondary to acute primary-angle closure. Clin Ophthalmol. 2013; 7:1233–1238

[172] Wanichwecharungruang B, Chantra S. Non-arteritic anterior ischaemic optic neuropathy associated with neovascular glaucoma. BMJ Case Rep. 2009; 2009:pii:bcr07.2008.0483

[173] Sugahara M, Fujimoto T, Shidara K, Inoue K, Wakakura M. A case of anterior ischemic optic neuropathy associated with uveitis. Clin Ophthalmol. 2013; 7:1023–1026

[174] Balachandran C, Millar MJ, Murali R, Bulliard C, Malcolm CM, Maloof A. Malignant optic glioma presenting as an acute anterior optic neuropathy. Retin Cases Brief Rep. 2009; 3(2):156–160

[175] Shen B, MacIntosh PW. Posterior vitreous detachment associated with non-arteritic ischaemic optic neuropathy. Neuroophthalmology. 2016; 40(5): 234–236

[176] Ganssauge M, Wilhelm H, Bartz-Schmidt KU, Aisenbrey S. Non-arteritic anterior ischemic optic neuropathy (NA-AION) after intravitreal injection of bevacizumab (Avastin) for treatment of angoid streaks in pseudoxanthoma elasticum. Graefes Arch Clin Exp Ophthalmol. 2009; 247(12):1707–1710

[177] Golnik KC, Newman SA. Anterior ischemic optic neuropathy associated with macrocytic anemia. J Clin Neuroophthalmol. 1990; 10(4):244–247

[178] Kacer B, Hattenbach LO, Hörle S, Scharrer I, Kroll P, Koch F. Central retinal vein occlusion and nonarteritic ischemic optic neuropathy in 2 patients with mild iron deficiency anemia. Ophthalmologica. 2001; 215(2):128–131

[179] Kawasaki A, Purvin VA, Burgett RA. Hyperhomocysteinaemia in young patients with non-arteritic anterior ischaemic optic neuropathy. Br J Ophthalmol. 1999; 83(11):1287–1290

[180] Pianka P, Almog Y, Man O, Goldstein M, Sela BA, Loewenstein A. Hyperhomocystinemia in patients with nonarteritic anterior ischemic optic neuropathy, central retinal artery occlusion, and central retinal vein occlusion. Ophthalmology. 2000; 107(8):1588–1592

[181] Weger M, Stanger O, Deutschmann H, et al. Hyperhomocyst(e)inaemia, but not MTHFR C677T mutation, as a risk factor for non-arteritic ischaemic optic neuropathy. Br J Ophthalmol. 2001; 85(7):803–806

[182] Aziz A, Conway MD, Robertson HJ, Espinoza LR, Wilson WA. Acute optic neuropathy and transverse myelopathy in patients with antiphospholipid antibody syndrome: favorable outcome after treatment with anticoagulants and glucocorticoids. Lupus. 2000; 9(4):307–310

[183] Fry CL, Carter JE, Kanter MC, Tegeler CH, Tuley MR. Anterior ischemic optic neuropathy is not associated with carotid artery atherosclerosis. Stroke. 1993; 24(4):539–542

[184] Galetta SL, Plock GL, Kushner MJ, Wyszynski RE, Brucker AJ. Ocular thrombosis associated with antiphospholipid antibodies. Ann Ophthalmol. 1991; 23(6):207–212

[185] Reino S, Muñoz-Rodriguez FJ, Cervera R, Espinosa G, Font J, Ingelmo M. Optic neuropathy in the "primary" antiphospholipid syndrome: report of a case and review of the literature. Clin Rheumatol. 1997; 16(6):629–631

[186] Srinivasan S, Fern A, Watson WH, McColl MD. Reversal of nonarteritic anterior ischemic optic neuropathy associated with coexisting primary antiphospholipid syndrome and Factor V Leiden mutation. Am J Ophthalmol. 2001; 131(5):671–673

[187] Worrall BB, Moazami G, Odel JG, Behrens MM. Anterior ischemic optic neuropathy and activated protein C resistance. A case report and review of the literature. J Neuroophthalmol. 1997; 17(3):162–165

[188] Bertram B, Remky A, Arend O, Wolf S, Reim M. Protein C, protein S, and antithrombin III in acute ocular occlusive diseases. Ger J Ophthalmol. 1995; 4(6):332–335

[189] Titlic M, Karaman K, Andelinovic S. Anterior ischemic optic neuropathy comorbid with Factor V Leiden and PAI-1 4G/5G mutation. Bratisl Lek Listy (Tlacene Vyd). 2009; 110(3):192–194

[190] Schockman S, Glueck CJ, Hutchins RK, Patel J, Shah P, Wang P. Diagnostic ramifications of ocular vascular occlusion as a first thrombotic event associated with factor V Leiden and prothrombin gene heterozygosity. Clin Ophthalmol. 2015; 9:591–600

[191] Maramattom BV. Anterior ischemic optic neuropathy as a manifestation of HELLP syndrome. Case Rep Crit Care. 2014; 2014:671976

[192] Sawada A, Oie S, Mochizuki K, Yamamoto T. Anterior ischemic optic neuropathy in patient with hereditary spherocytosis and coexisting angioid streaks. Eur J Ophthalmol. 2012; 26:0

[193] Giuffre G. Hematological risk factors for anterior ischemic optic neuropathy. Neuro-ophthalmology. 1990; 10(4):197–203

[194] Talks SJ, Chong NHV, Gibson JM, Dodson PM. Fibrinogen, cholesterol and smoking as risk factors for non-arteritic anterior ischaemic optic neuropathy. Eye (Lond). 1995; 9(Pt 1):85–88

[195] Ohte A, Kimura T, Kimura W, et al. A case of optic disc infarction due to lupus anticoagulant. Nippon Ganka Kiyo. 1995; 46:783–787

[196] Rue KS, Hirsch LK, Sadun AA. Impending anterior ischemic optic neuropathy with elements of retinal vein occlusion in a patient on interferon for polycythemia vera. Clin Ophthalmol. 2012; 6:1763–1765

[197] Tönz MS, Rigamonti V, Iliev ME. Simultaneous, bilateral anterior ischemic optic neuropathy (AION) in polycythemia vera: a case report. Klin Monatsbl Augenheilkd. 2008; 225(5):504–506

[198] Perlman JI, Forman S, Gonzalez ER. Retrobulbar ischemic optic neuropathy associated with sickle cell disease. J Neuroophthalmol. 1994; 14(1):45–48

[199] Killer HE, Huber A, Portman C, Forrer A, Flammer J. Bilateral anterior ischemic optic neuropathy in a patient with autoimmune thrombocytopenia. Eur J Ophthalmol. 2000; 10(2):180–182

[200] Horton JC. Embolic cilioretinal artery occlusion with atherosclerosis of the ipsilateral carotid artery. Retina. 1995; 15(5):441–444

[201] Gupta A, Jalali S, Bansal RK, Grewal SP. Anterior ischemic optic neuropathy and branch retinal artery occlusion in cavernous sinus thrombosis. J Clin Neuroophthalmol. 1990; 10(3):193–196

[202] Dosso A, Safran AB, Sunaric G, Burger A. Anterior ischemic optic neuropathy in Graves' disease. J Neuroophthalmol. 1994; 14(3):170–174

[203] Purvin VA. Anterior ischemic optic neuropathy secondary to interferon alfa. Arch Ophthalmol. 1995; 113(8):1041–1044

[204] Tang RA. Interferon: friend or foe? Arch Ophthalmol. 1995; 113(8):987

[205] Fraunfelder FW, Fraunfelder FT. Interferon alfa-associated anterior ischemic optic neuropathy. Ophthalmology. 2011; 118(2):408–11.e1, 2

[206] Wei YH, Wang IH, Woung LC, Jou JR. Anterior ischemic optic neuropathy associated with pegylated interferon therapy for chronic hepatitis C. Ocul Immunol Inflamm. 2009; 17(3):191–194

[207] Vardizer Y, Linhart Y, Loewenstein A, Garzozi H, Mazawi N, Kesler A. Interferon-alpha-associated bilateral simultaneous ischemic optic neuropathy. J Neuroophthalmol. 2003; 23(4):256–259

[208] Cestari DM, Lessell S, Mantopoulos D. Early diagnosis of subclinical interferon alpha-associated optic neuropathy using fluorescein angiography. J Neuroophthalmol. 2015; 35(3):280–283

[209] Chiari M, Manzoni GC, Van de Geijn EJ. Ischemic optic neuropathy after sumatriptan in a migraine with aura patient. Headache. 1994; 34(4):237–238 (letter)

[210] Schönhöfer PS, Werner B, Tröger U. Ocular damage associated with proton pump inhibitors. BMJ. 1997; 314(7097):1805

[211] Mäntyjärvi M, Tuppurainen K, Ikäheimo K. Ocular side effects of amiodarone. Surv Ophthalmol. 1998; 42(4):360–366

[212] Fivgas GD, Newman NJ. Anterior ischemic optic neuropathy following the use of a nasal decongestant. Am J Ophthalmol. 1999; 127(1):104–106

[213] Cunningham AV, Smith KH. Anterior ischemic optic neuropathy associated with viagra. J Neuroophthalmol. 2001; 21(1):22–25

[214] Egan R, Pomeranz H. Sildenafil (Viagra) associated anterior ischemic optic neuropathy. Arch Ophthalmol. 2000; 118(2):291–292

[215] Pomeranz HD, Smith KH, Hart WM, Jr, Egan RA. Sildenafil-associated nonarteritic anterior ischemic optic neuropathy. Ophthalmology. 2002; 109 (3):584–587

[216] Thurtell MJ, Tomsak RL. Nonarteritic anterior ischemic optic neuropathy with PDE-5 inhibitors for erectile dysfunction. Int J Impot Res. 2008; 20(6): 537–543

[217] Bosley TM, Abu-Amero KK, Ozand PT. Mitochondrial DNA nucleotide changes in non-arteritic ischemic optic neuropathy. Neurology. 2004; 63(7): 1305–1308

[218] Scherer RW, Feldon SE, Levin L, et al. Ischemic Optic Neuropathy Decompression Trial Research Group. Visual fields at follow-up in the Ischemic Optic Neuropathy Decompression Trial: evaluation of change in pattern defect and severity over time. Ophthalmology. 2008; 115(10):1809–1817

[219] Fingert JH, Grassi MA, Janutka JC, et al. Mitochondrial variant G4132A is associated with familial non-arteritic anterior ischemic optic neuropathy in one large pedigree. Ophthalmic Genet. 2007; 28(1):1–7

[220] Guyer DR, Green WR, Schachat AP, Bastacky S, Miller NR. Bilateral ischemic optic neuropathy and retinal vascular occlusions associated with lymphoma and sepsis. Clinicopathologic correlation. Ophthalmology. 1990; 97(7):882–888

[221] Neri A, Rubino P, Macaluso C, Gandolfi SA. Light-chain amyloidosis mimicking giant cell arteritis in a bilateral anterior ischemic optic neuropathy case. BMC Ophthalmol. 2013; 13:82

[222] Kawasaki A, Purvin VA, Tang R. Bilateral anterior ischemic optic neuropathy following influenza vaccination. J Neuroophthalmol. 1998; 18(1):56–59

[223] Parsons JT, Bova FJ, Fitzgerald CR, Mendenhall WM, Million RR. Radiation optic neuropathy after megavoltage external-beam irradiation: analysis of time-dose factors. Int J Radiat Oncol Biol Phys. 1994; 30(4):755–763

[224] Haider S, Astbury NJ, Hamilton DV. Optic neuropathy in uraemic patients on dialysis. Eye (Lond). 1993; 7(Pt 1):148–151

[225] Korzets Z, Zeltzer E, Rathaus M, Manor R, Bernheim J. Uremic optic neuropathy. A uremic manifestation mandating dialysis. Am J Nephrol. 1998; 18(3):240–242

[226] Winkelmayer WC, Eigner M, Berger O, Grisold W, Leithner C. Optic neuropathy in uremia: an interdisciplinary emergency. Am J Kidney Dis. 2001; 37(3):E23

[227] Gadkari SS, Ladi DS, Gupta S, Gandhi VH, Patel MV. Traumatic ischaemic optic neuropathy (a case report). J Postgrad Med. 1991; 37(3):179–180

[228] Kaiserman I, Frucht-Pery J. Anterior ischemic optic neuropathy after a trans-Atlantic airplane journey. Am J Ophthalmol. 2002; 133(4):581–583

[229] Sadun F, Wang M, Levin LB, Feldon S. Familial nonarteritic ischemic optic neuropathy. Presented at the Annual meeting of the North American Neuro-Ophthalmology Society, 1996

[230] Wang MY, Sadun F, Levin LB, LaBree L, Feldon SE. Occurrence of familial nonarteritic anterior ischemic optic neuropathy in a case series. J Neuroophthalmol. 1999; 19(2):144–147

[231] Hayreh SS, Fingert JH, Stone E, Jacobson DM. Familial non-arteritic anterior ischemic optic neuropathy. Graefes Arch Clin Exp Ophthalmol. 2008; 246(9):1295–1305

[232] Beck RW. Optic neuritis or anterior ischemic optic neuropathy? Arch Ophthalmol. 1992; 110(10):1357

[233] Parsa CF, Muci-Mendoza R, Hoyt WF. Anterior ischemic optic neuropathy in a disc with a cup: an exception to the rule. J Neuroophthalmol. 1998; 18(3):169–170

[234] Hayreh SS, Podhajsky PA, Zimmerman B. Ipsilateral recurrence of nonarteritic anterior ischemic optic neuropathy. Am J Ophthalmol. 2001; 132(5):734–742

[235] Boone MI, Massry GG, Frankel RA, Holds JB, Chung SM. Visual outcome in bilateral nonarteritic anterior ischemic optic neuropathy. Ophthalmology. 1996; 103(8):1223–1228

[236] Beri M, Klugman MR, Kohler JA, Hayreh SS. Anterior ischemic optic neuropathy. VII. Incidence of bilaterality and various influencing factors. Ophthalmology. 1987; 94(8):1020–1028

[237] WuDunn D, Zimmerman K, Sadun AA, Feldon SE. Comparison of visual function in fellow eyes after bilateral nonarteritic anterior ischemic optic neuropathy. Ophthalmology. 1997; 104(1):104–111

[238] Kupersmith MJ, Frohman L, Sanderson M, et al. Aspirin reduces the incidence of second eye NAION: a retrospective study. J Neuroophthalmol. 1997; 17(4):250–253

[239] Hayreh SS, Zimmerman MB. Bilateral nonarteritic anterior ischemic optic neuropathy: comparison of visual outcome in the two eyes. J Neuroophthalmol. 2013; 33(4):338–343

[240] Aiello AL, Sadun AA, Feldon SE. Spontaneous improvement of progressive anterior ischemic optic neuropathy: report of two cases. Arch Ophthalmol. 1992; 110(9):1197–1199

[241] Barrett DA, Glaser JS, Schatz NJ, Winterkorn JMS. Spontaneous recovery of vision in progressive anterior ischemic optic neuropathy. J Clin Neuroophthalmol. 1992; 12(4):219–225

[242] Movsas T, Kelman SE, Elman MJ, et al. The natural course of non-arteritic ischemic optic neuropathy. (abstract). Invest Ophthalmol Vis Sci. 1991; 42 (Suppl):951

[243] Lee YC, Wang JH, Huang TL, Tsai RK. Increased risk of stroke in patients with nonarteritic anterior ischemic optic neuropathy: a nationwide retrospective cohort study. Am J Ophthalmol. 2016; 170:183–189

[244] Yao F, Wan P, Su Y, Liao R, Zhu W. Impaired systemic vascular endothelial function in patients with non-arteritic anterior ischaemic optic neuropathy. Graefes Arch Clin Exp Ophthalmol. 2016; 254(5):977–981

[245] Lee AG. Prothrombotic and vascular risk factors in nonarteritic anterior ischemic optic neuropathy. Ophthalmology. 1999; 106(12):2231

[246] Felekis T, Kolaitis NI, Kitsos G, Vartholomatos G, Bourantas KL, Asproudis I. Thrombophilic risk factors in the pathogenesis of non-arteritic anterior ischemic optic neuropathy patients. Graefes Arch Clin Exp Ophthalmol. 2010; 248(6):877–884

[247] Arnold AC, Hepler RS, Lieber M, Alexander JM. Hyperbaric oxygen therapy for nonarteritic anterior ischemic optic neuropathy. Am J Ophthalmol. 1996; 122(4):535–541

[248] Katz DM, Trobe JD. Is there treatment for nonarteritic anterior ischemic optic neuropathy. Curr Opin Ophthalmol. 2015; 26(6):458–463

[249] Yee RD, Selky AK, Purvin VA. Outcomes of surgical and nonsurgical management of nonarteritic ischemic optic neuropathy. Trans Am Ophthalmol Soc. 1993; 91:227–240, discussion 240–243

[250] Hayreh SS, Jonas JB, Zimmerman MB. Nonarteritic anterior ischemic optic neuropathy and tobacco smoking. Ophthalmology. 2007; 114(4):804–809

[251] Nagy V, Facsko A, Takacs L, et al. Activated protein C resistance in anterior ischaemic optic neuropathy. Acta Ophthalmol Scand. 2004; 82(2):140–143

[252] Polat O, Yavaş GF, İnan S, İnan ÜÜ. Neutrophil-to-lymphocyte ratio as a marker in patients with non-arteritic anterior ischemic optic neuropathy. Balkan Med J. 2015; 32(4):382–387

[253] Sakai T, Shikishima K, Matsushima M, Tsuneoka H. Endothelin-1 in ischemic optic neuropathy. Ophthalmology. 2008; 115(7):1262

[254] Guyer DR, Miller NR, Auer CL, Fine SL. The risk of cerebrovascular and cardiovascular disease in patients with anterior ischemic optic neuropathy. Arch Ophthalmol. 1985; 103(8):1136–1142

[255] Guyer DR, Miller NR, Enger CL, Fine SL. Incidence of subcortical lesions not increased in nonarteritic ischemic optic neuropathy on magnetic resonance imaging. Am J Ophthalmol. 1988; 105(3):324–325

[256] Hasanreisoglu M, Robenshtok E, Ezrahi D, Stiebel-Kalish H. Do patients with non-arteritic ischemic optic neuritis have increased risk for cardiovascular and cerebrovascular events? Neuroepidemiology. 2013; 40(3):220–224

[257] Arnold AC, Hepler RS, Hamilton DR, Lufkin RB. Magnetic resonance imaging of the brain in nonarteritic ischemic optic neuropathy. J Neuroophthalmol. 1995; 15(3):158–160

[258] Kosmorsky G, Straga J, Knight C, Dagirmanjian A, Davis DA. The role of transcranial Doppler in nonarteritic ischemic optic neuropathy. Am J Ophthalmol. 1998; 126(2):288–290

[259] Fraser CL. Obstructive sleep apnea and optic neuropathy: is there a link? Curr Neurol Neurosci Rep. 2014; 14(8):465

[260] Ghaleh Bandi MF, Naserbakht M, Tabasi A, Marghaiezadeh A, Riazee Esfahani M, Golzarian Z. Obstructive sleep apnea syndrome and non-arteritic anterior ischemic optic neuropathy: a case control study. Med J Islam Repub Iran. 2015; 29:300

[261] Botelho PJ, Johnson LN, Arnold AC. The effect of aspirin on the visual outcome of nonarteritic anterior ischemic optic neuropathy. Am J Ophthalmol. 1996; 121(4):450–451

[262] Beck RW, Hayreh SS, Podhajsky PA, Tan ES, Moke PS. Aspirin therapy in nonarteritic anterior ischemic optic neuropathy. Am J Ophthalmol. 1997; 123(2):212–217

[263] Sanderson M, Kupersmith M, Frohman L, et al. Aspirin reduces anterior ischemic optic neuropathy in the second eye. ARVO abstracts. Invest Ophthalmol Vis Sci. 1995; 36:S196

[264] Roth GJ, Calverley DC. Aspirin, platelets, and thrombosis: theory and practice. Blood. 1994; 83(4):885–898

[265] Nicholson JD, Leiba H, Goldenberg-Cohen N. Translational preclinical research may lead to improved medical management of non-arteritic anterior ischemic optic neuropathy. Front Neurol. 2014; 5:122

[266] Hayreh SS. Ischemic optic neuropathies - where are we now? Graefes Arch Clin Exp Ophthalmol. 2013; 251(8):1873–1884

[267] Peeler C, Cestari DM. Non-arteritic anterior ischemic optic neuropathy (NAION): A review and update on animal models. Semin Ophthalmol. 2016; 31(1–2):99–106

[268] Johnson LN, Guy ME, Krohel GB, Madsen RW. Levodopa may improve vision loss in recent-onset, nonarteritic anterior ischemic optic neuropathy. Ophthalmology. 2000; 107(3):521–526

[269] Cox TA, Beck RW, Ferris FL, Hayreh SS. Does levodopa improve visual function in NAION? Ophthalmology. 2000; 107(8):1431–1438

[270] Simsek T, Eryilmaz T, Acaroglu G. Efficacy of levodopa and carbidopa on visual function in patients with non-arteritic anterior ischaemic optic neuropathy. Int J Clin Pract. 2005; 59(3):287–290

[271] Lyttle DP, Johnson LN, Margolin EA, Madsen RW. Levodopa as a possible treatment of visual loss in nonarteritic anterior ischemic optic neuropathy. Graefes Arch Clin Exp Ophthalmol. 2016; 254(4):757–764

[272] Razeghinejad MR, Nowroozzadeh MH, Eghbal MH. Levodopa and other pharmacologic interventions in ischemic and traumatic optic neuropathies and amblyopia. Clin Neuropharmacol. 2016; 39(1):40–48

[273] Hayreh SS, Zimmerman MB. Non-arteritic anterior ischemic optic neuropathy: role of systemic corticosteroid therapy. Graefes Arch Clin Exp Ophthalmol. 2008; 246(7):1029–1046

[274] Rebolleda G, Pérez-López M, Casas-LLera P, Contreras I, Muñoz-Negrete FJ. Visual and anatomical outcomes of non-arteritic anterior ischemic optic neuropathy with high-dose systemic corticosteroids. Graefes Arch Clin Exp Ophthalmol. 2013; 251(1):255–260

[275] Kinori M, Ben-Bassat I, Wasserzug Y, Chetrit A, Huna-Baron R. Visual outcome of mega-dose intravenous corticosteroid treatment in non-arteritic anterior ischemic optic neuropathy - retrospective analysis. BMC Ophthalmol. 2014; 14:62

[276] Pakravan M, Sanjari N, Esfandiari H, Pakravan P, Yaseri M. The effect of high-dose steroids, and normobaric oxygen therapy, on recent onset non-arteritic

anterior ischemic optic neuropathy: a randomized clinical trial. Graefes Arch Clin Exp Ophthalmol. 2016; 254(10):2043–2048

[277] Radoi C, Garcia T, Brugniart C, Ducasse A, Arndt C. Intravitreal triamcinolone injections in non-arteritic anterior ischemic optic neuropathy. Graefes Arch Clin Exp Ophthalmol. 2014; 252(2):339–345

[278] Jonas JB, Spandau UH, Harder B, Sauder G. Intravitreal triamcinolone acetonide for treatment of acute nonarteritic anterior ischemic optic neuropathy. Graefes Arch Clin Exp Ophthalmol. 2007; 245(5): 749–750

[279] Sohn BJ, Chun BY, Kwon JY. The effect of an intravitreal triamcinolone acetonide injection for acute nonarteritic anterior ischemic optic neuropathy. Korean J Ophthalmol. 2009; 23(1):59–61

[280] Yaman A, Selver OB, Saatci AO, Soylev MF. Intravitreal triamcinolone acetonide injection for acute non-arteritic anterior ischaemic optic neuropathy. Clin Exp Optom. 2008; 91(6):561–564

[281] Kaderli B, Avci R, Yucel A, Guler K, Gelisken O. Intravitreal triamcinolone improves recovery of visual acuity in nonarteritic anterior ischemic optic neuropathy. J Neuroophthalmol. 2007; 27(3):164–168

[282] Modarres M, Falavarjani KG, Nazari H, et al. Intravitreal erythropoietin injection for the treatment of non-arteritic anterior ischaemic optic neuropathy. Br J Ophthalmol. 2011; 95(7):992–995

[283] Bennett JL, Thomas S, Olson JL, Mandava N. Treatment of nonarteritic anterior ischemic optic neuropathy with intravitreal bevacizumab. J Neuroophthalmol. 2007; 27(3):238–240

[284] Rootman DB, Gill HS, Margolin EA. Intravitreal bevacizumab for the treatment of nonarteritic anterior ischemic optic neuropathy: a prospective trial. Eye (Lond). 2013; 27(4):538–544

[285] Saatci AO, Taskin O, Selver OB, Yaman A, Bajin MS. Efficacy of intravitreal ranibizumab injection in acute nonarteritic ischemic optic neuropathy: a long-term follow up. Open Ophthalmol J. 2013; 7:58–62

[286] Huang TL, Chang CH, Chang SW, Lin KH, Tsai RK. Efficacy of intravitreal injections of antivascular endothelial growth factor agents in a rat model of anterior ischemic optic neuropathy. Invest Ophthalmol Vis Sci. 2015; 56(4): 2290–2296

[287] Ramunni A, Giancipoli G, Saracino A, et al. LDL-apheresis in acute anterior ischemic optic neuropathy. Int J Artif Organs. 2004; 27(4):337–341

[288] Ramunni A, Giancipoli G, Guerriero S, et al. LDL-apheresis accelerates the recovery of nonarteritic acute anterior ischemic optic neuropathy. Ther Apher Dial. 2005; 9(1):53–58

[289] Ramunni A, Ranieri G, Giancipoli G, et al. Is the efficacy of LDL apheresis in ischemic optic neuropathy linked to a reduction in endothelial activation markers? Blood Purif. 2006; 24(4):405–412

[290] Guerriero S, Giancipoli G, Cantatore A, et al. LDL apheresis in the treatment of non-arteritic ischaemic optic neuropathy: a 6-month follow-up study. Eye (Lond). 2009; 23(6):1343–1344

[291] Schönfeld CL, Fischer M, Distelmaier P, et al. Recovery of visual function after administration of dabigatran etexilate. Case Rep Ophthalmol. 2014; 5(2): 262–266

[292] Zhu W, Liao R, Chen Y, Liu L, Zhang Y. Effect of enhanced extracorporeal counterpulsation in patients with non-arteritic anterior ischaemic optic neuropathy. Graefes Arch Clin Exp Ophthalmol. 2015; 253(1):127–133

[293] Yang Y, Zhang H, Yan Y, Gui Y. Clinical study in patients with ocular ischemic diseases treated with enhanced external counterpulsation combined with drugs. Mol Med Rep. 2013; 7(6):1845–1849

[294] Ellenberger C, Jr, Burde RM, Keltner JL. Acute optic neuropathy. Treatment with diphenylhydantoin. Arch Ophthalmol. 1974; 91(6):435–438

[295] Pakravan M, Sanjari N, Esfandiari H, Pakravan P, Yaseri M. The effect of high-dose steroids, and normobaric oxygen therapy, on recent onset non-arteritic anterior ischemic optic neuropathy: a randomized clinical trial. Graefes Arch Clin Exp Ophthalmol. 2016; 254(10):2043–2048

[296] Opre Opremcak E, Bruce R, Lomeo M, et al. Radial optic neurotomy for central retinal vein occlusion: a retrospective pilot study of 11 consecutive cases. Retina. 2001; 21:408–415

[297] Pinxten I, Stalmans P. Radial optic neurotomy as a treatment for AION secondary to optic disc drusen. GMS Ophthalmol Cases. 2014; 4:18–21

[298] Soheilian M, Koochek A, Yazdani S, Peyman GA. Transvitreal optic neurotomy for nonarteritic anterior ischemic optic neuropathy. Retina. 2003; 23(5):692–697

[299] Modarres M, Sanjari MS, Falavarjani KG. Vitrectomy and release of presumed epipapillary vitreous traction for treatment of nonarteritic anterior ischemic optic neuropathy associated with partial posterior vitreous detachment. Ophthalmology. 2007; 114(2):340–344

[300] Lee MS, Foroozan R, Kosmorsky GS. Posterior vitreous detachment in AION. Ophthalmology. 2009; 116(3):597–597.e1

[301] Lovelace K, O'Donnell T, Enzenauer RW. Anterior ischemic optic neuropathy. Ophthalmology. 2007; 114(12):2368–, author reply 2368–2369

[302] Soheilian M, Yazdani S. Ischemic optic neuropathy. Ophthalmology. 2007; 114(11):2102–2103, author reply 2103–2104

[303] Goldenberg-Cohen N, Dadon-Bar-El S, Hasanreisoglu M, et al. Possible neuroprotective effect of brimonidine in a mouse model of ischaemic optic neuropathy. Clin Experiment Ophthalmol. 2009; 37(7):718–729

[304] Danylkova NO, Alcala SR, Pomeranz HD, McLoon LK. Neuroprotective effects of brimonidine treatment in a rodent model of ischemic optic neuropathy. Exp Eye Res. 2007; 84(2):293–301

[305] Wilhelm B, Lüdtke H, Wilhelm H, BRAION Study Group. Efficacy and tolerability of 0.2% brimonidine tartrate for the treatment of acute non-arteritic anterior ischemic optic neuropathy (NAION): a 3-month, double-masked, randomised, placebo-controlled trial. Graefes Arch Clin Exp Ophthalmol. 2006; 244(5):551–558

[306] Fazzone HE, Kupersmith MJ, Leibmann J. Does topical brimonidine tartrate help NAION? Br J Ophthalmol. 2003; 87(9):1193–1194

[307] Parisi V, Coppola G, Ziccardi L, Gallinaro G, Falsini B. Cytidine-5'-diphosphocholine (Citicoline): a pilot study in patients with non-arteritic ischaemic optic neuropathy. Eur J Neurol. 2008; 15(5):465–474

[308] Sanjari N, Pakravan M, Nourinia R, et al. Intravitreal injection of a rho-kinase inhibitor (fasudil) for recent-onset nonanterior ischemic optic neuropathy. J Clin Pharmacol. 2016; 56(6):749–753

[309] Solano EC, Kornbrust DJ, Beaudry A, Foy JW, Schneider DJ, Thompson JD. Toxicological and pharmacokinetic properties of QPI-1007, a chemically modified synthetic siRNA targeting caspase 2 mRNA, following intravitreal injection. Nucleic Acid Ther. 2014; 24(4):258–266

[310] Quark Pharmaceuticals. Phase 2/3, randomized, double-masked, sham-controlled trial of QPI-1007 in subjects with acute nonarteritic anterior ischemic optic neuropathy (NAION). Available at: http://clinicaltrials.gov/ct2/show/NCT02341560. Accessed May 28, 2017

[311] Giri S, Rattan R, Singh AK, Singh I. The 15-deoxy-delta12,14-prostaglandin J2 inhibits the inflammatory response in primary rat astrocytes via down-regulating multiple steps in phosphatidylinositol 3-kinase-Akt-NF-kappaB-p300 pathway independent of peroxisome proliferator-activated receptor gamma. J Immunol. 2004; 173(8):5196–5208

[312] Touitou V, Johnson MA, Guo Y, Miller NR, Bernstein SL. Sustained neuroprotection from a single intravitreal injection of PGJ2 in a rodent model of anterior ischemic optic neuropathy. Invest Ophthalmol Vis Sci. 2013; 54(12):7402–7409

[313] Miller NR, Johnson MA, Nolan T, Guo Y, Bernstein AM, Bernstein SL. Sustained neuroprotection from a single intravitreal injection of PGJ2 in a nonhuman primate model of nonarteritic anterior ischemic optic neuropathy. Invest Ophthalmol Vis Sci. 2014; 55(11):7047–7056

[314] Kelman SE, Elman MJ. Optic nerve sheath decompression for nonarteritic ischemic optic neuropathy improves multiple visual function measurements. Arch Ophthalmol. 1991; 109(5):667–671

[315] Manor RS. Nonarteritic ischemic optic neuropathy in identical female twins: improvement of visual outcome in one by optic nerve decompression. (letter). Arch Ophthalmol. 1990; 108(8):1067–1068

[316] Sergott RC, Savino PJ, Bosley TM. Optic nerve sheath decompression: a clinical review and proposed pathophysiologic mechanism. Aust N Z J Ophthalmol. 1990; 18(4):365–373

[317] Flaharty PM, Sergott RC, Lieb W, Bosley TM, Savino PJ. Optic nerve sheath decompression may improve blood flow in anterior ischemic optic neuropathy. Ophthalmology. 1993; 100(3):297–302, discussion 303–305

[318] Glaser JS, Teimory M, Schatz NJ. Optic nerve sheath fenestration for progressive ischemic optic neuropathy. Results in second series consisting of 21 eyes. Arch Ophthalmol. 1994; 112(8):1047–1050

[319] Jablons MM, Glaser JS, Schatz NJ, Siatkowski RM, Tse DT, Kronish JW. Optic nerve sheath fenestration for treatment of progressive ischemic optic neuropathy. Results in 26 patients. Arch Ophthalmol. 1993; 111(1):84–87

[320] McHenry JG, Spoor TC. Optic nerve sheath fenestration for treatment of progressive ischemic optic neuropathy. Arch Ophthalmol. 1993; 111(12): 1601–1602

[321] McHenry JG, Spoor TC. The efficacy of optic nerve sheath decompression for anterior ischemic optic neuropathy and other optic neuropathies. Am J Ophthalmol. 1993; 116(2):254–256

[322] Mutlukan E, Cullen JF. Can empty sella syndrome be mistaken for a progressive form of nonarteritic ischemic optic neuropathy? Arch Ophthalmol. 1990; 108(8):1066–1067

[323] Sadun AA. The efficacy of optic nerve sheath decompression for anterior ischemic optic neuropathy and other optic neuropathies. Am J Ophthalmol. 1993; 115(3):384–389

[324] Spoor TC, McHenry JG, Lau-Sickon L. Progressive and static nonarteritic ischemic optic neuropathy treated by optic nerve sheath decompression. Ophthalmology. 1993; 100(3):306–311

[325] Wall M, Newman SA. Optic nerve sheath decompression for the treatment of progressive nonarteritic ischemic optic neuropathy. Am J Ophthalmol. 1991; 112(6):741–742

[326] Wilson WB. Does optic nerve sheath decompression help progressive ischemic optic neuropathy? Arch Ophthalmol. 1990; 108(8):1065–1066

[327] Ischemic Optic Neuropathy Decompression Trial Research Group. Ischemic Optic Neuropathy Decompression Trial: twenty-four-month update. Arch Ophthalmol. 2000; 118(6):793–798

[328] Beck RW. Optic nerve sheath fenestration for anterior ischemic optic neuropathy? The answer is in. (editorial). J Neuroophthalmol. 1995; 15(2):61–62

[329] Lessell S. Surgery for ischemic optic neuropathy. Arch Ophthalmol. 1995; 113(3):273–274

[330] Smith DB. Ischemic optic neuropathy decompression trial. JAMA. 1995; 274(8):612

5 Arteritic Anterior Ischemic Optic Neuropathy and Giant Cell Arteritis

Alec L. Amram

Abstract

Giant cell arteritis is an inflammatory vasculopathy of the elderly, and one of the most common manifestations is anterior ischemic optic neuropathy (AION). Arteritic anterior ischemic optic neuropathy (A-AION) is characterized by acute, painful loss of vision in one or both eyes and should be differentiated from the nonarteritic form of AION (NA-AION). This chapter discusses the clinical pathway for diagnosing and treating giant cell arteritis. The differences and similarities between NAION and A-AION are discussed.

Keywords: arteritic ischemic optic neuropathy, giant cell arteritis, temporal arteritis, anterior ischemic optic neuropathy, temporal artery biopsy

5.1 Introduction

Giant cell (temporal or cranial) arteritis (GCA) is an inflammatory vasculopathy of the elderly that affects medium- to large-sized arteries. GCA may present with numerous systemic and ocular manifestations.[1,2,3,4,5,6,7,8,9,10,11,12,13,14,15,16,17,18,19,20,21,22,23,24,25,26,27,28,29,30,31,32,33,34,35,36,37,38,39] Here we concentrate on the ocular manifestations, diagnosis, and treatment of GCA. Less emphasis is placed on nonocular involvement by GCA.

5.2 What Clinical Features Suggest Giant Cell Arteritis?

GCA usually causes visual loss due to anterior ischemic optic neuropathy (AION). All patients older than 50 years with AION should be suspected of having GCA. The index of suspicion is greater with increasing numbers of typical features of GCA listed in Box 5.1.[1,2,3,4,5,6,7,9,10,11,12,13,14,15,16,18,19,20,22,23,24,26,27,28,29,30,31,32,33,34,36,37,38,39,40,41,42]

Box 5.1 Typical features of giant cell arteritis

- Age greater than 50 years (median 75 years).
- Acute, often severe, visual loss (usually AION).
- Unilateral or bilateral visual loss (higher incidence of bilateral than nonarteritic [NA]-AION).
- Pallid swelling of the optic nerve (may be "chalk white").
- Optic atrophy eventually (usually in 6 to 8 weeks) often with end-stage optic disc appearance of cupping with pallor and loss of neuroretinal rim.[20,43,44]
- Constitutional signs and symptoms.
  - Headache (4–100%).
  - Scalp or temporal artery tenderness (28–91%).
  - Weight loss (16–76%).
  - Jaw claudication (4–67%).[45]
  - Anorexia (14–69%)

- Fever (low grade) and diaphoresis.[46]
- Proximal muscle aches or weakness (28–86%).
- Polymyalgia rheumatica.
- Morning stiffness lasting 30 minutes or more.
- Proximal joint pain (e.g., shoulders, hips, neck, or torso).
- Fatigue and malaise (12–97%).
- Leg claudication (2–43%).
- Elevated erythrocyte sedimentation rate (ESR; usually > 50 mm/hour by the Westergren method).
- Temporal artery biopsy (TAB) positive.

5.3 Is the Clinical Suspicion for GCA High?

In 1990, the American College of Rheumatology analyzed 214 patients with GCA (196 proven by positive TAB) and compared them with 593 patients with other forms of vasculitis.[47]

In their analysis of 33 criteria, the highest sensitivity criteria for GCA were the following:
1. Age older than 50 years (mean age 69 years, 90% > 60 years).
2. Westergren ESR greater than 50 mm/hour.
3. Abnormal TAB.

The highest specificity clinical criteria were the following:
1. Jaw and/or tongue claudication.
2. Visual abnormalities (e.g., AION, amaurosis, optic atrophy).
3. Temporal artery abnormalities (e.g., decreased pulse, tenderness, or nodules).

If at least three or more criteria of the following five were met, the specificity of diagnosis was 91.2% and the sensitivity was 93.5%:
1. Age older than 50 years.
2. New headache (localized).
3. Temporal artery abnormality (see above).
4. Elevated ESR (> 50 mm/hour).
5. Abnormal TAB (e.g., necrotizing arteritis, multinucleated giant cells).

One of these diagnostic criteria (positive TAB) makes the diagnosis with high specificity and is the "gold standard" for diagnosis. Fernandez-Herlihy increased the specificity for diagnosis of GCA by defining symptom clusters, for example, jaw claudication with any of the following[48]:
1. Recent headaches and scalp tenderness.
2. Scalp tenderness and ESR greater than 50 mm/hour.
3. Visual symptoms and ESR greater than 50 mm/hour.

A specificity of 90 to 100% could be obtained if the cluster included elevated ESR, scalp tenderness, jaw claudication, recent visual changes, polymyalgia rheumatica, and a good response to steroid therapy. A 94.8% sensitivity and 100% specificity were obtained if the symptom cluster included new-onset headache, jaw claudication, and abnormal temporal artery examination.[28] Vilaseca et al found that simultaneous jaw claudication, abnormal temporal arteries on examination, and new headache had a specificity of 94.8% for positive TAB.[49] Chmelewski et al compared the initial clinical features of 30 patients with positive TAB and 68 with negative TAB.[50] TAB-positive patients had significantly increased incidence of headache (93 vs. 62%) and jaw claudication (50 vs. 18%). Jaw claudication had a specificity of 56% as a differentiating feature, but the specificity of headache was low (40%). Hayreh et al reported that jaw claudication (p = 0.001) and neck pain (mostly in the occipital and back parts of the neck; p = 0.0003) were significant indicators of a positive TAB independent of ESR and age, and that these clinical signs were more highly correlated to a positive TAB than anorexia, weight loss, fever, and scalp tenderness.[51] Hayreh et al felt that the odds of a positive TAB were 9.0 times greater with jaw claudication, 3.3 times greater with neck pain, 3.2 times greater with a C-reactive protein (CRP) > 2.45 mg/dL, 2.1 times greater with an ESR of 47 to 107 mm/hour, 2.7 times greater with an ESR > 107 mm/hour, and 2.0 times greater when the patient was older than 75 years (compared with age below 75 years). The typical features of GCA are listed earlier in the chapter.

Acute visual loss is reported in 7 to 60% (average 36%) of patients with GCA. Although the usual cause of visual loss in GCA is AION or central retinal artery occlusion (CRAO),[41,52,53] cilioretinal artery occlusion, ocular ischemic syndrome, posterior ischemic optic neuropathy (PION), choroidal ischemia, or rarely occipital lobe ischemia may also occur.[54,55] In a prospective study of 170 patients with biopsy-proven GCA, 85 (50%) presented with ocular involvement.[19] The ocular findings in this study are outlined in ▶ Table 5.1.

Although visual loss and AION in GCA tend to be more severe than that seen in NA-AION,[19] the lack of severe visual loss is not a differentiating feature. Patients with AION in GCA may have little or no visual loss. On the other hand, very severe visual loss with AION is a "red flag" for GCA. In a study by Hayreh et al, 54% of patients with arteritic AION had initial visual acuity of

counting fingers to no light perception (compared to 26% of patients with NA-AION). Light perception was present in 29% and no light perception in 4% of AION due to GCA.[20] Therefore, massive early visual loss in AION is suggestive of GCA. Up to 25% of GCA patients have visual acuities of 20/40 or better and 20% of NA-AION patients have initial visual acuities of counting fingers or worse.[57] See Boxes 5.2 and 5.3 for additional features of giant cell arteritis.

Box 5.2 Clinical features favoring arteritic AION over NA-AION

- Elderly patients with constitutional symptoms (especially scalp tenderness or jaw claudication).
- Polymyalgia rheumatica.
- Elevated ESR and/or CRP.
- Amaurosis fugax—likely transient optic nerve ischemia rather than retinal ischemia.[19,41,58]
- Ocular findings[19,20,51,55,57]:
  ○ PION.
  ○ Cup-to-disc ratio greater than 0.2 in fellow eye.
  ○ Early massive or bilateral simultaneous visual loss.
  ○ Markedly pallid optic disc edema (chalky white in 68.7%).
  ○ End-stage optic disc appearance of cupping[59] (seen in 92% of eyes with arteritic AION vs. 2% of eyes with NA-AION).[43]
  ○ Fluorescein angiography findings of choroidal nonperfusion or delayed choroidal filling (indocyanine green angiography provides no additional information).[36,57,60,61,62]
  ○ AION associated with choroidal nonfilling.
  ○ Simultaneous AION with nonembolic cilioretinal artery occlusion.
  ○ Simultaneous AION with choroidal or retinal infarction.

Box 5.3 Other less common ocular features of GCA

- Visual loss:
  ○ Transient visual loss.[19,41,63]
  ○ Alternating transient visual loss.[64]
  ○ Alternating transient visual loss induced by bright light.[65]
  ○ Posture-related retinal ischemia.
  ○ Bilateral transient visual loss with change in posture due to vertebrobasilar involvement.[66]
  ○ Bilateral transient visual loss with change in posture due to impending AION.[66]
  ○ Nonembolic branch or central retinal artery occlusion.[16,19,41,54,67,68]
  ○ Combined central retinal artery and vein occlusion.
  ○ Ophthalmic artery occlusion.
  ○ Ophthalmic artery microembolism.[69]
  ○ Choroidal or retinal ischemia.[16,70,71]
  ○ Cotton-wool spots.[19,63,72,73]
  ○ General anesthesia–induced ischemic optic neuropathy.
  ○ Pre- and perichiasmal ischemia and visual field defects.
  ○ Postchiasmal ischemic visual field defects (rare).
- Anterior segment involvement
  ○ Anterior segment ischemia[74]:
  ○ Episcleritis and scleritis.

Table 5.1 Ocular findings in 85 patients with biopsy-proven GCA[56] and ocular involvement

Finding	Number of patients (%)
Ocular symptoms	
• Visual loss of varying severity	83 (97.7%)
• Amaurosis fugax	26 (30.6%)
• Diplopia	5 (5.9%)
• Eye pain	7 (8.2%)
Ocular signs	
• AION	69 (81.2%)
• Central retinal artery occlusion	12 (14.1%)
• Cilioretinal artery occlusion	12 (14.1%)
• Posterior ION	6 (7.1%)
• Ocular ischemic syndrome	1 (1.2%)

Abbreviations: AION, anterior ischemic optic neuropathy; GCA, giant cell arteritis; ION, ischemic optic neuropathy.
Note: n = 85 with ocular involvement.

- ○ Iritis.
- ○ Panuveitis.[75]
- ○ Conjunctivitis.
- ○ Glaucoma (e.g., acute angle closure glaucoma).[76]
- ○ Uveitic glaucoma.[77]
- ○ Transient bilateral corneal edema.
- ○ Acute hypotony.
- ○ Marginal corneal ulceration.[77]
- Autonomic pupil abnormalities:
  - ○ Tonic pupil.
  - ○ Light-near dissociation.
  - ○ Horner syndrome.[78]
  - ○ Miosis.
  - ○ Mydriasis.
- Diplopia:
  - ○ Orbital ischemia.
  - ○ Ophthalmoplegia[79] due to ischemia to cranial nerves III, IV, and/or VI.[10,80,81]
  - ○ Brainstem ischemia (rare).
  - ○ Internuclear ophthalmoplegia.[82,83,84,85,86]
  - ○ Internuclear ophthalmoplegia with facial nerve palsy ("eight-and-a-half syndrome").[84]
  - ○ One-and-a-half syndrome.[65]
  - ○ Nystagmus.
  - ○ Subjective diplopia by history.
  - ○ Transient diplopia with or without ptosis.[19,41]
  - ○ Divergence insufficiency.[87]
  - ○ Transient oculomotor synkinesis.
- Laboratory measures of ischemia:
  - ○ Color Doppler hemodynamics[88]:
    - – Decreased ocular pulse.
    - – Decreased ocular pulse amplitudes.
- Orbital involvement:
  - ○ Orbital pseudotumor.[89,90,91,92,93]
  - ○ Orbital infarction.[89,91,94]
  - ○ Ocular ischemic syndrome[19,95,96,97]; may be bilateral.[95]
  - ○ Reversible bruit.
  - ○ Optic nerve enhancement on magnetic resonance imaging (MRI; may help in differentiation from NA-AION).[98]

The differential diagnosis for these ocular conditions (especially unexplained diplopia, retinal or choroidal ischemia, central retinal artery occlusion without visible emboli, or transient visual loss in an older patient) should include GCA. Goldberg reviewed the literature in 1983 on ocular motor paresis in GCA and found ocular muscle involvement was reported in 59 patients.[99] The duration of symptoms was transitory to several months. Many cases had other signs to suggest GCA (e.g., headache, scalp tenderness, optic nerve, or retinal involvement). The diplopia was often transient, variable, and sometimes not associated with motility examination abnormalities. The optic nerve or central retinal artery involvement followed within several days in many patients. Graham described 10 GCA patients with ophthalmoplegia (four pupil-sparing third nerve palsies, four sixth nerve palsies, and two multiple ocular motor nerve palsies).[100] Bondeson described a patient with pupil-sparing third nerve palsy secondary to GCA.[80] Brilakis and Lee reviewed 18 previous reports (81 patients) of diplopia with GCA.[101] Of these 81

patients, 60 (74%) had other signs and symptoms of GCA and 21 (26%) had insufficient clinical information to determine if other signs and symptoms of GCA were present. In a prospective trial evaluating isolated third, fourth, and sixth cranial nerve palsies, Tamhankar et al describe three patients with sixth cranial nerve palsies who were diagnosed with GCA on the basis of elevated ESR, CRP, and positive temporal artery biopsies who had no symptoms of GCA apart from diplopia.[102]

Liu et al noted that transient monocular blindness (18% of patients) and transient diplopia (15% of patients) were the most common premonitory visual complaint in GCA.[41] Hayreh also described transient diplopia in 5.9% of patients with GCA[19] and noted that all of the extraocular muscles and the levator palpebrae superioris are supplied by more than one and up to five vascular branches of the ophthalmic artery, except for the inferior oblique (with only one branch). This collateral vascular supply may explain the usual transient nature of diplopia in GCA, which is thought to be due to ischemia of one or more of the extraocular muscles due to arteritic occlusion of one or more of the muscular arteries.[103]

We do not routinely obtain an ESR on patients with transient or persistent diplopia without systemic signs of GCA in whom there is a clear alternative etiology (e.g., other vasculopathic risk factors). Nevertheless, we consider the diagnosis of GCA in all patients older than 55 years with unexplained diplopia (class III, level U). It is our current practice to evaluate for GCA in elderly patients with diplopia that is ill defined or transient or if there are other signs or symptoms of GCA (class III, level U).

Caselli and Hunder reviewed the neurologic aspects of GCA and emphasized the often under-recognized fact that GCA affects the aortic arch and its branches, not just the superficial temporal arteries. Although GCA does not cause a widespread intracranial vasculitis, it may involve the cervicocephalic arteries including the carotid artery and vertebral arteries.[104] Less commonly recognized systemic findings of GCA are listed below in Box 5.4.

Box 5.4 Less commonly recognized systemic findings of GCA

- Large vessel involvement[105,106]:
  - ○ Carotid siphon.
  - ○ Bruits.[107]
  - ○ Facial artery.[108]
  - ○ Pain on palpation of external carotid artery.[109]
  - ○ Occipital artery pain and occipital neuralgia.[110]
  - ○ Subclavian or axillary artery.[111]
  - ○ Aortitis or aortic rupture.[112,113,114,115,116,117,118]
  - ○ Aortic aneurysm.[119,120]
  - ○ Limb claudication or gangrene.[121,122,123]
  - ○ Upper or lower limb ischemia.[124]
  - ○ Unilateral distal extremity swelling and edema.[125]
  - ○ Raynaud phenomenon.[126]
- Neurologic features:
  - ○ Central nervous system arteritis.[104,107,120,127,128,129]
  - ○ Acute encephalopathy.[127,130]
  - ○ Aseptic meningitis.
  - ○ Cerebellar infarction.[131]
  - ○ Diabetes insipidus.

- ○ Occipital infarction and cortical blindness.
- ○ Multifocal dural enhancement and enhancement of temporalis muscles on MRI.[132]
- ○ Myelopathy[107]:
  - – Cervical radiculopathy.[133]
  - – Quadriplegia.[134]
  - – Transverse myelopathy.
  - – Spinal cord infarction.[135]
- ○ Seizures.
- ○ Transient ischemic attacks.[107]
- ○ Tremor.
- ○ Dysarthria precipitated by chewing or prolonged talking.[136]
- ○ Numb chin syndrome.[137]
- ○ Proximal muscle weakness with skeletal muscle vasculitis.[138]
- ○ Brainstem[139,140]:
  - – Ataxia, nystagmus, upgaze palsy.
  - – Lateral medullary syndrome.[141]
  - – Vertebrobasilar involvement.[142]
- ○ Acute confusional states.[107,127]
- ○ Cluster headache.[143]
- ○ Peripheral neuropathies[107]:
  - – Sciatic neuropathy.
  - – Carpal tunnel syndrome.[144]
- ○ Vernet's syndrome (affection of ninth, tenth, and eleventh cranial nerves due to ischemia of ascending pharyngeal artery).[145]
- Neuropsychiatric syndromes:
  - ○ Hallucinations.
  - ○ Depression.
  - ○ Behavioral changes.
  - ○ Psychosis and confusion.
- Neuro-otologic symptoms.[107]
  - ○ Deafness.[107,129]
  - ○ Tinnitus.
  - ○ Vertigo.
- Pain syndromes (headache, neck pain, backache).[104,146]
- Respiratory tract[147,148,149]:
  - ○ Cough.[150,151]
  - ○ Hoarseness.
  - ○ Diaphragmatic weakness.[152]
  - ○ Tongue ischemia.[107]
- Seronegative polyarthritis.
- Coronary arteritis and myocardial infarction.[153]
- Visceral involvement:
  - ○ Renal involvement.[154]
  - ○ Visceral angiitis.
  - ○ Liver involvement.[81,155]
  - ○ Small bowel infarction.[156]
  - ○ Pericardial effusion.[157]
  - ○ Tongue necrosis.[158]
  - ○ Submandibular swelling.[159]
  - ○ Secondary amyloidosis.[160,161]
- Ischemic skin lesions[162] and scalp necrosis.[163,164,165,166]
- Association with parvovirus B19 infection.[167,168]
- Mortality[169,170]:
  - ○ Myocardial infarction and mesenteric infarction.

5.4 Is the ESR Always Elevated in GCA?

Although the ESR is often elevated in GCA,[171,172] patients with biopsy-proven GCA may have a normal ESR (2–30%).[16,41,51,110,171,173,174,175,176,177,178,179,180,181,182,183] GCA can be seen in the context of normal ESR, normal CRP, or normal ESR, and normal CRP.[181,182] Cullen found an average ESR of 84 mm/hour in TAB-proven GCA.[184] Not only is ESR useful in screening for disease, but the value itself can aid in risk stratification for ocular complications. Higher values increase the risk of severe vision loss.[185,186]

5.5 What Is the Normal Value for an ESR?

The ESR rises with increasing age. The Westergren method is preferred over the Wintrobe method because of the more limited scale of the Wintrobe ESR. Boyd and Hoffbrand reported a Westergren normal ESR of 40 mm/hour for persons older than 65 years.[187] Böttiger and Svedberg felt that 30 mm/hour for women and 20 mm/hour for men were reasonable limits.[188] Hayreh concluded that a patient with an ESR > 40 mm/hour should be considered to "suffer from temporal arteritis, unless proven otherwise."

Miller et al measured Westergren ESR in 27,912 adults aged 20 to 65 years.[189] None of the subjects were anemic. A series of curves of ESR versus age were derived for men and women with maximum values for 98% of the population. An empiric formula (98% curve) for deriving the maximum normal ESR is listed as follows[190]: for men, age divided by 2; for women, age + 10 divided by 2. A recent retrospective study confirmed this rule still applies in patients over age 65.[191]

Hayreh et al suggested a cut-off criterion for an elevated ESR of 33 mm/hour for men and 35 mm/hour for women with a sensitivity and specificity of 92%.[51] In addition, the ESR value at the time of diagnosis may not correlate with the clinical features or prognosis for visual loss in GCA. Other markers (e.g., CRP, von Willebrand factor) have also been proposed in the evaluation of GCA. Jacobson and Slamovits found an inverse correlation between ESR and hematocrit and felt that the "ESR may not reliably indicate active disease in a patient with a normal hematocrit."[192] Finally, it should be emphasized that the diagnosis of GCA is a clinical diagnosis. If the clinical suspicion for GCA is high, TAB and treatment with empiric prednisone should begin regardless of the initial ESR value.

5.6 Are There Other Tests for the Diagnosis of GCA?

Another acute-phase reactant, CRP, is a useful predictor for GCA.[51,182,183,193] Hayreh et al felt that an elevated CRP (above 2.45 mg/dL) was more sensitive (100%) than the ESR (92%) for the detection of GCA, and that a CRP combined with an ESR gave the best specificity for diagnosis (97%).[51]

The following hematologic tests have been reported in association with GCA, but are of uncertain significance (Box 5.5).

Box 5.5 Hematologic tests reported in association with GCA

- Anticardiolipin antibodies.[194,195,196]
- Antineutrophilic antibodies.[196,197]
- Mild to moderate normochromic, normocytic anemia.[198]
- Elevated white blood cell count and platelet count.
- Thrombocytosis.[199,200]
- Elevated acute-phase reactant proteins (e.g., fibrinogen, von Willebrand factor).[201]
- Abnormal plasma viscosity.[202,203]
- Serum protein electrophoresis abnormalities.
- Hepatic dysfunction.
- Elevated endothelin-1 plasma levels.[204]
- Multiple immunologic abnormalities.[197,205,206,207,208,209,210,211]
- Immune complexes:
  - T-cell abnormalities.
  - Immunohistochemical abnormalities.
  - HLA-DR4 and HLA-DR3.[212,213]

Anticardiolipin antibodies were present at the onset in 19 of 40 patients with GCA and polymyalgia rheumatica.[195] In 56% of these patients, these antibodies disappeared during steroid treatment. Thrombocytosis has also been advocated for as a useful predictor of positive TAB in several retrospective trials.[183,199,214]

Several imaging modalities are being evaluated for their utility in the diagnosis of GCA. High-resolution contrast-enhanced MRI can often demonstrate inflammation of cranial arteries and temporalis muscles in patients with suspected GCA and has been advocated for biopsy segment selection and diagnosis.[215,216,217,218,219,220] Ultrasound of superficial temporal, occipital, ophthalmic, vertebral, carotid, and axillary arteries has been evaluated as a noninvasive diagnostic technique with mixed results.[220,221,222,223,224,225,226,227,228,229,230,231,232,233,234,235,236] Large-vessel fluorodeoxyglucose (FDG) uptake in positron emission tomography may have a role in GCA diagnosis as well with the added benefit of potential discovery of occult neoplastic or inflammatory disorders.[237,238,239,240,241]

5.7 Is a TAB Necessary in a Patient with a High Clinical Suspicion for GCA? Should a Unilateral or Bilateral TAB Be Performed?

TAB is a relatively easy and safe procedure to perform with low morbidity. Complications of TAB include infection, chronic skin ulceration, transient brow droop, hemorrhage, damage to the facial nerve, and, rarely, stroke.[242,243,244,245] TAB should be avoided in patients with known carotid artery occlusion or history of superior temporal artery to middle cerebral artery bypass, as this usually insignificant artery can become a source of intracranial blood supply in some cases. Several authors have

reported various biopsy techniques.[56,246,247] Temporal arteries that are difficult to locate may require the use of intraoperative Doppler for localization.[248] Hall et al performed 134 TABs; and 46 (34%) showed GCA.[249] Of the 88 TABs (66%) that were normal (over a 70-month follow-up period), only 8 patients required steroid therapy. Thus, a negative TAB predicted the absence of steroid therapy requirement in 91% and helped determine the appropriate treatment in 94% of cases. These and other authors thought that a TAB should be done before patients are committed to long-term corticosteroid therapy[249] because of the associated significant side effects of chronic steroid use including cushingoid features, hypertension, diabetes, osteoporosis, compression fractures (up to 25% of patients), gastritis, peptic ulcers, steroid myopathy, steroid psychosis, and fluid retention requiring diuretics.[250] Using a clinical decision analysis approach, Nadeau concluded that when steroid complications were likely, a TAB was useful even with "fairly high pre-biopsy probabilities of disease."[189] In addition, Hedges et al thought that no laboratory test (i.e., ESR) or frequently observed symptom or sign of GCA alone or in combination with other findings (e.g., jaw claudication) had the diagnostic specificity or sensitivity of the TAB.[251]

Patients with a negative unilateral TAB in whom there is a strong clinical suspicion (see clinical features and symptom clusters, discussed earlier) for GCA should be considered for a contralateral TAB.[23,252] To minimize costs, some authors have advocated that a frozen section be performed on the symptomatic-side TAB and, if it is normal, proceed at the same sitting with a contralateral TAB.[253]

Ponge et al analyzed 200 patients, all of whom underwent bilateral TAB, all of which were preceded by Doppler flow studies. Forty-two TABs were positive, 20 bilaterally and 22 unilaterally.[254] In their analysis, they discovered that four patients with GCA would not have been diagnosed if only a unilateral TAB had been performed. Unilaterally positive TABs have been demonstrated in 8 to 14% of retrospective bilateral TAB series.[253] Hall and Hunder retrospectively reviewed 652 TABs at Mayo Clinic.[253] Of these, 234 (36%) revealed GCA, and 193 (82%) were positive on unilateral TAB. Bilateral TABs were performed in 41 cases (18%) because frozen section was normal on the first TAB. Of the 193 unilateral TABs, frozen section was abnormal in 188 and normal in 5. Thus, 86% of the 234 cases would have been diagnosed by unilateral TAB alone and 14% were diagnosed only because a TAB was performed on the contralateral side. Hayreh et al reported 76 of 363 patients who underwent a second TAB because of a strong clinical index of suspicion for GCA.[21] Seven of these 76 patients had a positive contralateral TAB. Of the remaining 257 patients with a negative TAB, none developed signs of GCA on follow-up and these authors thought that this was indicative that a second TAB would not have been positive.

Boyev et al performed a retrospective study to determine the utility of unilateral versus bilateral TABs in detecting the pathologic changes of GCA.[255] Of 908 specimens examined from 758 patients, 300 specimens were simultaneous bilateral biopsies from 150 patients, 72 specimens were bilateral sequential biopsies from 36 patients, and the remaining 536 specimens were unilateral biopsies from 536 patients. Of the 186 patients who had bilateral simultaneous or nonsimultaneous biopsies, 176 had identical diagnoses on both sides. In four patients, no artery was obtained on one side. In each of the remaining six patients, five of whom had bilateral simultaneous biopsies and one of whom had bilateral sequential biopsies performed 8 days apart, the biopsy specimen from one side was interpreted as showing only arteriosclerotic changes with no evidence of active or healed arteritis, whereas the other specimen was interpreted as showing either probable healed arteritis (three specimens) or possible early arteritis (three cases). In none of the six patients with differing diagnoses between the two sides was one side interpreted as showing definite, active GCA. Five of six patients were subsequently determined to have GCA, based on a combination of clinical findings, ESR, and response to treatment with corticosteroids. The authors concluded that performing simultaneous or sequential TABs improves the diagnostic yield in at least 3% of cases of GCA, whereas in 97% of cases the two specimens show the same findings. Thus, in patients in whom only one artery can be biopsied, there is a high probability of obtaining the correct diagnosis. Nevertheless, although the improvement in diagnostic yield of bilateral TABs is low, the consequences of both delayed diagnosis and treatment of GCA as well as the use of systemic corticosteroids in patients who do not have GCA are of such severity that consideration should be given to performing bilateral TABs in patients suspected of having the disease.

Pless et al reviewed 60 bilateral TAB results and reported a 5% chance of obtaining a positive biopsy result on one side and a negative biopsy result on the other side,[256] whereas Danesh-Meyer et al found a 1% discordance among 91 bilateral TABs.[243] Danesh-Meyer et al performed a meta-analysis of existing literature and concluded that the overall chance of discordance is about 4%.[243] They suggest that "consideration of simultaneous bilateral TABs appears to be a safe and prudent approach for diagnosis of GCA,"[243] and Pless et al suggest that "it is reasonable to biopsy both sides at the same session in order to increase the likelihood of achievement of a correct diagnosis."[256] In editorials following the papers of Danesh-Meyer et al and Pless et al, the following suggestions were noted:

1. Miller suggested that bilateral TABs should be considered in all patients in whom the diagnosis of GCA is suspected. "The biopsies can be simultaneous or sequential."[245]

2. Lessell suggests that "it makes sense to routinely perform bilateral biopsies or to biopsy the other side if the first side has a negative result in patients whose symptoms, signs, and laboratory results point to the diagnosis of giant cell arteritis."[257]

3. Savino suggests that "performance of bilateral TAB, with or without the aid of frozen sections, appears to be the safest strategy."[258]

We perform unilateral TAB in all patients (classes II–III, level C). If the pre-TAB index of suspicion for GCA is low, then we do not perform a second TAB. If the pre-TAB index of suspicion for GCA is high, then we consider a contralateral TAB. In the cases of moderate suspicion, we individualize the decision for contralateral TAB (class III, level C). In cases where the patient cannot or will not undergo biopsy, counseling and treatment plan are made on an individual basis and the index of suspicion for disease. If clinical suspicion is high enough to warrant TAB, then it is often frequently high enough to also initiate empiric steroid therapy until obtaining pathological biopsy results.

TAB has a variable sensitivity for GCA in the literature ranging from 56 to 93%.[28,259] The sensitivity improves to 85 to 90% when clear criteria for negative TAB are established.[151] Skip lesions may occur pathologically (even in bilateral TAB) and may produce a false-negative rate of at least 4 to 5%.[260] A large segment TAB of a length of at least 2 to 5 cm is often recommended,[260,261,262,263] but other authors have found that even TAB as short as 4 mm (if serially sectioned properly at 1-mm segments and with a minimum of nine sections from each segment) may result in a less than 1% false-negative rate (99% probability of detecting any evidence of GCA).[264] Short-length TAB, insufficient sectioning (0.25–0.5 mm cross-sections through the entire specimen are recommended),[265] and variability in the quality and availability of good ophthalmic pathologic interpretation of specimens contribute to a high false-negative rate of 9 to 61%.[28] In addition, although steroid therapy may produce a false-negative result, TABs may be performed up to a few weeks (or more) of starting steroid treatment.[266,267] Posttreatment TABs produce characteristic histopathological changes that can be detected reliably; occasionally, TAB may be positive even after 6 months of prednisone treatment.[268] Thus, even in the setting of a negative unilateral (or bilateral) TAB, the patient with a high clinical suspicion for GCA should be treated with continued empiric corticosteroids (oral prednisone 80–120 mg/d). Consideration could be given to a third biopsy of other arteries (e.g., occipital, facial, or frontal artery) if the clinical suspicion for GCA remains high and pathologic confirmation is desired.[269,270] We have rarely had to resort to a third biopsy (class IV, level U). It should also be noted that TABs may occasionally reveal etiologies other than GCA (e.g., sarcoidosis or granulomatosis with polyangiitis) for temporal artery vasculitis[271,272] and a tender superficial temporal artery and decreased pulse on palpation may occur with intimal fibrosis.[273] In a patient thought to have arteritic posterior ION, a TAB revealed lung adenocarcinoma as a cause for the optic neuropathy.[274]

5.8 What Is the Evaluation for a Patient with a Moderate Clinical Suspicion for GCA?

Patients with moderate clinical suspicion for GCA should undergo an ESR and a TAB (classes II–III, level B). Unfortunately, constitutional symptoms and signs may be absent in up to 21.2% of cases ("occult" GCA).[20,41,275] In a study of 85 patients with biopsy-proven GCA, occult GCA occurred in 18 patients (21.5%).[20] Ocular symptoms in these patients with occult GCA included visual loss in 18 patients (100%), amaurosis fugax in 6 (33.3%), diplopia in 2 (11.1%), and eye pain in 1 (5.6%), whereas ocular ischemia lesions included AION in 17 (94.4%), central retinal artery occlusion in 2 (11.1%), and cilioretinal artery occlusion in 2 (11.1%). If the ESR is elevated, and if a unilateral TAB is negative, then a contralateral TAB should be performed. Alternatively, a frozen section of the TAB on the symptomatic side could be performed and, if negative, a simultaneous contralateral TAB is done.[253] If both TABs are negative, alternative etiologies of the elevated ESR should be considered, such as infections, connective tissue disease, renal disease (especially nephrotic syndrome and uremia),[276] malignant neoplasm (21% of negative TAB were cancer in the Hedges series), diabetes mellitus,[251] and diffuse disseminated atheroembolism.[277]

If the ESR (and/or CRP) are normal, a unilateral TAB is negative, and the patient has few or nonspecific constitutional symptoms, then the steroid therapy can be tapered or a contralateral TAB can be performed. If both TABs are negative, the steroids can be tapered.

5.9 What Is the Evaluation of the Patient with a Low Clinical Suspicion for GCA?

In patients with low clinical suspicion for GCA (e.g., typical AION in a known vasculopathic patient with no constitutional signs or symptoms), alternative etiologies (e.g., infection, inflammation, collagen vascular disease, underlying malignancy, diabetes) for a high or even borderline high ESR should be investigated.[251] Bedell and Bush suggested that patients with markedly elevated ESR (i.e., ESR > 100 mm/hour) should be evaluated for underlying disease.[278] Based in part on these recommendations, we suggest the evaluation outlined in Box 5.6 for patients with an elevated ESR and a low clinical suspicion for GCA.

> **Box 5.6 Evaluation outline for patients with an elevated ESR and a low clinical suspicion for GCA**
>
> - Complete blood count with differential.
> - Blood urea nitrogen and creatinine.
> - Alkaline phosphatase.
> - Serum protein electrophoresis.
> - Serum cholesterol.
> - Pregnancy test.
> - Chest radiography.
> - Consider mammogram and other evaluation for underlying malignancy.
> - Urine analysis.
> - Purified protein derivative (ppd), control skin testing, and/or interferon gamma release assay (IGRA).
> - Guaiac tests of stools (six determinations).

In patients with a low clinical suspicion for GCA and an elevated ESR, a unilateral TAB could be performed and, if negative, no further evaluation or treatment for GCA is needed (class III, level C).

5.10 What Is the Preferred Treatment Regimen for GCA?

Untreated GCA may result in significant visual loss in one or both eyes. Therefore, it is imperative that corticosteroid therapy begin immediately upon clinical suspicion of GCA (class II, level B) to prevent visual loss (i.e., before TAB and laboratory confirmation). Most authors have recommended an initial dose of oral prednisone of 1.0 to 1.5 mg/kg (60–100 mg/day) class III,

level C).[29,91,279,280,281] Although some authors[3] have reported that an initial lower dose of 40 mg/day may be adequate to control clinical symptoms,[29] patients with visual loss probably require higher doses. Some anecdotal cases of visual improvement have been reported following intravenous (IV) corticosteroids for patients with visual loss and GCA.[10,27,31,41] Many patients note improvement in symptoms within 1 to 2 days of starting steroid therapy, but other patients may continue to experience symptoms of GCA including visual loss despite adequate corticosteroid therapy.[3,41,282,283] A rapid or premature reduction of steroid therapy in GCA may also precipitate visual loss.[184] Occasionally, new AION may occur in patients on "adequate" doses of corticosteroids.[283] Hwang et al reported a patient who developed bilateral ocular ischemic syndrome despite corticosteroid treatment.[97]

Jover et al reported a randomized, double-blind, placebo-controlled study comparing corticosteroids alone versus corticosteroids combined with methotrexate in 42 patients with new-onset GCA.[284] The prednisone plus methotrexate group experienced fewer relapses than the prednisone with placebo group, whereas the rate and severity of adverse events were similar in both groups. The authors suggested that methotrexate plus corticosteroids is a safe alternative to corticosteroids alone for GCA and is more effective in controlling disease.[284] A meta-analysis of drug effectiveness in GCA referenced a marginal benefit of adjunctive methotrexate with respect to relapse,[285] but individual trials have reported conflicting results regarding methotrexate's ability to control disease activity, reduce relapse rate, and reduce corticosteroid dose and toxicity.[286,287]

Staunton et al described a patient with GCA whose clinical condition deteriorated steadily with signs suggesting an evolving vertebrobasilar stroke during corticosteroid treatment.[288] The authors theorized that the clinical deterioration might have actually been induced by the initiation of the corticosteroids.

Low-dose aspirin has been evaluated as a concomitant treatment in GCA, but its safety and efficacy are lacking in evidence from randomized controlled trials; its use should be guided by traditional cardiovascular risk factors.[289,290,291]

5.11 Should Oral or Intravenous Corticosteroids Be Used for GCA?

Liu et al reported a 34% chance of visual improvement after corticosteroid therapy. Additional visual loss occurred in 7 of 41 (17%) patients despite corticosteroids.[41] Three patients experienced fellow-eye involvement after oral therapy, but none of those treated with IV steroids developed fellow-eye involvement. Based on these results, these authors recommended IV therapy (methylprednisolone 250 mg four times daily for 3–5 days) in patients with visual loss due to GCA.[41]

Matzkin et al reported visual recovery in two patients with central retinal artery occlusions due to GCA after treatment with high-dose IV methylprednisolone.[27] Other authors have described anecdotal cases of visual improvement following IV corticosteroids for patients with visual loss and GCA.[3,10,27,31,41] Well-controlled prospective data on oral versus IV corticosteroids are limited,[53,292] but one double-blind, placebo-controlled, randomized prospective clinical trial found that initial treatment with IV glucocorticoid led to higher rates of eventual sustained remission and more rapid tapering of oral glucocorticoids.[293] Cornblath and Eggenberger reviewed charts from two centers and reviewed all previously reported cases of GCA treated with IV methylprednisolone.[292] Four patients with GCA exhibited severe progressive visual loss after at least 48 hours of high-dose IV methylprednisolone, and a fifth patient had further loss in one eye and improvement in the other eye after 24 hours of treatment. They noted that in previous reports of IV methylprednisolone for GCA, 4 patients lost vision and 14 patients recovered vision. They concluded that the results of IV methylprednisolone treatment of patients with visual loss from GCA are similar to the results of treatment with oral corticosteroids, with IV methylprednisolone treatment being more costly and having a small risk of sudden death. In a retrospective study, Chan et al reported visual acuity improvement in 21 of 73 (29%) patients treated promptly with oral or IV corticosteroids.[294] There was an increased likelihood of improved vision in the group given IV corticosteroids (40%) compared with those who received oral steroids (13%). Patients with GCA treated with oral or IV corticosteroids can have visual loss in a previously involved eye or an uninvolved eye, or can have visual recovery.[295] Nevertheless, we favor IV steroids in patients with severe visual loss of less than 48 hours' duration due to GCA, especially if there is bilateral involvement, if the patient is monocular, or if the patient has lost vision during oral steroid therapy (class III, level C).[57,296]

The visual prognosis after AION or CRAO due to GCA is poor, but significant visual improvement after steroid therapy has been reported in a small percentage of patients.[3,9,10,27,41,53,294] Aiello et al reviewed 245 patients over a 5-year period at the Mayo Clinic.[3] Of these 245 patients, 34 (14%) permanently lost vision due to GCA. After 5 years, the probability of visual loss after starting steroid therapy (oral) was 1%. These authors reviewed an additional 857 patients from the literature. Of these 857 patients, 174 (20%) lost vision due to GCA, and 31 of these 174 patients had visual loss or progression on steroid therapy. Kupersmith et al studied 22 patients with GCA, 7 of whom (9 eyes) had ischemic optic nerve injury.[297] Four eyes had improved visual acuity of two lines or more within 1 year of starting corticosteroids, and no patient developed visual loss as the steroids were reduced. At 1 year, visual acuity, contrast sensitivity, color vision, and threshold perimetry were not significantly different from 4- to 5-week determinations. At 1 year, no significant cataractous or glaucomatous changes were noted. The authors concluded that patients with GCA-related visual loss can improve with treatment (starting doses 60–1,000 mg/day with reduction to daily doses of 40–50 mg/day given for 4–6 weeks) and that gradual reduction of dose thereafter, as clinically permitted, did not result in delayed visual loss. There were no significant dose-related ophthalmic complications.

Gonzalez-Gay et al noted visual involvement in 69 of 239 patients with GCA with predictors of permanent visual loss including transient visual loss, jaw claudications, normal liver enzymes, and absence of constitutional syndrome.[140] Partial improvement of vision was noted in eight patients, with the only predictor of improvement being early corticosteroid treatment (oral or IV) within the first day of visual loss.

Consultation with an internist or rheumatologist is recommended for the detection of constitutional signs, monitoring of ESR, and management of steroid therapy and potential side effects in patients with GCA.[28] Hunder emphasized that the goal of therapy is to use the lowest dose of steroid over the shortest period of time to adequately control the symptoms of GCA.[23] Unfortunately, the dosage and duration of therapy are variable among patients and must be determined on an individual and empirical basis.[23,298] Gradual tapering of the steroid while monitoring for recurrent symptoms or ESR elevation is a typical approach. Many patients can be tapered off steroids within 1 year, but some patients (especially those with neurologic or other systemic symptoms) may require prolonged (years) or indefinite therapy. Recurrences may also occur years later. Turner et al reported a normalization of the ESR in 87% of 47 patients within 4 weeks of treatment.[299] Huston et al reported a duration of steroid treatment of 1 to 77 months (median 7 months).[300] Cullen and Coleiro felt that an ESR of less than 20 mm/hour was a desirable goal.[301] Delecoeuillerie et al reported a mean duration of therapy of 30.9 months in 210 patients,[302] but Andersson et al reported an average duration of 5 to 6 years.[303,304] Tapering of steroids is equally important as starting therapy in GCA because the risk of fracture is increased sixfold and that of cataract formation fourfold after 5 years of steroid therapy.[305] Recurrent symptoms and/or ESR elevation may prompt increasing the steroid dosage, but clinical symptoms may be a better indicator than the ESR alone.[171] As corticosteroid doses are lowered, the ESR may rise and, if it increases to above normal rates, the tapering schedule may be interrupted for 2 to 4 weeks to allow stabilization of the ESR. Although a rise in the ESR is often associated with clinical recurrence of GCA, ischemic complications may occur on steroid therapy despite a stable ESR. Steroid therapy every other day does not sufficiently control disease activity.[306]

5.12 If Major Steroid Complications Occur, Therapy Is Prolonged, or the Disease Is Still Active, What Should Be Done?

A repeat TAB could be considered, but it subjects the patient to a second surgical procedure. In addition, as already stated, a negative TAB (first or second), especially after prolonged steroid therapy, does not exclude GCA. Nevertheless, Cohen reported 13 patients with known GCA and a rising ESR with any attempt at tapering steroid therapy.[307] Nine of these patients underwent a second TAB and one of those had a third TAB to determine if active GCA was present histologically or whether the ESR was elevated due to alternative etiologies. Steroid-related complications (e.g., cushingoid appearance, melena, hematuria, and osteoporosis) had developed in nine patients. Five of the 10 second TABs (50%) continued to show active inflammation, and patients were continued on steroid therapy, whereas the 5 (50%) patients with inactive TAB were tapered off steroids.

Patients with significant contraindications to steroid therapy, those who fail steroid therapy,[308] and those who develop steroid complications may benefit from other immunosuppressive agents. Steroid derivatives such as deflazacort[309] and other immunosuppressive regimens such as cyclophosphamide, azathioprine, dapsone, and cyclosporine have been employed in GCA, but there is little controlled clinical data regarding their efficacy in GCA.[310,311,312] Two trials investigating the additive effect of cyclosporine compared to corticosteroids alone in patients with GCA failed to demonstrate steroid-sparing benefit.[313,314] Several authors[285,286,287,315,316,317] have reported variable responses to methotrexate in addition to steroid therapy in GCA, and this agent can be a useful steroid-sparing medication for GCA in some circumstances. In addition, De Silva and Hazleman reported the use of azathioprine in a double-blind, placebo-controlled study. There was a statistically significant reduction in mean prednisolone dose after 52 weeks in the azathioprine-treated group.[318] Recently, biologics including infliximab, etanercept, adalimumab, and tocilizumab have been evaluated with mixed results; infliximab and adalimumab did not demonstrate clinical benefit,[319,320,321] and trials involving etanercept were too small to draw conclusions.[322,323] Tocilizumab combined with prednisone showed better efficacy and allowed earlier tapering of steroids. It is now FDA-approved for the treatment of GCA based on the randomized clinical trial.[324] Patients with GCA on angiotensin II receptor blockers were found to have lower relapse rates, more prolonged disease-free survival, and quicker reduction of prednisone maintenance dose in one noninterventional prospective cohort trial.[325]

When used, nonsteroid immunosuppressants are typically employed to allow more rapid or sustained tapering of steroids. Corticosteroid therapy must be maintained until the immunosuppressant can reach therapeutic effect, which may be weeks or months. Often, rheumatology consultation is sought to provide input on the appropriate choice of immunosuppressant agent, and to oversee the administration of the therapy.

Our approach to the patient with GCA is outlined in ► Fig. 5.1.

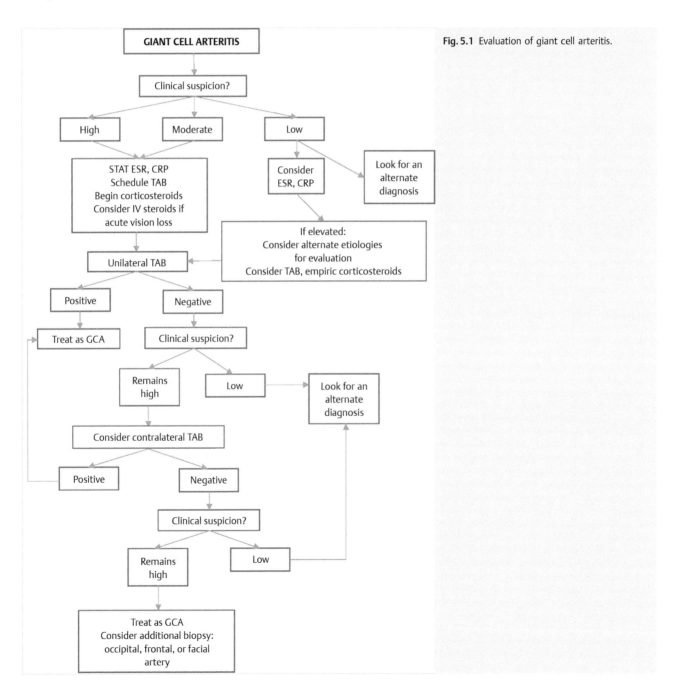

Fig. 5.1 Evaluation of giant cell arteritis.

References

[1] AbuRrahma AF, Thaxton L. Temporal arteritis: diagnostic and therapeutic considerations. Am Surg. 1996; 62(6):449–451

[2] Aburahma AF, Witsberger TA. Diagnosing giant cell temporal arteritis. W V Med J. 1992; 88(5):188–193

[3] Aiello PD, Trautmann JC, McPhee TJ, Kunselman AR, Hunder GG. Visual prognosis in giant cell arteritis. Ophthalmology. 1993; 100(4):550–555

[4] Astion ML, Wener MH, Thomas RG, Hunder GG, Bloch DA. Application of neural networks to the classification of giant cell arteritis. Arthritis Rheum. 1994; 37(5):760–770

[5] Barton JJ, Corbett JJ. Neuro-ophthalmologic vascular emergencies in the elderly. Clin Geriatr Med. 1991; 7(3):525–548

[6] Berlit P. Clinical and laboratory findings with giant cell arteritis. J Neurol Sci. 1992; 111(1):1–12

[7] Buchbinder R, Detsky AS. Management of suspected giant cell arteritis: a decision analysis. J Rheumatol. 1992; 19(8):1220–1228

[8] Cid MC, Font C, Oristrell J, et al. Association between strong inflammatory response and low risk of developing visual loss and other cranial ischemic complications in giant cell (temporal) arteritis. Arthritis Rheum. 1998; 41 (1):26–32

[9] Clearkin L, Caballero J. Recovery of visual function in anterior ischemic optic neuropathy due to giant cell arteritis. Am J Med. 1992; 92(6):703–704

[10] Diamond JP. Treatable blindness in temporal arteritis. Br J Ophthalmol. 1991; 75(7):432

[11] Diamond JP. IV steroid treatment of giant cell arteritis. Ophthalmology. 1993; 100(3):291–292

[12] DiBartolomeo AG, Brick JE. Giant cell arteritis and polymyalgia rheumatica. Postgrad Med. 1992; 91(2):107–109, 112

[13] Evans JM, Vukov LF, Hunder GG. Polymyalgia rheumatica and giant cell arteritis in emergency department patients. Ann Emerg Med. 1993; 22(10): 1633–1635

[14] Gabriel SE, O'Fallon WM, Achkar AA, Lie JT, Hunder GG. The use of clinical characteristics to predict the results of temporal artery biopsy among patients with suspected giant cell arteritis. J Rheumatol. 1995; 22(1):93–96

[15] Gaynes BI. Occult giant cell arteritis: a diagnosis of suspicion. J Am Optom Assoc. 1994; 65(8):564–571

[16] Glutz von Blotzheim S, Borruat FX. Neuro-ophthalmic complications of biopsy-proven giant cell arteritis. Eur J Ophthalmol. 1997; 7(4):375–382

[17] Grosser SJ, Reddy RK, Tomsak RL, Katzin WE. Temporal arteritis in African Americans. Neuro-ophth. 1999; 21(1):25–31

[18] Hayreh SS. Ophthalmic features of giant cell arteritis. Baillieres Clin Rheumatol. 1991; 5(3):431–459

[19] Hayreh SS, Podhajsky PA, Zimmerman B. Ocular manifestations of giant cell arteritis. Am J Ophthalmol. 1998; 125(4):509–520

[20] Hayreh SS, Podhajsky PA, Zimmerman B. Occult giant cell arteritis: ocular manifestations. Am J Ophthalmol. 1998; 125(4):521–526

[21] Heathcote JG. Update in pathology: temporal arteritis and its ocular manifestations. Can J Ophthalmol. 1999; 34(2):63–68

[22] Hellmann DB. Immunopathogenesis, diagnosis, and treatment of giant cell arteritis, temporal arteritis, polymyalgia rheumatica, and Takayasu's arteritis. Curr Opin Rheumatol. 1993; 5(1):25–32

[23] Hunder GG. Giant cell (temporal) arteritis. Rheum Dis Clin North Am. 1990; 16(2):399–409

[24] Kachroo A, Tello C, Bais R, Panush RS. Giant cell arteritis: diagnosis and management. Bull Rheum Dis. 1996; 45(5):2–5

[25] Kattah JC, Mejico L, Chrousos GA, Zimmerman LE, Manz HJ. Pathologic findings in a steroid-responsive optic nerve infarct in giant-cell arteritis. Neurology. 1999; 53(1):177–180

[26] Kyle V, Hazleman BL. The clinical and laboratory course of polymyalgia rheumatica/giant cell arteritis after the first two months of treatment. Ann Rheum Dis. 1993; 52(12):847–850

[27] Matzkin DC, Slamovits TL, Sachs R, Burde RM. Visual recovery in two patients after intravenous methylprednisolone treatment of central retinal artery occlusion secondary to giant-cell arteritis. Ophthalmology. 1992; 99 (1):68–71

[28] Mizen TR. Giant cell arteritis: diagnostic and therapeutic considerations. Ophthalmol Clin North Am. 1991; 4:547–556

[29] Myles AB, Perera T, Ridley MG. Prevention of blindness in giant cell arteritis by corticosteroid treatment. Br J Rheumatol. 1992; 31(2):103–105

[30] Nordborg E, Bengtsson BA. Epidemiology of biopsy-proven giant cell arteritis (GCA). J Intern Med. 1990; 227(4):233–236

[31] Postel EA, Pollock SC. Recovery of vision in a 47-year-old man with fulminant giant cell arteritis. J Clin Neuroophthalmol. 1993; 13(4):262–270

[32] Pountain G, Hazleman B. ABC of rheumatology. Polymyalgia rheumatica and giant cell arteritis. BMJ. 1995; 310(6986):1057–1059

[33] Rousseau P. Giant cell arteritis. Arch Fam Med. 1994; 3(7):628–632

[34] Salvarani C, Gabriel SE, O'Fallon WM, Hunder GG. The incidence of giant cell arteritis in Olmsted County, Minnesota: apparent fluctuations in a cyclic pattern. Ann Intern Med. 1995; 123(3):192–194

[35] Schmidt D, Löffler KU. Temporal arteritis. Comparison of histological and clinical findings. Acta Ophthalmol (Copenh). 1994; 72(3):319–325

[36] Siatkowski RM, Gass JDM, Glaser JS, Smith JL, Schatz NJ, Schiffman J. Fluorescein angiography in the diagnosis of giant cell arteritis. Am J Ophthalmol. 1993; 115(1):57–63

[37] Sonnenblick M, Nesher G, Friedlander Y, Rubinow A. Giant cell arteritis in Jerusalem: a 12-year epidemiological study. Br J Rheumatol. 1994; 33(10): 938–941

[38] Stevens RJ, Hughes RA. The aetiopathogenesis of giant cell arteritis. Br J Rheumatol. 1995; 34(10):960–965

[39] Weinberg DA, Savino PJ, Sergott RC, Bosley TM. Giant cell arteritis. Corticosteroids, temporal artery biopsy, and blindness. Arch Fam Med. 1994; 3(7):623–627

[40] Goh KY, Lim TH. Giant cell arteritis causing bilateral sequential anterior ischaemic optic neuropathy: a case report. Singapore Med J. 2000; 41(1): 32–33

[41] Liu GT, Glaser JS, Schatz NJ, Smith JL. Visual morbidity in giant cell arteritis. Clinical characteristics and prognosis for vision. Ophthalmology. 1994; 101 (11):1779–1785

[42] González-López JJ, González-Moraleja J, Burdaspal-Moratilla A, Rebolleda G, Núñez-Gómez-Álvarez MT, Muñoz-Negrete FJ. Factors associated to temporal artery biopsy result in suspects of giant cell arteritis: a retrospective, multicenter, case-control study. Acta Ophthalmol. 2013; 91 (8):763–768

[43] Danesh-Meyer HV, Savino PJ, Sergott RC. The prevalence of cupping in end-stage arteritic and nonarteritic anterior ischemic optic neuropathy. Ophthalmology. 2001; 108(3):593–598

[44] Hayreh SS, Jonas JB. Optic disc morphology after arteritic anterior ischemic optic neuropathy. Ophthalmology. 2001; 108(9):1586–1594

[45] Lee AG. A case report. Jaw claudication: a sign of giant cell arteritis. J Am Dent Assoc. 1995; 126(7):1028–1029

[46] Fife A, Dorrell L, Snow MH, Ong EL. Giant cell arteritis: a cause of pyrexia of unknown origin. Scott Med J. 1994; 39(4):114–115

[47] Hunder GG, Bloch DA, Michel BA, et al. The American College of Rheumatology 1990 criteria for the classification of giant cell arteritis. Arthritis Rheum. 1990; 33(8):1122–1128

[48] Fernandez-Herlihy L. Temporal arteritis: clinical aids to diagnosis. J Rheumatol. 1988; 15(12):1797–1801

[49] Vilaseca J, González A, Cid MC, Lopez-Vivancos J, Ortega A. Clinical usefulness of temporal artery biopsy. Ann Rheum Dis. 1987; 46(4):282–285

[50] Chmelewski WL, McKnight KM, Agudelo CA, Wise CM. Presenting features and outcomes in patients undergoing temporal artery biopsy. A review of 98 patients. Arch Intern Med. 1992; 152(8):1690–1695

[51] Hayreh SS, Podhajsky PA, Raman R, Zimmerman B. Giant cell arteritis: validity and reliability of various diagnostic criteria. Am J Ophthalmol. 1997; 123(3):285–296

[52] Charness ME, Liu GT. Central retinal artery occlusion in giant cell arteritis: treatment with nitroglycerin. Neurology. 1991; 41(10):1698–1699

[53] Clearkin LG. IV steroids for central retinal artery occlusion in giant-cell arteritis. Ophthalmology. 1992; 99(10):1482–1484

[54] Miller NR. Walsh and Hoyt's Clinical Neuro-ophthalmology. 4th ed. Baltimore, MD: Williams & Wilkins; 1991:2601–2627

[55] Sadda SR, Nee M, Miller NR, Biousse V, Newman NJ, Kouzis A. Clinical spectrum of posterior ischemic optic neuropathy. Am J Ophthalmol. 2001; 132(5):743–750

[56] Hedges TR, III. The importance of temporal artery biopsy in the diagnosis of giant cell arteritis. Arch Ophthalmol. 1992; 110(10):1377

[57] Hayreh SS. Anterior ischaemic optic neuropathy. Differentiation of arteritic from non-arteritic type and its management. Eye (Lond). 1990; 4(Pt 1):25–41

[58] Ronchetto F. Transient monocular blindness in a patient with giant-cell arteritis. Pathogenetic and therapeutic considerations. Recenti Prog Med. 1992; 83(4):241–242

[59] Orgül S, Gass A, Flammer J. Optic disc cupping in arteritic anterior ischemic optic neuropathy. Ophthalmologica. 1994; 208(6):336–338

[60] Mack HG, O'Day J, Currie JN. Delayed choroidal perfusion in giant cell arteritis. J Clin Neuroophthalmol. 1991; 11(4):221–227

[61] Segato T, Piermarocchi S, Midena E. The role of fluorescein angiography in the interpretation of optic nerve head diseases. Metab Pediatr Syst Ophthalmol (1985). 1990; 13(2–4):111–114

[62] Valmaggia C, Speiser P, Bischoff P, Niederberger H. Indocyanine green versus fluorescein angiography in the differential diagnosis of arteritic and nonarteritic anterior ischemic optic neuropathy. Retina. 1999; 19(2): 131–134

[63] Thystrup J, Knudsen GM, Mogensen AM, Fledelius HC. Atypical visual loss in giant cell arteritis. Acta Ophthalmol (Copenh). 1994; 72(6):759–764

[64] Finelli PF. Alternating amaurosis fugax and temporal arteritis. Am J Ophthalmol. 1997; 123(6):850–851

[65] Galetta SL, Balcer LJ, Liu GT. Giant cell arteritis with unusual flow-related neuro-ophthalmologic manifestations. Neurology. 1997; 49(5):1463–1465

[66] Diego M, Margo CE. Postural vision loss in giant cell arteritis. J Neuroophthalmol. 1998; 18(2):124–126

[67] Fineman MS, Savino PJ, Federman JL, Eagle RC, Jr. Branch retinal artery occlusion as the initial sign of giant cell arteritis. Am J Ophthalmol. 1996; 122(3):428–430

[68] Wein FB, Miller NR. Unilateral central retinal artery occlusion followed by contralateral anterior ischemic optic neuropathy in giant cell arteritis. Retina. 2000; 20(3):301–303

[69] Schäuble B, Wijman CAC, Koleini B, Babikian VL. Ophthalmic artery microembolism in giant cell arteritis. J Neuroophthalmol. 2000; 20(4): 273–275

[70] Quillen DA, Cantore WA, Schwartz SR, Brod RD, Sassani JW. Choroidal nonperfusion in giant cell arteritis. Am J Ophthalmol. 1993; 116(2):171–175

[71] Slavin ML, Barondes MJ. Visual loss caused by choroidal ischemia preceding anterior ischemic optic neuropathy in giant cell arteritis. Am J Ophthalmol. 1994; 117(1):81–86

[72] MacLeod JD, Rizk SN. Cotton-wool spots in giant cell arteritis. Eye (Lond). 1993; 7(Pt 5):715–716

[73] Melberg NS, Grand MG, Dieckert JP, et al. Cotton-wool spots and the early diagnosis of giant cell arteritis. Ophthalmology. 1995; 102(11):1611–1614

[74] Birt CM, Slomovic A, Motolko M, Buncic R. Anterior segment ischemia in giant cell arteritis. Can J Ophthalmol. 1994; 29(2):93–94

[75] Rajesh CV, Cole M. Panuveitis as a presenting feature of giant cell arteritis. Br J Ophthalmol. 2000; 84(3):340

[76] Kranemann CF, Buys YM. Acute angle-closure glaucoma in giant cell arteritis. Can J Ophthalmol. 1997; 32(6):389–391

[77] Tomsak RL. Handbook of Treatment in Neuro-ophthalmology. Newton, MA: Butterworth-Heinemann; 1997

[78] Pascual-Sedano B, Roig C. Horner's syndrome due to giant cell arteritis. Neuroophthalmology. 1998; 20:75–77

[79] Goadsby PJ, Mossman S. Giant cell arteritis and ophthalmoplegia. Aust N Z J Med. 1991; 21(6):930

[80] Bondeson J, Asman P. Giant cell arteritis presenting with oculomotor nerve palsy. Scand J Rheumatol. 1997; 26(4):327–328

[81] Killer HE, Holtz DJ, Kaiser HJ, Laeng RH. Diplopia, ptosis, and hepatitis as presenting signs and symptoms of giant cell arteritis. Br J Ophthalmol. 2000; 84(11):1319–1320

[82] Ahmad I, Zaman M. Bilateral internuclear ophthalmoplegia: an initial presenting sign of giant cell arteritis. J Am Geriatr Soc. 1999; 47(6):734–736

[83] Askari A, Jolobe OM, Shepherd DI. Internuclear ophthalmoplegia and Horner's syndrome due to presumed giant cell arteritis. J R Soc Med. 1993; 86(6):362

[84] Eggenberger E. Eight-and-a-half syndrome: one-and-a-half syndrome plus cranial nerve VII palsy. J Neuroophthalmol. 1998; 18(2):114–116

[85] Johnston JL, Thomson GT, Sharpe JA, Inman RD. Internuclear ophthalmoplegia in giant cell arteritis. J Neurol Neurosurg Psychiatry. 1992; 55(1):84–85

[86] Trend P, Graham E. Internuclear ophthalmoplegia in giant-cell arteritis. J Neurol Neurosurg Psychiatry. 1990; 53(6):532–533

[87] Jacobson DM. Divergence insufficiency revisited: natural history of idiopathic cases and neurologic associations. Arch Ophthalmol. 2000; 118 (9):1237–1241

[88] Ho AC, Sergott RC, Regillo CD, et al. Color Doppler hemodynamics of giant cell arteritis. Arch Ophthalmol. 1994; 112(7):938–945

[89] Chertok P, Leroux JL, Le Marchand M, Aboukrat P, Alary JC, Blotman F. Orbital pseudo-tumor in temporal arteritis revealed by computerized tomography. Clin Exp Rheumatol. 1990; 8(6):587–589

[90] de Heide LJ, Talsma MA. Giant-cell arteritis presenting as an orbital pseudotumor. Neth J Med. 1999; 55(4):196–198

[91] Laidlaw DA, Smith PEM, Hudgson P. Orbital pseudotumour secondary to giant cell arteritis: an unreported condition. BMJ. 1990; 300(6727):784

[92] Lee AG, Tang RA, Feldon SE, et al. Orbital presentations of giant cell arteritis. Graefes Arch Clin Exp Ophthalmol. 2001; 239(7):509–513

[93] Looney BD. Unilateral proptosis resulting from giant-cell arteritis. J Am Optom Assoc. 1999; 70(7):443–449

[94] Borruat FX, Bogousslavsky J, Uffer S, Klainguti G, Schatz NJ. Orbital infarction syndrome. Ophthalmology. 1993; 100(4):562–568

[95] Casson RJ, Fleming FK, Shaikh A, James B. Bilateral ocular ischemic syndrome secondary to giant cell arteritis. Arch Ophthalmol. 2001; 119(2): 306–307

[96] Hamed LM, Guy JR, Moster ML, Bosley T. Giant cell arteritis in the ocular ischemic syndrome. Am J Ophthalmol. 1992; 113(6):702–705

[97] Hwang JM, Girkin CA, Perry JD, Lai JC, Miller NR, Hellmann DB. Bilateral ocular ischemic syndrome secondary to giant cell arteritis progressing despite corticosteroid treatment. Am J Ophthalmol. 1999; 127(1):102–104

[98] Lee AG, Eggenberger ER, Kaufman DI, Manrique C. Optic nerve enhancement on magnetic resonance imaging in arteritic ischemic optic neuropathy. J Neuroophthalmol. 1999; 19(4):235–237

[99] Goldberg RT. Ocular muscle paresis and cranial arteritis–an unusual case. Ann Ophthalmol. 1983; 15(3):240–243

[100] Graham E. Survival in temporal arteritis. Trans Ophthalmol Soc U K. 1980; 100(Pt 1):108–110

[101] Brilakis HS, Lee AG. Ophthalmoplegia in treated polymyalgia rheumatica and healed giant cell arteritis. Strabismus. 1998; 6(2):71–75

[102] Tamhankar MA, Biousse V, Ying GS, et al. Isolated third, fourth, and sixth cranial nerve palsies from presumed microvascular versus other causes: a prospective study. Ophthalmology. 2013; 120(11):2264–2269

[103] Hayreh SS. Ocular manifestations of giant cell arteritis (reply to correspondence). Am J Ophthalmol. 1998; 126:742–744

[104] Caselli RJ, Hunder GG. Neurologic aspects of giant cell (temporal) arteritis. Rheum Dis Clin North Am. 1993; 19(4):941–953

[105] Butt Z, Cullen JF, Mutlukan E. Pattern of arterial involvement of the head, neck, and eyes in giant cell arteritis: three case reports. Br J Ophthalmol. 1991; 75(6):368–371

[106] Lambert M, Weber A, Boland B, De Plaen JF, Donckier J. Large vessel vasculitis without temporal artery involvement: isolated form of giant cell arteritis? Clin Rheumatol. 1996; 15(2):174–180

[107] Caselli RJ, Hunder GG, Whisnant JP. Neurologic disease in biopsy-proven giant cell (temporal) arteritis. Neurology. 1988; 38(3):352–359

[108] Achkar AA, Lie JT, Gabriel SE, Hunder GG. Giant cell arteritis involving the facial artery. J Rheumatol. 1995; 22(2):360–362

[109] Gonzalez-Gay MA, Garcia-Porrua C. Carotid tenderness: an ominous sign of giant cell arteritis? Scand J Rheumatol. 1998; 27(2):154–156

[110] Jundt JW, Mock D. Temporal arteritis with normal erythrocyte sedimentation rates presenting as occipital neuralgia. Arthritis Rheum. 1991; 34(2):217–219

[111] Ninet JP, Bachet P, Dumontet CM, Du Colombier PB, Stewart MD, Pasquier JH. Subclavian and axillary involvement in temporal arteritis and polymyalgia rheumatica. Am J Med. 1990; 88(1):13–20

[112] Evans JM, O'Fallon WM, Hunder GG. Increased incidence of aortic aneurysm and dissection in giant cell (temporal) arteritis. A population-based study. Ann Intern Med. 1995; 122(7):502–507

[113] Gersbach P, Läng H, Kipfer B, Meyer R, Schüpbach P. Impending rupture of the ascending aorta due to giant cell arteritis. Eur J Cardiothorac Surg. 1993; 7(12):667–670

[114] Lagrand WK, Hoogendoorn M, Bakker K, te Velde J, Labrie A. Aortoduodenal fistula as an unusual and fatal manifestation of giant-cell arteritis. Eur J Vasc Endovasc Surg. 1996; 11(4):502–503

[115] Lie JT. Aortic and extracranial large vessel giant cell arteritis: a review of 72 cases with histopathologic documentation. Semin Arthritis Rheum. 1995; 24(6):422–431

[116] Liu G, Shupak R, Chiu BK. Aortic dissection in giant-cell arteritis. Semin Arthritis Rheum. 1995; 25(3):160–171

[117] Mitnick HJ, Tunick PA, Rotterdam H, Esposito R. Antemortem diagnosis of giant cell aortitis. J Rheumatol. 1990; 17(5):708–711

[118] Richardson MP, Lever AM, Fink AM, Dixon AK, Hazleman BL. Survival after aortic dissection in giant cell arteritis. Ann Rheum Dis. 1996; 55(5):332–333

[119] Hamano K, Gohra H, Katoh T, et al. An ascending aortic aneurysm caused by giant cell arteritis: report of a case. Surg Today. 1999; 29(9):957–959

[120] Imakita M, Yutani C, Ishibashi-Ueda H. Giant cell arteritis involving the cerebral artery. Arch Pathol Lab Med. 1993; 117(7):729–733

[121] Desmond J, Hussain ST, Colin JF. Giant cell arteritis as a cause of intermittent claudication. Hosp Med. 1999; 60(4):302

[122] Lie JT, Tokugawa DA. Bilateral lower limb gangrene and stroke as initial manifestations of systemic giant cell arteritis in an African-American. J Rheumatol. 1995; 22(2):363–366

[123] Walz-Leblanc BA, Ameli FM, Keystone EC. Giant cell arteritis presenting as limb claudication. Report and review of the literature. J Rheumatol. 1991; 18(3):470–472

[124] García Vázquez JM, Carreira JM, Seoane C, Vidal JJ. Superior and inferior limb ischaemia in giant cell arteritis: angiography follow-up. Clin Rheumatol. 1999; 18(1):61–65

[125] Kontoyianni A, Maragou M, Alvanou E, Kappou I, Dantis P. Unilateral distal extremity swelling with pitting oedema in giant cell arteritis. Clin Rheumatol. 1999; 18(1):82–84

[126] Mallia C, Coleiro B, Crockford M, Ellul B. Raynaud's phenomenon caused by giant cell arteritis. A case report. Adv Exp Med Biol. 1999; 455:517–520

[127] Caselli RJ. Giant cell (temporal) arteritis: a treatable cause of multi-infarct dementia. Neurology. 1990; 40(5):753–755

[128] Husein AM, Haq N. Cerebral arteritis with unusual distribution. Clin Radiol. 1990; 41(5):353–354

[129] Reich KA, Giansiracusa DF, Strongwater SL. Neurologic manifestations of giant cell arteritis. Am J Med. 1990; 89(1):67–72

[130] Tomer Y, Neufeld MY, Shoenfeld Y. Coma with triphasic wave pattern in EEG as a complication of temporal arteritis. Neurology. 1992; 42(2):439–440

[131] Mclean CA, Gonzales MF, Dowling JP. Systemic giant cell arteritis and cerebellar infarction. Stroke. 1993; 24(6):899–902

[132] Joelson E, Ruthrauff B, Ali F, Lindeman N, Sharp FR. Multifocal dural enhancement associated with temporal arteritis. Arch Neurol. 2000; 57(1):119–122

[133] Rivest D, Brunet D, Desbiens R, Bouchard JP. C-5 radiculopathy as a manifestation of giant cell arteritis. Neurology. 1995; 45(6):1222–1224

[134] Brennan MJ, Sandyk R. Reversible quadriplegia in a patient with giant-cell arteritis. S Afr Med J. 1982; 62(3):81–82

[135] Galetta SL, Balcer LJ, Lieberman AP, Syed NA, Lee JM, Oberholtzer JC. Refractory giant cell arteritis with spinal cord infarction. Neurology. 1997; 49(6):1720–1723

[136] Lee CC, Su WW, Hunder GG. Dysarthria associated with giant cell arteritis. J Rheumatol. 1999; 26(4):931–932

[137] Généreau T, Lortholary O, Biousse V, Guillevin L. Numb chin syndrome as first sign of temporal arteritis. J Rheumatol. 1999; 26(6):1425–1426

[138] Lacomis D, Giuliani MJ, Wasko MC, Oddis CV. Giant cell arteritis presenting with proximal weakness and skeletal muscle vasculitis. Muscle Nerve. 1999; 22(1):142–144

[139] Dick AD, Millar A, Johnson N. Brainstem vascular accidents and cranial arteritis. Scott Med J. 1991; 36(3):85

[140] González-Gay MA, Blanco R, Rodríguez-Valverde V, et al. Permanent visual loss and cerebrovascular accidents in giant cell arteritis: predictors and response to treatment. Arthritis Rheum. 1998; 41(8):1497–1504

[141] Shanahan EM, Hutchinson M, Hanley SD, Bresnihan B. Giant cell arteritis presenting as lateral medullary syndrome. Rheumatology (Oxford). 1999; 38(2):188–189

[142] Sheehan MM, Keohane C, Twomey C. Fatal vertebral giant cell arteritis. J Clin Pathol. 1993; 46(12):1129–1131

[143] Jiménez-Jiménez FJ, García-Albea E, Zurdo M, Martínez-Onsurbe P, Ruiz de Villaespesa A. Giant cell arteritis presenting as cluster headache. Neurology. 1998; 51(6):1767–1768

[144] Dennis RH, II, Ransome JR. Giant cell arteritis presenting as a carpal tunnel syndrome. J Natl Med Assoc. 1996; 88(8):524–525

[145] Gout O, Viala K, Lyon-Caen O. Giant cell arteritis and Vernet's syndrome. Neurology. 1998; 50(6):1862–1864

[146] Swartz NG, Beck RW, Savino PJ, et al. Pain in anterior ischemic optic neuropathy. J Neuroophthalmol. 1995; 15(1):9–10

[147] Gur H, Ehrenfeld M, Izsak E. Pleural effusion as a presenting manifestation of giant cell arteritis. Clin Rheumatol. 1996; 15(2):200–203

[148] Rischmueller M, Davies RP, Smith MD. Three year follow-up of a case of giant cell arteritis presenting with a chronic cough and upper limb ischaemic symptoms. Br J Rheumatol. 1996; 35(8):800–802

[149] Zenone T, Souquet PJ, Bohas C, Vital Durand D, Bernard JP. Unusual manifestations of giant cell arteritis: pulmonary nodules, cough, conjunctivitis and otitis with deafness. Eur Respir J. 1994; 7(12):2252–2254

[150] Lim KH, Liam CK, Vasudevan AE, Wong CM. Giant cell arteritis presenting as chronic cough and prolonged fever. Respirology. 1999; 4(3):299–301

[151] Olopade CO, Sekosan M, Schraufnagel DE. Giant cell arteritis manifesting as chronic cough and fever of unknown origin. Mayo Clin Proc. 1997; 72(11):1048–1050

[152] Burton EA, Winer JB, Barber PC. Giant cell arteritis of the cervical radicular vessels presenting with diaphragmatic weakness. J Neurol Neurosurg Psychiatry. 1999; 67(2):223–226

[153] Freddo T, Price M, Kase C, Goldstein MP. Myocardial infarction and coronary artery involvement in giant cell arteritis. Optom Vis Sci. 1999; 76(1):14–18

[154] Lin JL, Hsueh S. Giant cell arteritis induced renal artery aneurysm. Clin Nephrol. 1995; 43(1):66–68

[155] Ilan Y, Ben-Chetrit E. Liver involvement in giant cell arteritis. Clin Rheumatol. 1993; 12(2):219–222

[156] Phelan MJ, Kok K, Burrow C, Thompson RN. Small bowel infarction in association with giant cell arteritis. Br J Rheumatol. 1993; 32(1):63–65

[157] Pedro-Botet J, Coll J, López MJ, Grau JM. Pericardial effusion and giant cell arteritis. Br J Rheumatol. 1996; 35(2):194–195

[158] Llorente Pendás S, De Vicente Rodríguez JC, González García M, Junquera Gutierrez LM, López Arranz JS. Tongue necrosis as a complication of temporal arteritis. Oral Surg Oral Med Oral Pathol. 1994; 78(4):448–451

[159] Ruiz-Masera JJ, Alamillos-Granados FJ, Dean-Ferrer A, et al. Submandibular swelling as the first manifestation of giant cell arteritis. Report of a case. J Craniomaxillofac Surg. 1995; 23(2):119–121

[160] Altiparmak MR, Tabak F, Pamuk ON, Pamuk GE, Mert A, Aktuğlu Y. Giant cell arteritis and secondary amyloidosis: the natural history. Scand J Rheumatol. 2001; 30(2):114–116

[161] Stebbing J, Buetens O, Hellmann D, Stone J. Secondary amyloidosis associated with giant cell arteritis/polymyalgia rheumatica. J Rheumatol. 1999; 26(12):2698–2700

[162] Hansen BL, Junker P. Giant cell arteritis presenting with ischaemic skin lesions of the neck. Br J Rheumatol. 1995; 34(12):1182–1184

[163] Botella-Estrada R, Sammartín O, Martínez V, Campos S, Aliaga A. Magnetic resonance angiography in the diagnosis of a case of giant cell arteritis manifesting as scalp necrosis. Arch Dermatol. 1999; 135(7):769–771

[164] Currey J. Scalp necrosis in giant cell arteritis and review of the literature. Br J Rheumatol. 1997; 36(7):814–816

[165] Rudd JC, Fineman MS, Sergott RC, Eagle RC, Jr. Ischemic scalp necrosis preceding loss of visual acuity in giant cell arteritis. Arch Ophthalmol. 1998; 116(12):1690–1691

[166] Dudenhoefer EJ, Cornblath WT, Schatz MP. Scalp necrosis with giant cell arteritis. Ophthalmology. 1998; 105(10):1875–1878

[167] Gabriel SE, Espy M, Erdman DD, Bjornsson J, Smith TF, Hunder GG. The role of parvovirus B19 in the pathogenesis of giant cell arteritis: a preliminary evaluation. Arthritis Rheum. 1999; 42(6):1255–1258

[168] Staud R, Corman LC. Association of parvovirus B19 infection with giant cell arteritis. Clin Infect Dis. 1996; 22(6):1123

[169] Bisgård C, Sloth H, Keiding N, Juel K. Excess mortality in giant cell arteritis. J Intern Med. 1991; 230(2):119–123

[170] Matteson EL, Gold KN, Bloch DA, Hunder GG. Long-term survival of patients with giant cell arteritis in the American College of Rheumatology giant cell arteritis classification criteria cohort. Am J Med. 1996; 100(2):193–196

[171] Brittain GP, McIlwaine GG, Bell JA, Gibson JM. Plasma viscosity or erythrocyte sedimentation rate in the diagnosis of giant cell arteritis? Br J Ophthalmol. 1991; 75(11):656–659

[172] Weinstein A, Del Giudice J. The erythrocyte sedimentation rate–time honored and tradition bound. J Rheumatol. 1994; 21(7):1177–1178

[173] Brigden M. The erythrocyte sedimentation rate. Still a helpful test when used judiciously. Postgrad Med. 1998; 103(5):257–262, 272–274

[174] Ellis JD, Munro P, McGettrick P. Blindness with a normal erythrocyte sedimentation rate in giant cell arteritis. Br J Hosp Med. 1994; 52(7):358–359

[175] Grodum E, Petersen HA. Temporal arteritis with normal erythrocyte sedimentation rate. J Intern Med. 1990; 227(4):279–280

[176] Litwin MS, Henderson DR, Kirkham B. Normal sedimentation rates and giant cell arteritis. Arch Intern Med. 1992; 152(1):209

[177] Neish PR, Sergent JS. Giant cell arteritis. A case with unusual neurologic manifestations and a normal sedimentation rate. Arch Intern Med. 1991; 151(2):378–380

[178] Salvarani C, Hunder GG. Giant cell arteritis with low erythrocyte sedimentation rate: frequency of occurence in a population-based study. Arthritis Rheum. 2001; 45(2):140–145

[179] Wise CM, Agudelo CA, Chmelewski WL, McKnight KM. Temporal arteritis with low erythrocyte sedimentation rate: a review of five cases. Arthritis Rheum. 1991; 34(12):1571–1574

[180] Zweegman S, Makkink B, Stehouwer CD. Giant-cell arteritis with normal erythrocyte sedimentation rate: case report and review of the literature. Neth J Med. 1993; 42(3–4):128–131

[181] Laria A, Zoli A, Bocci M, Castri F, Federico F, Ferraccioli GF. Systematic review of the literature and a case report informing biopsy-proven giant cell arteritis (GCA) with normal C-reactive protein. Clin Rheumatol. 2012; 31(9):1389–1393

[182] Parikh M, Miller NR, Lee AG, et al. Prevalence of a normal C-reactive protein with an elevated erythrocyte sedimentation rate in biopsy-proven giant cell arteritis. Ophthalmology. 2006; 113(10):1842–1845

[183] Walvick MD, Walvick MP. Giant cell arteritis: laboratory predictors of a positive temporal artery biopsy. Ophthalmology. 2011; 118(6):1201–1204

[184] Cullen JF. Occult temporal arteritis. A common cause of blindness in old age. Br J Ophthalmol. 1967; 51(8):513–525

[185] Lopez-Diaz MJ, Llorca J, Gonzalez-Juanatey C, Peña-Sagredo JL, Martin J, Gonzalez-Gay MA. The erythrocyte sedimentation rate is associated with the development of visual complications in biopsy-proven giant cell arteritis. Semin Arthritis Rheum. 2008; 38(2):116–123

[186] Diaz VA, DeBroff BM, Sinard J. Comparison of histopathologic features, clinical symptoms, and erythrocyte sedimentation rates in biopsy-positive temporal arteritis. Ophthalmology. 2005; 112(7):1293–1298

[187] Boyd RV, Hoffbrand BI. Erythrocyte sedimentation rate in elderly hospital in-patients. BMJ. 1966; 1(5492):901–902

[188] Böttiger LE, Svedberg CA. Normal erythrocyte sedimentation rate and age. BMJ. 1967; 2(5544):85–87

[189] Miller A, Green M, Robinson D. Simple rule for calculating normal erythrocyte sedimentation rate. Br Med J (Clin Res Ed). 1983; 286(6361):266

[190] Sox HC, Jr, Liang MH. The erythrocyte sedimentation rate. Guidelines for rational use. Ann Intern Med. 1986; 104(4):515–523

[191] Nishisako H, et al. Investigation on prediction formulae for calculating erythrocyte sedimentation rate. J Gen Fam Med. 2017 May 2;18(3):146–147. doi: 10.1002/jgf2.1. eCollection 2017 Jun.

[192] Jacobson DM, Slamovits TL. Erythrocyte sedimentation rate and its relationship to hematocrit in giant cell arteritis. Arch Ophthalmol. 1987; 105 (7):965–967

[193] Kermani TA, Schmidt J, Crowson CS, et al. Utility of erythrocyte sedimentation rate and C-reactive protein for the diagnosis of giant cell arteritis. Semin Arthritis Rheum. 2012; 41(6):866–871

[194] Kerleau JM, Lévesque H, Delpech A, et al. Prevalence and evolution of anticardiolipin antibodies in giant cell arteritis during corticosteroid therapy. A prospective study of 20 consecutive cases. Br J Rheumatol. 1994; 33(7):648–650

[195] Manna R, Latteri M, Cristiano G, Todaro L, Scuderi F, Gasbarrini G. Anticardiolipin antibodies in giant cell arteritis and polymyalgia rheumatica: a study of 40 cases. Br J Rheumatol. 1998; 37(2):208–210

[196] McHugh NJ, James IE, Plant GT. Anticardiolipin and antineutrophil antibodies in giant cell arteritis. J Rheumatol. 1990; 17(7):916–922

[197] Bosch X, Font J, Mirapeix E, Cid MC, Revert L, Ingelmo M. Antineutrophil cytoplasmic antibodies in giant cell arteritis. J Rheumatol. 1991; 18(5):787–788

[198] Weiss LM, Gonzalez E, Miller SB, Agudelo CA. Severe anemia as the presenting manifestation of giant cell arteritis. Arthritis Rheum. 1995; 38 (3):434–436

[199] Gonzalez-Alegre P, Ruiz-Lopez AD, Abarca-Costalago M, Gonzalez-Santos P. Increment of the platelet count in temporal arteritis: response to therapy and ischemic complications. Eur Neurol. 2001; 45(1):43–45

[200] Lincoff NS, Erlich PD, Brass LS. Thrombocytosis in temporal arteritis rising platelet counts: a red flag for giant cell arteritis. J Neuroophthalmol. 2000; 20(2):67–72

[201] Pountain GD, Calvin J, Hazleman BL. Alpha 1-antichymotrypsin, C-reactive protein and erythrocyte sedimentation rate in polymyalgia rheumatica and giant cell arteritis. Br J Rheumatol. 1994; 33(6):550–554

[202] Gudmundsson M, Nordborg E, Bengtsson BA, Bjelle A. Plasma viscosity in giant cell arteritis as a predictor of disease activity. Ann Rheum Dis. 1993; 52(2):104–109

[203] Orrell RW, Johnson MH. Plasma viscosity and the diagnosis of giant cell arteritis. Br J Clin Pract. 1993; 47(2):71–72

[204] Pache M, Kaiser HJ, Haufschild T, Lübeck P, Flammer J. Increased endothelin-1 plasma levels in giant cell arteritis: a report on four patients. Am J Ophthalmol. 2002; 133(1):160–162

[205] Radda TM, Pehamberger H, Smolen J, Menzel J. Ocular manifestation of temporal arteritis. Immunological studies. Arch Ophthalmol. 1981; 99(3):487–488

[206] Salvarani C, Macchioni P, Zizzi F, et al. Epidemiologic and immunogenetic aspects of polymyalgia rheumatica and giant cell arteritis in northern Italy. Arthritis Rheum. 1991; 34(3):351–356

[207] Wawryk SO, Ayberk H, Boyd AW, Rode J. Analysis of adhesion molecules in the immunopathogenesis of giant cell arteritis. J Clin Pathol. 1991; 44(6):497–501

[208] Weyand CM, Bartley GB. Giant cell arteritis: new concepts in pathogenesis and implications for management. Am J Ophthalmol. 1997; 123(3):392–395

[209] Weyand CM, Goronzy JJ. Giant cell arteritis as an antigen-driven disease. Rheum Dis Clin North Am. 1995; 21(4):1027–1039

[210] Weyand CM, Hicok KC, Hunder GG, Goronzy JJ. The HLA-DRB1 locus as a genetic component in giant cell arteritis. Mapping of a disease-linked sequence motif to the antigen binding site of the HLA-DR molecule. J Clin Invest. 1992; 90(6):2355–2361

[211] Weyand CM, Schönberger J, Oppitz U, Hunder NN, Hicok KC, Goronzy JJ. Distinct vascular lesions in giant cell arteritis share identical T cell clonotypes. J Exp Med. 1994; 179(3):951–960

[212] Combe B, Sany J, Le Quellec A, Clot J, Eliaou JF. Distribution of HLA-DRB1 alleles of patients with polymyalgia rheumatica and giant cell arteritis in a Mediterranean population. J Rheumatol. 1998; 25(1):94–98

[213] Gros F, Maillefert JF, Behin A, et al. Giant cell arteritis with ocular complications discovered simultaneously in two sisters. Clin Rheumatol. 1998; 17(1):58–61

[214] Foroozan R, Danesh-Meyer H, Savino PJ, Gamble G, Mekari-Sabbagh ON, Sergott RC. Thrombocytosis in patients with biopsy-proven giant cell arteritis. Ophthalmology. 2002; 109(7):1267–1271

[215] Bley TA, Wieben O, Uhl M, Thiel J, Schmidt D, Langer M. High-resolution MRI in giant cell arteritis: imaging of the wall of the superficial temporal artery. AJR Am J Roentgenol. 2005; 184(1):283–287

[216] Veldhoen S, Klink T, Geiger J, et al. MRI displays involvement of the temporalis muscle and the deep temporal artery in patients with giant cell arteritis. Eur Radiol. 2014; 24(11):2971–2979

[217] Franke P, Markl M, Heinzelmann S, et al. Evaluation of a 32-channel versus a 12-channel head coil for high-resolution post-contrast MRI in giant cell arteritis (GCA) at 3 T. Eur J Radiol. 2014; 83(10):1875–1880

[218] Bley TA, Weiben O, Uhl M, et al. Assessment of the cranial involvement pattern of giant cell arteritis with 3 T magnetic resonance imaging. Arthritis Rheum. 2005; 52(8):2470–2477

[219] Klink T, Geiger J, Both M, et al. Giant cell arteritis: diagnostic accuracy of MR imaging of superficial cranial arteries in initial diagnosis-results from a multicenter trial. Radiology. 2014; 273(3):844–852

[220] Bley TA, Reinhard M, Hauenstein C, et al. Comparison of duplex sonography and high-resolution magnetic resonance imaging in the diagnosis of giant cell (temporal) arteritis. Arthritis Rheum. 2008; 58(8):2574–2578

[221] Salvarani C, Silingardi M, Ghirarduzzi A, et al. Is duplex ultrasonography useful for the diagnosis of giant-cell arteritis? Ann Intern Med. 2002; 137(4):232–238

[222] Pfadenhauer K, Weber H. Duplex sonography of the temporal and occipital artery in the diagnosis of temporal arteritis. A prospective study. J Rheumatol. 2003; 30(10):2177–2181

[223] Karassa FB, Matsagas MI, Schmidt WA, Ioannidis JP. Meta-analysis: test performance of ultrasonography for giant-cell arteritis. Ann Intern Med. 2005; 142(5):359–369

[224] Germanò G, Muratore F, Cimino L, et al. Is colour duplex sonography-guided temporal artery biopsy useful in the diagnosis of giant cell arteritis? A randomized study. Rheumatology (Oxford). 2015; 54(3):400–404

[225] Muratore F, Boiardi L, Restuccia G, et al. Comparison between colour duplex sonography findings and different histological patterns of temporal artery. Rheumatology (Oxford). 2013; 52(12):2268–2274

[226] LeSar CJ, Meier GH, DeMasi RJ, et al. The utility of color duplex ultrasonography in the diagnosis of temporal arteritis. J Vasc Surg. 2002; 36 (6):1154–1160

[227] Czihal M, Zanker S, Rademacher A, et al. Sonographic and clinical pattern of extracranial and cranial giant cell arteritis. Scand J Rheumatol. 2012; 41(3):231–236

[228] Pérez López J, Solans Laqué R, Bosch Gil JA, Molina Cateriano C, Huguet Redecilla P, Vilardell Tarrés M. Colour-duplex ultrasonography of the temporal and ophthalmic arteries in the diagnosis and follow-up of giant cell arteritis. Clin Exp Rheumatol. 2009; 27(1) Suppl 52:S77–S82

[229] Murgatroyd H, Nimmo M, Evans A, MacEwen C. The use of ultrasound as an aid in the diagnosis of giant cell arteritis: a pilot study comparing histological features with ultrasound findings. Eye (Lond). 2003; 17(3): 415–419

[230] Schmidt WA, Gromnica-Ihle E. Incidence of temporal arteritis in patients with polymyalgia rheumatica: a prospective study using colour Doppler ultrasonography of the temporal arteries. Rheumatology (Oxford). 2002; 41 (1):46–52

[231] Reinhard M, Schmidt D, Hetzel A. Color-coded sonography in suspected temporal arteritis-experiences after 83 cases. Rheumatol Int. 2004; 24(6): 340–346

[232] Ball EL, Walsh SR, Tang TY, Gohil R, Clarke JM. Role of ultrasonography in the diagnosis of temporal arteritis. Br J Surg. 2010; 97(12):1765–1771

[233] Arida A, Kyprianou M, Kanakis M, Sfikakis PP. The diagnostic value of ultrasonography-derived edema of the temporal artery wall in giant cell arteritis: a second meta-analysis. BMC Musculoskelet Disord. 2010; 11:44

[234] Pfadenhauer K, Weber H. Giant cell arteritis of the occipital arteries–a prospective color coded duplex sonography study in 78 patients. J Neurol. 2003; 250(7):844–849

[235] Black R, Roach D, Rischmueller M, Lester SL, Hill CL. The use of temporal artery ultrasound in the diagnosis of giant cell arteritis in routine practice. Int J Rheum Dis. 2013; 16(3):352–357

[236] García-García J, Ayo-Martín Ó, Argandoña-Palacios L, Segura T. Vertebral artery halo sign in patients with stroke: a key clue for the prompt diagnosis of giant cell arteritis. Stroke. 2011; 42(11):3287–3290

[237] Blockmans D, de Ceuninck L, Vanderschueren S, Knockaert D, Mortelmans L, Bobbaers H. Repetitive 18F-fluorodeoxyglucose positron emission tomography in giant cell arteritis: a prospective study of 35 patients. Arthritis Rheum. 2006; 55(1):131–137

[238] Hooisma GA, Balink H, Houtman PM, Slart RH, Lensen KD. Parameters related to a positive test result for FDG PET(/CT) for large vessel vasculitis: a multicenter retrospective study. Clin Rheumatol. 2012; 31(5):861–871

[239] Walter MA, Melzer RA, Schindler C, Müller-Brand J, Tyndall A, Nitzsche EU. The value of [18F]FDG-PET in the diagnosis of large-vessel vasculitis and the assessment of activity and extent of disease. Eur J Nucl Med Mol Imaging. 2005; 32(6):674–681

[240] Besson FL, Parienti JJ, Bienvenu B, et al. Diagnostic performance of 18F-fluorodeoxyglucose positron emission tomography in giant cell arteritis: a systematic review and meta-analysis. Eur J Nucl Med Mol Imaging. 2011; 38 (9):1764–1772

[241] Belhocine T, Blockmans D, Hustinx R, Vandevivere J, Mortelmans L. Imaging of large vessel vasculitis with (18)FDG PET: illusion or reality? A critical review of the literature data. Eur J Nucl Med Mol Imaging. 2003; 30(9): 1305–1313

[242] Bhatti MT, Goldstein MH. Facial nerve injury following superficial temporal artery biopsy. Dermatol Surg. 2001; 27(1):15–17

[243] Danesh-Meyer HV, Savino PJ, Eagle RC, Jr, Kubis KC, Sergott RC. Low diagnostic yield with second biopsies in suspected giant cell arteritis. J Neuroophthalmol. 2000; 20(3):213–215

[244] Haist SA. Stroke after temporal artery biopsy. Mayo Clin Proc. 1985; 60(8): 538

[245] Miller NR. Giant cell arteritis. J Neuroophthalmol. 2000; 20(3):219–220

[246] Clearkin LG, Watts MT. How to perform a temporal artery biopsy. Br J Hosp Med. 1991; 46(3):172–174

[247] Tomsak RL. Superficial temporal artery biopsy. A simplified technique. J Clin Neuroophthalmol. 1991; 11(3):202–204

[248] Beckman RL, Hartmann BM. The use of a Doppler flow meter to identify the course of the temporal artery. J Clin Neuroophthalmol. 1990; 10(4):304

[249] Hall S, Persellin S, Lie JT, O'Brien PC, Kurland LT, Hunder GG. The therapeutic impact of temporal artery biopsy. Lancet. 1983; 2(8361):1217–1220

[250] Nesher G, Sonnenblick M, Friedlander Y. Analysis of steroid related complications and mortality in temporal arteritis: a 15-year survey of 43 patients. J Rheumatol. 1994; 21(7):1283–1286

[251] Hedges TR, III, Gieger GL, Albert DM. The clinical value of negative temporal artery biopsy specimens. Arch Ophthalmol. 1983; 101(8):1251–1254

[252] Coppeto JR, Monteiro M. Diagnosis of highly occult temporal arteritis by repeat temporal artery biopsies. Neuroophthalmology. 1990; 10:217–218

[253] Hall S, Hunder GG. Is temporal artery biopsy prudent? Mayo Clin Proc. 1984; 59(11):793–796

[254] Ponge T, Barrier JH, Grolleau JY, Ponge A, Vlasak AM, Cottin S. The efficacy of selective unilateral temporal artery biopsy versus bilateral biopsies for diagnosis of giant cell arteritis. J Rheumatol. 1988; 15(6):997–1000

[255] Boyev LR, Miller NR, Green WR. Efficacy of unilateral versus bilateral temporal artery biopsies for the diagnosis of giant cell arteritis. Am J Ophthalmol. 1999; 128(2):211–215

[256] Pless M, Rizzo JF, III, Lamkin JC, Lessell S. Concordance of bilateral temporal artery biopsy in giant cell arteritis. J Neuroophthalmol. 2000; 20(3):216–218

[257] Lessell S. Bilateral temporal artery biopsies in giant cell arteritis. J Neuroophthalmol. 2000; 20(3):220–221

[258] Savino PJ. Giant cell arteritis. J Neuroophthalmol. 2000; 20(3):221

[259] Gonzalez-Gay MA, Garcia-Porrua C, Llorca J, Gonzalez-Louzao C, Rodriguez-Ledo P. Biopsy-negative giant cell arteritis: clinical spectrum and predictive factors for positive temporal artery biopsy. Semin Arthritis Rheum. 2001; 30 (4):249–256

[260] Klein RG, Campbell RJ, Hunder GG, Carney JA. Skip lesions in temporal arteritis. Mayo Clin Proc. 1976; 51(8):504–510

[261] Goslin BJ, Chung MH. Temporal artery biopsy as a means of diagnosing giant cell arteritis: is there over-utilization? Am Surg. 2011; 77(9):1158–1160

[262] Breuer GS, Nesher R, Nesher G. Effect of biopsy length on the rate of positive temporal artery biopsies. Clin Exp Rheumatol. 2009; 27(1) Suppl 52: S10–S13

[263] Sharma NS, Ooi JL, McGarity BH, Vollmer-Conna U, McCluskey P. The length of superficial temporal artery biopsies. ANZ J Surg. 2007; 77(6):437–439

[264] Chambers WA, Bernardino VB. Specimen length in temporal artery biopsies. J Clin Neuroophthalmol. 1988; 8:121–125

[265] McDonnell PJ, Moore GW, Miller NR, Hutchins GM, Green WR. Temporal arteritis. A clinicopathologic study. Ophthalmology. 1986; 93(4):518–530

[266] Achkar AA, Lie JT, Hunder GG, O'Fallon WM, Gabriel SE. How does previous corticosteroid treatment affect the biopsy findings in giant cell (temporal) arteritis? Ann Intern Med. 1994; 120(12):987–992

[267] To KW, Enzer YR, Tsiaras WG. Temporal artery biopsy after one month of corticosteroid therapy. Am J Ophthalmol. 1994; 117(2):265–267

[268] Guevara RA, Newman NJ, Grossniklaus HE. Positive temporal artery biopsy 6 months after prednisone treatment. Arch Ophthalmol. 1998; 116(9):1252–1253

[269] Kattah JC, Cupps T, Manz HJ, el Khodary A, Caputy A. Occipital artery biopsy: a diagnostic alternative in giant cell arteritis. Neurology. 1991; 41(6):949–950

[270] Weems JJ, Jr. Diagnosis of giant cell arteritis by occipital artery biopsy. Am J Med. 1992; 93(2):231–232

[271] Levy MH, Margo CE. Temporal artery biopsy and sarcoidosis. Am J Ophthalmol. 1994; 117(3):409–410

[272] Nishino H, DeRemee RA, Rubino FA, Parisi JE. Wegener's granulomatosis associated with vasculitis of the temporal artery: report of five cases. Mayo Clin Proc. 1993; 68(2):115–121

[273] Petzold A, Plant GT, Scaravilli F. Rapidly developing intimal fibrosis mimicking giant cell arteritis. Br J Ophthalmol. 2002; 86(1):114–115

[274] Bhatti MT, Furman J, Gupta S, Tabandeh H, Monshizadeh R. Superficial temporal artery biopsy diagnostic for lung carcinoma. Am J Ophthalmol. 2001; 132(1):135–138

[275] Desmet GD, Knockaert DC, Bobbaers HJ. Temporal arteritis: the silent presentation and delay in diagnosis. J Intern Med. 1990; 227(4):237–240

[276] Gruener G, Merchut MP. Renal causes of elevated sedimentation rate in suspected temporal arteritis. J Clin Neuroophthalmol. 1992; 12(4):272–274

[277] Coppeto JR, Lessell S, Lessell IM, et al. Diffuse disseminated atheroembolism. Three cases with neuro-ophthalmic manifestations. Arch Ophthalmol. 1984; 102(2):225–228

[278] Bedell SE, Bush BT. Erythrocyte sedimentation rate. From folklore to facts. Am J Med. 1985; 78(6, Pt 1):1001–1009

[279] Lundberg I, Hedfors E. Restricted dose and duration of corticosteroid treatment in patients with polymyalgia rheumatica and temporal arteritis. J Rheumatol. 1990; 17(10):1340–1345

[280] Weisman MH. Corticosteroids in the treatment of rheumatologic diseases. Curr Opin Rheumatol. 1995; 7(3):183–190

[281] Proven A, Gabriel SE, Orces C, O'Fallon WM, Hunder GG. Glucocorticoid therapy in giant cell arteritis: duration and adverse outcomes. Arthritis Rheum. 2003; 49(5):703–708

[282] Evans JM, Batts KP, Hunder GG. Persistent giant cell arteritis despite corticosteroid treatment. Mayo Clin Proc. 1994; 69(11):1060–1061

[283] Rauser M, Rismondo V. Ischemic optic neuropathy during corticosteroid therapy for giant cell arteritis. Arch Ophthalmol. 1995; 113(6):707–708

[284] Jover JA, Hernández-García C, Morado IC, Vargas E, Bañares A, Fernández-Gutiérrez B. Combined treatment of giant-cell arteritis with methotrexate and prednisone. a randomized, double-blind, placebo-controlled trial. Ann Intern Med. 2001; 134(2):106–114

[285] Yates M, Loke YK, Watts RA, MacGregor AJ. Prednisolone combined with adjunctive immunosuppression is not superior to prednisolone alone in terms of efficacy and safety in giant cell arteritis: meta-analysis. Clin Rheumatol. 2014; 33(2):227–236

[286] Hoffman GS, Cid MC, Hellmann DB, et al. International Network for the Study of Systemic Vasculitides. A multicenter, randomized, double-blind, placebo-controlled trial of adjuvant methotrexate treatment for giant cell arteritis. Arthritis Rheum. 2002; 46(5):1309–1318

[287] Mahr AD, Jover JA, Spiera RF, et al. Adjunctive methotrexate for treatment of giant cell arteritis: an individual patient data meta-analysis. Arthritis Rheum. 2007; 56(8):2789–2797

[288] Staunton H, Stafford F, Leader M, O'Riordain D. Deterioration of giant cell arteritis with corticosteroid therapy. Arch Neurol. 2000; 57(4):581–584

[289] Nesher G, Berkun Y, Mates M, Baras M, Rubinow A, Sonnenblick M. Low-dose aspirin and prevention of cranial ischemic complications in giant cell arteritis. Arthritis Rheum. 2004; 50(4):1332–1337

[290] Mollan SP, Sharrack N, Burdon MA, Denniston AK. Aspirin as adjunctive treatment for giant cell arteritis. Cochrane Database Syst Rev. 2014; 8(8): CD010453

[291] Martínez-Taboada VM, López-Hoyos M, Narvaez J, Muñoz-Cacho P. Effect of antiplatelet/anticoagulant therapy on severe ischemic complications in patients with giant cell arteritis: a cumulative meta-analysis. Autoimmun Rev. 2014; 13(8):788–794

[292] Cornblath WT, Eggenberger ER. Progressive visual loss from giant cell arteritis despite high-dose intravenous methylprednisolone. Ophthalmology. 1997; 104(5):854–858

[293] Mazlumzadeh M, Hunder GG, Easley KA, et al. Treatment of giant cell arteritis using induction therapy with high-dose glucocorticoids: a double-blind, placebo-controlled, randomized prospective clinical trial. Arthritis Rheum. 2006; 54(10):3310–3318

[294] Chan CCK, Paine M, O'Day J. Steroid management in giant cell arteritis. Br J Ophthalmol. 2001; 85(9):1061–1064

[295] Costa MM, Romeu JC, da Silva P, de Queiroz V. Successful treatment of ischaemic optic neuropathy secondary to giant cell arteritis with intravenous pulse of methylprednisolone. Clin Rheumatol. 1995; 14(6):713–714

[296] Clearkin LG, Watzkin SC, Burde RM, Sachs R. IV steroids for central retinal artery occlusion in giant-cell arteritis. Ophthalmology. 1992; 99(10):1482–1484

[297] Kupersmith MJ, Langer R, Mitnick H, et al. Visual performance in giant cell arteritis (temporal arteritis) after 1 year of therapy. Br J Ophthalmol. 1999; 83(7):796–801

[298] Hayreh SS, Zimmerman B, Kardon RH. Visual improvement with corticosteroid therapy in giant cell arteritis. Report of a large study and review of literature. Acta Ophthalmol Scand. 2002; 80(4):355–367

[299] Turner RG, Henry J, Friedmann AI, et al. Giant cell arteritis. Postgrad Med J. 1974; 50:265–269

[300] Huston KA, Hunder GG, Lie JT, Kennedy RH, Elveback LR. Temporal arteritis: a 25-year epidemiologic, clinical, and pathologic study. Ann Intern Med. 1978; 88(2):162–167

[301] Cullen JF, Coleiro JA. Ophthalmic complications of giant cell arteritis. Surv Ophthalmol. 1976; 20(4):247–260

[302] Delecoeuillerie G, Joly P, Cohen de Lara A, Paolaggi JB. Polymyalgia rheumatica and temporal arteritis: a retrospective analysis of prognostic features and different corticosteroid regimens (11 year survey of 210 patients). Ann Rheum Dis. 1988; 47(9):733–739

[303] Andersson R, Malmvall BE, Bengtsson BA. Long-term survival in giant cell arteritis including temporal arteritis and polymyalgia rheumatica. A follow-up study of 90 patients treated with corticosteroids. Acta Med Scand. 1986; 220(4):361–364

[304] Andersson R, Malwall B, Bengtsson BA. Long-term corticosteroid treatment in giant cell arteritis. Acta Med Scand. 1986; 220(5):465–469

[305] Robb-Nicholson C, Chang RW, Anderson S, et al. Diagnostic value of the history and examination in giant cell arteritis: a clinical pathological study of 81 temporal artery biopsies. J Rheumatol. 1988; 15(12):1793–1796

[306] Hunder GG, Sheps SG, Allen GL, Joyce JW. Daily and alternate-day corticosteroid regimens in treatment of giant cell arteritis: comparison in a prospective study. Ann Intern Med. 1975; 82(5):613–618

[307] Cohen DN. Temporal arteritis: improvement in visual prognosis and management with repeat biopsies. Trans Am Acad Ophthalmol Otolaryngol. 1973; 77(1):OP74–OP85

[308] Wilke WS, Hoffman GS. Treatment of corticosteroid-resistant giant cell arteritis. Rheum Dis Clin North Am. 1995; 21(1):59–71

[309] Cimmino MA, Moggiana G, Montecucco C, Caporali R, Accardo S. Long term treatment of polymyalgia rheumatica with deflazacort. Ann Rheum Dis. 1994; 53(5):331–333

[310] de Vita S, Tavoni A, Jeracitano G, Gemignani G, Dolcher MP, Bombardieri S. Treatment of giant cell arteritis with cyclophosphamide pulses. J Intern Med. 1992; 232(4):373–375

[311] Loock J, Henes J, Kötter I, et al. Treatment of refractory giant cell arteritis with cyclophosphamide:a retrospective analysis of 35 patients from three centres. Clin Exp Rheumatol. 2012; 30(1) Suppl 70:S70–S76

[312] de Boysson H, Boutemy J, Creveuil C, et al. Is there a place for cyclophosphamide in the treatment of giant-cell arteritis? A case series and systematic review. Semin Arthritis Rheum. 2013; 43(1):105–112

[313] Schaufelberger C, Andersson R, Nordborg E. No additive effect of cyclosporin A compared with glucocorticoid treatment alone in giant cell arteritis: results of an open, controlled, randomized study. Br J Rheumatol. 1998; 37 (4):464–465

[314] Schaufelberger C, Möllby H, Uddhammar A, Bratt J, Nordborg E. No additional steroid-sparing effect of cyclosporine A in giant cell arteritis. Scand J Rheumatol. 2006; 35(4):327–329

[315] Hernández-García C, Soriano C, Morado C, et al. Methotrexate treatment in the management of giant cell arteritis. Scand J Rheumatol. 1994; 23(6):295–298

[316] Langford CA, Sneller MC, Hoffman GS. Methotrexate use in systemic vasculitis. Rheum Dis Clin North Am. 1997; 23(4):841–853

[317] van der Veen MJ, Dinant HJ, van Booma-Frankfort C, van Albada-Kuipers GA, Bijlsma JW. Can methotrexate be used as a steroid sparing agent in the treatment of polymyalgia rheumatica and giant cell arteritis? Ann Rheum Dis. 1996; 55(4):218–223

[318] De Silva M, Hazleman BL. Azathioprine in giant cell arteritis/polymyalgia rheumatica: a double-blind study. Ann Rheum Dis. 1986; 45(2):136–138

[319] Hoffman GS, Cid MC, Rendt-Zagar KE, et al. Infliximab-GCA Study Group. Infliximab for maintenance of glucocorticosteroid-induced remission of giant cell arteritis: a randomized trial. Ann Intern Med. 2007; 146(9):621–630

[320] Visvanathan S, Rahman MU, Hoffman GS, et al. Tissue and serum markers of inflammation during the follow-up of patients with giant-cell arteritis–a prospective longitudinal study. Rheumatology (Oxford). 2011; 50(11):2061–2070

[321] Seror R, Baron G, Hachulla E, et al. Adalimumab for steroid sparing in patients with giant-cell arteritis: results of a multicentre randomised controlled trial. Ann Rheum Dis. 2014; 73(12):2074–2081

[322] Salvarani C, Magnani L, Catanoso M, et al. Tocilizumab: a novel therapy for patients with large-vessel vasculitis. Rheumatology (Oxford). 2012; 51(1): 151–156

[323] Martínez-Taboada VM, Rodríguez-Valverde V, Carreño L, et al. A double-blind placebo controlled trial of etanercept in patients with giant cell arteritis and corticosteroid side effects. Ann Rheum Dis. 2008; 67(5):625–630

[324] Stone JH, Tuckwell K, Dimonaco S, Klearman M, Aringer M, Blockmans D, et al. Trial of tocilizumab in giant-cell arteritis. N Engl J Med 2017;377:317–328. doi: 10.1056/NEJMoa1613849

[325] Alba MA, García-Martínez A, Prieto-González S, et al. Treatment with angiotensin II receptor blockers is associated with prolonged relapse-free survival, lower relapse rate, and corticosteroid-sparing effect in patients with giant cell arteritis. Semin Arthritis Rheum. 2014; 43(6):772–777

6 Traumatic Optic Neuropathy

Stacy V. Smith

Abstract

Traumatic optic neuropathy is optic nerve damage from impact injury to the head, face, or orbit. Patients typically experience vision loss associated with an ipsilateral relative afferent pupillary defect and develop optic atrophy with time. This chapter discusses the clinical pathways for the evaluation and treatment of traumatic optic neuropathy, reviewing the literature in detail.

Keywords: traumatic optic neuropathy, optic atrophy, craniofacial trauma, traumatic vision loss

- Hemorrhage:
  - Retrobulbar with increased intraorbital pressure.
  - Subperiosteal hematoma.
  - Optic nerve sheath hematoma.
- Disrupted vascular supply:
  - Vascular injury.
  - Vasospasm.
  - Ischemia.
  - Infarction.

6.1 What Is the Traumatic Optic Neuropathy?

Traumatic optic neuropathy (TON) is a clinical diagnosis that presents with typical clinical features (Box 6.1). The incidence of TON after craniofacial trauma is probably 2 to 5%. Multiple mechanisms have been proposed in TON. Box 6.2 lists the major theories for pathogenesis of TON.

Box 6.1 Clinical features of traumatic optic neuropathy

- History of direct or indirect impact injury to the head, face, or orbit.
- Vision loss:
  - Unilateral or bilateral.
  - Variable loss of visual acuity (range 20/20 to no light perception).
  - Variable loss of visual field.
- Pupil:
  - Relative afferent pupillary defect if injury is unilateral or bilateral but asymmetric.
- Optic disc:
  - Commonly normal on initial examination; less commonly swollen optic nerve.[1,2]
  - Eventual ipsilateral optic atrophy.
- Exclusion of other etiologies of visual loss in the setting of trauma:
  - Open globe.
  - Traumatic cataract.
  - Vitreous hemorrhage.
  - Retinal detachment.

Box 6.2 Proposed mechanisms of traumatic optic neuropathy[3,4,5,6,7,8]

- Direct mechanical injury:
  - Laceration.
  - Optic nerve contusion, edema, and swelling.
  - Avulsion or transection.
- Bone fragment or fracture (compressive lesion).

6.2 What Is the Evaluation of Traumatic Optic Neuropathy?

Once the clinical diagnosis of TON is made, neuroimaging should be performed if possible. The incidence of visible canal fracture in TON is variable and does not correlate well with the severity of visual loss.[6,9,10] Computed tomography (CT) may be the best imaging study for the evaluation of TON, detailed examination for bone fractures, evaluation of bone anatomy,[9] and detection of acute hemorrhage.[10,11] However, some fractures may not be visible on the CT scan.[12] Crowe et al described a case of an intrasheath and intrachiasmal hemorrhage and delayed visual loss.[13] Chou et al in 1996 summarized the literature on TON from 1922 to 1990 and reported optic canal fracture in 92 of 431 cases (21%).[14]

The role of magnetic resonance imaging (MRI) in TON has yet to be clearly defined.[15] Yang et al reports that diffusion tensor imaging sequences can be used to track the optic nerve fiber bundle and identify disrupted nerve fiber signals on the side of the injured nerve.[16] However, MRI is generally not available in the acute setting and is less useful than CT imaging for the detection of acute hemorrhage, canal fractures, and bone anatomy (class III, level C).

Pattern visual evoked potentials (VEPs) can assess the electrophysiologic function of the optic nerve after injury. While not routinely used in the assessment of TON, it may be useful in cases where the history and complaint do not match the clinical examination findings (e.g., patients with nonorganic overlay). Ikejiri et al assessed pattern VEPs in patients with TON and optic neuritis, and found that TON patients demonstrated significantly lower mean amplitudes, as well as a delay of peak latency.[17] Agarwal and Mahapatra found that recovery of the VEP indicated a good visual prognosis, although patients did not return to baseline visual status.[18]

In patients with TON, the disc develops atrophy over time due to axon loss. Optical coherence tomography (OCT) allows for quantitative measurement of the optic nerve head and retinal thickness. In addition, retinal nerve fiber layer (RNFL) and macular thickness measurements also show thinning due to axon loss in TON. The RNFL thinning appeared to be more pronounced and to occur earlier compared to the macular thinning according to a small study by Cunha et al.[19]

6.3 What Is the Treatment of Traumatic Optic Neuropathy?

The natural history of TON is not well defined, but up to 20 to 38% of untreated patients may improve over time. Hughes described 56 cases of untreated TON, of which 44% were permanently blind and 16% gained useful vision.[20] The literature on medical and surgical treatment of TON is difficult to summarize accurately because of the variations in clinical presentation, treatment modalities (e.g., steroids alone, steroids with surgery, surgery alone), surgical techniques and approaches, study inclusion criteria, and outcome measures, and because of recruitment bias and small sample sizes (classes III–IV, level U). Several early studies, such as Cook et al and Chou et al, suggested that treatment led to a higher rate of visual recovery, whereas others showed no difference compared to observation alone.[14,21,22]

The only randomized, double-blind, placebo-controlled trial for steroids showed no difference from placebo therapy in 31 male patients.[23] Initial visual acuity was a prognostic factor for improvement in final visual acuity, as was visual recovery within the first 48 hours. There was no relation between orbital wall fracture and visual recovery, but a high rate of fractures (80%) may have confounded this result. Also, there was no association with age and visual recovery, but over 75% of the cases were older than 40 years in this trial.[23] Other recent studies have shown that better initial vision on presentation, lack of orbital fracture and/or hemorrhage, earlier presentation, and younger age may be supportive of an improved outcome, regardless of the type of intervention.[24,25,26]

The most recent studies and meta-analyses of the literature continue to show no significant difference between steroids, surgery, steroids and surgery, and observation alone.[23,24,25,27,28] In addition, the corticosteroid randomization after significant head injury (CRASH) trial found that high-dose steroids in significant head trauma are associated with an increased risk of death or severe disability.[29,30] TON occurs in the setting of significant head trauma in many cases, and thus the use of steroids in these cases would be contraindicated. Similarly, surgical treatment poses its own risks relative to the unproven benefits, and may be hazardous in patients with multiple other injuries or an unstable condition. Cochrane reviews of both steroids and surgical treatment of TON recommended that each case be assessed on an individual basis and that proper informed consent be obtained before initiating any therapy.[31,32] Randomized clinical trials were recommended to further evaluate the treatment options.

Newer treatments have been suggested, but lack sufficient data to support their recommendation at this time (classes I–IV, level U): oral levodopa, adenosine disodium, vitamin B1 (thiamine), vitamin B12, nerve growth factor, coenzyme A, triphosphate acid glycosides, red sage root, recombinant human erythropoietin, and transcorneal electrical stimulation.[26,33,34,35,36]

A retrospective review of pediatric and adolescent patients by Goldenberg-Cohen et al found that this population experiences TON from similar mechanisms as adults, and that there was no evidence that treatment led to an improved visual outcome.[37]

6.4 If Corticosteroids Are Used, What Is the Standard Dose?

Although the mainstay of medical treatment for TON has been corticosteroids, there is no prospective well-controlled study (i.e., no class I evidence) to support the efficacy of treatment or the validity of the various steroid preparations, dosages, or duration of therapy.[4,7,38,39] There has only been one small randomized trial, and the results showed that steroids and observation had similar outcomes.[23] Also, the recent CRASH trial data raise the question of whether steroids could have an increased risk of death or disability.[29,30] However, without any other effective treatment to offer in a patient with acute and severe vision loss, a trial of corticosteroids can still be considered if there are no other contraindications (i.e., severe head trauma, gastrointestinal disease, uncontrolled diabetes mellitus).

Anderson et al proposed dexamethasone 3 to 5 mg/kg/day for all patients with TON and advocated surgery for patients with delayed visual loss who failed medical treatment or those with initial visual improvement, followed by worsening despite medical treatment.[38] Three of six patients (50%) had visual recovery after steroids, and four patients underwent transethmoidal-sphenoidal decompression with return of vision in one case (25%). Seiff reported a nonconsecutive, nonrandomized retrospective series of 36 patients with TON.[10] Eighteen patients experienced visual improvement, including 5 of 15 (33%) patients who did not receive corticosteroids, and 13 of 21 (62%) patients treated with dexamethasone 1 mg/kg/day. This difference was not found to be statistically significant. Spoor et al reported an uncontrolled, nonconsecutive, retrospective series of 22 eyes in 21 patients with TON.[40] Of these 21 patients, 8 received intravenous (IV) dexamethasone 20 mg every 6 hours and 13 received IV methylprednisolone (MP) 30 mg/kg load, followed by 15 mg/kg every 6 hours. Visual improvement occurred in 7 of 9 patients in the dexamethasone group, and 12 of the 13 patients in the MP group. Chuenkongkaew and Chirapapaisan also compared the response of TON to IV dexamethasone versus IV MP.[41] Forty-four patients were randomized to either dexamethasone 0.7 mg/kg, followed by 0.35 mg/kg every 6 hours for 72 hours or MP 30 mg/kg bolus, followed by 5.4 mg/kg/h continuous infusion for 72 hours. Both groups received prednisone 1 mg/kg for 2 weeks after the IV steroid. The rate of improvement was the same between the two groups with 8 of 24 (33.3%) patients in the dexamethasone group and 7 of 20 (35%) patients in the MP group demonstrating vision improvement of two lines or better on the Snellen chart.[41] Lessell described 33 cases of TON. Vision improved in 5 of 25 untreated cases, 1 of 4 treated with corticosteroids, and 3 of 4 treated with transethmoidal decompression.[42] Kitthaweesin and Yospaiboon[43] performed a randomized, double-blind study comparing dexamethasone and MP in 20 patients with TON. There were no significant differences in visual improvement between the two groups. Chen et al reviewed 30 cases of TON.[44] Thirteen of 21 cases treated with IV MP improved and patients with vision better than light perception had a better prognosis.

The first National Acute Spinal Cord Injury Study (NASCIS 1)[45] was a non–placebo-controlled study that concluded there was no beneficial effect of MP 1,000 mg bolus, followed by 1,000 mg/day for 10 days ("high dose") compared with MP 100 mg bolus, then 100 mg/day for 10 days ("standard dose"). NASCIS 2 was a multi-center, placebo-controlled, randomized, double-masked study of acute spinal cord injury that showed that treatment within 8 hours with MP 30 mg/kg bolus, followed by 5.4 mg/kg/hour for 24 hours resulted in significant improvement in motor and sensory function compared to placebo. MP delivered after 8 hours did not improve neurologic outcome. It was thought that MP in the 15 to 30 mg/kg dose range had a different pharmacologic effect on central nervous system (CNS) injury parameters including blood flow, calcium homeostasis, energy metabolism, and clinical outcome.[45,46] The traditional dose calculation for an equivalent dose of dexamethasone compared with MP has been based on the glucocorticoid potency of 5:1. Steinsapir and Goldberg emphasized in 1994 that the potency ratio of dexamethasone to MP in CNS injury may be closer to 2:1 and therefore that dexamethasone 15 mg/kg may be required (compared to the dose of 3–6 mg/kg recommended by Anderson and other authors) for adequate treatment of TON.[6] In a more recent review, Steinsapir[47] questioned the evidence that high-dose MP is beneficial in TON and this have been raised by others as well.[24,25,27,31] In one study using a crush injury model in rats, there was a dose-dependent decrease in the number of axons in the MP-treated animals compared with saline-treated controls.[48]

6.5 What Is the Surgical Treatment of Traumatic Optic Neuropathy?

Multiple surgical approaches (e.g., lateral facial, transantral, transconjunctival/intranasal endoscopic, sublabial transnasal, transfrontal, transethmoidal, or a combination of these approaches, extracranial vs. intracranial, etc.) and surgical indications have been offered for the treatment of TON. Unfortunately, there is no well-controlled prospective class I data to support the use of any one surgical approach to the optic nerve over another.[6,11,49,50,51,52,53,54,55,56,57,58,59,60,61] The most recent Cochrane review found the wide range of interventions made it difficult to compare the studies as a group. Based on the relatively high rate of spontaneous visual recovery, the lack of evidence that surgical decompression provides any additional benefit, and the multiple definite risks of surgery, they recommended that each case be assessed individually until there is randomized, prospective data to further guide the decision.[32]

Several articles have suggested that TON is much more common in Japan and more responsive to surgical treatment. Fukado reported 460 canal fractures on stereoscopic radiography of the optic canal in 500 patients with loss of vision following head trauma.[62,63] Of 400 patients who underwent transethmoidal canal decompression, almost 100% had improvement. Several authors have raised serious questions about these studies, including the validity of the diagnostic criteria for canal fracture, the lack of complete ocular examination data including visual field information, the paucity of bilateral cases, the high percentage of improvement after surgery, and the suspiciously high frequency of canal fracture.[64] Niho et al reported an 80% success rate in 25 patients with TON and transsphenoidal decompression of the canal.[65] Matsuzaki et al reported optic canal fractures in 52% of

33 patients with TON.[66] Vision improved in 36% of the 11 cases undergoing surgical decompression of the canal (8 transcranial and 3 transethmoidal). Vision improved in 50% of the 22 patients treated medically with prednisone (40–100 mg/day for 5–7 days), mannitol, and urokinase (if perineural hematoma was suspected). Fujitani et al reported 110 cases of TON, of which 43 cases underwent medical therapy with prednisone 60 mg/day and 70 eyes underwent transethmoidal decompression. The medically treated group had a 44% improvement rate versus a 47% improvement rate after surgery.[67] Mine et al studied 34 patients with indirect TON.[68] Twelve cases (13 eyes) underwent surgery and 24 patients (24 eyes) were managed without surgery. When initial visual acuity was hand motions or better, vision improved significantly more in patients with surgery than in those without surgery. Age and optic canal fracture did not affect visual improvement or influence the decision for or against surgery.

Joseph et al reported 14 patients in a retrospective, nonconsecutive study with TON treated with transethmoidal–sphenoidal canal decompression and dexamethasone pre- and postoperatively. Eleven of the 14 patients improved, including 3 of 5 patients who presented with no light perception (NLP) vision.[53] Luxenberger et al retrospectively studied 14 patients who underwent optic nerve decompression surgery (within 48 hours in 67%) and megadose corticosteroid therapy and noted improvement in 7 patients (50%).[57] However, in this study there was no formal measurement of initial vision, the definition of visual improvement was not stated, and the length of follow-up was not stated. Li et al reported the results of 45 consecutive patients treated with extracranial optic nerve decompression after at least 12 to 24 hours of corticosteroid therapy without improvement and noted visual improvement in 32 patients after surgery (71%).[69] Wang et al[70] reviewed 61 consecutive, nonrandomized patients with TON. There was no significant difference in visual improvement in patients treated with surgical versus nonsurgical means. NLP vision, however, or the presence of an orbital fracture (presumably a marker of more severe trauma), were poor prognostic indicators. In this series, 29 of 34 patients (85%) with orbital fractures presented with NLP. Lübben et al[71] reported a retrospective analysis of 65 cases of TON who underwent optic nerve decompression. Thirteen of their 65 patients were comatose and the surgical indication for TON was based on the finding of a canal or orbital apex lesion. We generally do not recommend surgery for comatose patients who cannot provide visual information. Kountakis et al[72] performed a retrospective review of TON treated with endoscopic optic nerve decompression. Eleven of 34 patients treated with high-dose steroids improved and 23 did not improve. Of these 23 patients, 17 underwent endoscopic optic nerve decompression and 14 of 17 (82%) had improved visual acuity. These authors suggested that patients with visual acuity better than 20/200 had a better prognosis with steroids alone than patients with worse than 20/400 visual acuity.

The data for surgical outcomes in TON have often been confounded by the fact that most patients receive steroids prior to surgery, or studies compare steroid therapy alone to steroids and surgery. Ropposch et al retrospectively reviewed TON cases who underwent optic nerve decompression surgery with or without steroids.[24] Steroids were used in 21 of 42 cases with 29% of patients showing improvements; 8 of 15 patients (53%)

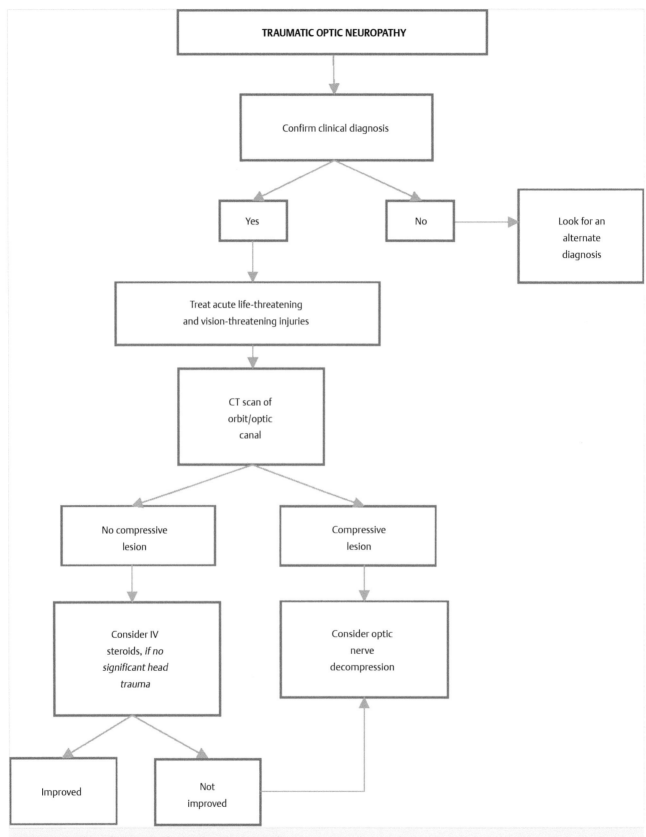

Fig. 6.1 Evaluation and treatment of traumatic optic neuropathy.

who did not receive any steroids had visual improvement (6 cases had insufficient documentation to determine if steroids had been used). The difference between the two groups was not significant, and the authors concluded that the steroids provided no additional benefit on visual outcome.[24] While there was no evidence in this retrospective review to support steroid administration with surgery, we still cannot draw any conclusions to the efficacy of surgery itself due to a lack of a control group who received no intervention.

Gupta et al evaluated early versus late surgical intervention for TON in the pediatric population in a prospective study. The authors concluded that earlier intervention led to better visual outcomes, but this trial had numerous limitations including lack of randomization and a control group, and small sample size.[73] Other studies have not found any evidence that treatment alters outcome in the pediatric population, much like the adult data.[37,74]

Unfortunately, until a randomized, prospective, double-masked, placebo-controlled clinical trial is performed, the treatment of TON will remain controversial (classes II–III, level U).[75,76]

The approach to TON is outlined in ▶ Fig. 6.1.

References

[1] Brodsky MC, Wald KJ, Chen S, Weiter JJ. Protracted posttraumatic optic disc swelling. Ophthalmology. 1995; 102(11):1628–1631

[2] Sullivan G, Helveston EM. Optic atrophy after seemingly trivial trauma. Arch Ophthalmol. 1969; 81(2):159–161

[3] Aitken P, Sofferman R. Traumatic optic neuropathy. Ophthalmol Clin North Am. 1991; 4:479–490

[4] Mauriello JA, DeLuca J, Krieger A, Schulder M, Frohman L. Management of traumatic optic neuropathy–a study of 23 patients. Br J Ophthalmol. 1992; 76 (6):349–352

[5] Miller NR. The management of traumatic optic neuropathy. Arch Ophthalmol. 1990; 108(8):1086–1087

[6] Steinsapir KD, Goldberg RA. Traumatic optic neuropathy. Surv Ophthalmol. 1994; 38(6):487–518

[7] Volpe N, Lessel S, Kline L. Traumatic optic neuropathy: diagnosis and management. Int Ophthalmol Clin. 1991; 31:142–156

[8] Wolin MJ, Lavin PJ. Spontaneous visual recovery from traumatic optic neuropathy after blunt head injury. Am J Ophthalmol. 1990; 109(4):430–435

[9] Goldberg RA, Hannani K, Toga AW. Microanatomy of the orbital apex. Computed tomography and microcryoplaning of soft and hard tissue. Ophthalmology. 1992; 99(9):1447–1452

[10] Seiff SR. High dose corticosteroids for treatment of vision loss due to indirect injury to the optic nerve. Ophthalmic Surg. 1990; 21(6):389–395

[11] Knox BE, Gates GA, Berry SM. Optic nerve decompression via the lateral facial approach. Laryngoscope. 1990; 100(5):458–462

[12] Yang QT, Zhang GH, Liu X, Ye J, Li Y. The therapeutic efficacy of endoscopic optic nerve decompression and its effects on the prognoses of 96 cases of traumatic optic neuropathy. J Trauma Acute Care Surg. 2012; 72(5):1350–1355

[13] Crowe NW, Nickles TP, Troost BT, Elster AD. Intrachiasmal hemorrhage: a cause of delayed post-traumatic blindness. Neurology. 1989; 39(6):863–865

[14] Chou PI, Sadun AA, Chen YC, et al. Clinical experiences in the management of traumatic optic neuropathy. Neuro-ophthalmology. 1996; 18:325–336

[15] Takehara S, Tanaka T, Uemura K, et al. Optic nerve injury demonstrated by MRI with STIR sequences. Neuroradiology. 1994; 36(7):512–514

[16] Yang QT, Fan YP, Zou Y, et al. Evaluation of traumatic optic neuropathy in patients with optic canal fracture using diffusion tensor magnetic resonance imaging: a preliminary report. ORL J Otorhinolaryngol Relat Spec. 2011; 73 (6) Spec:301–307

[17] Ikejiri M, Adachi-Usami E, Mizota A, Tsuyama Y, Miyauchi O, Suehiro S. Pattern visual evoked potentials in traumatic optic neuropathy. Ophthalmologica. 2002; 216(6):415–419

[18] Agarwal A, Mahapatra AK. Visual outcome in optic nerve injury patients without initial light perception. Indian J Ophthalmol. 1999; 47(4):233–236

[19] Cunha LP, Costa-Cunha LV, Malta RF, Monteiro ML. Comparison between retinal nerve fiber layer and macular thickness measured with OCT detecting progressive axonal loss following traumatic optic neuropathy. Arq Bras Oftalmol. 2009; 72(5):622–625

[20] Hughes B. Indirect injury of the optic nerves and chiasma. Bull Johns Hopkins Hosp. 1962; 111:98–126

[21] Cook MW, Levin LA, Joseph MP, Pinczower EF. Traumatic optic neuropathy. A meta-analysis. Arch Otolaryngol Head Neck Surg. 1996; 122(4):389–392

[22] Levin LA, Beck RW, Joseph MP, Seiff S, Kraker R. The treatment of traumatic optic neuropathy: the International Optic Nerve Trauma Study. Ophthalmology. 1999; 106(7):1268–1277

[23] Entezari M, Rajavi Z, Sedighi N, Daftarian N, Sanagoo M. High-dose intravenous methylprednisolone in recent traumatic optic neuropathy; a randomized double-masked placebo-controlled clinical trial. Graefes Arch Clin Exp Ophthalmol. 2007; 245(9):1267–1271

[24] Ropposch T, Steger B, Meço C, et al. The effect of steroids in combination with optic nerve decompression surgery in traumatic optic neuropathy. Laryngoscope. 2013; 123(5):1082–1086

[25] Yang WG, Chen CT, Tsay PK, de Villa GH, Tsai YJ, Chen YR. Outcome for traumatic optic neuropathy–surgical versus nonsurgical treatment. Ann Plast Surg. 2004; 52(1):36–42

[26] Peng A, Li Y, Hu P, Wang Q. Endoscopic optic nerve decompression for traumatic optic neuropathy in children. Int J Pediatr Otorhinolaryngol. 2011; 75(8):992–998

[27] Yip CC, Chng NW, Au Eong KG, Heng WJ, Lim TH, Lim WK. Low-dose intravenous methylprednisolone or conservative treatment in the management of traumatic optic neuropathy. Eur J Ophthalmol. 2002; 12(4):309–314

[28] Hsieh CH, Kuo YR, Hung HC, Tsai HH, Jeng SF. Indirect traumatic optic neuropathy complicated with periorbital facial bone fracture. J Trauma. 2004; 56(4):795–801

[29] Roberts I, Yates D, Sandercock P, et al. CRASH trial collaborators. Effect of intravenous corticosteroids on death within 14 days in 10008 adults with clinically significant head injury (MRC CRASH trial): randomised placebo-controlled trial. Lancet. 2004; 364(9442):1321–1328

[30] Edwards P, Arango M, Balica L, et al. CRASH trial collaborators. Final results of MRC CRASH, a randomised placebo-controlled trial of intravenous corticosteroid in adults with head injury-outcomes at 6 months. Lancet. 2005; 365(9475):1957–1959

[31] Yu-Wai-Man P, Griffiths PG. Steroids for traumatic optic neuropathy. Cochrane Database Syst Rev. 2013; 2013(6):CD006032

[32] Yu-Wai-Man P, Griffiths PG. Surgery for traumatic optic neuropathy. Cochrane Database Syst Rev. 2013; 6:CD005024

[33] Razeghinejad MR, Rahat F, Bagheri M. Levodopa-carbidopa may improve vision loss in indirect traumatic optic neuropathy. J Neurotrauma. 2010; 27 (10):1905–1909

[34] Zhong Y, Shen X, Liu X, Cheng Y. The early effect of nerve growth factor in the management of serious optic nerve contusion. Clin Exp Optom. 2010; 93(6):466–470

[35] Fujikado T, Morimoto T, Matsushita K, Shimojo H, Okawa Y, Tano Y. Effect of transcorneal electrical stimulation in patients with nonarteritic ischemic optic neuropathy or traumatic optic neuropathy. Jpn J Ophthalmol. 2006; 50 (3):266–273

[36] Kashkouli MB, Study Director. Traumatic Optic Neuropathy Treatment Trial (TONTT). ClinicalTrials.gov Identifier: NCT01783847. Available at: https://www.clinicaltrials.gov/ct2/show/nct01783847. Accessed March 29, 2016

[37] Goldenberg-Cohen N, Miller NR, Repka MX. Traumatic optic neuropathy in children and adolescents. J AAPOS. 2004; 8(1):20–27

[38] Anderson RL, Panje WR, Gross CE. Optic nerve blindness following blunt forehead trauma. Ophthalmology. 1982; 89(5):445–455

[39] Lam BL, Weingeist TA. Corticosteroid-responsive traumatic optic neuropathy. Am J Ophthalmol. 1990; 109(1):99–101

[40] Spoor TC, Hartel WC, Lensink DB, Wilkinson MJ. Treatment of traumatic optic neuropathy with corticosteroids. Am J Ophthalmol. 1990; 110(6):665–669

[41] Chuenkongkaew W, Chirapapaisan N. A prospective randomized trial of megadose methylprednisolone and high dose dexamethasone for traumatic optic neuropathy. J Med Assoc Thai. 2002; 85(5):597–603

[42] Lessell S. Indirect optic nerve trauma. Arch Ophthalmol. 1989; 107(3):382–386

[43] Kitthaweesin K, Yospaiboon Y. Dexamethasone and methylprednisolone in treatment of indirect traumatic optic neuropathy. J Med Assoc Thai. 2001; 84 (5):628–634

[44] Chen HY, Tsai RK, Wang HZ. Intravenous methylprednisolone in treatment of traumatic optic neuropathy. Kaohsiung J Med Sci. 1998; 14(9):577–583

[45] Bracken MB, Holford TR. Effects of timing of methylprednisolone or naloxone administration on recovery of segmental and long-tract neurological function in NASCIS 2. J Neurosurg. 1993; 79(4):500–507

[46] Bracken MB, Shepard MJ, Collins WF, et al. A randomized, controlled trial of methylprednisolone or naloxone in the treatment of acute spinal-cord injury. Results of the Second National Acute Spinal Cord Injury Study. N Engl J Med. 1990; 322(20):1405–1411

[47] Steinsapir KD. Traumatic optic neuropathy. Curr Opin Ophthalmol. 1999; 10(5):340–342

[48] Steinsapir KD, Goldberg RA, Sinha S, Hovda DA. Methylprednisolone exacerbates axonal loss following optic nerve trauma in rats. Restor Neurol Neurosci. 2000; 17(4):157–163

[49] Anand VK, Sherwood C, Al-Mefty O. Optic nerve decompression via transethmoid and supraorbital approaches. Oper Tech Otolaryngol–Head Neck Surg. 1991; 2:157–166

[50] Salazar Fernandez CI, Rollon A, Gonzalez Padilla JD. Posttraumatic amaurosis with partial return of visual acuity. J Oral Maxillofac Surg. 1994; 52(10):1077–1079

[51] Friedman M. Optic nerve decompression. Oper Tech Otolaryngol–Head Neck Surg. 1991; 2:149

[52] Girard BC, Bouzas EA, Lamas G, Soudant J. Visual improvement after transethmoid-sphenoid decompression in optic nerve injuries. J Clin Neuroophthalmol. 1992; 12(3):142–148

[53] Joseph MP, Lessell S, Rizzo J, Momose KJ. Extracranial optic nerve decompression for traumatic optic neuropathy. Arch Ophthalmol. 1990; 108(8):1091–1093

[54] Kuppersmith RB, Alford EL, Patrinely JR, Lee AG, Parke RB, Holds JB. Combined transconjunctival/intranasal endoscopic approach to the optic canal in traumatic optic neuropathy. Laryngoscope. 1997; 107(3):311–315

[55] Levin LA, Joseph MP, Rizzo JF, III, Lessell S. Optic canal decompression in indirect optic nerve trauma. Ophthalmology. 1994; 101(3):566–569

[56] Li KK, Teknos TN, Lai A, Lauretano A, Terrell J, Joseph MP. Extracranial optic nerve decompression: a 10-year review of 92 patients. J Craniofac Surg. 1999; 10(5):454–459

[57] Luxenberger W, Stammberger H, Jebeles JA, Walch C. Endoscopic optic nerve decompression: the Graz experience. Laryngoscope. 1998; 108(6):873–882

[58] Chen CT, Chen YR. Endoscopic orbital surgery. Atlas Oral Maxillofac Surg Clin North Am. 2003; 11(2):179–208

[59] Yang Y, Wang H, Shao Y, Wei Z, Zhu S, Wang J. Extradural anterior clinoidectomy as an alternative approach for optic nerve decompression: anatomic study and clinical experience. Neurosurgery. 2006; 59(4) Suppl 2: ONS253–ONS262, discussion ONS262

[60] Chen CT, Huang F, Tsay PK, et al. Endoscopically assisted transconjunctival decompression of traumatic optic neuropathy. J Craniofac Surg. 2007; 18(1):19–26, discussion 27–28

[61] Li HB, Shi JB, Cheng L, Yun O, Xu G. Salvage optic nerve decompression for traumatic blindness under nasal endoscopy: risk and benefit analysis. Clin Otolaryngol. 2007; 32(6):447–451

[62] Fukado Y. Results in 350 cases of surgical decompression of the optic nerve. Trans Ophthalmol Soc N Z. 1973; 25:96–99

[63] Fukado Y. Results in 400 cases of surgical decompression of the optic nerve. Mod Probl Ophthalmol. 1975; 14:474–481

[64] Kennerdell JS, Amsbaugh GA, Myers EN. Transantral-ethmoidal decompression of optic canal fracture. Arch Ophthalmol. 1976; 94(6):1040–1043

[65] Niho S, Niho M, Niho K. Decompression of the optic canal by the transethmoidal route and decompression of the superior orbital fissure. Can J Ophthalmol. 1970; 5(1):22–40

[66] Matsuzaki H, Kunita M, Kawai K. Optic nerve damage in head trauma: clinical and experimental studies. Jpn J Ophthalmol. 1982; 26(4):447–461

[67] Fujitani T, Inoue K, Takahashi T, Ikushima K, Asai T. Indirect traumatic optic neuropathy–visual outcome of operative and nonoperative cases. Jpn J Ophthalmol. 1986; 30(1):125–134

[68] Mine S, Yamakami I, Yamaura A, et al. Outcome of traumatic optic neuropathy. Comparison between surgical and nonsurgical treatment. Acta Neurochir (Wien). 1999; 141(1):27–30

[69] Li KK, Teknos TN, Lai A, Lauretano AM, Joseph MP. Traumatic optic neuropathy: result in 45 consecutive surgically treated patients. Otolaryngol Head Neck Surg. 1999; 120(1):5–11

[70] Wang BH, Robertson BC, Girotto JA, et al. Traumatic optic neuropathy: a review of 61 patients. Plast Reconstr Surg. 2001; 107(7):1655–1664

[71] Lübben B, Stoll W, Grenzebach U. Optic nerve decompression in the comatose and conscious patients after trauma. Laryngoscope. 2001; 111(2):320–328

[72] Kountakis SE, Maillard AA, El-Harazi SM, Longhini L, Urso RG. Endoscopic optic nerve decompression for traumatic blindness. Otolaryngol Head Neck Surg. 2000; 123(1, Pt 1):34–37

[73] Gupta AK, Gupta AK, Gupta A, Malhotra SK. Traumatic optic neuropathy in pediatric population: early intervention or delayed intervention? Int J Pediatr Otorhinolaryngol. 2007; 71(4):559–562

[74] Mahapatra AK, Tandon DA. Traumatic optic neuropathy in children: a prospective study. Pediatr Neurosurg. 1993; 19(1):34–39

[75] Berestka JS, Rizzo JF, III. Controversy in the management of traumatic optic neuropathy. Int Ophthalmol Clin. 1994; 34(3):87–96

[76] Pomeranz HD, Rizzo JF, Lessell S. Treatment of traumatic optic neuropathy. Int Ophthalmol Clin. 1999; 39(1):185–194

7 Papilledema

Murtaza M. Mandviwala, Alec L. Amram, and Mohammed Rigi

Abstract

Papilledema is a term preferably reserved for optic disc edema due to increased intracranial pressure. It must be differentiated from other causes of optic disc edema and pseudopapilledema (e.g., disc drusen). This chapter discusses the clinical pathways of papilledema diagnosis and evaluation, as well as the diagnosis and management of pseudotumor cerebri and idiopathic intracranial hypertension. The literature is reviewed in detail.

Keywords: optic disc edema, papilledema, pseudopapilledema, pseudotumor cerebri, idiopathic intracranial hypertension

7.1 What Is the Definition of Papilledema?

While the term *papilledema* is frequently applied to optic disc swelling from any cause, it should only be used clinically to describe disc swelling resulting from increased intracranial pressure. This term should be used judiciously to avoid inappropriate or unnecessary testing resulting from miscommunication.

Other forms of optic disc swelling should be named in accordance with their underlying local or systemic etiologies (e.g., optic neuritis, anterior ischemic optic neuropathy, etc.). It is usually not possible to determine the etiology of disc swelling from the ophthalmoscopic appearance of the disc alone. The history and neuro-ophthalmologic examination, especially the visual fields, are necessary to reach a diagnosis. It is also important to note that optic disc swelling may not develop if optic atrophy is present. For example, in patients with prior "band" or "bow-tie" atrophy of the optic nerve due to a suprasellar mass, disc swelling may affect only the superior and inferior aspects of the nerve ("twin peaks papilledema").[1]

The symptoms associated with optic disc swelling depend on the underlying etiology. In general, swollen optic discs from any cause may be associated with transient visual obscurations (see Chapter 8).[2] These are typically unilateral or bilateral dimming or blacking out of vision that usually lasts seconds and may be precipitated by changes in posture (e.g., bending or straightening).

7.2 What Are the Features that Distinguish Real Papilledema from Pseudopapilledema?

True disc swelling must be distinguished from pseudopapilledema (e.g., anomalously elevated discs caused by optic nerve head drusen).[3] Pseudopapilledema is a relatively common finding and optic disc drusen are among the most frequent etiologies. Drusen of the disc may be obvious, tiny, or buried. Other disc anomalies that may be mistaken for papilledema include small, "crowded" hyperopic discs and tilted or anomalous discs. With pseudopapilledema, the peripapillary nerve fiber layer is normal, venous pulsations are usually present, there is no vascular engorgement or hemorrhages, there are no cotton-

wool spots, and the discs do not leak dye on fluorescein angiography. Myelinated nerve fibers may occasionally resemble disc swelling but are characterized by a white feathery nerve fiber layer appearance. Hyaloid traction on the optic disc and epipapillary glial tissue may occasionally also be mistaken for disc swelling. Ophthalmoscopic criteria that help distinguish pseudopapilledema from true papilledema include the following[4]:

1. An absent central cup with a small disc diameter.
2. Vessels arising from the central apex of the disc.
3. Anomalous branching of vessels (e.g., bifurcations, trifurcations) with increased number of disc vessels.
4. Visible "glow" of drusen seen with disc transillumination.
5. Irregular optic disc margins with derangement of peripapillary retinal pigment epithelium.
6. Absence of superficial capillary telangiectasia on the optic disc head.
7. No hemorrhages (although subretinal hemorrhages may occur with disc drusen).
8. No exudates or cotton-wool spots.

7.3 What Evaluation Is Necessary for Optic Disc Drusen?

Most cases of pseudopapilledema can be diagnosed clinically and simply documented photographically. In difficult cases, further testing may be useful in the diagnosis of drusen. Disc drusen may show autofluorescence noted prior to injection of fluorescein angiography dye. Although generally not required for the diagnosis, computed tomography (CT) may demonstrate the calcified drusen as a hyperdense lesion in the optic nerve. Buried drusen may also be visible as a hyperreflective echo on orbital ultrasound.

Kurz-Levin and Landau retrospectively reviewed 142 patients (261 eyes) with suspected optic disc drusen.[3] Evaluations included B-scan echography, orbital CT scan, and/or preinjection control photography for autofluorescence. Thirty-six of the 261 eyes were evaluated using all three techniques, and drusen of the optic nerve head were diagnosed in 21 eyes. B-scan ultrasonography was positive in all 21 eyes. Nine cases had positive CT scans findings, and 10 had positive preinjection control photographs. In 82 eyes with suspected buried drusen of the optic nerve head, B-scan echography showed drusen in 39 eyes, compared with 15 eyes in which drusen were shown using preinjection control photography. No drusen were seen on preinjection control photography or CT scan that were missed on B-scan echography. The authors concluded that drusen of the optic nerve head are diagnosed most reliably using B-scan echography compared with both preinjection control photography and CT scans. Preinjection control photography is usually positive when there are visible drusen of the optic disc, and therefore its clinical use is limited. Likewise, CT scan is an expensive and less sensitive test for the detection of buried drusen of the optic nerve head.

In a recent retrospective study, authors determined that orbital ultrasonography is 90% sensitive in detecting papilledema but less specific (79%) in differentiating pseudopapilledema from papilledema in a subset of adult patients referred to a neuro-ophthalmology service for evaluation of suspected papilledema over a 14-year period.[5] They considered ultrasound positive when the optic nerve sheath diameter was ≥ 3.3 mm along with a positive 30-degree test, and concluded that orbital ultrasound is a valuable ancillary test for guiding further management in patients with atypical optic nerve elevation. Similar but lower sensitivity and specificity (85 and 63% respectively) has been obtained for ultrasonography in a subset of a pediatric patients.[6]

In addition, optical coherence tomography (OCT) is emerging as another clinical imaging modality[7] that may be utilized in differentiating these two conditions. Investigators have shown promising results using spectral domain OCT (SD-OCT) as a diagnostic modality to detect buried disc drusen.[8,9,10,11,12,13] OCT may prove valuable as a complementary tool to distinguish buried disc drusen (appearing as the "boot sign") from papilledema and has further implications in monitoring papilledema using reliable parameters. We recommend B-scan ultrasonography for the detection of buried drusen as the initial diagnostic study (class III, level C).

The Idiopathic Intracranial Hypertension Treatment Trial (IIHTT) used SD-OCT to monitor the papilledema in 89 patients diagnosed with idiopathic intracranial hypertension (IIH) over a 6-month period.[7,14] The results showed that although OCT can quantitatively measure papilledema in IIH patients over time, certain eyes had algorithm failure in the commercial software resulting in increased average retinal nerve fiber layer (RNFL) thickness, total retinal thickness (TRT), and optic nerve head (ONH) volume. OCT can be used in conjunction with the Frisén scale to monitor papilledema over time.

Features helpful in differentiating true optic disc edema from pseudodisc edema (e.g., buried disc drusen) are outlined in ▶ Table 7.1.

7.4 Is the Disc Swelling Caused by Optic Neuropathy or Papilledema?

Disc swelling due to raised intracranial pressure (i.e., papilledema) is usually bilateral and symmetric in both eyes. Unilateral disc swelling is most commonly caused by local pathology

within the optic nerve or orbit. Unilateral papilledema, however, can occur, although most of these cases are actually bilateral but asymmetric.[15,16,17,18,19,20] If one optic nerve is atrophic, it may not swell, and unilateral papilledema may occur from increased intracranial pressure (e.g., Foster Kennedy syndrome).[21] These optic neuropathies are discussed in Chapters 1 through 6. Processes causing optic neuropathy associated with disc swelling are usually unilateral, but may be bilateral. Other processes that may mimic papilledema and that may present with bilateral optic disc swelling with little or no visual acuity impairment, color vision loss, or visual field defects and normal intracranial pressure are listed in Box 7.1 and Box 7.2.

Box 7.1 Optic neuropathies associated with disc edema

- Infectious (e.g., infectious optic neuritis, meningitis, neuroretinitis, uveitis-associated disc edema, cat-scratch disease, Lyme disease).
- Demyelinating (e.g., multiple sclerosis).
- Inflammatory (e.g., systemic lupus erythematosus, sarcoidosis).[22]
- Vascular (e.g., arteritic and nonarteritic anterior ischemic optic neuropathy, diabetic papillopathy, central retinal vein occlusion, and carotid-cavernous sinus fistula).
- Infiltrative (e.g., carcinomatous meningitis, sarcoidosis).
- Compressive (e.g., neoplastic, thyroid ophthalmopathy).
- Hereditary (e.g., Leber hereditary optic neuropathy).
- Traumatic (rare).
- Paraneoplastic optic neuropathy.
- Mechanical (e.g., hypotony).
- Chronic respiratory disease.[23]

Box 7.2 Etiologies of optic disc edema with normal visual function

- Hypertensive optic neuropathy and retinopathy.
- Blood dyscrasias (e.g., anemia, polycythemia, dysproteinemia).
- Cyanotic congenital heart disease.
- Sleep apnea.[24]
- Spinal cord tumors.
- Acute inflammatory demyelinating polyradiculopathy (AIDP) and chronic inflammatory demyelinating polyradiculopathy (CIDP).[25]
- Peripheral neuropathy, organomegaly, endocrinopathy, monoclonal gammopathy, and skin changes (POEMS).
- Crow-Fukase syndrome.[26,27]
- Hypoparathyroidism (primary or surgically induced).[28]
- Uremia.
- Hypoxemia.

Table 7.1 Differentiating true optic disc edema from pseudopapilledema

Optic disc edema	Pseudopapilledema
Disc vasculature obscured	Disc margin vasculature clear
Elevation of peripapillary NFL	Elevation confined to disc
Obscured peripapillary NFL	Sharp peripapillary NFL
Venous congestion	No venous congestion
Exudates/cotton-wool spots	No exudates/cotton-wool spots
Loss of cup late	Small cupless disc
Normal disc vessels	Anomalous disc vessels
No circumpapillary light reflex	Crescent circumpapillary light reflex
Absent venous pulsations	With or without spontaneous venous pulsations

Abbreviation: NFL, nerve fiber layer.

Certain inflammatory or infectious processes, such as syphilis, sarcoidosis, HIV-associated meningoradiculitis, and viral meningoencephalitis that affect the meninges, may cause optic disc swelling due to perineuritis.[29,30,31] Cat-scratch disease and Lyme disease may also cause bilateral disc edema with normal visual fields and vision.[32,33,34]

7.5 What Are the Clinical Features of Papilledema?

Papilledema most often occurs in both eyes. During the early stages, visual acuity and color vision is usually preserved. Occasionally, transient vision loss lasting seconds may occur due to the edema causing transient optic nerve ischemia, thereby obscuring the vision. Similarly, visual field defects such as enlarged blind spots, generalized constriction, glaucomatous-like defects, and nasal peripheral constriction can also be seen. Fluorescein angiography can reveal early disc capillary dilation, dye leakage, microaneurysm formation, or late leakage of dye beyond the disc margins. Increased fluid in the optic nerve sheath can often be seen on neuroimaging or with echography in patients with papilledema. Afferent pupillary defects are usually not seen unless the patient has severe, asymmetric disc edema. The stages of papilledema and the Frisén papilledema grading scale are outlined in Box 7.3 and Box 7.4, respectively.

Box 7.3 The stages of papilledema

- Early papilledema.
  - Minimal disc hyperemia with capillary dilation.
  - Early opacification of nerve fiber layer (peripapillary retina loses its superficial linear and curvilinear light reflex and appears red without luster).
  - Early swelling of disc.
  - Absence of venous pulsations.
  - Peripapillary retinal nerve fiber layer hemorrhage.
- Fully developed papilledema
  - Engorged and tortuous retinal veins.
  - May have splinter hemorrhages at or adjacent to the disc margin.
  - Disc surface grossly elevated.
  - Surface vessels become obscured by now opaque nerve fiber layer.
  - May have cotton-wool spots.
  - Paton's lines (circumferential retinal folds) or choroidal folds.
  - May have exudates (e.g., macular star or hemistar).
  - May have hemorrhages or fluid in the macula that may decrease vision.
  - In acute cases (e.g., subarachnoid hemorrhage), subhyaloid hemorrhages may occur that may break into vitreous (Terson's syndrome).
  - Rarely macular or peripapillary subretinal neovascularization.
- Chronic papilledema
  - Hemorrhages and exudates slowly resolve.
  - Central cup, which is initially retained even in severe cases, ultimately becomes obliterated.
  - Initial disc hyperemia changes to a milky gray.
  - Small hard exudates that are refractile and drusen-like may appear on disc surface.
  - Visual field loss including nerve fiber layer defects may develop.
  - Optociliary "shunt" (collaterals) vessels may develop.
- Atrophic papilledema (pale disc edema)
  - Optic disc pallor with nerve fiber bundle visual field defects.
  - Retinal vessels become narrow and sheathed.
  - Occasional pigmentary changes or choroidal folds in macula.
  - Selective loss of peripheral axons while sparing central axons (usually preservation of good central visual acuity).

Box 7.4 Frisén papilledema grading system[35,36,37]

- Stage 0:
  - Normal optic disc.
- Stage 1:
  - Incomplete C-shaped peripapillary halo with temporal gap.*
  - Normal temporal disc margin.
  - No elevation of the disc borders.
  - Disruption of the normal radial nerve fiber layer arrangement with grayish opacity accentuating nerve fiber bundles.
- Stage 2:
  - Complete peripapillary halo.*
  - Elevation of nasal border.
- Stage 3:
  - Peripapillary halo—irregular outer fringe with finger-like extensions.
  - Elevation of all borders.
  - Increased diameter of the optic nerve head.
  - Obscuration of one or more segments of major blood vessels leaving the disc.*
- Step 4:
  - Peripapillary halo.
  - Obscuration of all borders.
  - Elevation of entire nerve head, including the optic cup.
  - Total obscuration of a segment of a major blood vessel on the disc.*
- Stage 5:
  - Partial obscuration of all blood vessels on the disc head with total obscuration of at least on major blood vessel.*

*Defining feature of each stage.

7.6 What Studies Should Be Performed to Investigate the Patient with Papilledema?

All patients with papilledema require a thorough neurologic and neuro-ophthalmologic history and physical examination.

In all patients with bilateral optic disc swelling, the blood pressure should be evaluated for possible malignant hypertension.[38,39] The presence of cotton-wool spots with papilledema may be an indicator of hypertension as the underlying etiology.[40] Blood dyscrasia should be considered if there are other suggestive retinal vascular findings (e.g., incomplete or complete central retinal vein occlusion with optic disc edema). Neuroimaging is required in all patients (class II, level B).

CT imaging is the preferred study in evaluating acute vascular processes (e.g., subarachnoid, epidural, subdural, or intracerebral hemorrhage, acute infarction) or in acute head trauma (e.g., assess for fracture, acute bleed). CT scan may be used in patients with contraindications to magnetic resonance imaging (MRI; e.g., pacemakers, metallic clips in head, metallic foreign bodies). Otherwise, MRI is the modality of choice in papilledema. MR venography can be performed concurrent to the MRI to evaluate for venous obstruction. If neuroimaging shows no structural lesion or hydrocephalus, then lumbar puncture is warranted. Studies should include an accurate opening pressure, cerebrospinal fluid (CSF) cell count and differential, glucose, protein, cytology, venereal disease research laboratory test, and appropriate studies for microbial agents.

Patients with a history of a ventriculoperitoneal shunt for hydrocephalus may develop papilledema, visual loss, or signs of a dorsal midbrain syndrome (see Chapter 14) due to shunt failure. Usually CT or MRI reveals recurrence of hydrocephalus. Shunt malfunction may occur without ventriculomegaly, perhaps due to poor ventricular compliance and "stiff ventricles."[38,41,42] Thus, shunt revision is indicted when there are signs or symptoms of increased intracranial pressure, even if ventriculomegaly is absent, to prevent deterioration of visual function and potentially irreversible visual loss.

7.7 What Is the Pseudotumor Cerebri Syndrome?

Pseudotumor cerebri (PTC) is a syndrome of increased intracranial pressure with papilledema, transient visual obscurations, visual field changes, diplopia, pulsatile tinnitus, and headaches. Although first described in the late 1800s, physicians could not accurately diagnose the condition until the advent ventriculography in 1918.[43] While many cases are idiopathic, there are a number of secondary causes and risk factors for the syndrome even after a "real" tumor is ruled out, such as systemic diseases, drugs, and intracranial or extracranial venous obstruction (see Box 7.5).

Box 7.5 Syndromes causing increased intracranial pressure

- Primary causes:
  - Idiopathic intracranial hypertension.
- Secondary causes and risk factors:
  - Venous abnormalities:
    - Cerebral venous sinus thrombosis.
    - Bilateral jugular vein thrombosis or surgical ligation.
    - Increased right heart pressure.
    - Superior vena cava syndrome.
    - Cerebral arteriovenous malformation (AVM).[44]
    - Arteriovenous fistulas.
    - Decreased CSF absorption (e.g., previous intracranial infection or hemorrhage).
  - Medications and exposures:
    - Antibiotics: tetracycline,[45,46,47,48] minocycline,[48,49,50,51,52,53] doxycycline,[48] nalidixic acid,[47,54] sulfa drugs, nitrofurantoin, penicillin, ofloxacin,[55] ciprofloxacin.[56]

- Vitamin A and retinoids: hypervitaminosis A,[47,48,52,57,58,59,60] hypovitaminosis A,[61] isotretinoin,[48] all-*trans*-retinoic acid (ATRA) or tretinoin,[62,63,64,65,66,67,68,69] etretinate, excessive liver ingestion.
- Hormones: human growth hormone,[70,71,72,73,74,75,76] levothyroxine,[77,78,79] leuprorelin acetate,[80] levonorgestrel (Norplant system), anabolic steroids,[47] oxytocin,[81] beta-human chorionic gonadotropin,[82] danazol.[83,84]
- Withdrawal from chronic corticosteroids.[47,85,86]
- Chemotherapy/immunotherapy: cytosine arabinoside[87,88,89] cyclosporine,[90] arsenic trioxide.[91]
- Amiodarone.[92,93]
- Phenytoin.
- Ketamine.
- Nonsteroidal anti-inflammatory medications (ketoprofen, indomethacin) in Bartter's syndrome.[94]
- Lithium.[95,96,97]
- Lindane.
- Chlordecone (insecticide).[98]
- Medical conditions:
  - Endocrine disorders and alterations.
    - Addison disease.[99,100,101]
    - Hypoparathyroidism and pseudohypoparathyroidism.[102]
    - Hypothyroidism.
    - Hyperthyroidism.[103]
    - Pregnancy (including ectopic pregnancy) and postpartum.[104,105,106,107]
    - Cushing disease and postpituitary surgery for Cushing disease.[108]
    - Polycystic ovarian syndrome.[109]
    - Rickets.[110,111]
    - Familial hypomagnesemia-hypercalcuria.[112]
  - Hypercapnia:
    - Sleep apnea.[113]
    - Pickwickian syndrome.[114]
  - Renal failure.[47,115,116]
  - Renal or bone marrow transplantation.[117,118,119,120]
  - Turner syndrome.
  - Down syndrome.
  - Cystic fibrosis.[47,121,122,123]
  - Reye syndrome.
  - Mucopolysaccharidoses.[124]
  - Post-occipitocervical arthrodesis and immobilization in a halo vest.[125]
  - Balloon venoplasty and urokinase infusion.[126]
  - Chiari I malformation.[127]
  - Guillain-Barre syndrome.[128]
  - Chronic inflammatory demyelinating polyradiculoneuropathy (CIDP).[129,130,131]
  - Multiple sclerosis.[132]
  - Crohn disease.[47]
  - Peripheral nerve sheath tumor of thigh.[133]
  - Familial PTC .[134,135,136]
  - Infections and inflammatory diseases:
    - Cryptococcal meningitis.[137]
    - HIV infection and AIDS.[138,139,140,141]
    - Lyme disease.[47,142]
    - Typhoid fever.[143,144]
    - Familial Mediterranean fever.[145]

- Trichinosis.
- Varicella zoster.
- Otitis media.[47]
- Mastoiditis.
- Acute purulent sinusitis.[146]
- Neurosarcoidosis.[147,148,149]
- Tolosa-Hunt syndrome.[150]
- Behçet syndrome.[104,151,152,153]
- Systemic lupus erythematosus.[47,104,154,155,156,157,158]

○ Hematologic abnormalities and malignancies (hypercoagulable states):
- Iron-deficiency anemia.[47,159]
- Pernicious anemia and other megaloblastic anemias.[160]
- Thrombocythemia and thrombocytosis.[161,162]
- Cryofibrinogenemia.
- Abnormal fibrinogen or increased serum fibrinogen.[161]
- Cryoglobulinemia.
- Hodgkin disease.
- Leukemia.[163,164]
- Myeloma.[165]
- Protein S deficiency.[104]
- Activated protein C resistance.[166]
- Antithrombin III deficiency[104,161]
- Anticardiolipin antibodies.[167]
- Hemophilia A (factor VIII deficiency).[168]
- Multicentric angiofollicular lymph node hyperplasia.[169]
- Paroxysmal nocturnal hemoglobinuria.[170]
- Thrombocytopenic purpura.
- Polycythemia.[161]

Source: Adapted from Friedman et al.[171]

Obstruction or impairment of intracranial venous drainage may result in cerebral edema with increased intracranial pressure and papilledema. Tumors that occlude the posterior portion of the superior sagittal sinus or other cerebral venous sinuses may cause increased intracranial pressure. Septic or aseptic thrombosis or ligation of the cavernous sinus, lateral sinus, sigmoid sinus, or superior sagittal sinus may mimic PTC.[95,104,172,173,174,175,176,177,178] A patient with neurofibromatosis type 2 developed papilledema from obstruction of cerebrospinal outflow at the arachnoid granulations by diffuse convexity meningiomatosis.[179] Keiper et al noted that 5 of 107 patients who underwent suboccipital craniotomy or translabyrinthine craniectomy developed PTC.[180] In each patient, the transverse sinus on the treated side was thrombosed, and patency of the contralateral sinus was confirmed on MRI. PTC has also been described after AVM embolization.[181] Sluggish flow in a venous varix after embolization, resulting in thrombosis propagation to the vein of Galen, was the proposed mechanism. Ligation of one or both jugular veins (e.g., radical neck dissection), thrombosis of a central intravenous catheter in the chest or neck, subclavian vein catheterization and arteriovenous fistula, superior vena cava syndrome, or a glomus jugular tumor impairing venous drainage may also cause increased intracranial pressure. Osteopetrosis causing obstruction of venous outflow at the jugular foramen has also been reported.[177,182,183,184] Venous sinus thrombosis may be the mechanism for PTC reported in several conditions,

including systemic lupus erythematosus, essential thrombocythemia, protein S deficiency, antithrombin III deficiency, the antiphospholipid antibody syndrome, activated protein C resistance, paroxysmal nocturnal hemoglobinuria, Behçet disease, meningeal sarcoidosis, lymphoma, hypervitaminosis A, mastoiditis, and trichinosis.[104,147,148,152,166,170,175,185,186,187,188] In fact, elevated intracranial venous pressure is thought by some authors to be the universal mechanism of PTC of varying etiologies, including idiopathic PTC.[174,189,190] Higgins et al presented a case of PTC thought to be secondary to bilateral transverse sinus stenosis discovered on venography that was treated successfully by inserting a self-expanding stent across the stenosis in the right transverse sinus.[191] These authors suggest that the transverse sinus pathology was not due to thrombosis but instead an idiopathic bilateral narrowing of the transverse sinuses.

Biousse et al noted that cerebral venous thrombosis (CVT) can present with all the classic criteria for idiopathic PTC including normal CT imaging and CSF contents.[185] Of 160 consecutive patients with CVT, 59 patients (37%) presented with isolated intracranial hypertension. Neuroimaging revealed involvement of more than one venous sinus in 35 patients (59%); CT imaging was normal in 27 of 50 patients (54%). The superior sagittal sinus was involved in 32 patients (54%; isolated in 7) and the lateral sinus in 47 (80%; isolated in 17). The straight sinus was thrombosed in eight patients, cortical veins were involved in two patients, and deep cerebral veins in three, always in association with thrombosis in the superior sagittal sinus or lateral sinuses. Lumbar puncture was performed in 44 patients and showed elevated opening pressure in 25 of 32 (78%) and abnormal CSF contents in 11 (25%). Etiologic risk factors included local causes (7), surgery (1), inflammatory disease (18), infection (2), cancer (1), postpartum (1), coagulopathies (11), and oral contraception (7). The cause was unknown in 11 cases (19%). Anticoagulants were used in 41 of 59 patients (69%), steroids or acetazolamide in 26 (44%), therapeutic lumbar puncture in 44 (75%), and surgical shunt in 1. Three patients had optic atrophy with severe visual loss, 1 died from carcinomatous meningitis, and 55 (93%) had complete recovery (although visual field testing was not systematically performed). The authors emphasized that MRI and MR venography should be considered in presumed isolated intracranial hypertension.

Among the 59 patients with isolated increased intracranial hypertension, 33 (56%) were female, but the authors did not record the patients' weights. They noted, however, that being a young, obese woman does not protect a patient from developing CVT, and therefore should not be used on an individual basis to rule out CVT. When MRI is not available, the authors suggest that conventional angiography be performed and, indeed, in another prospective study of 24 patients with apparently idiopathic PTC, angiography disclosed CVT in six patients.[192] Increased blood flow and venous hypertension have also been implicated as the mechanism of papilledema noted in some patients with cerebral AVMs, especially dural AVMs and fistulas.[172,193,194,195,196,197,198,199] Thus, we consider MR venography (and, in selected cases, MR angiography or even formal angiography) to investigate the possibility of venous sinus occlusion in patients with PTC, especially in patients with features not typical for idiopathic PTC (e.g., in thin patients, men, and the elderly persons; class III, level C). However, we found

MR venography to be normal in 22 consecutive obese females with idiopathic PTC.[200]

King et al found that when transducer-measured intracranial venous pressure is high in patients with idiopathic PTC, reduction of CSF pressure by removal of CSF predictably lowers the venous sinus pressure, indicating that the increased venous pressure in idiopathic PTC is caused by the elevated intracranial pressure and not the reverse.[201] This study indicates that the increased venous pressure in idiopathic PTC patients is caused by the elevated intracranial pressure and not the reverse. The idiopathic narrowing of the venous sinuses bilaterally noted in the case of PTC described by Higgins et al may conceivably have been transverse sinus compression from increased intracranial pressure.[191] Thus, venous occlusive disease and elevated venous pressure may not be the mechanism of PTC in most idiopathic cases.

Many systemic diseases, drugs, vitamin deficiencies and excesses, pregnancy, and hereditary conditions have been associated with the PTC syndrome (secondary PTC). These reported etiologies are listed in Box 7.5. In general, many of these reported associations may be coincidental and anecdotal. Of those listed in Box 7.5, the etiologies most firmly associated with PTC include drugs and systemic diseases.[202] The drugs or drug conditions associated with PTC include vitamin A products, steroid use or withdrawal, lithium, antibiotics, and certain hormone therapies. Systemic diseases or syndromes associated with PTC include Behçet disease, renal failure, Addison disease, hypoparathyroidism, systemic lupus erythematosus, and sarcoidosis (most of these likely cause PTC syndrome by venous sinus obstruction or impairment of venous sinus drainage).

7.8 What Is Idiopathic Intracranial Hypertension?

Primary PTC without an identified underlying cause is known as idiopathic intracranial hypertension (IIH), in order to distinguish it from secondary, nonidiopathic causes of the PTC syndrome (Box 7.4). The modified Dandy criteria for IIH include (1) normal neuroimaging studies (usually MRI/MRV); (2) normal CSF contents; (3) elevated opening pressure; and (4) signs and symptoms related only to increased intracranial pressure (e.g., headache, papilledema, nonlocalizing sixth nerve palsy). The disease typically affects obese women of childbearing age.[202, 203,204,205,206,207,208,209,210] Approximately 10 to 15% of cases are male,[211] and, when it occurs in children, there is usually no gender preference,[47,212,213,214] although in some series girls outnumber boys.[215] Children with PTC, especially younger children, are less likely to be obese than adults with PTC.[47,212,213] Even though men with PTC are less likely to be obese than women, they tend to be more obese than controls.[211] In a study from Israel, 18 of 134 patients with idiopathic PTC were men and 25% of the men were significantly overweight, as compared to 78% of the women.[216] The occurrence of PTC in a man, especially a thin man, should raise the possibility of venous occlusive disease or a secondary PTC syndrome. African American men appear to be at greater risk of visual loss. The incidence of idiopathic PTC is approximately 1 or 2 per 100,000, with a higher incidence in obese women between the ages of 15 and 44 years (4–21 per 100,000).[206,217,218] Friedman and Jacobson

proposed revised diagnostic criteria for idiopathic intracranial hypertention that is commonly used in clinical practice (Box 7.6).[219]

Box 7.6 Diagnostic criteria for idiopathic intracranial hypertension[37]

- Increased intracranial pressure must be documented in an alert and oriented patient without localizing neurologic findings (except for cranial nerve VI palsy).
- Spinal fluid pressures between 200 and 250 mm H_2O may occur normally in obese patients, and when elevated spinal fluid pressure is suspected, confirmation requires values greater than 250 mm H_2O.[220]
- The CSF should have normal contents (including protein and glucose) with no cytologic abnormalities; occasionally, the CSF protein level may be low.
- Neuroimaging (MR imaging with and without contrast and possibly MR venography) should be normal with no evidence of hydrocephalus, mass lesion, meningeal enhancement, or venous occlusive disease; neuroimaging may often show the following, which may be helpful in establishing the diagnosis of PTC (percentages from Brodsky and Vaphiades[221]):
  - Flattening of the posterior sclera (80% of patients).
  - Distention of perioptic subarachnoid space (50% of patients).
  - Enhancement (with gadolinium) of the prelaminar optic nerve (45% of patients).
  - Empty sella (70% of patients).
  - Intraocular protrusion of the prelaminar optic nerve (30% of patients).
  - Vertical tortuosity of the orbital optic nerve (40% of patients).[221,222,223,224]
- No secondary cause (secondary PTC) is evident.

7.9 What Are the Risk Factors and Clinical Characteristics of Idiopathic Pseudotumor Cerebri?

The most important risk factors for the development of idiopathic PTC include female sex, obesity, and recent moderate weight gain (5–15% of body weight) with or without obesity.[202, 225,226,227] Several conditions previously associated with idiopathic PTC are no more common in PTC than in controls. In a retrospective case–control study of 40 patients with idiopathic PTC and 39 age- and sex-matched controls, all forms of menstrual abnormalities, incidence of pregnancy, antibiotic use, and oral contraceptive use were equal in both groups.[202] In another study comparing 50 PTC patients with 100 age-matched controls, iron-deficiency anemia, thyroid dysfunction, pregnancy, antibiotic intake, and the use of oral contraceptives were no more common in PTC patients than in controls.[225]

The reason that obesity predisposes to PTC is unclear. Central obesity may raise intra-abdominal pressure, which increases pleural pressure and cardiac filling pressure, including central venous pressure, leading to increased intracranial venous pressure and increased intracranial pressure.[228] As noted earlier, elevated intracranial venous pressure is thought by some authors to be the universal mechanism of PTC of various etiologies, including idiopathic PTC. However, the study of King et al cited earlier indicated that the increased venous pressure in idiopathic PTC is caused by the elevated intracranial pressure and not the reverse.[201] Idiopathic PTC may share a common pathogenesis with orthostatic edema, a condition in which there is evidence of dependent edema after prolonged standing.[229] Seventy-seven percent of PTC patients had evidence of peripheral edema and 80% had significant orthostatic retention of sodium and water. Excretions of a standard saline load and of a tap water load were significantly impaired in the upright posture in the PTC patients with orthostatic edema compared to lean and obese but otherwise normal subjects. Orthostatic retention of water and sodium and consequent edema is similar in patients with idiopathic PTC and orthostatic edema. This suggests that these two disorders may have a common pathogenesis.

Elevated vitamin A levels have been noted in patients with idiopathic PTC.[230] Serum retinol concentrations were significantly higher in patients with idiopathic PTC compared to controls,[231] even after adjusting for age and body mass index. Patients may ingest an abnormally large amount of vitamin A, metabolize it abnormally, or be unusually sensitive to its effects. Alternatively, elevated levels of serum retinol may reflect an epiphenomenon of another variable not measured or a nonspecific effect of elevated retinol binding capacity.[230]

Endocrinologic abnormalities may be more common in men with PTC.[232] In a study of eight men with PTC, two had abnormal estradiol levels, four had abnormal follicle-stimulating hormone and luteinizing hormone levels, and seven had low testosterone levels.[232]

7.10 What Are the Symptoms of Pseudotumor Cerebri?

The most common symptoms of PTC include headache, transient visual obscurations, pulsatile tinnitus, and diplopia.[202,210,225] In a prospective study of 50 idiopathic PTC patients (92% women; mean age, 32 years; 92% obese), symptoms included headache (94%), transient visual obscurations (68%), intracranial noises (58%), sustained visual loss (26%), photopsia (54%), diplopia (38%), and retrobulbar pain (44%).[210] Headaches associated with PTC may be constant or intermittent, and in 93% of patients they are reported to be the most severe headache ever experienced by the patient.[233] The headache is often described as pulsatile, and precipitated by position changes. It may awaken the patient at night and many patients note transient relief with lumbar puncture.[233] Pain in a cervical nerve root distribution (possibly from a dilated nerve root sleeve) or retroocular pain with eye movement, uncommon with other headache disorders, may help differentiate this headache syndrome.[233] There is no clear correlation between CSF pressure and headache severity, and many patients continue to experience headaches after the CSF pressure normalizes. Transient visual obscurations last seconds, may be unilateral or bilateral, and are often related to changes in posture. They do not correlate with the degree of intracranial hypertension or the extent of disc swelling, and are not considered to be harbingers of permanent visual loss.[204,225] Intracranial noises are common with

PTC and are perhaps due to the transmission of intensified vascular pulsations via CSF under high pressure to the walls of the venous sinuses.[234] This pulsatile tinnitus may be audible to others.[235] In fact, PTC without papilledema has been reported in patients with pulsatile tinnitus.[236,237] Diplopia is often mild and usually due to a sixth cranial nerve palsy, presumably a nonlocalizing sign of raised intracranial pressure.

In a study of 101 patients with PTC, other minor symptoms included neck stiffness in 31 patients, distal extremity paresthesias in 31, tinnitus in 27, joint pains in 13, low back pain in 13, and gait instability in 4 patients.[238] These minor symptoms resolved promptly upon lowering of the intracranial pressure. Stiff neck and strabismus may be the most common presenting symptoms in children with PTC.[213] Sleep-related breathing problems are common in PTC patients and may be a risk factor.[239] Patients with idiopathic PTC are significantly more affected by hardships associated with health problems than age- and weight-matched controls and have higher levels of depression and anxiety.[240] Other rare and exceptional clinical abnormalities that have been described in patients with PTC include fourth cranial nerve palsy,[241,242] third cranial nerve palsy, sixth cranial nerve palsy (unilateral) without papilledema,[243] bilateral sixth and fourth cranial nerve palsies,[244] skew deviation, complete external ophthalmoplegia,[245] bilateral total internal and external ophthalmoplegia, internuclear ophthalmoplegia with vertical gaze paresis with or without ptosis,[245,246] vertical gaze palsy,[245] divergence insufficiency,[247] sensory exotropia or comitant esotropia in children,[213] ptosis,[245] lid retraction,[245] trigeminal neuropathy,[248] unilateral or bilateral facial nerve palsy,[249,250,251] hemifacial spasm,[251,252,253] CSF rhinorrhea,[254,255] transient partial pituitary deficiency,[256] and fatal tonsillar herniation after lumbar puncture.[257] Furthermore, patients with PTC have also been described with atypical ophthalmoscopic findings and visual abnormalities, such as visual field loss despite resolution of papilledema,[258] gaze-evoked amaurosis,[259] acquired hyperopia with choroidal folds,[260,261] coexistence with optic nerve head drusen,[262] optociliary collateral vessels,[263] acute visual loss secondary to anterior ischemic optic neuropathy, acute visual loss due to central retinal artery occlusion, acute visual loss due to branch retinal artery occlusion,[85,264] acute visual loss due to central retinal vein occlusion,[265] and visual loss (occasionally acute) due to macular disease including chorioretinal striae, pigmentary disturbances, exudates, macular edema, nerve fiber layer hemorrhages, subretinal hemorrhages from neovascular membranes, or subretinal scars.[85,261,266,267]

7.11 What Are the Signs of Pseudotumor Cerebri?

Papilledema is present in most cases of PTC. It may be asymmetric, rarely unilateral, and even occasionally absent.[15,237,243, 268,269,270,271,272,273,274] In one series, 10% of 478 patients with PTC had asymmetric papilledema, and visual loss was most pronounced in the eye with the higher grade of papilledema.[274] If optic atrophy is present unilaterally, disc swelling will be unilateral in the opposite eye, thus mimicking the Foster Kennedy syndrome.[273] In the patient described by Saito et al with unilateral disc swelling as a manifestation of PTC related to cyclosporin therapy for leukemia, the right disc was thought to be spared because of leukemic infiltration causing constriction of the optic nerve sheath.[271] If no papilledema is evident, there is no risk of visual loss no matter how high the intracranial pressure is; however, the severity of papilledema cannot predict the severity of visual loss. Isolated elevated intracranial pressure without papilledema may present as chronic daily headache. Quattrone et al investigated 114 consecutive patients with chronic daily headache with MR venography and found that 11 (9.6%) had cerebral venous sinus thrombosis affecting one or both transverse sinuses and half of these patients had isolated intracranial hypertension without papilledema.[275]

Visual field loss is the major cause of morbidity in PTC.[204,210,276] Visual acuity loss and optic atrophy are late sequelae of papilledema and may occur in some patients. Hypertension and recent weight gain have been reported to be significant risk factors for visual loss.[204] The patient is often unaware of peripheral visual field dysfunction and Snellen acuity testing is a poor indicator of early visual deficit in PTC. Papilledema causes optic nerve fiber loss that results in field constriction and nerve fiber bundle defects similar to those seen in glaucoma, disc drusen, and anterior ischemic optic neuropathy, suggesting a shared ischemic or mechanical mechanism.[204,210,277] Any nerve fiber layer visual field defect can be observed in a patient with disc edema.[278] Optic nerve diameter changes on ultrasound in PTC are associated with perimetric threshold loss; PTC functional deficits may thus be related to the degree of optic nerve sheath distention resulting from increased CSF pressure.[279] Blind spot enlargement is commonly encountered and is more a reflection of disc swelling itself as opposed to optic nerve damage. Corbett et al demonstrated that blind spot enlargement is in part a refractive scotoma due to peripapillary hyperopia caused by the disc edema.[280] Acute visual acuity loss is rare but may occur by the mechanisms listed above (e.g., anterior ischemic optic neuropathy, retinal artery or vein occlusion, or subretinal hemorrhage from neovascular membranes). The frequency of visual field loss and acuity loss with PTC is variable, but in one study field loss was noted in 75% of eyes tested using manual perimetry and 78% of eyes using automated threshold perimetry.[281] Motion perimetry abnormalities correlate well with static perimetry abnormalities in patients with PTC and indeed may identify nerve fiber bundle defects not detected with conventional perimetry.[282,283] Contrast sensitivity testing is also a relatively sensitive means of assessing optic nerve damage in patients with PTC.[284] Rowe and Sarkies, however, noted that visual field testing, as opposed to visual acuity and contrast sensitivity testing, is the most sensitive indicator of visual loss in PTC patients.[285] Perimetry, fundus examination (i.e., Frisén's grading), and OCT used in combination provide accurate and repeatable measurements on which to determine the progression of the condition.

7.12 What Is the Evaluation of Pseudotumor Cerebri?

All patients with PTC require a thorough history, especially regarding medication use, pregnancy, recent or current illnesses, and recent changes in weight. Most cases do not require laboratory evaluation (class II, level C). Some patients may require blood work (e.g., sedimentation rate, complete blood count, syphilis serology, calcium, phosphate, creatinine, and electrolytes). Complete ophthalmologic examination typically includes formal perimetry (e.g., Goldmann and/or automated) and OCT of the optic nerve. Secondary causes of PTC should especially be considered in men, in thin patients, and in patients younger than 15 years or older than 45 years (atypical PTC).

Cognard et al noted that dural arteriovenous fistulas may present with isolated intracranial hypertension, mimicking idiopathic PTC, and endorsed cerebral angiography to evaluate for their presence in all patients with PTC.[196] Biousse et al noted that CVT may present with PTC and that this diagnosis should be considered even in women with the typical body habitus of idiopathic PTC.[185] In another prospective study of 24 patients with apparently idiopathic PTC, angiography disclosed CVT in six patients.[192] We recommend that patients with PTC undergo MRI of the head (class II–III, level B) with MR venography to evaluate for venous occlusive disease. We recommend cerebral angiography only in select cases (class III, level C). If venous occlusive disease is discovered, then evaluation for a hypercoagulable state and vasculitis should be performed (class III, level C).

7.13 What Is the Treatment for Pseudotumor Cerebri?

PTC treatment has two major goals: the alleviation of symptoms and preservation of visual function. We suggest a management plan, adapted from that recommended by Lee and Wall,[277] and updated in a recent review (see Box 7.5).[286] In summary, patients should be screened for secondary causes of intracranial hypertension and treated accordingly, and where possible, causative agents should be eliminated.[48] Conditions that predispose to CVS thrombosis and associated complications need to be addressed and anticoagulant therapy should be considered if evaluation confirms a CVS thrombosis.[287] In cases where no cause can be identified, intracranial hypertension can be managed with medical or surgical treatment. Weight loss and diuretics are the mainstay of treatment[288] and surgery is reserved for patients who are intolerant or noncompliant with maximal medical therapy.[286] Effective headache management is an important component of treatment as well. Many patients with secondary PTC also benefit from similar interventions to decrease intracranial pressure while also managing the underlying etiology.

7.14 What Is the Medical Management of Pseudotumor Cerebri?

Some patients require no treatment if symptoms are minimal and visual function remains intact. Patients may fail to notice visual field defects, and should be followed up and closely monitored for signs of visual impairment using formal perimetry. Combined pharmacotherapy, weight loss, and diet constitute medical therapy, with weight loss being the most effective long-term therapy.

7.14.1 Weight Loss

Weight reduction, including surgically induced weight reduction in morbidly obese patients, may reduce intracranial pressure and associated papilledema.[289,290,291,292,293,294] It should be emphasized that even a modest amount of weight loss (5–15% of total body weight) often improves signs and symptoms.[295] Johnson et al noted that approximately 6% of weight loss was associated with resolution of marked papilledema in obese PTC patients.[289] Similarly, Sinclair et al documented a reduction in intracranial pressure in PTC patients treated with daily 425 kcal/day diet for 3 months.[296] These authors concluded that weight loss improves headache and ICP control.

In another study, nine patients placed on a salt-restricted, rapid weight reduction rice diet showed improvement in papilledema (mean weight 261 pounds before treatment and 187 pounds after treatment).[292] In another study, all eight morbidly obese patients with PTC who underwent bariatric surgery had complete resolution of their papilledema. There was resolution or marked reduction in headache, resolution of tinnitus, and a decrease in CSF pressure from a mean of 353 to a mean of 168 mm of H_2O following a mean weight loss of 57 kg when measured at 34 months after surgery.[293] In another study of 24 severely obese women with IIH, 23 were treated by gastric bypass surgery and 1 underwent laparoscopic adjustable gastric binding.[297] At 1 year after surgery, 19 patients lost an average of 45 ± 12 kg, which was 71% ± 18% of their excess weight. Five patients were lost to follow-up and four were followed up for less than 1 year after their surgery. Surgically induced weight loss was associated with resolution of headache and pulsatile tinnitus in all but one patient within 4 months of the procedure. Of the 19 patients not lost to follow-up, 2 regained the weight with recurrence of their headache and pulsatile tinnitus. The authors concluded that bariatric surgery should be considered the "procedure of choice for severely obese patients with PTC and is shown to have a much higher rate of success than CSF-peritoneal shunting. .. as well as providing resolution of additional obesity comorbidity."[297] A recent review of the published literature concluded that bariatric surgery in obese PTC patients may help resolve symptoms and improve visual outcomes (class IV evidence).[294] Analysis of the pooled data from 11 studies showed that 56 (92%) of 61 patients reported resolution of their symptoms and 34 (97%) of 35 patients had documented resolution of papilledema in the postoperative period. On average, the decrease in CSF pressure of 254 mm H_2O was found in 13 patients who had their pre- and postoperative CSF pressure recorded. Complete or near-complete resolution of visual field deficits was found in 11 (92%) of 12 patients who underwent visual field testing pre- and postoperatively using formal perimetry.

In a retrospective study, Kupersmith et al noted that weight reduction sped recovery from PTC in women but may not have definitely improved final visual outcome.[290] Kupersmith et al later noted that weight reduction was associated with a more rapid recovery of papilledema and visual field dysfunction in patients with IIH (weight loss ≥ 2.5 kg during any 3-month interval in the study).[291]

The Idiopathic Intracranial Hypertension Treatment Trial (IIHTT), the first large, randomized, double-masked, placebo-controlled trial of medical treatment for IIH, showed that acetazolamide combined with weight loss was safe and effective in IIH patients with mild visual loss at presentation.[288] All subjects participated in a weight loss program, and received either acetazolamide or placebo therapy. Although the acetazolamide group demonstrated significantly greater improvement in mean perimetry deviation and quality of life at 6-month follow-up, the placebo group also showed significant improvement, indicating the importance of weight loss in the treatment of IIH.[288]

Studies have reported a possible link between PTC and obstructive sleep apnea, especially in obese patients. PTC patients should be screened for obstructive sleep apnea and treated appropriately, given the significant morbidity associated with this condition.

7.14.2 Medications

Medications commonly used for PTC include carbonic anhydrase inhibitors (e.g., acetazolamide), loop diuretics, and topiramate. Acetazolamide in addition to low-sodium weight reduction diet is widely used as a first-line therapy in patients with mild to moderate visual loss. As mentioned earlier, results of the IIHTT showed that acetazolamide combined with weight loss was effective in IIH patients.[288] The combination therapy resulted in a significant but small (0.71 dB) improvement of the Humphrey visual field mean deviation versus diet alone, even when the results were controlled for the greater weight loss seen in the acetazolamide group. Similar to the IIHTT protocol, patients are typically started on 500 mg of oral acetazolamide twice daily, and the dose is titrated upward as tolerated if papilledema and symptoms persist, or downward if side effects develop. Acetazolamide in doses up to 2 to 4 g per day has proven effective in some patients with IIH,[298] and this was also the maximum dose used in IIHTT patients.[288] The IIHTT also showed that acetazolamide is safe and generally well tolerated up to 4 g per day.[299] Acetazolamide use should be avoided if possible during pregnancy, especially before 20 weeks, due to potential teratogenic effects demonstrated in animal studies. The teratogenic effect in humans is not well established, so risk versus benefit must be considered in the individual patient. Caloric restriction and diuretic use in general are relatively contraindicated during pregnancy. Other carbonic anhydrase inhibitors, such as methazolamide, are often used in acetazolamide-intolerant patients, but their efficacy has not been proven.

Furosemide as a second-line alternative is used in patients who cannot tolerate, are noncompliant with, or fail acetazolamide therapy. Furosemide inhibits CSF production and may have an additive effect with acetazolamide. The suggested initial dose is 20 mg twice daily, increasing the dose to as much as 40 mg three times daily when needed. The use of furosemide as monotherapy has not been systematically studied. In one report of eight children treated with combined therapy of acetazolamide and furosemide, all patients had a rapid clinical response with resolution of papilledema, reduction in the mean CSF pressure after the first week of treatment, and normalization of pressure within 6 weeks of starting therapy.[298]

Topiramate, a drug commonly used in the management of primary headache disorders, has shown similar efficacy to acetazolamide for treatment of mild to moderate PTC. However, the small randomized treatment trial that provided the evidence lacked a placebo control group.[300] Another weakness of the study was that the patients were alternately assigned to the treatments without a matching process. Topiramate causes some weight loss that may prove beneficial to PTC patients. It may also prove advantageous in managing coexisting headaches in these patients.

Weaker diuretics such as thiazides, glycerol, and digoxin appear to be less effective, but have been used with anecdotal success.[301] Förderreuther and Straube reported using intravenous indomethacin to transiently decrease CSF pressure in seven patients,[302] although indomethacin and other nonsteroidal anti-inflammatory agents have been reported as possible causes of increased intracranial pressure.[94]

Corticosteroids may initially be efficacious, but associated complications, including weight gain in the chronic treatment of an obese patient population and the associated risk of rebound PTC, have resulted in most clinicians avoiding their use.[303] Liu et al treated four patients with acute, severe visual loss associated with PTC with a combination of high-dose methylprednisolone (250 mg four times per day for 5 days followed by an oral taper), acetazolamide, and ranitidine.[85] In addition to severe disc edema, one patient had a serous detachment of both maculae and lipid deposition, one had unilateral macular star, and one had a monocular branch retinal artery occlusion. These three patients experienced rapid and lasting improvement in visual acuity, visual fields, papilledema, and symptoms, whereas the fourth patient did not improve and required optic nerve sheath fenestration (ONSF). The authors suggested this combination treatment for patients with acute, severe visual loss associated with florid papilledema and suggested surgical treatment if no immediate improvement occurs.[85]

7.15 What About Repeated Lumbar Punctures?

Repeated lumbar punctures have never been systematically studied for the treatment of PTC. As these procedures are uncomfortable, of questionable benefit, and potentially associated with complications (e.g., infection, CSF leak, intraspinal epidermoid tumors),[220] we feel that they should not be performed therapeutically, except perhaps to reduce CSF pressure while waiting for a definitive surgical procedure or medical improvement and with PTC in pregnancy (class III, level C). In patients with fulminant PTC, a temporary lumbar drain can serve as a temporizing measure until definitive surgical intervention can take place.

7.16 What Is the Surgical Management of Pseudotumor Cerebri?

Consider surgical intervention for PTC when maximum medical therapy fails and there is a threat of severe or permanent visual dysfunction without prompt intervention.[303] The indications for surgical therapy, as suggested by Corbett and Thompson, are outlined in Box 7.7.[303] The procedures performed include CSF diversion (lumboperitoneal shunt [LPS] or ventricular peritoneal shunt [VPS]), ONSF and venous sinus stenting. One of the earliest surgical treatments was subtemporal decompression,

which is now uncommon but might still be considered for IIH refractory to other medical and surgical management.[304] The procedure of choice often depends on availability and expertise at the center, as well as the preferences of the surgeon and patient. Various authorities have vehemently advocated one or the other procedure, but no prospective study has compared the efficacy of each procedure. The existing evidence is derived solely from observational and retrospective studies and is insufficient to inform treatment decisions.[286,305,306,307] A recent analysis of pooled data from several studies suggests an overall similar improved visual outcome in surgically treated PTC patients, but a higher rate of periprocedural complications in those treated with shunts.[305] The analysis also shows that CSF diversion procedures and endovascular stent placement have the added advantage of improving headaches (modest effect).

Box 7.7 Management of IIH

- Confirm clinical diagnosis (diagnosis of exclusion).
- Encourage weight reduction:
  - 10% of body weight and/or achievement of BMI < 30.
- Medical treatment recommendations:
  - Acetazolamide (e.g., starting at 500 mg twice daily and titrating up to 4 g per day)[288] if no contraindications
  - Consider furosemide (Lasix) if acetazolamide intolerant.
  - Other medications have not been proven but may indeed be useful (e.g., topiramate, methazolamide).
  - Avoid corticosteroids if possible (cause weight gain and other side effects).
- Treat headache symptomatically.
- Consider diagnosis of and treat associated sleep apnea.

If fail, intolerant to, or noncompliant with maximal medical therapy:
- Surgical treatment options
  - CSF diversion:
    - Lumboperitoneal shunt
    - Ventriculoperitoneal shunt
  - Optic nerve sheath fenestration.
  - Cerebral venous sinus stenting.
- Indications for surgery:
  - New visual field defect.*
  - Enlargement of previously existing visual field defect.*
  - Reduced visual acuity not due to macular edema.
  - Presence of severe visual loss (20/40 or worse) in one or both eyes at the time of initial examination.
  - Anticipated hypotension induced by treatment of high blood pressure or renal dialysis.
  - Psychosocial reasons, such as patient's inability to perform visual field studies, noncompliance with medications, or itinerant lifestyle.
- Follow-up visit intervals:
  - Return monthly until disc edema resolved, then usually every several months.
  - Perform formal visual fields and complete eye exam.

*Blind spot enlargement should not be considered significant visual loss.

Note: Usually avoid diuretics and caloric restriction if pregnant.

7.16.1 Cerebrospinal Fluid Diversion

Shunting procedures (LPS and VPS) can be performed to treat PTC in selected patients whose visual function declines despite maximal medical therapy. CSF diversion can relieve headache, diplopia, and papilledema, and can reverse visual loss.[308,309,310,311,312,313,314,315] This procedure may also be performed in pregnancy.[107]

A recent review and 10-year follow-up of PTC patients undergoing CSF diversion (LPS in 49 patients vs. VPS in 4) revealed significant improvement of papilledema (44%), but also the persistence of headaches (79%) at 2 years. Thus, persistent headache alone in an IIH patient is not a sufficient indication for surgical intervention. In addition, shunts had to be revised in half of the patients consistent with the analysis by Eggenberger et al[310] and 30% required multiple revisions.[316] However, when patent, shunts may improve headaches in PTC patients, as demonstrated by two smaller studies reporting headache improvement (78–86%) in association with lower revision rates (27–35%).[317,318]

An LPS obviates the need for an intracranial procedure (ventricular shunt) and spares the patient from associated risks (e.g., intracranial hemorrhage), but an LPS is more likely to require revision, or conversion to a ventricular shunt.[319,320] A retrospective review of 42 PTC patients (79 LPS vs. 36 VPS) by McGirt et al reported 2.5-fold increased risk of LP shunt revision mainly due to increased risk (3-fold) of LPS obstruction as opposed to ventricular shunts.[320] Similarly, in a retrospective review of 25 patients by Abubaker et al, a higher revision rate for LPS (60%) was reported compared with 30% for VPS.[319] This trend was corroborated in a retrospective review of 36 PTC patients undergoing LPS, VPS, or both. Authors reported more complications and first-time revisions in patients with LPS, but found no difference in headache or visual outcomes between the groups.[321]

It remains to be established whether this difference in efficacy is accurate given the unequal number of lumboperitoneal and ventricular shunts performed to date. Historically, LP shunts have been performed more often than ventricular shunts due to the difficulty in placing ventricular catheters in ventricles that are classically "slit-like" in PTC patients. However, ventricular shunts have been increasingly performed and the advent of stereotactic neuronavigation has contributed to this increase.[322]

Eggenberger et al retrospectively studied 27 patients with PTC treated with at least one LPS to ascertain the efficacy of this treatment.[310] The indication for LPS was intractable headache in 18 patients (67%) and progressive optic neuropathy in 14 patients (52%). Visual function returned to normal in both eyes of six patients, showed no change in either eye in four patients, and improved in at least one eye in the remaining four. Four patients had unilateral and one had bilateral sixth nerve palsies; all completely resolved postsurgery. The average duration of follow-up for this population was 77 months (mean 47 months). A functioning LPS was successful in alleviating symptoms in all patients studied and no patient with a functioning shunt complained of shunt-related symptoms, such as low-pressure headache or abdominal pain, within 2 months after surgery.

A major complication of LPS surgery is shunt failure requiring revision. The authors concluded that placement of an LPS is a satisfactory treatment for the majority of patients with PTC who require surgical therapy for the disorder even though some patients require multiple revisions. LPS failure is common, and most shunt failures occur within 2 to 3 months of the initial LPS (cumulative risk, 37%)[310] A patient with PTC who undergoes LPS placement and who maintains a functioning shunt for more than 1 year has a lower risk of requiring a shunt revision over subsequent years.[310] Patients undergoing LPS placement, however, also need careful follow-up after their procedure because of the possibility of late failures. LPS failure has been successfully treated by repeat LPS, VPS, or by ONSF.

Rosenberg et al reviewed the efficacy of cerebrospinal diversion procedures for PTC in patients from six different institutions.[314] Thirty-seven patients underwent a total of 73 LPS and 10 VPS. Only 14 patients remained "'cured" after a single surgical procedure. The average time between shunt insertion and shunt replacement was 9 months, although 64% of the shunts lasted less than 6 months. Shunt failure (recurrent papilledema or increased CSF pressure on lumbar puncture) (55%) and low-pressure headaches (21%) were the most common indications for reoperation. Other reasons for shunt replacement included infection, abdominal pain, radicular pain, operative complications, and CSF leak. The vision of most patients improved (13) or stabilized (13) postoperatively. However, three patients who had initially improved subsequently lost vision, six had a postoperative decrease in vision, two patients improved in one eye but worsened postoperatively in the other, and four lost vision despite apparently adequate shunt function. Shunt failure with relapse of PTC occurred as late as 7 years after insertion. The authors concluded that CSF diversion procedures have a significant failure rate as well as a high frequency of side effects. Johnston et al reported 36 patients who, during follow-up, required a total of 85 shunting procedures with an overall complication rate of 52% and a failure rate of 48%.[311]

Burgett et al retrospectively analyzed clinical data from 30 patients who underwent LPS for PTC and found LPS to be an effective means of acutely lowering intracranial pressure.[309] Symptoms of increased intracranial pressure improved in 82% of patients, and five patients (29%) demonstrated total resolution of all symptoms. Among 14 patients with impaired visual acuity, 10 (71%) improved by at least two Snellen lines. Worsening of vision occurred in only one eye. Of 28 eyes with abnormal Goldmann perimetry, 18 (64%) improved and none worsened. The incidence of serious complications was low, but the major drawback was a need for frequent revisions in a few patients (30 patients underwent a total of 126 revisions with the mean revision rate of 4.2 per patient). The authors suggested that LPS should be considered the first surgical procedure for patients with PTC with severe visual loss at presentation or with intractable headache (with or without visual loss). After shunting, it is important to identify patients who are shunt intolerant.[309]

Thus, CSF diversion procedures are often effective in controlling PTC, and although placement of the shunt is generally safe, any operation performed under general anesthesia carries inherent risk, and there is at least one perioperative death reported following LPS.[323] Shunt obstruction is the most common complication[309,310,314,324] followed by secondary intracranial hypotension caused by excessive drainage of the CSF via the LPS.[309,310,311,312,314,324,325] Symptoms of intracranial hypotension include nausea and vomiting, nuchal rigidity, disturbances of vision, vertigo, tinnitus, and reduced hearing (the last three are thought to be due to a decreased intra-labyrinthine pressure gradient across the cochlear aqueduct). Complications of LPS include shunt obstruction,[309,310,314,324] intracranial hypotension,[279,309,310,311,312,314,324] CSF leak, lumbar radiculopathy,[310,311,312,314,325] shunt or disc space infection,[310,311,312,314,326] abdominal pain, bowel perforation, migration or dislocation of the peritoneal end of the catheter,[310,314,324] tonsillar herniation (symptomatic or asymptomatic) and syringomyelia,[196,324,327] subdural hemorrhage, visual loss from retinal ischemia, bilateral visual loss and simultagnosia from bilateral parieto-occipital infarction related to rupture of a previously asymptomatic intracranial aneurysm,[328] and death.[323] Complications of VPS include shunt failure,[41] shunt overdrainage,[329] shunt migration,[330,331,332] shunt obstruction, intracranial hemorrhage, intracranial infection, stroke, seizure, cerebral CSF cyst,[333] ascites, peritonitis, bowel perforation,[334] hernia,[335] bladder perforation,[336] isolated left homonymous hemianopia secondary to a pericatheter cyst,[337] and volvulus. Both VPS and LPS carry a risk of postprocedure headaches that must be considered when approaching a patient with already-intractable headaches.

7.16.2 Optic Nerve Sheath Fenestration

Optic nerve sheath fenestration has been proven to prevent deterioration in vision and, in some cases, improve visual function in patients with PTC.[85,103,261,263,267,338,339,340,341,342,343,344,345,346,347,348,349,350,351,352] A recent meta-analysis by Lai et al indicated that ONSF improves visual acuity, headache, and papilledema in 36.5, 70, and 90% of reported cases, respectively.[305] For example, in one study 26 patients underwent 40 ONSFs for relief of visual loss or to preserve vision (16 unilateral and 12 bilateral operations).[353] Papilledema resolved or was strikingly reduced in 24 of 28 patients. The other four patients had gliotic discs (two patients) or were followed up for only a short time. Visual acuity improved in 12 of 40 eyes and remained the same in 22 of 40 eyes. In six eyes, visual acuity decreased. Visual fields improved in 21 of 40 eyes and remained the same in 10 eyes; five of the 10 eyes that did not change had poor vision before surgery. Eight eyes in five patients continued to lose acuity postoperatively. An additional two eyes developed visual field loss with preserved visual acuity. In another study, 23 patients with chronic papilledema had ONSF and 21 of the 23 patients demonstrated improvement in visual function.[349] Twelve of 21 patients with bilateral visual loss had improved visual function bilaterally after unilateral surgery, and 6 of 21 patients needed bilateral surgery. ONSF improved vision in six patients who failed to recover vision after LPS.

Kelman et al performed ONSF on 17 patients with severe visual acuity or field loss.[343] Postoperatively, visual acuity improved or stabilized in 33 of 34 eyes (97%) and the visual fields improved in 20 of 21 eyes that underwent surgery. Kelman et al also performed ONSF in 12 patients (16 eyes) with functioning LPS and progressive visual loss,[344] and all patients demonstrated improvement in visual function. Liu et al reported a woman with PTC treated with an LPS who developed acute pallid disc swelling with peripapillary hemorrhages and visual acuity of no light perception (NLP) OD and 20/70 OS in association with LPS failure.[354] The patient underwent ONSF and LPS revision and her visual acuity improved to 20/20 OU and her papilledema resolved. Pearson et al operated upon nine

patients (14 eyes) and visual function significantly improved or stabilized in all but one patient.[348] Goh et al described 29 eyes of patients with IIH who underwent ONSF for visual loss following failure of acetazolamide treatment.[355] Visual acuity and visual fields were compared before and after shunt placement (within 1 and 6 months). Mean follow-up was 15.7 months (ranging from 1 to 50 months). Visual acuity improved in 4 eyes (14%), was unchanged in 22 eyes (76%), and worsened in 3 eyes (10%). Visual fields improved in 10 eyes (48%), remained unchanged in 8 eyes (38%), and worsened in 3 eyes (14%) with 6 eyes lost to follow-up. There were four repeat surgeries, one of which led to vision loss in one eye.

Banta et al reported 158 ONSFs in 86 patients with PTC with visual loss despite medical treatment.[356] Visual acuity stabilized or improved in 148 of 158 eyes (94%) and visual fields stabilized or improved in 71 of 81 eyes (88%). Surgical complications, most often benign and transient, occurred in 39 of 86 patients. Diplopia occurred in 30 patients, with 87% resolving spontaneously (2 patients required prismatic correction and 2 other patients underwent subsequent strabismus surgery). Only one eye in one patient had permanent severe visual loss (count fingers acuity) secondary to an operative complication (presumed traumatic optic neuropathy). One patient had total ophthalmoplegia and blindness after surgery (orbital apex compression syndrome) that completely resolved over 1 month with steroid therapy. Visual loss occurred in 16 of 158 (10%) eyes after initially successful primary ONSF with time from surgery to failure variable (up to 5 years postoperatively). No specific risk factors were identified that had predisposed patients to ONSF failure. Nine eyes in six patients underwent repeat ONSF for progressive visual loss after an initially successful ONSF. The only complication encountered on repeat ONSF was transient diplopia in two patients. Two patients who underwent repeat ONSF required a CSF diversion procedure to halt progressive visual loss and two patients with stable visual function after repeat ONSF required CSF diversion procedures for intractable headaches. Three patients with progressive visual loss after initially successful primary ONSF underwent CSF diversion procedures instead of repeat ONSF. After ONSF, many patients initially had symptomatic improvement of headaches, but only 8 of 61 (13%) patients with headache as a presenting symptom had subjective improvement in this study. Nine patients underwent CSF diversion procedures for intractable headaches after ONSF despite stable visual parameters. The authors noted that the patient population with a significant headache component would likely benefit from an initial CSF diversion procedure. The authors concluded that ONSF is a safe and effective means of stabilizing visual acuity and visual fields in patients with PTC with progressive visual loss despite maximum medical therapy.

Mittra et al examined changes in color Doppler imaging before and after ONSF for PTC.[347] Their results suggest that some of the visual loss from chronic papilledema may be due to ischemia, and worsening visual acuity correlates with greater impairment of the retrobulbar circulation. Reversal of this ischemic process may be one of the mechanisms by which ONSF improves visual function.

Talks et al reported 24 patients with PTC who required ONSF.[261] Twenty-one of the 48 eyes (44%) had macular changes including choroidal folds (nine patients), circumferential (Paton's) lines (four), nerve fiber layer hemorrhages (three), macular stars (five), macular edema (six), retinal pigment epithelial changes (four), and subretinal hemorrhage leading to a macular scar (one). Significant visual loss attributable to the macular changes was found in five eyes in the short term and three eyes in the long term. The two eyes that improved had macular stars; of the three eyes that did not improve, two had retinal pigment epithelial changes and one had subretinal hemorrhage leading to a macular scar. The authors concluded that the majority of macular changes in PTC patients resolve and do not add to visual loss from optic nerve damage. Patients with marked macular edema, however, are at greatest risk for permanent visual loss and should be considered for early surgical treatment.

ONSF has also been effective in children with PTC.[345] Of 12 patients younger than 16 years with PTC, 67% had improved visual acuity and 33% had improved visual fields, but 17% had worsening of visual acuity and visual fields postoperatively.[345]

Headaches may be relieved in over half of the patients with PTC undergoing ONSF.[303] For example, with unilateral decompression, headaches were improved or were relieved in 13 of 17 patients in one series[349] and in 10 of 16 patients in another study,[303] whereas while 91% of patients (10/11) had relief of headache after ONSF in a third study.[357] ONSF may also relieve papilledema and improve vision when performed on patients with PTC secondary to occlusion of the dural sinuses.[342,347]

Some reports have suggested that ONSF is more effective and associated with fewer complications than CSF diversion.[341,349] Because of these reports, many physicians favor ONSF for the majority of patients with PTC who require surgery.[310] Long-term follow-up data suggests, however, that ONSF may not be as effective as originally claimed. Approximately one-third of patients undergoing ONSF will not experience headache relief and only about 75% of ONSFs appear to be functioning 6 months after surgery. The probability of an ONSF remaining functional steadily decreases such that 66% are functioning at 12 months, 55% at 3 years, 38% at 5 years, and 16% at 6 years after surgery.[350] As such, these patients must have their visual function monitored for years following surgery as deterioration may indicate ONSF failure and require repeat procedures. Although patients may be treated with a second ONSF after initial failure, eyes that have more than one ONSF are less likely to improve after surgery and more likely to experience significant vascular complications than eyes that undergo a single surgery.[358] Up to 33% of patients undergoing ONSF for PTC who show initial improvement in visual function later show deterioration in visual field and acuity.[350,351] In a study of the long-term effectiveness of ONSF for PTC, Spoor and McHenry reviewed 32 series of postoperative visual fields in patients who were undergoing ONSF for PTC who had stable visual acuity and four or more fields during 6 to 60 months of follow-up.[350] The authors then extended the review to include all patients (54 patients, 75 eyes) who underwent ONSF for PTC and were evaluated with serial automated perimetry. Thirty-six percent of eyes showed improvement of visual function, whereas an equal number of eyes experienced deterioration (32%) or stabilization (32%) of visual function after an initially successful ONSF. The probability of failure from 3 to 5 years was 0.35 by life-table analysis. The authors concluded that ONSF effectively stabilizes or improves visual function in the majority of patients with PTC and visual loss. It may fail at any time after surgery, however,

and patients need routine follow-up with automated perimetry to detect deterioration of visual function. Some of these late failures may be prevented by improved operative techniques.[349,351] Also, Acheson et al reported 14 patients (11 with IIH and 3 with dural venous sinus occlusion) who underwent eight unilateral and six bilateral ONSFs.[338] Visual acuity and fields either improved or stabilized in 17 out of 20 eyes while three deteriorated. Of the eight patients undergoing unilateral surgery, the other eye remained stable in seven and deteriorated in one. Four patients required ONSF despite previous shunting or subtemporal decompression. Five patients required shunting or subtemporal decompression after ONSF because of persistent headache in three cases and for uncontrolled visual failure in two cases. No patient lost vision as a direct complication of surgery.

Thus, vision can be saved after shunt failure, and in other cases may be maintained without the need for a shunt. However, shunting may still be required after ONSF. Mauriello et al reviewed the records of 108 patients with PTC who underwent ONSF and who showed visual loss within 1 month of surgery.[346] Five patients, including two with renal failure and hypertension, had visual loss within 1 month of ONSF. The first had an abrupt decrease in vision 6 days after ONSF, and in this patient a vessel on the nerve sheath bled into the surgical site. After high-dose intravenous (IV) steroids failed to improve vision, emergency LPS resulted in full visual recovery. An apparent infectious optic neuropathy developed in the second patient 3 days after surgery. After 72 hours of IV antibiotics, visual acuity improved from 20/600 to 20/15. The other three patients had gradual visual loss after ONSF, which stabilized after LPS placement. These authors reviewed ONSF failures in the literature and showed that four of seven patients with abrupt visual loss within the first 2 weeks of ONSF had no improvement in vision despite various treatments, including shunts. The series of Corbett et al of 40 ONSFs in 28 patients included six patients who lost vision within the first 2 weeks of surgery.[341] Only one of these six patients had return of vision, and this patient had a dramatic decrease of vision from 20/30 in the involved eye to NLP 3 hours postoperatively due to retrobulbar hemorrhage, with acuity improving to 20/20 after surgical drainage of the retrobulbar hematoma. The other five patients had no visual recovery despite LPS, continuous lumbar drainage, and repeat ONSF in one patient who had intrasheath hemorrhage due to coughing (this patient went from 20/30 to 20/200 10 days postoperatively). Intravenous steroids appeared to enhance visual recovery in one patient of Flynn et al who went from 20/400 to NLP 5 hours postoperatively but who improved to 20/800 after intravenous dexamethasone.[359] Mauriello et al concluded that avoidance of bleeding during ONSF may prevent fibrous occlusion of the surgical site and that patients with no identifiable cause for visual loss after ONSF who do not respond to IV steroids should be evaluated for emergent LPS placement.[346] Also, postoperative infectious optic neuropathy should be considered in the differential of abrupt visual loss after ONSF. If ONSF fails, the authors favor LPS rather than repeat ONSF.

Numerous complications have also been reported following ONSF.[341,358,359,360,361] Plotnik and Kosmorsky reported postoperative complications in 15 of the 38 eyes (39%) undergoing ONSF.[358] Temporary motility disorders (due to direct extraocular muscle damage or damage to their associated nerves and/or

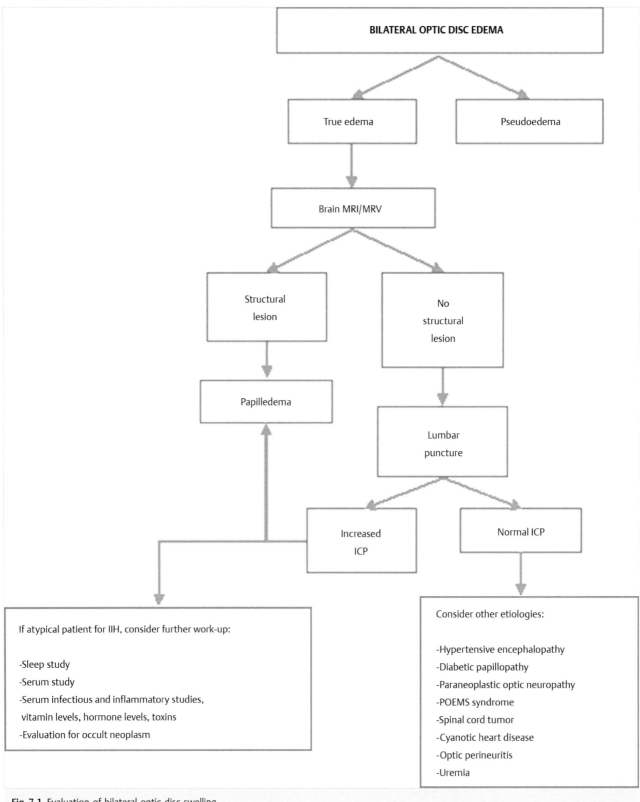

Fig. 7.1 Evaluation of bilateral optic disc swelling.

vasculature) occurred in 29% and all resolved, the longest taking 9 weeks. Pupillary dysfunction occurred in four eyes (11%) and consisted of sectoral tonic pupils (due to damage to short ciliary nerves or their blood supply causing iris sphincter palsy) that lasted 2 to 8 weeks in three eyes but persisted in one eye for 12 weeks. Four eyes (11%) had postoperative vascular complications, including two with central retinal artery occlusions, one superotemporal branch retinal artery occlusion, and one episode of transient outer retinal ischemia. Both eyes with central retinal artery occlusions had poor visual outcomes and eyes that had undergone prior ONSF were significantly more likely to have vascular complications than those without a previous operation. The incidence of vascular complications was 67% in eyes that had undergone prior ONSF and 6% in those that had never undergone ONSF. Additional complications reported with ONSF are listed in Box 7.8.

Box 7.8 Complications of optic nerve sheath fenestration[340,341,356,358,359,360,361]

- Ocular motility disorders (e.g., temporary horizontal motility disorder caused by disinsertion of the medial rectus muscle or combined third and sixth nerve palsies).
- Transient or permanent diffuse or sectorial tonic pupils.
- Conjunctival blebs with dellen formation.
- Chemosis.
- Chorioretinal scar from excessive traction on the globe.
- Peripapillary hemorrhages thought to be secondary to short ciliary vessel injury.
- Orbital hemorrhage.
- Trauma to the optic nerve.
- Myelinated nerve fibers (noted 5 months and 6 years postoperatively, thought to be stimulated by trauma associated with surgery).
- Microhyphemas.
- Orbital apex syndrome.
- Subconjunctival Tenon's cysts.
- Streptococcal corneal ulcers.
- Dacryocystitis.
- Intraoperative angle closure glaucoma.
- Deterioration of visual function, transient blindness, choroidal infarction (fundus changes with choroidal infarction may not be evident for several weeks after operation).
- Central or branch retinal artery occlusion.
- Death.

7.16.3 Venous Sinus Stenting

Venous sinus stenting is a relatively new intervention that has piqued the interest of many investigators. Increased application of magnetic resonance venography (MRV) and cerebral angiography has led to the identification of stenotic dural sinuses in some PTC patients. Farb et al used high-resolution MRV to show stenotic dural sinuses in more than 90% of 29 PTC patients as opposed to 7% of 59 controls.[362] Riggeal et al observed bilateral transverse sinus stenosis in 90% of 51 patients and concluded that the degree and location of venous sinus stenosis does not

predict clinical outcomes.[363] It is uncertain whether the stenotic venous sinus is the cause or effect of intracranial hypertension in PTC. However, some authors have reported favorable outcomes using dural sinus stenting to treat these patients. Puffer et al meta-analyzed the pooled data of 143 patients who had a stent placed in the focal area of sinus stenosis (with documented pressure gradient across); visual symptoms, headaches, and papilledema improved in 88, 97, and 87%, respectively.[364] Similar rates of improvement were reported poststenting in a meta-analysis of 19 studies and 207 patients by Teleb et al; headaches, papilledema, and pulsatile tinnitus, improved in 81, 87, and 95% of the time, respectively.[365] However, authors failed to specify the interval between the intervention and the reported outcomes and to control for bias that might arise when the effect of natural history of IIH is unaccounted for. It is known that IIH can be self-limited and may resolve within months in some patients.[366]

Despite favorable results overall, life-threatening complications may rarely occur, most notably intracranial hemorrhage requiring emergent neurosurgery.[367] Poststenting, patients typically require dual-antiplatelet therapy for longer than 3 months that might limit the use of this intervention in some. Endovascular stenting can be complicated by restenosis, in-stent stenosis, stent migration, or sinus perforation.[367] One retrospective analysis of 15 studies reported an overall complication rate of 6%.[364] The largest cohort of 52 PTC patients had retreatment of 12% due to restenosis.[316] In another retrospective study, 13% required VPS despite stenting due to persistent refractory headache.[368] Further studies are warranted to determine the role of dural sinus stenting in treating patients with PTC.

The evaluation of the patient with optic disc swelling is summarized in ▸ Fig. 7.1.

References

[1] Ing EB, Leavitt JA, Younge BR. Papilledema following bowtie optic atrophy. Arch Ophthalmol. 1996; 114(3):356–357

[2] Sadun AA, Currie JN, Lessell S. Transient visual obscurations with elevated optic discs. Ann Neurol. 1984; 16(4):489–494

[3] Kurz-Levin MM, Landau K. A comparison of imaging techniques for diagnosing drusen of the optic nerve head. Arch Ophthalmol. 1999; 117(8):1045–1049

[4] Glaser JS. Neuro-ophthalmology. 2nd ed. Philadelphia, PA: JP Lippincott; 1990:106

[5] Carter SB, Pistilli M, Livingston KG, et al. The role of orbital ultrasonography in distinguishing papilledema from pseudopapilledema. Eye (Lond). 2014; 28(12):1425–1430

[6] Neudorfer M, Ben-Haim MS, Leibovitch I, Kesler A. The efficacy of optic nerve ultrasonography for differentiating papilloedema from pseudopapilloedema in eyes with swollen optic discs. Acta Ophthalmol. 2013; 91(4):376–380

[7] Auinger P, Durbin M, Feldon S, et al. OCT Sub-Study Committee for NORDIC Idiopathic Intracranial Hypertension Study Group. Baseline OCT measurements in the idiopathic intracranial hypertension treatment trial, part II: correlations and relationship to clinical features. Invest Ophthalmol Vis Sci. 2014; 55(12):8173–8179

[8] Johnson LN, Diehl ML, Hamm CW, Sommerville DN, Petroski GF. Differentiating optic disc edema from optic nerve head drusen on optical coherence tomography. Arch Ophthalmol. 2009; 127(1):45–49

[9] Kulkarni KM, Pasol J, Rosa PR, Lam BL. Differentiating mild papilledema and buried optic nerve head drusen using spectral domain optical coherence tomography. Ophthalmology. 2014; 121(4):959–963

[10] Merchant KY, Su D, Park SC, et al. Enhanced depth imaging optical coherence tomography of optic nerve head drusen. Ophthalmology. 2013; 120(7):1409–1414

[11] Lee KM, Woo SJ, Hwang JM. Differentiation of optic nerve head drusen and optic disc edema with spectral-domain optical coherence tomography. Ophthalmology. 2011; 118(5):971–977

[12] Sarac O, Tasci YY, Gurdal C, Can I. Differentiation of optic disc edema from optic nerve head drusen with spectral-domain optical coherence tomography. J Neuroophthalmol. 2012; 32(3):207–211

[13] Bassi ST, Mohana KP. Optical coherence tomography in papilledema and pseudopapilledema with and without optic nerve head drusen. Indian J Ophthalmol. 2014; 62(12):1146–1151

[14] Auinger P, Durbin M, Feldon S, et al. OCT Sub-Study Committee for NORDIC Idiopathic Intracranial Hypertension Study Group. Baseline OCT measurements in the idiopathic intracranial hypertension treatment trial, part I: quality control, comparisons, and variability. Invest Ophthalmol Vis Sci. 2014; 55(12):8180–8188

[15] Chari C, Rao NS. Benign intracranial hypertension–its unusual manifestations. Headache. 1991; 31(9):599–600

[16] Huna-Baron R, Landau K, Rosenberg M, Warren FA, Kupersmith MJ. Unilateral swollen disc due to increased intracranial pressure. Neurology. 2001; 56(11):1588–1590

[17] Killer HE, Flammer J. Unilateral papilledema caused by a fronto-temporo-parietal arachnoid cyst. Am J Ophthalmol. 2001; 132(4):589–591

[18] Lepore FE. Unilateral and highly asymmetric papilledema in pseudotumor cerebri. Neurology. 1992; 42(3, Pt 1):676–678

[19] Strominger MB, Weiss GB, Mehler MF. Asymptomatic unilateral papilledema in pseudotumor cerebri. J Clin Neuroophthalmol. 1992; 12(4):238–241

[20] To KW, Warren FA. Unilateral papilledema in pseudotumor cerebri. Arch Ophthalmol. 1990; 108(5):644–645

[21] Watnick RL, Trobe JD. Bilateral optic nerve compression as a mechanism for the Foster Kennedy syndrome. Ophthalmology. 1989; 96(12):1793–1798

[22] Sherman MD, Own KH. Interstitial nephritis and uveitis syndrome presenting with bilateral optic disk edema. Am J Ophthalmol. 1999; 127(5):609–610

[23] O'Halloran HS, Berger JR, Baker RS, Lee WB, Pearson PA, Ryan S. Optic nerve edema as a consequence of respiratory disease. Neurology. 1999; 53(9):2204–2205

[24] Purvin VA, Kawasaki A, Yee RD. Papilledema and obstructive sleep apnea syndrome. Arch Ophthalmol. 2000; 118(12):1626–1630

[25] Morrison KE, Davies PT. Chronic inflammatory demyelinating polyneuropathy presenting with headache and papilledema. Headache. 1999; 39(4):299–300

[26] Bolling JP, Brazis PW. Optic disk swelling with peripheral neuropathy, organomegaly, endocrinopathy, monoclonal gammopathy, and skin changes (POEMS syndrome). Am J Ophthalmol. 1990; 109(5):503–510

[27] Wong VA, Wade NK. POEMS syndrome: an unusual cause of bilateral optic disk swelling. Am J Ophthalmol. 1998; 126(3):452–454

[28] McLean C, Lobo R, Brazier JD. Optic disc involvement in hypocalcaemia with hypoparathyroidism: papilloedema or optic neuropathy? Neuroophthalmology. 1998; 20(3):117–124

[29] Hykin PG, Spalton DJ. Bilateral perineuritis of the optic nerves. J Neurol Neurosurg Psychiatry. 1991; 54(4):375–376

[30] Nakamura N, Hara R, Kimura R, et al. Optic perineuritis not associated with syphilitic infection. Neuro-ophthalmology. 1999; 21:135–145

[31] Prevett MC, Plant GT. Intracranial hypertension and HIV associated meningoradiculitis. J Neurol Neurosurg Psychiatry. 1997; 62(4):407–409

[32] Bafna S, Lee AG. Bilateral optic disc edema and multifocal retinal lesions without loss of vision in cat scratch disease. Arch Ophthalmol. 1996; 114(8):1016–1017

[33] Fedorowski JJ, Hyman C. Optic disk edema as the presenting sign of Lyme disease. Clin Infect Dis. 1996; 23(3):639–640

[34] Rothermel H, Hedges TR, III, Steere AC. Optic neuropathy in children with Lyme disease. Pediatrics. 2001; 108(2):477–481

[35] Friedman DI. Papilledema and pseudotumor cerebri. Ophthalmol Clin North Am. 2001; 14(1):129–147, ix

[36] Scott CJ, Kardon RH, Lee AG, Frisén L, Wall M. Diagnosis and grading of papilledema in patients with raised intracranial pressure using optical coherence tomography vs clinical expert assessment using a clinical staging scale. Arch Ophthalmol. 2010; 128(6):705–711

[37] Fischer WS, Wall M, McDermott MP, Kupersmith MJ, Feldon SE, NORDIC Idiopathic Intracranial Hypertension Study Group. Photographic reading center of the idiopathic intracranial hypertension treatment trial (IIHTT): methods and baseline results. Invest Ophthalmol Vis Sci. 2015; 56(5):3292–3303

[38] Lee AG. Visual loss as the manifesting symptom of ventriculoperitoneal shunt malfunction. Am J Ophthalmol. 1996; 122(1):127–129

[39] Lee AG, Beaver HA. Acute bilateral optic disk edema with a macular star figure in a 12-year-old girl. Surv Ophthalmol. 2002; 47(1):42–49

[40] Wall M. Optic disk edema with cotton-wool spots. Surv Ophthalmol. 1995; 39(6):502–508

[41] Katz DM, Trobe JD, Muraszko KM, Dauser RC. Shunt failure without ventriculomegaly proclaimed by ophthalmic findings. J Neurosurg. 1994; 81(5):721–725

[42] Newman NJ. Bilateral visual loss and disc edema in a 15-year-old girl. Surv Ophthalmol. 1994; 38(4):365–370

[43] Bandyopadhyay S. Pseudotumor cerebri. Arch Neurol. 2001; 58(10):1699–1701

[44] Verm A, Lee AG. Bilateral optic disk edema with macular exudates as the manifesting sign of a cerebral arteriovenous malformation. Am J Ophthalmol. 1997; 123(3):422–424

[45] Cuddihy J. Case report of benign inter-cranial hypertension secondary to tetracycline. Ir Med J. 1994; 87(3):90

[46] Gardner K, Cox T, Digre KB. Idiopathic intracranial hypertension associated with tetracycline use in fraternal twins: case reports and review. Neurology. 1995; 45(1):6–10

[47] Scott IU, Siatkowski RM, Eneyni M, Brodsky MC, Lam BL. Idiopathic intracranial hypertension in children and adolescents. Am J Ophthalmol. 1997; 124(2):253–255

[48] Friedman DI. Medication-induced intracranial hypertension in dermatology. Am J Clin Dermatol. 2005; 6(1):29–37

[49] Chiu AM, Chuenkongkaew WL, Cornblath WT, et al. Minocycline treatment and pseudotumor cerebri syndrome. Am J Ophthalmol. 1998; 126(1):116–121

[50] Donnet A, Dufour H, Graziani N, Grisoli F. Minocycline and benign intracranial hypertension. Biomed Pharmacother. 1992; 46(4):171–172

[51] Lewis PA, Kearney PJ. Pseudotumor cerebri induced by minocycline treatment for acne vulgaris. Acta Derm Venereol. 1997; 77(1):83

[52] Moskowitz Y, Leibowitz E, Ronen M, Aviel E. Pseudotumor cerebri induced by vitamin A combined with minocycline. Ann Ophthalmol. 1993; 25(8):306–308

[53] Torres M, May E, Watanabe F, et al. Intracranial hypertension associated with minocycline. Presented at the 23rd Annual Meeting of the North American Neuro Ophthalmology Society, Keystone, Colorado, February 9–13, 1997

[54] Mukherjee A, Dutta P, Lahiri M, Sinha S, Mitra AK, Bhattacharya SK. Benign intracranial hypertension after nalidixic acid overdose in infants. Lancet. 1990; 335(8705):1602

[55] Getenet JC, Croisile B, Vighetto A, et al. Idiopathic intracranial hypertension after ofloxacin treatment. Acta Neurol Scand. 1993; 87(6):503–504

[56] Winrow AP, Supramaniam G. Benign intracranial hypertension after ciprofloxacin administration. Arch Dis Child. 1990; 65(10):1165–1166

[57] Alemayehu W. Pseudotumor cerebri (toxic effect of the "magic bullet"). Ethiop Med J. 1995; 33(4):265–270

[58] Donahue SP. Recurrence of idiopathic intracranial hypertension after weight loss: the carrot craver. Am J Ophthalmol. 2000; 130(6):850–851

[59] Sharieff GQ, Hanten K. Pseudotumor cerebri and hypercalcemia resulting from vitamin A toxicity. Ann Emerg Med. 1996; 27(4):518–521

[60] Sirdofsky M, Kattah J, Macedo P. Intracranial hypertension in a dieting patient. J Neuroophthalmol. 1994; 14(1):9–11

[61] Panozzo G, Babighian S, Bonora A. Association of xerophthalmia, flecked retina, and pseudotumor cerebri caused by hypovitaminosis A. Am J Ophthalmol. 1998; 125(5):708–710

[62] Chen HY, Tsai RK, Huang SM. ATRA-induced pseudotumour cerebri–one case report. Kaohsiung J Med Sci. 1998; 14(1):58–60

[63] Mahmoud HH, Hurwitz CA, Roberts WM, Santana VM, Ribeiro RC, Krance RA. Tretinoin toxicity in children with acute promyelocytic leukaemia. Lancet. 1993; 342(8884):1394–1395

[64] Naderi S, Nukala S, Marruenda F, Kudarvalli P, Koduri PR. Pseudotumour cerebri in acute promyelocytic leukemia: improvement despite continued ATRA therapy. Ann Hematol. 1999; 78(7):333–334

[65] Schroeter T, Lanvers C, Herding H, Suttorp M. Pseudotumor cerebri induced by all-trans-retinoic acid in a child treated for acute promyelocytic leukemia. Med Pediatr Oncol. 2000; 34(4):284–286

[66] Selleri C, Pane F, Notaro R, et al. All-trans-retinoic acid (ATRA) responsive skin relapses of acute promyelocytic leukaemia followed by ATRA-induced pseudotumour cerebri. Br J Haematol. 1996; 92(4):937–940

[67] Varadi G, Lossos A, Or R, Kapelushnik J, Nagler A. Successful allogeneic bone marrow transplantation in a patient with ATRA-induced pseudotumor cerebri. Am J Hematol. 1995; 50(2):147–148

[68] Visani G, Bontempo G, Manfroi S, Pazzaglia A, D'Alessandro R, Tura S. All-trans-retinoic acid and pseudotumor cerebri in a young adult with acute promyelocytic leukemia: a possible disease association. Haematologica. 1996; 81(2):152–154

[69] Yokokura M, Hatake K, Komatsu N, Kajitani H, Miura Y. Toxicity of tretinoin in acute promyelocytic leukaemia. Lancet. 1994; 343(8893):361–362

[70] Alison L, Hobbs CJ, Hanks HG, Butler G. Non-organic failure to thrive complicated by benign intracranial hypertension during catch-up growth. Acta Paediatr. 1997; 86(10):1141–1143

[71] Blethen SL. Complications of growth hormone therapy in children. Curr Opin Pediatr. 1995; 7(4):466–471

[72] Francois I, Casteels I, Silberstein J, Casaer P, de Zegher F. Empty sella, growth hormone deficiency and pseudotumour cerebri: effect of initiation, withdrawal and resumption of growth hormone therapy. Eur J Pediatr. 1997; 156(1):69–70

[73] Koller EA, Stadel BV, Malozowski SN. Papilledema in 15 renally compromised patients treated with growth hormone. Pediatr Nephrol. 1997; 11(4):451–454

[74] Malozowski S, Tanner LA, Wysowski DK, Fleming GA, Stadel BV. Benign intracranial hypertension in children with growth hormone deficiency treated with growth hormone. J Pediatr. 1995; 126(6):996–999

[75] Maneatis T, Baptista J, Connelly K, Blethen S. Growth hormone safety update from the National Cooperative Growth Study. J Pediatr Endocrinol Metab. 2000; 13 Suppl 2:1035–1044

[76] Rogers AH, Rogers GL, Bremer DL, McGregor ML. Pseudotumor cerebri in children receiving recombinant human growth hormone. Ophthalmology. 1999; 106(6):1186–1189, discussion 1189–1190

[77] Campos SP, Olitsky S. Idiopathic intracranial hypertension after L-thyroxine therapy for acquired primary hypothyroidism. Clin Pediatr (Phila). 1995; 34(6):334–337

[78] Misra M, Khan GM, Rath S. Eltroxin induced pseudotumour cerebri–a case report. Indian J Ophthalmol. 1992; 40(4):117

[79] Raghavan S, DiMartino-Nardi J, Saenger P, Linder B. Pseudotumor cerebri in an infant after L-thyroxine therapy for transient neonatal hypothyroidism. J Pediatr. 1997; 130(3):478–480

[80] Arber N, Shirin H, Fadila R, Melamed E, Pinkhas J, Sidi Y. Pseudotumor cerebri associated with leuprorelin acetate. Lancet. 1990; 335(8690):668

[81] Mayer-Hubner B. Pseudotumour cerebri from intranasal oxytocin and excessive fluid intake. Lancet. 1996; 347(9001):623

[82] Haller JS, Meyer DR, Cromie W, Fagles N, Hayes S. Pseudotumor cerebri following beta-human chorionic gonadotropin hormone treatment for undescended testicles. Neurology. 1993; 43(2):448–449

[83] Fanous M, Hamed LM, Margo CE. Pseudotumor cerebri associated with danazol withdrawal. JAMA. 1991; 266(9):1218–1219

[84] Pears J, Sandercock PA. Benign intracranial hypertension associated with danazol. Scott Med J. 1990; 35(2):49

[85] Liu GT, Kay MD, Bienfang DC, Schatz NJ. Pseudotumor cerebri associated with corticosteroid withdrawal in inflammatory bowel disease. Am J Ophthalmol. 1994; 117(3):352–357

[86] Sakamaki Y, Nakamura R, Uchida M, Saito T, Okajima S. A case of pseudotumor cerebri following glucocorticoid therapy in which warfarin prevented recurrence. Jpn J Med. 1990; 29(5):566–570

[87] Evers JP, Jacobson RJ, Pincus J, Zwiebel JA. Pseudotumour cerebri following high-dose cytosine arabinoside. Br J Haematol. 1992; 80(4):559–560

[88] Fort JA, Smith LD. Pseudotumor cerebri secondary to intermediate-dose cytarabine HCl. Ann Pharmacother. 1999; 33(5):576–578

[89] Sacchi S, Kantarjian HM, Freireich EJ, et al. Unexpected high incidence of severe toxicities associated with alpha interferon, low-dose cytosine arabinoside and all-trans retinoic acid in patients with chronic myelogenous leukemia. Leuk Lymphoma. 1999; 35(5–6):483–489

[90] Cruz OA, Fogg SG, Roper-Hall G. Pseudotumor cerebri associated with cyclosporine use. Am J Ophthalmol. 1996; 122(3):436–437

[91] Galm O, Fabry U, Osieka R. Pseudotumor cerebri after treatment of relapsed acute promyelocytic leukemia with arsenic trioxide. Leukemia. 2000; 14(2):343–344

[92] Ahmad S. Amiodarone and reversible benign intracranial hypertension. Cardiology. 1996; 87(1):90

[93] Borruat FX, Regli F. Pseudotumor cerebri as a complication of amiodarone therapy. Am J Ophthalmol. 1993; 116(6):776–777

[94] Konomi H, Imai M, Nihei K, Kamoshita S, Tada H. Indomethacin causing pseudotumor cerebri in Bartter's syndrome. N Engl J Med. 1978; 298(15):855

[95] Ames D, Wirshing WC, Cokely HT, Lo LL. The natural course of pseudotumor cerebri in lithium-treated patients. J Clin Psychopharmacol. 1994; 14(4):286–287

[96] Dommisse J. Pseudotumor cerebri associated with lithium therapy in two patients. J Clin Psychiatry. 1991; 52(5):239

[97] Levine SH, Puchalski C. Pseudotumor cerebri associated with lithium therapy in two patients. J Clin Psychiatry. 1990; 51(6):251–253

[98] Verderber L, Lavin P, Wesley R. Pseudotumour cerebri and chronic benzene hexachloride (lindane) exposure. J Neurol Neurosurg Psychiatry. 1991; 54(12):1123

[99] Alexandrakis G, Filatov V, Walsh T. Pseudotumor cerebri in a 12-year-old boy with Addison's disease. Am J Ophthalmol. 1993; 116(5):650–651

[100] Condulis N, Germain G, Charest N, Levy S, Carpenter TO. Pseudotumor cerebri: a presenting manifestation of Addison's disease. Clin Pediatr (Phila). 1997; 36(12):711–713

[101] Leggio MG, Cappa A, Molinari M, Corsello SM, Gainotti G. Pseudotumor cerebri as presenting syndrome of Addisonian crisis. Ital J Neurol Sci. 1995; 16(6):387–389

[102] Madan Mohan P, Noushad TP, Sarita P, Abdu Rahiman P, Girija AS. Hypoparathyroidism with benign intracranial hypertension. J Assoc Physicians India. 1993; 41(11):752–753

[103] Adams C, Dean HJ, Israels SJ, Patton A, Fewer DH. Primary hypothyroidism with intracranial hypertension and pituitary hyperplasia. Pediatr Neurol. 1994; 10(2):166–168

[104] Daif A, Awada A, al-Rajeh S, et al. Cerebral venous thrombosis in adults. A study of 40 cases from Saudi Arabia. Stroke. 1995; 26(7):1193–1195

[105] Koppel BS, Kaunitz AM, Tuchman AJ. Pseudotumor cerebri following eclampsia. Eur Neurol. 1990; 30(1):6–8

[106] McDonnell GV, Patterson VH, McKinstry S. Cerebral venous thrombosis occurring during an ectopic pregnancy and complicated by intracranial hypertension. Br J Clin Pract. 1997; 51(3):194–197

[107] Shapiro S, Yee R, Brown H. Surgical management of pseudotumor cerebri in pregnancy: case report. Neurosurgery. 1995; 37(4):829–831

[108] Parfitt VJ, Dearlove JC, Savage D, Griffith HB, Hartog M. Benign intracranial hypertension after pituitary surgery for Cushing's disease. Postgrad Med J. 1994; 70(820):115–117

[109] Au Eong KG, Hariharan S, Chua EC, et al. Idiopathic intracranial hypertension, empty sella turcica and polycystic ovary syndrome–a case report. Singapore Med J. 1997; 38(3):129–130

[110] Alpan G, Glick B, Peleg O, Eyal F. Pseudotumor cerebri and coma in vitamin D–dependent rickets. Clin Pediatr (Phila). 1991; 30(4):254–256

[111] Salaria M, Poddar B, Parmar V. Rickets presenting as pseudotumour cerebri and seizures. Indian J Pediatr. 2001; 68(2):181

[112] Gregoric A, Bracic K, Novljan G, Marcun-Varda N. Pseudotumor cerebri in a child with familial hypomagnesemia-hypercalciuria. Pediatr Nephrol. 2000; 14(3):269–270

[113] Lee AG, Golnik K, Kardon R, Wall M, Eggenberger E, Yedavally S. Sleep apnea and intracranial hypertension in men. Ophthalmology. 2002; 109(3):482–485

[114] Wolin MJ, Brannon WL. Disk edema in an overweight woman. Surv Ophthalmol. 1995; 39(4):307–314

[115] Chang D, Nagamoto G, Smith WE. Benign intracranial hypertension and chronic renal failure. Cleve Clin J Med. 1992; 59(4):419–422

[116] Guy J, Johnston PK, Corbett JJ, Day AL, Glaser JS. Treatment of visual loss in pseudotumor cerebri associated with uremia. Neurology. 1990; 40(1):28–32

[117] Avery R, Jabs DA, Wingard JR, Vogelsang G, Saral R, Santos G. Optic disc edema after bone marrow transplantation. Possible role of cyclosporine toxicity. Ophthalmology. 1991; 98(8):1294–1301

[118] Katz B. Disk edema subsequent to renal transplantation. Surv Ophthalmol. 1997; 41(4):315–320

[119] Obeid T, Awada A, Huraib S, Quadri K, Abu-Romeh S. Pseudotumor cerebri in renal transplant recipients: a diagnostic challenge. J Nephrol. 1997; 10(5):258–260

[120] Sheth KJ, Kivlin JD, Leichter HE, Pan CG, Multauf C. Pseudotumor cerebri with vision impairment in two children with renal transplantation. Pediatr Nephrol. 1994; 8(1):91–93

[121] Bikangaga P, Canny GJ. Benign intracranial hypertension in infants with cystic fibrosis. Arch Pediatr Adolesc Med. 1996; 150(5):551–552

[122] Lucidi V, Di Capua M, Rosati P, Papadatou B, Castro M. Benign intracranial hypertension in an older child with cystic fibrosis. Pediatr Neurol. 1993; 9(6):494–495

[123] Nasr SZ, Schaffert D. Symptomatic increase in intracranial pressure following pancreatic enzyme replacement therapy for cystic fibrosis. Pediatr Pulmonol. 1995; 19(6):396–397

[124] Sheridan M, Johnston I. Hydrocephalus and pseudotumour cerebri in the mucopolysaccharidoses. Childs Nerv Syst. 1994; 10(3):148–150

[125] Daftari TK, Heller JG, Newman NJ. Pseudotumor cerebri after occipitocervical arthrodesis and immobilization in a halo vest. A case report. J Bone Joint Surg Am. 1995; 77(3):455–458

[126] Kollar C, Parker G, Johnston I. Endovascular treatment of cranial venous sinus obstruction resulting in pseudotumor syndrome. Report of three cases. J Neurosurg. 2001; 94(4):646–651

[127] Milhorat TH, Chou MW, Trinidad EM, et al. Chiari I malformation redefined: clinical and radiographic findings for 364 symptomatic patients. Neurosurgery. 1999; 44(5):1005–1017

[128] Weiss GB, Bajwa ZH, Mehler MF. Co-occurrence of pseudotumor cerebri and Guillain-Barré syndrome in an adult. Neurology. 1991; 41(4):603–604

[129] Fantin A, Feist RM, Reddy CV. Intracranial hypertension and papilloedema in chronic inflammatory demyelinating polyneuropathy. Br J Ophthalmol. 1993; 77(3):193

[130] Kaufman DI. Peripheral demyelinating and axonal disorders. In: Miller NR, Newman NJ, eds. Walsh and Hoyt's Clinical Neuro-ophthalmology. 5th ed. Baltimore, MD: Williams & Wilkins; 1998:5677–5719

[131] Midroni G, Dyck PJ. Chronic inflammatory demyelinating polyradiculoneuropathy: unusual clinical features and therapeutic responses. Neurology. 1996; 46(5):1206–1212

[132] Newman NJ, Selzer KA, Bell RA. Association of multiple sclerosis and intracranial hypertension. J Neuroophthalmol. 1994; 14(4):189–192

[133] Hills C, Sohn RS. Peripheral nerve sheath tumor presents as idiopathic intracranial hypertension. Neurology. 1998; 50(1):308–309

[134] Fujiwara S, Sawamura Y, Kato T, Abe H, Katusima H. Idiopathic intracranial hypertension in female homozygous twins. J Neurol Neurosurg Psychiatry. 1997; 62(6):652–654

[135] Kharode C, McAbee G, Sherman J, Kaufman M. Familial intracranial hypertension: report of a case and review of the literature. J Child Neurol. 1992; 7(2):196–198

[136] Santinelli R, Tolone C, Toraldo R, Canino G, De Simone A, D'Avanzo M. Familial idiopathic intracranial hypertension with spinal and radicular pain. Arch Neurol. 1998; 55(6):854–856

[137] Graybill JR, Sobel J, Saag M, et al. The NIAID Mycoses Study Group and AIDS Cooperative Treatment Groups. Diagnosis and management of increased intracranial pressure in patients with AIDS and cryptococcal meningitis. Clin Infect Dis. 2000; 30(1):47–54

[138] Gross FJ, Mindel JS. Pseudotumor cerebri and Guillain-Barré syndrome associated with human immunodeficiency virus infection. Neurology. 1991; 41(11):1845–1846

[139] Javeed N, Shaikh J, Jayaram S. Recurrent pseudotumor cerebri in an HIV-positive patient. AIDS. 1995; 9(7):817–819

[140] Schwarz S, Husstedt IW, Georgiadis D, Reichelt D, Zidek W. Benign intracranial hypertension in an HIV-infected patient: headache as the only presenting sign. AIDS. 1995; 9(6):657–658

[141] Traverso F, Stagnaro R, Fazio B. Benign intracranial hypertension associated with HIV infection. Eur Neurol. 1993; 33(3):191–192

[142] Kan L, Sood SK, Maytal J. Pseudotumor cerebri in Lyme disease: a case report and literature review. Pediatr Neurol. 1998; 18(5):439–441

[143] Moodley M, Coovadia HM. Benign intracranial hypertension in typhoid fever. A case report. S Afr Med J. 1990; 78(10):608–609

[144] Vargas JA, García-Merino A, Rodríguez E, Villagra A. Pseudotumor cerebri complicating typhoid fever. Eur Neurol. 1990; 30(6):345–346

[145] Gökalp HZ, Başkaya MK, Aydin V. Pseudotumor cerebri with familial Mediterranean fever. Clin Neurol Neurosurg. 1992; 94(3):261–263

[146] Kumar RK, Ghali M, Dragojevic F, Young F. Papilloedema secondary to acute purulent sinusitis. J Paediatr Child Health. 1999; 35(4):396–398

[147] Akova YA, Kansu T, Duman S. Pseudotumor cerebri secondary to dural sinus thrombosis in neurosarcoidosis. J Clin Neuroophthalmol. 1993; 13(3):188–189

[148] Pelton RW, Lee AG, Orengo-Nania SD, Patrinely JR. Bilateral optic disk edema caused by sarcoidosis mimicking pseudotumor cerebri. Am J Ophthalmol. 1999; 127(2):229–230

[149] Redwood MD, Winer JB, Rossor M. Neurosarcoidosis presenting as benign intracranial hypertension. Eur Neurol. 1990; 30(5):282–283

[150] Nezu A, Kimura S, Osaka H. Tolosa-Hunt syndrome with pseudotumor cerebri. Report of an unusual case. Brain Dev. 1995; 17(3):216–218

[151] Bosch JA, Valdes M, Solans R, Montalban J, Vilardell M. Skin hyper-reactivity in patients with benign intracranial hypertension as an early manifestation of Behçet's disease. Br J Rheumatol. 1995; 34(2):184

[152] Farah S, Al-Shubaili A, Montaser A, et al. Behçet's syndrome: a report of 41 patients with emphasis on neurological manifestations. J Neurol Neurosurg Psychiatry. 1998; 64(3):382–384

[153] Kansu T, Kansu E, Zileli T, Kirkali P. Neuro-ophthalmologic manifestations of Behçet's disease. Neuroophthalmology. 1991; 11(1):7–11

[154] Chaves-Carballo E, Dabbagh O, Bahabri S. Pseudotumor cerebri and leukoencephalopathy in childhood lupus. Lupus. 1999; 8(1):81–84

[155] Chevalier X, de Bandt M, Bourgeois P, Kahn MF. Primary Sjögren's syndrome preceding the presentation of systemic lupus erythematosus as a benign intracranial hypertension syndrome. Ann Rheum Dis. 1992; 51(6):808–809

[156] Green L, Vinker S, Amital H, et al. Pseudotumor cerebri in systemic lupus erythematosus. Semin Arthritis Rheum. 1995; 25(2):103–108

[157] Horoshovski D, Amital H, Katz M, Shoenfeld Y. Pseudotumour cerebri in SLE. Clin Rheumatol. 1995; 14(6):708–710

[158] Vachvanichsanong P, Dissaneewate P, Vasikananont P. Pseudotumor cerebri in a boy with systemic lupus erythematosus. Am J Dis Child. 1992; 146(12):1417–1419

[159] Tugal O, Jacobson R, Berezin S, et al. Recurrent benign intracranial hypertension due to iron deficiency anemia. Case report and review of the literature. Am J Pediatr Hematol Oncol. 1994; 16(3):266–270

[160] van Gelder T, van Gemert HM, Tjiong HL. A patient with megaloblastic anaemia and idiopathic intracranial hypertension. Case history. Clin Neurol Neurosurg. 1991; 93(4):321–322

[161] Sussman J, Leach M, Greaves M, Malia R, Davies-Jones GA. Potentially prothrombotic abnormalities of coagulation in benign intracranial hypertension. J Neurol Neurosurg Psychiatry. 1997; 62(3):229–233

[162] Tehindrazanarivelo A, Bousser MG. Possible benign intracranial hypertension and essential thrombocythaemia. J Neurol Neurosurg Psychiatry. 1990; 53(9):981

[163] Guymer RH, Cairns JD, O'Day J. Benign intracranial hypertension in chronic myeloid leukemia. Aust N Z J Ophthalmol. 1993; 21(3):181–185

[164] Saitoh S, Momoi MY, Gunji Y. Pseudotumor cerebri manifesting as a symptom of acute promyelocytic leukemia. Pediatr Int. 2000; 42(1):97–99

[165] Wasan H, Mansi JL, Benjamin S, Powles R, Cunningham D. Myeloma and benign intracranial hypertension. BMJ. 1992; 304(6828):685

[166] Provenzale JM, Barboriak DP, Ortel TL. Dural sinus thrombosis associated with activated protein C resistance: MR imaging findings and proband identification. AJR Am J Roentgenol. 1998; 170(2):499–502

[167] Kesler A, Ellis MH, Reshef T, Kott E, Gadoth N. Idiopathic intracranial hypertension and anticardiolipin antibodies. J Neurol Neurosurg Psychiatry. 2000; 68(3):379–380

[168] Jacome DE. Idiopathic intracranial hypertension and hemophilia A. Headache. 2001; 41(6):595–598

[169] Feigert JM, Sweet DL, Coleman M, et al. Multicentric angiofollicular lymph node hyperplasia with peripheral neuropathy, pseudotumor cerebri, IgA dysproteinemia, and thrombocytosis in women. A distinct syndrome. Ann Intern Med. 1990; 113(5):362–367

[170] Hauser D, Barzilai N, Zalish M, Oliver M, Pollack A. Bilateral papilledema with retinal hemorrhages in association with cerebral venous sinus thrombosis and paroxysmal nocturnal hemoglobinuria. Am J Ophthalmol. 1996; 122(4):592–593

[171] Friedman DI, Liu GT, Digre KB. Revised diagnostic criteria for the pseudotumor cerebri syndrome in adults and children. Neurology. 2013; 81(13):1159–1165

[172] Çelebisoy N, Seçil Y, Yüceyar N, Ertekin C. Occult cerebral vascular causes of pseudotumor cerebri. Neuroophthalmology. 1999; 21:157–163

[173] Couban S, Maxner CE. Cerebral venous sinus thrombosis presenting as idiopathic intracranial hypertension. CMAJ. 1991; 145(6):657–659

[174] Cremer PD, Thompson EO, Johnston IH, Halmagyi GM. Pseudotumor cerebri and cerebral venous hypertension. Neurology. 1996; 47(6):1602–1603

[175] Gironell A, Martí-Fàbregas J, Bello J, Avila A. Non-Hodgkin's lymphoma as a new cause of non-thrombotic superior sagittal sinus occlusion. J Neurol Neurosurg Psychiatry. 1997; 63(1):121–122

[176] Kim AW, Trobe JD. Syndrome simulating pseudotumor cerebri caused by partial transverse venous sinus obstruction in metastatic prostate cancer. Am J Ophthalmol. 2000; 129(2):254–256

[177] Lam BL, Schatz NJ, Glaser JS, Bowen BC. Pseudotumor cerebri from cranial venous obstruction. Ophthalmology. 1992; 99(5):706–712

[178] van den Brink WA, Pieterman H, Avezaat CJ. Sagittal sinus occlusion, caused by an overlying depressed cranial fracture, presenting with late signs and symptoms of intracranial hypertension: case report. Neurosurgery. 1996; 38 (5):1044–1046

[179] Thomas DA, Trobe JD, Cornblath WT. Visual loss secondary to increased intracranial pressure in neurofibromatosis type 2. Arch Ophthalmol. 1999; 117(12):1650–1653

[180] Keiper GL, Jr, Sherman JD, Tomsick TA, Tew JM, Jr. Dural sinus thrombosis and pseudotumor cerebri: unexpected complications of suboccipital craniotomy and translabyrinthine craniectomy. J Neurosurg. 1999; 91(2): 192–197

[181] Kollar CD, Johnston IH. Pseudotumour after arteriovenous malformation embolisation. J Neurol Neurosurg Psychiatry. 1999; 67(2):249

[182] Angeli SI, Sato Y, Gantz BJ. Glomus jugulare tumors masquerading as benign intracranial hypertension. Arch Otolaryngol Head Neck Surg. 1994; 120(11): 1277–1280

[183] Kiers L, King JO. Increased intracranial pressure following bilateral neck dissection and radiotherapy. Aust N Z J Surg. 1991; 61(6):459–461

[184] Siatkowski RM, Vilar NF, Sternau L, Coin CG. Blindness from bad bones. Surv Ophthalmol. 1999; 43(6):487–490

[185] Biousse V, Ameri A, Bousser MG. Isolated intracranial hypertension as the only sign of cerebral venous thrombosis. Neurology. 1999; 53(7):1537–1542

[186] Leker RR, Steiner I. Anticardiolipin antibodies are frequently present in patients with idiopathic intracranial hypertension. Arch Neurol. 1998; 55 (6):817–820

[187] Mokri B, Jack CR, Jr, Petty GW. Pseudotumor syndrome associated with cerebral venous sinus occlusion and antiphospholipid antibodies. Stroke. 1993; 24(3):469–472

[188] Orefice G, De Joanna G, Coppola M, Brancaccio V, Ames PR. Benign intracranial hypertension: a non-thrombotic complication of the primary antiphospholipid syndrome? Lupus. 1995; 4(4):324–326

[189] Karahalios DG, Rekate HL, Khayata MH, Apostolides PJ. Elevated intracranial venous pressure as a universal mechanism in pseudotumor cerebri of varying etiologies. Neurology. 1996; 46(1):198–202

[190] King JO, Mitchell PJ, Thomson KR, Tress BM. Cerebral venography and manometry in idiopathic intracranial hypertension. Neurology. 1995; 45 (12):2224–2228

[191] Higgins JN, Owler BK, Cousins C, Pickard JD. Venous sinus stenting for refractory benign intracranial hypertension. Lancet. 2002; 359(9302): 228–230

[192] Tehindrazanarivelo A, Evard S, Schaison M, et al. Prospective study of cerebral sinus venous thrombosis in patients presenting with benign intracranial hypertension. Cerebrovasc Dis. 1992; 2:22–27

[193] Adelman JU. Headaches and papilledema secondary to dural arteriovenous malformation. Headache. 1998; 38(8):621–623

[194] Chimowitz MI, Little JR, Awad IA, Sila CA, Kosmorsky G, Furlan AJ. Intracranial hypertension associated with unruptured cerebral arteriovenous malformations. Ann Neurol. 1990; 27(5):474–479

[195] Cockerell OC, Lai HM, Ross-Russell RW. Pseudotumour cerebri associated with arteriovenous malformations. Postgrad Med J. 1993; 69(814):637–640

[196] Cognard C, Casasco A, Toevi M, Houdart E, Chiras J, Merland JJ. Dural arteriovenous fistulas as a cause of intracranial hypertension due to impairment of cranial venous outflow. J Neurol Neurosurg Psychiatry. 1998; 65(3):308–316

[197] David CA, Peerless SJ. Pseudotumor syndrome resulting from a cerebral arteriovenous malformation: case report. Neurosurgery. 1995; 36(3): 588–590

[198] Martin TJ, Bell DA, Wilson JA. Papilledema in a man with an "occult" dural arteriovenous malformation. J Neuroophthalmol. 1998; 18(1):49–52

[199] Rosenfeld JV, Widaa HA, Adams CB. Cerebral arteriovenous malformation causing benign intracranial hypertension–case report. Neurol Med Chir (Tokyo). 1991; 31(8):523–525

[200] Lee AG, Brazis PW. Magnetic resonance venography in idiopathic pseudotumor cerebri. J Neuroophthalmol. 2000; 20(1):12–13

[201] King JO, Mitchell PJ, Thomson KR, Tress BM. Manometry combined with cervical puncture in idiopathic intracranial hypertension. Neurology. 2002; 58(1):26–30

[202] Ireland B, Corbett JJ, Wallace RB. The search for causes of idiopathic intracranial hypertension. A preliminary case-control study. Arch Neurol. 1990; 47(3):315–320

[203] Arseni C, Simoca I, Jipescu I, Leventi E, Grecu P, Sima A. Pseudotumor cerebri: risk factors, clinical course, prognostic criteria. Rom J Neurol Psychiatry. 1992; 30(2):115–132

[204] Corbett JJ, Savino PJ, Thompson HS, et al. Visual loss in pseudotumor cerebri. Follow-up of 57 patients from five to 41 years and a profile of 14 patients with permanent severe visual loss. Arch Neurol. 1982; 39(8):461–474

[205] Jain N, Rosner F. Idiopathic intracranial hypertension: report of seven cases. Am J Med. 1992; 93(4):391–395

[206] Kesler A, Gadoth N. Epidemiology of idiopathic intracranial hypertension in Israel. J Neuroophthalmol. 2001; 21(1):12–14

[207] Radhakrishnan K, Ahlskog JE, Garrity JA, Kurland LT. Idiopathic intracranial hypertension. Mayo Clin Proc. 1994; 69(2):169–180

[208] Soler D, Cox T, Bullock P, Calver DM, Robinson RO. Diagnosis and management of benign intracranial hypertension. Arch Dis Child. 1998; 78 (1):89–94

[209] Walker RW. Idiopathic intracranial hypertension: any light on the mechanism of the raised pressure? J Neurol Neurosurg Psychiatry. 2001; 71 (1):1–5

[210] Wall M, George D. Idiopathic intracranial hypertension. A prospective study of 50 patients. Brain. 1991; 114 Pt 1A:155–180

[211] Digre KB, Corbett JJ. Pseudotumor cerebri in men. Arch Neurol. 1988; 45(8): 866–872

[212] Balcer LJ, Liu GT, Forman S, et al. Idiopathic intracranial hypertension: relation of age and obesity in children. Neurology. 1999; 52(4):870–872

[213] Cinciripini GS, Donahue S, Borchert MS. Idiopathic intracranial hypertension in prepubertal pediatric patients: characteristics, treatment, and outcome. Am J Ophthalmol. 1999; 127(2):178–182

[214] Lessell S. Pediatric pseudotumor cerebri (idiopathic intracranial hypertension). Surv Ophthalmol. 1992; 37(3):155–166

[215] Gordon K. Pediatric pseudotumor cerebri: descriptive epidemiology. Can J Neurol Sci. 1997; 24(3):219–221

[216] Kesler A, Goldhammer Y, Gadoth N. Do men with pseudomotor cerebri share the same characteristics as women? A retrospective review of 141 cases. J Neuroophthalmol. 2001; 21(1):15–17

[217] Radhakrishnan K, Ahlskog JE, Cross SA, Kurland LT, O'Fallon WM. Idiopathic intracranial hypertension (pseudotumor cerebri). Descriptive epidemiology in Rochester, Minn, 1976 to 1990. Arch Neurol. 1993; 50(1):78–80

[218] Radhakrishnan K, Thacker AK, Bohlaga NH, Maloo JC, Gerryo SE. Epidemiology of idiopathic intracranial hypertension: a prospective and case-control study. J Neurol Sci. 1993; 116(1):18–28

[219] Friedman DI, Jacobson DM. Diagnostic criteria for idiopathic intracranial hypertension. Neurology. 2002; 59(10):1492–1495

[220] Corbett JJ, Mehta MP. Cerebrospinal fluid pressure in normal obese subjects and patients with pseudotumor cerebri. Neurology. 1983; 33(10):1386–1388

[221] Brodsky MC, Vaphiades M. Magnetic resonance imaging in pseudotumor cerebri. Ophthalmology. 1998; 105(9):1686–1693

[222] Gibby WA, Cohen MS, Goldberg HI, Sergott RC. Pseudotumor cerebri: CT findings and correlation with vision loss. AJR Am J Roentgenol. 1993; 160 (1):143–146

[223] Jacobson DM, Karanjia PN, Olson KA, Warner JJ. Computed tomography ventricular size has no predictive value in diagnosing pseudotumor cerebri. Neurology. 1990; 40(9):1454–1455

[224] Manfré L, Lagalla R, Mangiameli A, et al. Idiopathic intracranial hypertension: orbital MRI. Neuroradiology. 1995; 37(6):459–461

[225] Giuseffi V, Wall M, Siegel PZ, Rojas PB. Symptoms and disease associations in idiopathic intracranial hypertension (pseudotumor cerebri): a case-control study. Neurology. 1991; 41(2, Pt 1):239–244

[226] Rowe FJ, Sarkies NJ. The relationship between obesity and idiopathic intracranial hypertension. Int J Obes Relat Metab Disord. 1999; 23(1): 54–59

[227] Daniels AB, Liu GT, Volpe NJ, et al. Profiles of obesity, weight gain, and quality of life in idiopathic intracranial hypertension (pseudotumor cerebri). Am J Ophthalmol. 2007; 143(4):635–641

[228] Sugerman HJ, DeMaria EJ, Felton WL, III, Nakatsuka M, Sismanis A. Increased intra-abdominal pressure and cardiac filling pressures in obesity-associated pseudotumor cerebri. Neurology. 1997; 49(2):507–511

[229] Friedman DI, Streeten DH. Idiopathic intracranial hypertension and orthostatic edema may share a common pathogenesis. Neurology. 1998; 50 (4):1099–1104

[230] Jacobson DM, Berg R, Wall M, Digre KB, Corbett JJ, Ellefson RD. Serum vitamin A concentration is elevated in idiopathic intracranial hypertension. Neurology. 1999; 53(5):1114–1118

[231] Selhorst JB, Kulkantrakorn K, Corbett JJ, Leira EC, Chung SM. Retinol-binding protein in idiopathic intracranial hypertension (IIH). J Neuroophthalmol. 2000; 20(4):250–252

[232] Lee AG, Kardon RH, Wall M, Schlechte J. (2002). Endocrinologic abnormalities in pseudotumor cerebri in men. Presented at the 28th annual meeting of the North American Neuro-Ophthalmology Society. Copper Mountain, CO, February 9–14, 2002

[233] Wall M. The headache profile of idiopathic intracranial hypertension. Cephalalgia. 1990; 10(6):331–335

[234] Sismanis A, Butts FM, Hughes GB. Objective tinnitus in benign intracranial hypertension: an update. Laryngoscope. 1990; 100(1):33–36

[235] Biousse V, Newman NJ, Lessell S. Audible pulsatile tinnitus in idiopathic intracranial hypertension. Neurology. 1998; 50(4):1185–1186

[236] Felton WL, Sismanis A. Idiopathic intracranial hypertension without papilledema in patients with pulsatile tinnitus. Presented at the North American Neuro-Ophthalmology meeting, Tucson, AZ, 1995

[237] Wang SJ, Silberstein SD, Patterson S, Young WB. Idiopathic intracranial hypertension without papilledema: a case-control study in a headache center. Neurology. 1998; 51(1):245–249

[238] Round R, Keane JR. The minor symptoms of increased intracranial pressure: 101 patients with benign intracranial hypertension. Neurology. 1988; 38(9):1461–1464

[239] Marcus DM, Lynn J, Miller JJ, Chaudhary O, Thomas D, Chaudhary B. Sleep disorders: a risk factor for pseudotumor cerebri? J Neuroophthalmol. 2001; 21(2):121–123

[240] Kleinschmidt JJ, Digre KB, Hanover R. Idiopathic intracranial hypertension: relationship to depression, anxiety, and quality of life. Neurology. 2000; 54(2):319–324

[241] Lee AG. Fourth nerve palsy in pseudotumor cerebri. Strabismus. 1995; 3(2):57–59

[242] Speer C, Pearlman J, Phillips PH, Cooney M, Repka MX. Fourth cranial nerve palsy in pediatric patients with pseudotumor cerebri. Am J Ophthalmol. 1999; 127(2):236–237

[243] Krishna R, Kosmorsky GS, Wright KW. Pseudotumor cerebri sine papilledema with unilateral sixth nerve palsy. J Neuroophthalmol. 1998; 18(1):53–55

[244] Patton N, Beatty S, Lloyd IC. Bilateral sixth and fourth cranial nerve palsies in idiopathic intracranial hypertension. J R Soc Med. 2000; 93(2):80–81

[245] Friedman DI, Forman S, Levi L, Lavin PJ, Donahue S. Unusual ocular motility disturbances with increased intracranial pressure. Neurology. 1998; 50(6):1893–1896

[246] Friedman DI, Forman S, Levi L, et al. (Unusual ocular motility disturbances in pseudotumor cerebri. Presented at the 23rd annual meeting of the North American Neuro-Ophthalmology Society, Keystone, Colorado, February 9–13, 1997

[247] Jacobson DM. Divergence insufficiency revisited: natural history of idiopathic cases and neurologic associations. Arch Ophthalmol. 2000; 118(9):1237–1241

[248] Davenport RJ, Will RG, Galloway PJ. Isolated intracranial hypertension presenting with trigeminal neuropathy. J Neurol Neurosurg Psychiatry. 1994; 57(3):381

[249] Bakshi SK, Oak JL, Chawla KP, Kulkarni SD, Apte N. Facial nerve involvement in pseudotumor cerebri. J Postgrad Med. 1992; 38(3):144–145

[250] Capobianco DJ, Brazis PW, Cheshire WP. Idiopathic intracranial hypertension and seventh nerve palsy. Headache. 1997; 37(5):286–288

[251] Selky AK, Dobyns WB, Yee RD. Idiopathic intracranial hypertension and facial diplegia. Neurology. 1994; 44(2):357

[252] Benegas NM, Volpe NJ, Liu GT, Galetta SL. Hemifacial spasm and idiopathic intracranial hypertension. J Neuroophthalmol. 1996; 16(1):70

[253] Selky AK, Purvin VA. Hemifacial spasm. An unusual manifestation of idiopathic intracranial hypertension. J Neuroophthalmol. 1994; 14(4):196–198

[254] Camras LR, Ecanow JS, Abood CA. Spontaneous cerebrospinal fluid rhinorrhea in a patient with pseudotumor cerebri. J Neuroimaging. 1998; 8(1):41–42

[255] Clark D, Bullock P, Hui T, Firth J. Benign intracranial hypertension: a cause of CSF rhinorrhoea. J Neurol Neurosurg Psychiatry. 1994; 57(7):847–849

[256] De Paepe L, Abs R, Verlooy J, et al. Benign intracranial hypertension as a cause of transient partial pituitary deficiency. J Neurol Sci. 1993; 114(2):152–155

[257] Sullivan HC. Fatal tonsillar herniation in pseudotumor cerebri. Neurology. 1991; 41(7):1142–1144

[258] Golnik KC, Devoto TM, Kersten RC, Kulwin D. Visual loss in idiopathic intracranial hypertension after resolution of papilledema. Ophthal Plast Reconstr Surg. 1999; 15(6):442–444

[259] O'Duffy D, James B, Elston J. Idiopathic intracranial hypertension presenting with gaze-evoked amaurosis. Acta Ophthalmol Scand. 1998; 76(1):119–120

[260] Jacobson DM. Intracranial hypertension and the syndrome of acquired hyperopia with choroidal folds. J Neuroophthalmol. 1995; 15(3):178–185

[261] Talks SJ, Mossa F, Elston JS. The contribution of macular changes to visual loss in benign intracranial hypertension. Eye (Lond). 1998; 12(Pt 5):806–808

[262] Krasnitz I, Beiran I, Mezer E, Miller B. Coexistence of optic nerve head drusen and pseudotumor cerebri: a clinical dilemma. Eur J Ophthalmol. 1997; 7(4):383–386

[263] Brazier DJ, Sanders MD. Disappearance of optociliary shunt vessels after optic nerve sheath decompression. Br J Ophthalmol. 1996; 80(2):186–187

[264] Lam BL, Siatkowski RM, Fox GM, Glaser JS. Visual loss in pseudotumor cerebri from branch retinal artery occlusion. Am J Ophthalmol. 1992; 113(3):334–336

[265] Chern S, Magargal LE, Brav SS. Bilateral central retinal vein occlusion as an initial manifestation of pseudotumor cerebri. Ann Ophthalmol. 1991; 23(2):54–57

[266] Akova YA, Kansu T, Yazar Z, Atabay C, Karagöz Y, Duman S. Macular subretinal neovascular membrane associated with pseudotumor cerebri. J Neuroophthalmol. 1994; 14(4):193–195

[267] Carter SR, Seiff SR. Macular changes in pseudotumor cerebri before and after optic nerve sheath fenestration. Ophthalmology. 1995; 102(6):937–941

[268] Greenfield DS, Wanichwecharungruang B, Liebmann JM, Ritch R. Pseudotumor cerebri appearing with unilateral papilledema after trabeculectomy. Arch Ophthalmol. 1997; 115(3):423–426

[269] Marcelis J, Silberstein SD. Idiopathic intracranial hypertension without papilledema. Arch Neurol. 1991; 48(4):392–399

[270] Mathew NT, Ravishankar K, Sanin LC. Coexistence of migraine and idiopathic intracranial hypertension without papilledema. Neurology. 1996; 46(5):1226–1230

[271] Saito J, Kami M, Taniguchi F, et al. Unilateral papilledema after bone marrow transplantation. Bone Marrow Transplant. 1999; 23(9):963–965

[272] Suzuki H, Takanashi J, Kobayashi K, Nagasawa K, Tashima K, Kohno Y. MR imaging of idiopathic intracranial hypertension. AJNR Am J Neuroradiol. 2001; 22(1):196–199

[273] Tourn N, Sharpe JA. Pseudotumor cerebri mimicking Foster Kennedy syndrome. Neuro-ophthalmology. 1996; 16(1):55–57

[274] Wall M, White WN, II. Asymmetric papilledema in idiopathic intracranial hypertension: prospective interocular comparison of sensory visual function. Invest Ophthalmol Vis Sci. 1998; 39(1):134–142

[275] Quattrone A, Bono F, Oliveri RL, et al. Cerebral venous thrombosis and isolated intracranial hypertension without papilledema in CDH. Neurology. 2001; 57(1):31–36

[276] Wall M. Idiopathic intracranial hypertension: mechanisms of visual loss and disease management. Semin Neurol. 2000; 20(1):89–95

[277] Lee AG, Wall M. Papilledema: are we any nearer to a consensus on pathogenesis and treatment? Curr Neurol Neurosci Rep. 2012; 12(3):334–339

[278] Hedges TR, III, Legge RH, Peli E, Yardley CJ. Retinal nerve fiber layer changes and visual field loss in idiopathic intracranial hypertension. Ophthalmology. 1995; 102(8):1242–1247

[279] Salgarello T, Tamburrelli C, Falsini B, Giudiceandrea A, Colotto A. Optic nerve diameters and perimetric thresholds in idiopathic intracranial hypertension. Br J Ophthalmol. 1996; 80(6):509–514

[280] Corbett JJ, Jacobson DM, Mauer RC, Thompson HS. Enlargement of the blind spot caused by papilledema. Am J Ophthalmol. 1988; 105(3):261–265

[281] Wall M, George D. Visual loss in pseudotumor cerebri. Incidence and defects related to visual field strategy. Arch Neurol. 1987; 44(2):170–175

[282] Wall M, Montgomery EB. Using motion perimetry to detect visual field defects in patients with idiopathic intracranial hypertension: a comparison with conventional automated perimetry. Neurology. 1995; 45(6):1169–1175

[283] Wall M. Idiopathic intracranial hypertension. Semin Ophthalmol. 1995; 10(3):251–259

[284] Stavroua P, Honan WP. Contrast sensitivity in benign intracranial hypertension. Neuroophthalmology. 1997; 17:127–134

[285] Rowe FJ, Sarkies NJ. Assessment of visual function in idiopathic intracranial hypertension: a prospective study. Eye (Lond). 1998; 12(Pt 1):111–118

[286] Rigi M, Almarzouqi SJ, Morgan ML, Lee AG. Papilledema: epidemiology, etiology, and clinical management. Eye Brain. 2015; 7(5):47–57

[287] Saposnik G, Barinagarrementeria F, Brown RD, Jr, et al. American Heart Association Stroke Council and the Council on Epidemiology and Prevention. Diagnosis and management of cerebral venous thrombosis: a statement for healthcare professionals from the American Heart Association/American Stroke Association. Stroke. 2011; 42(4):1158–1192

[288] Wall M, McDermott MP, Kieburtz KD, et al. NORDIC Idiopathic Intracranial Hypertension Study Group Writing Committee. Effect of acetazolamide on visual function in patients with idiopathic intracranial hypertension and mild visual loss: the idiopathic intracranial hypertension treatment trial. JAMA. 2014; 311(16):1641–1651

[289] Johnson LN, Krohel GB, Madsen RW, March GA, Jr. The role of weight loss and acetazolamide in the treatment of idiopathic intracranial hypertension (pseudotumor cerebri). Ophthalmology. 1998; 105(12):2313–2317

[290] Kupersmith MJ, Gemell L, Turbin R, et al. Effect of weight loss on pseudotumor cerebri in women. Neurology. 1997; 48 Suppl:A386

[291] Kupersmith MJ, Gamell L, Turbin R, Peck V, Spiegel P, Wall M. Effects of weight loss on the course of idiopathic intracranial hypertension in women. Neurology. 1998; 50(4):1094–1098

[292] Newborg B. Pseudotumor cerebri treated by rice reduction diet. Arch Intern Med. 1974; 133(5):802–807

[293] Sugerman HJ, Felton WL, III, Salvant JB, Jr, Sismanis A, Kellum JM. Effects of surgically induced weight loss on idiopathic intracranial hypertension in morbid obesity. Neurology. 1995; 45(9):1655–1659

[294] Fridley J, Foroozan R, Sherman V, Brandt ML, Yoshor D. Bariatric surgery for the treatment of idiopathic intracranial hypertension. J Neurosurg. 2011; 114(1):34–39

[295] Wong R, Madill SA, Pandey P, Riordan-Eva P. Idiopathic intracranial hypertension: the association between weight loss and the requirement for systemic treatment. BMC Ophthalmol. 2007; 7:15

[296] Sinclair AJ, Burdon MA, Nightingale PG, et al. Low energy diet and intracranial pressure in women with idiopathic intracranial hypertension: prospective cohort study. BMJ. 2010; 341:c2701

[297] Sugerman HJ, Felton WL, III, Sismanis A, Kellum JM, DeMaria EJ, Sugerman EL. Gastric surgery for pseudotumor cerebri associated with severe obesity. Ann Surg. 1999; 229(5):634–640, discussion 640–642

[298] Schoeman JF. Childhood pseudotumor cerebri: clinical and intracranial pressure response to acetazolamide and furosemide treatment in a case series. J Child Neurol. 1994; 9(2):130–134

[299] ten Hove MW, Friedman DI, Patel AD, Irrcher I, Wall M, McDermott MP, NORDIC Idiopathic Intracranial Hypertension Study Group. Safety and tolerability of acetazolamide in the idiopathic intracranial hypertension treatment trial. J Neuroophthalmol. 2016; 36(1):13–19

[300] Celebisoy N, Gökçay F, Sirin H, Akyürekli O. Treatment of idiopathic intracranial hypertension: topiramate vs acetazolamide, an open-label study. Acta Neurol Scand. 2007; 116(5):322–327

[301] Goodwin JA. Treatment of idiopathic intracranial hypertension with digoxin. Ann Neurol. 1990; 28:248

[302] Förderreuther S, Straube A. Indomethacin reduces CSF pressure in intracranial hypertension. Neurology. 2000; 55(7):1043–1045

[303] Corbett JJ, Thompson HS. The rational management of idiopathic intracranial hypertension. Arch Neurol. 1989; 46(10):1049–1051

[304] Kessler LA, Novelli PM, Reigel DH. Surgical treatment of benign intracranial hypertension–subtemporal decompression revisited. Surg Neurol. 1998; 50 (1):73–76

[305] Lai LT, Danesh-Meyer HV, Kaye AH. Visual outcomes and headache following interventions for idiopathic intracranial hypertension. J Clin Neurosci. 2014; 21(10):1670–1678

[306] Spitze A, Malik A, Al-Zubidi N, Golnik K, Lee AG. Optic nerve sheath fenestration vs cerebrospinal diversion procedures: what is the preferred surgical procedure for the treatment of idiopathic intracranial hypertension failing maximum medical therapy? J Neuroophthalmol. 2013; 33(2):183–188

[307] Mukherjee N, Bhatti MT. Update on the surgical management of idiopathic intracranial hypertension. Curr Neurol Neurosci Rep. 2014; 14(3):438

[308] Angiari P, Corradini L, Corsi M, Merli GA. Pseudotumor cerebri. Lumbo-peritoneal shunt in long lasting cases. J Neurosurg Sci. 1992; 36(3):145–149

[309] Burgett RA, Purvin VA, Kawasaki A. Lumboperitoneal shunting for pseudotumor cerebri. Neurology. 1997; 49(3):734–739

[310] Eggenberger ER, Miller NR, Vitale S. Lumboperitoneal shunt for the treatment of pseudotumor cerebri. Neurology. 1996; 46(6):1524–1530

[311] Johnston I, Besser M, Morgan MK. Cerebrospinal fluid diversion in the treatment of benign intracranial hypertension. J Neurosurg. 1988; 69(2):195–202

[312] Johnston I, Paterson A, Besser M. The treatment of benign intracranial hypertension: a review of 134 cases. Surg Neurol. 1988; 69:195–202

[313] Lundar T, Nornes H. Pseudotumour cerebri-neurosurgical considerations. Acta Neurochir Suppl (Wien). 1990; 51:366–368

[314] Rosenberg ML, Corbett JJ, Smith C, et al. Cerebrospinal fluid diversion procedures in pseudotumor cerebri. Neurology. 1993; 43(6):1071–1072

[315] Rowe FJ. Assessment of visual function in idiopathic intracranial hypertension. Br J Neurosurg. 2011; 25(1):45–54

[316] Sinclair AJ, Kuruvath S, Sen D, Nightingale PG, Burdon MA, Flint G. Is cerebrospinal fluid shunting in idiopathic intracranial hypertension worthwhile? A 10-year review. Cephalalgia. 2011; 31(16):1627–1633

[317] El-Saadany WF, Farhoud A, Zidan I. Lumboperitoneal shunt for idiopathic intracranial hypertension: patients' selection and outcome. Neurosurg Rev. 2012; 35(2):239–243, discussion 243–244

[318] Toma AK, Dherijha M, Kitchen ND, Watkins LD. Use of lumboperitoneal shunts with the Strata NSC valve: a single-center experience. J Neurosurg. 2010; 113(6):1304–1308

[319] Abubaker K, Ali Z, Raza K, Bolger C, Rawluk D, O'Brien D. Idiopathic intra-cranial hypertension: lumboperitoneal shunts versus ventriculoperitoneal shunts–case series and literature review. Br J Neurosurg. 2011; 25(1):94–99

[320] McGirt MJ, Woodworth G, Thomas G, Miller N, Williams M, Rigamonti D. Cerebrospinal fluid shunt placement for pseudotumor cerebri-associated intractable headache: predictors of treatment response and an analysis of long-term outcomes. J Neurosurg. 2004; 101(4):627–632

[321] Tarnaris A, Toma AK, Watkins LD, Kitchen ND. Is there a difference in outcomes of patients with idiopathic intracranial hypertension with the choice of cerebrospinal fluid diversion site: a single centre experience. Clin Neurol Neurosurg. 2011; 113(6):477–479

[322] Tulipan N, Lavin PJ, Copeland M. Stereotactic ventriculoperitoneal shunt for idiopathic intracranial hypertension: technical note. Neurosurgery. 1998; 43 (1):175–176, discussion 176–177

[323] Eisenberg HM, Davidson RI, Shillito J, Jr. Lumboperitoneal shunts. Review of 34 cases. J Neurosurg. 1971; 35(4):427–431

[324] Chumas PD, Kulkarni AV, Drake JM, Hoffman HJ, Humphreys RP, Rutka JT. Lumboperitoneal shunting: a retrospective study in the pediatric population. Neurosurgery. 1993; 32(3):376–383, discussion 383

[325] Sell JJ, Rupp FW, Orrison WW, Jr. Iatrogenically induced intracranial hypotension syndrome. AJR Am J Roentgenol. 1995; 165(6):1513–1515

[326] Cabezudo JM, Olabe J, Bacci F. Infection of the intervertebral disc space after placement of a percutaneous lumboperitoneal shunt for benign intracranial hypertension. Neurosurgery. 1990; 26(6):1005–1008, discussion 1008–1009

[327] Chumas PD, Armstrong DC, Drake JM, et al. Tonsillar herniation: the rule rather than the exception after lumboperitoneal shunting in the pediatric population. J Neurosurg. 1993; 78(4):568–573

[328] Miller NR. Bilateral visual loss and simultagnosia after lumboperitoneal shunt for pseudotumor cerebri. J Neuroophthalmol. 1997; 17(1):36–38

[329] Khan QU, Wharen RE, Grewal SS, et al. Overdrainage shunt complications in idiopathic normal-pressure hydrocephalus and lumbar puncture opening pressure. J Neurosurg. 2013; 119(6):1498–1502

[330] Lyon K, Ban VS, Bedros N, Aoun SG, El Ahmadieh T, White J. Migration of a ventriculoperitoneal shunt into the pulmonary vasculature: case report, review of the literature, and surgical pearls. World Neurosurg. 2016; 92:585.e5–585.e11

[331] Singh S, Pant N, Kumar P, et al. Migration of ventriculoperitoneal shunt into a hernia sac: an unusual complication of ventriculoperitoneal shunt surgery in children. Pediatr Neurosurg. 2016; 51(3):154–157

[332] Lee BS, Vadera S, Gonzalez-Martinez JA. Rare complication of ventriculoperitoneal shunt. Early onset of distal catheter migration into scrotum in an adult male: Case report and literature review. Int J Surg Case Rep. 2015; 6C:198–202

[333] Kalovidouri A, Boto J, Vargas MI. Cerebral CSF cyst as a rare complication of ventriculoperitoneal shunt. J Neuroradiol. 2016; 43(4):303–305

[334] Bourm K, Pfeifer C, Zarchan A. Small bowel perforation: a rare complication of ventriculoperitoneal shunt placement. J Radiol Case Rep. 2016; 10(6):30–35

[335] Bonatti M, Vezzali N, Frena A, Bonatti G. Incisional hernia following ventriculoperitoneal shunt positioning. J Radiol Case Rep. 2016; 10(6):9–15

[336] Miranda ME, de Sousa MB, Tatsuo ES, Quites LV, Giannetti AV. Bladder perforation by ventriculoperitoneal shunt. Childs Nerv Syst. 2016; 32(12):2321–2326

[337] Watkins JD, Lee J, Van Engen MJ, Tibbs ML, Ellegala DB, Nicholas JS. Isolated left homonymous hemianopia secondary to a pericatheter cyst-a rare presentation of a ventriculoperitoneal shunt failure. J Neuroophthalmol. 2015; 35(1):60–64

[338] Acheson JF, Green WT, Sanders MD. Optic nerve sheath decompression for the treatment of visual failure in chronic raised intracranial pressure. J Neurol Neurosurg Psychiatry. 1994; 57(11):1426–1429

[339] Anderson RL, Flaharty PM. Treatment of pseudotumor cerebri by primary and secondary optic nerve sheath decompression. Am J Ophthalmol. 1992; 113(5):599–601

[340] Brourman ND, Spoor TC, Ramocki JM. Optic nerve sheath decompression for pseudotumor cerebri. Arch Ophthalmol. 1988; 106(10):1378–1383

[341] Corbett JJ, Nerad JA, Tse DT, Anderson RL. Results of optic nerve sheath fenestration for pseudotumor cerebri. The lateral orbitotomy approach. Arch Ophthalmol. 1988; 106(10):1391–1397

[342] Horton JC, Seiff SR, Pitts LH, Weinstein PR, Rosenblum ML, Hoyt WF. Decompression of the optic nerve sheath for vision-threatening papilledema caused by dural sinus occlusion. Neurosurgery. 1992; 31(2):203–211, discussion 211–212

[343] Kelman SE, Heaps R, Wolf A, Elman MJ. Optic nerve decompression surgery improves visual function in patients with pseudotumor cerebri. Neurosurgery. 1992; 30(3):391–395

[344] Kelman SE, Sergott RC, Cioffi GA, Savino PJ, Bosley TM, Elman MJ. Modified optic nerve decompression in patients with functioning lumboperitoneal shunts and progressive visual loss. Ophthalmology. 1991; 98(9):1449–1453

[345] Lee AG, Patrinely JR, Edmond JC. Optic nerve sheath decompression in pediatric pseudotumor cerebri. Ophthalmic Surg Lasers. 1998; 29(6):514–517

[346] Mauriello JA, Jr, Shaderowfsky P, Gizzi M, Frohman L. Management of visual loss after optic nerve sheath decompression in patients with pseudotumor cerebri. Ophthalmology. 1995; 102(3):441–445

[347] Mittra RA, Sergott RC, Flaharty PM, et al. Optic nerve decompression improves hemodynamic parameters in papilledema. Ophthalmology. 1993; 100(7):987–997

[348] Pearson PA, Baker RS, Khorram D, Smith TJ. Evaluation of optic nerve sheath fenestration in pseudotumor cerebri using automated perimetry. Ophthalmology. 1991; 98(1):99–105

[349] Sergott RC, Savino PJ, Bosley TM. Modified optic nerve sheath decompression provides long-term visual improvement for pseudotumor cerebri. Arch Ophthalmol. 1988; 106(10):1384–1390

[350] Spoor TC, McHenry JG. Long-term effectiveness of optic nerve sheath decompression for pseudotumor cerebri. Arch Ophthalmol. 1993; 111(5):632–635

[351] Spoor TC, McHenry JG, Shin DH. Long-term results using adjunctive mitomycin C in optic nerve sheath decompression for pseudotumor cerebri. Ophthalmology. 1995; 102(12):2024–2028

[352] Spoor TC, Ramocki JM, Madion MP, Wilkinson MJ. Treatment of pseudotumor cerebri by primary and secondary optic nerve sheath decompression. Am J Ophthalmol. 1991; 112(2):177–185

[353] Knight RS, Fielder AR, Firth JL. Benign intracranial hypertension: visual loss and optic nerve sheath fenestration. J Neurol Neurosurg Psychiatry. 1986; 49(3):243–250

[354] Liu GT, Volpe NJ, Schatz NJ, Galetta SL, Farrar JT, Raps EC. Severe sudden visual loss caused by pseudotumor cerebri and lumboperitoneal shunt failure. Am J Ophthalmol. 1996; 122(1):129–131

[355] Goh KY, Schatz NJ, Glaser JS. Optic nerve sheath fenestration for pseudotumor cerebri. J Neuroophthalmol. 1997; 17(2):86–91

[356] Banta JT, Farris BK. Pseudotumor cerebri and optic nerve sheath decompression. Ophthalmology. 2000; 107(10):1907–1912

[357] Kosmorsky GS, Boyle KA. Relief of headache after ONSD. 19th annual meeting of the North American Neuro-Ophthalmologic Society, Big Sky, Montana, 1993

[358] Plotnik JL, Kosmorsky GS. Operative complications of optic nerve sheath decompression. Ophthalmology. 1993; 100(5):683–690

[359] Flynn WJ, Westfall CT, Weisman JS. Transient blindness after optic nerve sheath fenestration. Am J Ophthalmol. 1994; 117(5):678–679

[360] Brodsky MC, Rettele GA. Protracted postsurgical blindness with visual recovery following optic nerve sheath fenestration. Arch Ophthalmol. 1997; 115(11):1473–1474

[361] Smith KH, Wilkinson JT, Brindley GO. Combined third and sixth nerve paresis following optic nerve sheath fenestration. J Clin Neuroophthalmol. 1992; 12(2):85–87, discussion 88

[362] Farb RI, Vanek I, Scott JN, et al. Idiopathic intracranial hypertension: the prevalence and morphology of sinovenous stenosis. Neurology. 2003; 60(9):1418–1424

[363] Riggeal BD, Bruce BB, Saindane AM, et al. Clinical course of idiopathic intracranial hypertension with transverse sinus stenosis. Neurology. 2013; 80(3):289–295

[364] Puffer RC, Mustafa W, Lanzino G. Venous sinus stenting for idiopathic intracranial hypertension: a review of the literature. J Neurointerv Surg. 2013; 5(5):483–486

[365] Teleb MS, Cziep ME, Lazzaro MA, Gheith A, Asif K, Remler B, Zaidata OO. Diopathic Intracranial Hypertension: A Systematic Analysis of Transverse Sinus Stenting. Interv Neurol. 2014 May; 2(3): 132–143. Published online 2014 Mar 25. doi: 10.1159/000357503. PMCID: PMC4080637. NIHMSID: NIHMS577907

[366] Bruce BB, Biousse V, Newman NJ. Update on idiopathic intracranial hypertension. Am J Ophthalmol. 2011; 152(2):163–169

[367] Ahmed R, Friedman DI, Halmagyi GM. Stenting of the transverse sinuses in idiopathic intracranial hypertension. J Neuroophthalmol. 2011; 31(4):374–380

[368] Fields JD, Javedani PP, Falardeau J, et al. Dural venous sinus angioplasty and stenting for the treatment of idiopathic intracranial hypertension. J Neurointerv Surg. 2013; 5(1):62–68

8 Transient Vision Loss

Austin S. Nakatsuka, Alec L. Amram, and Mohammad Obadah Nakawah

Abstract

Transient vision loss (including amaurosis fugax) can be a symptom of many different ophthalmological disorders. A detailed understanding of the features of the vision loss episodes, such as duration, frequency, provoking factors, and laterality, helps establish a diagnosis. This chapter discusses the clinical pathways for the evaluation and differential diagnosis of transient vision loss, as well as review the literature in detail.

Keywords: transient vision loss, transient visual obscuration, amaurosis fugax, transient ischemic attack, migraine aura

8.1 What Questions Should Be Asked of a Patient with Transient Visual Loss?

The most important questions that need to be addressed in the assessment of the patient with transient visual loss (TVL) include the following:

8.1.1 Is the visual loss monocular or binocular?

Monocular TVL implies disease of one eye, retina, optic nerve, orbit, ocular vascular supply (e.g., ipsilateral carotid artery, ophthalmic artery, central retinal artery), or migraine. Binocular TVL implies bilateral ocular disease, disease affecting bilateral ocular vasculature (e.g., bilateral carotid stenosis or vertebrobasilar ischemia), increased intracranial pressure with papilledema, or migraine.

8.1.2 What is the temporal profile of the visual loss?

For example, TVL in one eye lasting seconds is characteristic of transient obscurations of vision resulting from optic nerve ischemia or papilledema. Monocular TVL lasting 1 to 30 minutes is characteristic of TVL associated with vascular disease (e.g., carotid artery disease or retinal vasospasm).

8.1.3 What are the precipitants of the visual loss?

For example, patients with an intraorbital mass may develop TVL only in certain positions of gaze due to mass compression of the ipsilateral optic nerve or optic nerve vasculature (gaze-evoked amaurosis). Monocular or binocular TVL due to carotid disease may occur following bright light exposure (i.e., retinal claudication).

8.2 Are Optic Nerve (e.g., Disc Drusen) and Retinal Vessel Abnormalities Evident on Funduscopic Examination?

For example, the fundus exam may reveal papilledema in transient obscurations of vision, retinal emboli in carotid or cardiac disease, and disc anomalies in monocular TVL.

This chapter discusses various entities that may cause monocular or binocular TVL. Approaches to patients with monocular and binocular TVL are given in ▶ Fig. 8.1 and ▶ Fig. 8.2, respectively.

8.3 Does Monocular TVL Occur Only in Certain Positions of Gaze (Gaze-Evoked TVL)?

Patients who experience TVL evoked by eccentric position of gaze (gaze-evoked TVL) usually have an intraorbital mass that intermittently compresses the circulation to the optic nerve or retina.[1,2,3,4,5,6,7,8,9,10,11,12,13] The visual loss immediately improves when the direction of gaze is changed. The most common lesions accounting for this finding are orbital cavernous hemangiomas and optic nerve sheath meningiomas (18 and 35% of cases, respectively).[9] Other orbital lesions reported to produce this symptom include osteomas, neurofibromas, gliomas, medial rectus granular myoblastoma, metastases, varices, orbital trauma, thyroid eye disease, intracranial aneurysm,[7] and intraocular foreign body (buckshot pellet or nail gun injury[12]). The examination may be normal or show evidence of an optic neuropathy with an afferent pupillary defect, color vision impairment, disc edema, or retinochoroidal venous collateral vessels (often somewhat misleadingly referred to in the literature as "optociliary shunt vessels"). Other signs indicating the presence of an orbital tumor, such as proptosis, extraocular motility limitation, eyelid swelling, chemosis, and conjunctival congestion may be evident. Evaluation requires magnetic resonance imaging (MRI) or computed tomography (CT) scan of the orbit. Intermittent visual loss and exophthalmos may occur with bending over or the Valsalva maneuver.[14] Gaze-evoked monocular TVL has also been noted in patients with papilledema in pseudotumor cerebri.[15] It has been hypothesized that in an eccentric position of gaze, ischemic compression of a tense, dilated optic nerve sheath results in elevation of intrasheath pressure compromising blood flow to the retina or optic nerve.[15,16] The direction of amaurotic gaze does not reliably localize the lesion.[9] Four cases of gaze-evoked TVL were reported secondary to vitreopapillary traction, thought to be caused by transient visual phosphenes related to traction of the vitreous on superficial nerve fibers.[17] Thyroid orbitopathy can also cause gaze-evoked TVL through compressive optic disk ischemia.[18,19] Gaze-evoked TVL with optic neuropathy has also been reported in neurosarcoidosis,[20] and after orbital reconstruction with poor graft positioning.[21]

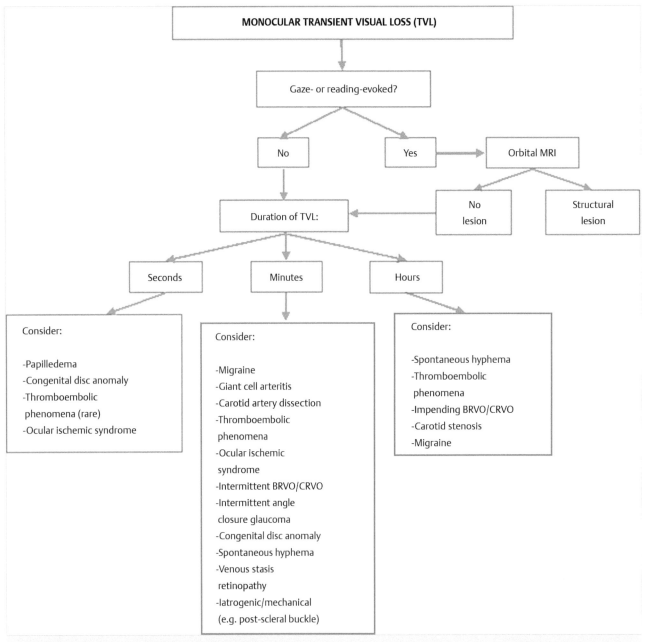

Fig. 8.1 Evaluation of monocular transient visual loss (TVL).

8.4 Does the Visual Loss Occur After Prolonged Reading (Reading-Evoked TVL)?

Reading may also induce monocular TVL. Manor et al described a 49-year-old man with a 5-year history of dimming of central vision in the left eye provoked only by reading.[22] An orbital apex tumor situated lateral to and above the optic nerve was found. This reading-evoked visual dimming may be a variant of gaze-evoked TVL. The optic nerve, displaced laterally and superiorly and stretched by the act of reading, may have been compressed between the tumor and the contracted inferior rectus muscle. Thus, orbital neuroimaging may be warranted in patients with reading-induced TVL.

Intermittent angle closure glaucoma may cause TVL, and reading-induced TVL has been reported in one case. O'Sullivan et al described a 66-year-old patient with episodes of monocular TVL lasting 3 minutes to several hours precipitated by reading, writing, or watching television.[23] Ophthalmologic exam was normal but 4 hours of reading induced corneal edema, a poorly reactive semidilated pupil, and a shallow anterior chamber with intraocular pressure of 50 mm Hg. The intermittent angle closure glaucoma and the patient's symptoms were treated successfully by iridotomies.

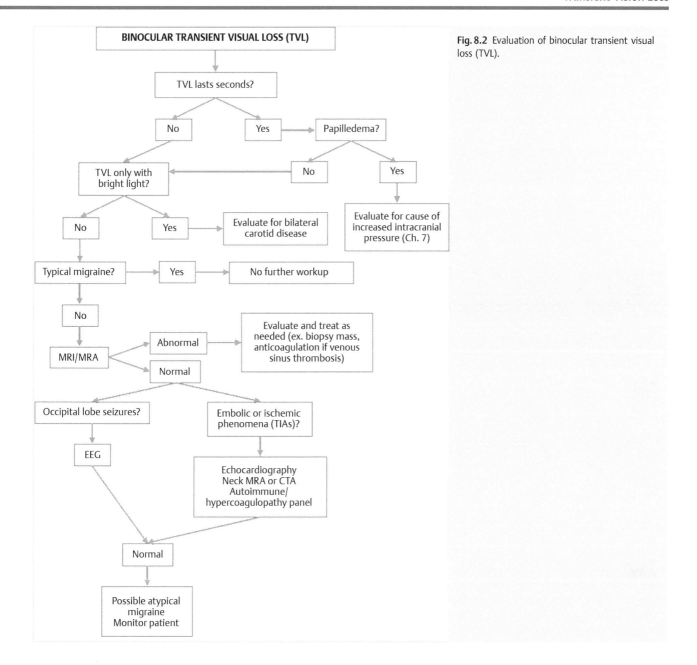

Fig. 8.2 Evaluation of binocular transient visual loss (TVL).

8.5 Do the Episodes of Monocular TVL Last Seconds?

Transient visual obscurations (TVO) are episodes of TVL lasting less than 60 seconds which typically occur in patients with papilledema.[24] These transient obscurations of vision may occur in one or both eyes (individually or simultaneously) and typically last only a few seconds, though in rare cases they may last for hours. Episodes may be precipitated by changes in position and are thought to be related to the effects of increased intracranial pressure on the flow of blood to the eye, perhaps where the central retinal artery penetrates the optic nerve sheath.[16]

Monocular TVO may occur in optic nerve sheath meningiomas unrelated to intracranial pressure. The pathogenesis of meningioma-related TVO is unknown and may be caused by

the effect of the meningioma on the central retinal artery where it enters the optic nerve.[16] TVO may also occur in an eye with congenital abnormalities of the optic disc, such as peripapillary staphyloma (see below) or optic disc drusen. A case of "ice-pick" headaches associated with monocular visual loss with scintillating scotoma lasting seconds has been described in a patient with a history of migraine with visual aura.[25] The patient was treated with oxygen inhalation and indomethacin with complete symptom resolution. Finally, carotid atherosclerotic disease may rarely cause very brief episodes of TVL, but more often last from 1 to 30 minutes.

An uncommon cause of monocular TVO was reported in a patient who noticed a "veil" lasting for seconds and relieved by blinking. The cause was found to be a periodic leak of aqueous over the corneal surface from a conjunctival filtration bleb.[26]

Patients with TVO first require ophthalmologic examination. If papilledema is evident (Chapter 7), an MRI scan of the brain is indicated to evaluate for intracranial mass lesions. If this study is normal, a lumbar puncture can be performed to investigate the possibility of infection or pseudotumor cerebri (idiopathic intracranial hypertension). Patients with disc drusen or other optic disc anomalies causing monocular TVL may require no further evaluation. If the patient has a cerebrospinal fluid shunt, evaluate the device for malfunctions such as obstruction, tubing fracture, or migration.[27] If there are signs of an optic neuropathy ipsilateral to the TVL (e.g., relative afferent pupillary defect and ipsilateral swollen or atrophic optic nerve), then MRI of the brain/orbit may be warranted to evaluate for the presence of a compressive lesion (e.g., optic nerve sheath meningioma) or signs of optic neuritis, which may produce monocular TVL lasting seconds to minutes.[28] Patients without apparent disc abnormalities should be screened for carotid atherosclerotic disease or other sources of emboli (see later in the chapter).

8.6 Do the Episodes of Monocular TVL Last Minutes?

Monocular TVL lasting 1 to 30 minutes (rarely an hour or more) is strongly suggestive of thromboembolic disease. Retinal emboli may arise from the heart, aorta, or carotid artery.[29,30] Patients often describe the TVL as a veil or shade descending or ascending over a portion of their visual field. Other patients complain of patchy vision loss ("Swiss cheese" pattern) or peripheral constriction with central visual sparing.[31] Some episodes of monocular TVL are accompanied by a sensation of color or other photopsias. These may be similar to migraine symptoms, consisting of showers of stationary flecks of light that disperse quickly.[31,32,33,34] Marshall and Meadows found that in 51 of 67 patients (76%), TVL episodes lasted 30 minutes or less, with 29 patients (43%) experiencing episodes lasting 5 minutes or less.[35] Pessin et al noted that attacks lasted less than 15 minutes in 30 of 33 patients, and in 14 patients (42%) the episodes lasted 5 minutes or less.[33] Among 35 patients evaluated by Goodwin et al, 22 patients (63%) had attacks lasting 5 minutes or less, 8 (23%) had episodes lasting 6 to 15 minutes, and 6 patients (17%) had episodes lasting more than 15 minutes.[32]

Patients with thromboembolic disease may demonstrate emboli within the retinal vessels. Emboli may be composed of clotted blood, fibrin, platelets, atheromatous tissue, white cells, calcium, infectious material (e.g., septic emboli), air, fat, tumor cells, amniotic fluid, or foreign materials (e.g., talc, artificial valve material, catheters, silicone, cornstarch, mercury, corticosteroids). The most common types of emboli seen in atherosclerotic disease of the aorta, carotid arteries, or cardiac disease include the following:

1. Cholesterol emboli (i.e., Hollenhorst plaques) are bright, glistening, yellow- or copper-colored fragments most often seen in peripheral arterioles in the temporal fundus. These emboli most often arise from atheromatous plaques in the aorta or carotid bifurcation.
2. Platelet-fibrin emboli are dull, white, gray, often elongated, and subject to fragmentation and distal movement. These emboli most often lodge at bifurcations of retinal vessels and

arise from the walls of atherosclerotic arteries or from the heart, especially from heart valves. They may also be seen in coagulopathies.
3. Calcific emboli tend to be large, ovoid or rectangular, and chalky white. These emboli often occur over or adjacent to the optic disc. They usually arise from cardiac (aortic or mitral) valves and less often from the aorta or carotid artery. Unlike cholesterol emboli, which often disappear within a few days, calcific emboli may remain permanently visible.

Sharma et al found that in the setting of acute retinal artery occlusion, the sensitivity and specificity of visible retinal emboli for the detection of hemodynamically significant carotid artery stenosis (defined as ≥ 60% stenosis on either side by Doppler ultrasonography) are 39 and 68%, respectively.[36] The presence of a visible embolus generated a likelihood ratio of 1.24, whereas the absence of a visible embolus generated a likelihood ratio of 0.88. The authors concluded that the presence of a visible embolus is a poor diagnostic test for the detection of hemodynamically significant carotid artery stenosis in the setting of acute retinal artery occlusion. Klein et al described the prevalence at baseline and the 5-year incidence of retinal emboli in the Beaver Dam Study. They reported the associated risk factors, the relationship of retinal emboli at baseline to stroke, and ischemic heart disease mortality in these patients. The study consisted of 4,926 patients, aged 43 to 86 years at presentation.[37] The prevalence of retinal emboli at baseline was 1.3% and the 5-year incidence was 0.9%. The prevalence of retinal emboli was associated with high pulse pressure, hypertension, diabetes mellitus, past and current smoking, cardiovascular disease, and the presence of retinopathy. Patients with retinal emboli had a significantly higher risk of dying with stroke than those without retinal emboli. In a study of 2,398 patients with suspected transient ischemic attack (TIA), 826 patients (34.5%) had transient visual symptoms, with monocular TVL being the most frequent TVS (36.3%).[34] Surprisingly, in a multicenter retrospective study of 464 patients done in Japan, only 13 patients (2.9%) presented with monocular TVL and were less likely to be brought to a specialized stroke center than those without these symptoms.[38]

TVL may also occur from ocular hypoperfusion rather than embolization. In some patients, monocular TVL may occur when the patient is exposed to bright light. These patients usually have severe ipsilateral carotid occlusive disease. Bilateral, simultaneous TVL induced by exposure to bright light may rarely occur with bilateral severe carotid stenosis or occlusion.[39] Light-induced TVL probably reflects the inability of a borderline ocular circulation to sustain the increased retinal metabolic activity associated with light exposure. Alternating TVL to bright light has also been described with giant cell arteritis (GCA).[40]

One prospective study assessed the clinical features of monocular TVL and the likelihood of atherosclerotic lesions of the internal carotid artery (ICA).[41] Of the 337 patients, 159 (47%) had a normal ipsilateral ICA, 33 (10%) had stenosis of less than 70%, 100 (30%) had stenosis of 70 to 99%, and 45 (13%) had complete ICA occlusion. An altitudinal onset or resolution of symptoms was associated with atherosclerotic lesions of the ipsilateral ICA. Severe (70–99%) stenosis was associated with TVL duration of 1 to 10 minutes and a speed of onset in seconds. ICA occlusion was associated with light-provoked attacks, altitudinal character, and the occurrence of more than 10 attacks.

TVL may also occur with carotid artery dissection. In a review of the clinical features of 146 patients with extracranial carotid artery dissection, 41 patients (28%) had monocular TVL. The TVL was painful in 31 cases, associated with a Horner syndrome in 13 cases, and described as "scintillations" or "flashing lights" (often related to postural changes suggesting choroidal hypoperfusion) in 23 cases.[42] Two of 23 patients with spontaneous carotid artery dissection experienced TVL; in one of these patients, TVL episodes were provoked by sitting up from a supine position.[43]

Postprandial TVL has also been described.[44] In one patient, episodes of splotchy visual loss occurred unilaterally on the left 1 hour after eating her largest meal of the day. The episodes lasted approximately 3 hours and were occasionally accompanied by numbness and weakness of the contralateral arm; she was found to have severe left-sided carotid stenosis. In a second patient, blotchy bilateral TVL episodes lasting 2 to 90 minutes were precipitated by eating or standing from a sitting or supine position. This patient was found to have complete occlusion of the right carotid artery and moderate stenosis of the left carotid artery. The authors proposed that postprandial visual loss may be a symptom of critical carotid stenosis, with retinal and choroidal hypoperfusion probably caused by a combination of mesenteric steal, decreased cardiac output, and abnormal vasomotor control.[44]

Venous stasis retinopathy secondary to severe carotid or ophthalmic artery occlusive disease (hypoperfusion retinopathy) may also be associated with TVL.[45] This syndrome is characterized by visual loss and ischemic retinal infarction often accompanied by signs of ciliary artery obstruction, pallor of the disc, and hypotony. Venous stasis retinopathy may simulate Purtscher retinopathy (multifocal retinal ischemia) and may present with a variety of fundus findings[45]:

1. Minimal or no ophthalmoscopic changes in some patients with monocular TVL.
2. Few widely scattered blot and dot hemorrhages with mild retinal vein dilation (venous stasis retinopathy) often seen in patients with minimal visual complaints.
3. Cotton-wool patches with dilation of the retinal arterial tree and retinal veins.
4. Retinal capillary changes including microaneurysms, cystoid macular edema, and angiographic evidence of capillary nonperfusion that may be confined to the area surrounding the horizontal raphe.
5. Large areas of peripheral capillary nonperfusion, retinal neovascularization, and hemorrhage.
6. Any branch or central retinal vein or artery occlusion.
7. Optic disc edema (ischemic optic neuropathy).
8. Fluorescein angiography showing diffuse retinal capillary telangiectasia, delayed retinal artery circulation time, late staining of the disc, and aggregations of microaneurysms around the preequatorial zone mimicking idiopathic juxtafoveal retinal telangiectasia.
9. Any of the above associated with panuveitis, neovascular glaucoma, and a rapidly progressing cataract (ocular ischemic syndrome).

Venous stasis retinopathy may be difficult to differentiate from central retinal vein occlusion (CRVO). Helpful differentiating features include the following:

1. Retinal vein caliber is irregular in venous stasis retinopathy.
2. Hemorrhages, microaneurysms, and capillary dilations are often peripheral (rather than posterior) in venous stasis retinopathy. Changes in CRVO are often diffuse (rather than peripheral).
3. Venous stasis retinopathy is not associated with disc edema or retinochoroidal collaterals (compared with CRVO).

The ocular ischemic syndrome[45,46,47,48] is a progressive disorder due to ocular hypoperfusion that may be associated with TVL and ocular discomfort or frank pain localized to the orbit and upper face often improved in horizontal positioning. Rubeosis iridis (i.e., neovascularization of the iris) in an older nondiabetic patient without evidence of venous obstructive disease or other predisposing diagnoses is suggestive of ocular ischemic syndrome. In persons older than 50 years with new-onset iritis, ocular ischemic syndrome should be considered. It is usually due to atherosclerotic carotid or ophthalmic artery disease. Less common causes for venous stasis retinopathy and ocular ischemic syndrome include GCA, carotid artery dissection, cavernous sinus thrombosis, Takayasu arteritis, fibromuscular dysplasia, mucormycosis, herpes zoster ophthalmicus, myelofibrosis, vasospasm, and aneurysm repair.[47,49,50,51,52,53,54,55,56,57,58,59] Hayreh reported 15% prevalence of amaurosis fugax in ocular ischemic syndrome in an investigation conducted at the University of Iowa.[60] Four of seven patients with maxillofacial arteriovenous malformations (AVMs) that had been treated previously with proximal ligation of the supplying external carotid artery had signs of ocular ischemia.[61] These four patients had significant ophthalmic artery supply by the malformations, suggesting that when the ophthalmic arterial blood supply is recruited, an ophthalmic artery "steal" phenomenon occurs, causing ocular ischemia. This "steal" may be precipitated or worsened by previous surgical proximal ligation of external carotid arterial branches that are potential collaterals with the ophthalmic artery but fail to occlude the arteriovenous shunt. There is some evidence to support improvement of symptoms with superficial temporal artery to middle cerebral artery bypass surgery in ocular ischemic syndrome (class III, level C).[48,62]

GCA can produce attacks of TVL lasting minutes to hours that may be indistinguishable from those produced by atherosclerotic disease (see Chapter 5).[63,64] TVL probably results from intermittent inflammatory occlusion of the ophthalmic, posterior ciliary, or central retinal arteries. A postural form of TVL has been described in GCA with tenuous optic disc perfusion.[65] Alternating monocular TVL may occur with GCA[66] and may be induced by bright light (i.e., retinal claudication).[40]

TVL may also occur in association with antiphospholipid antibodies, hyperviscosity and hypercoagulable states, polycythemia vera, systemic lupus erythematosus (SLE), and hepatitis C–associated cryoglobulinemic vasculitis. AVMs may steal, divert, or reduce blood flow in the ophthalmic artery (ophthalmic steal syndrome).[67,68,69,70,71] The TVL may alternate from eye to eye. Donders et al noted that TVL occurred in 6% of patients with SLE.[68] Half of those patients had TVL alternating TVL. Furthermore, there was no relationship between TVL and the presence of antiphospholipid antibodies or livedo reticularis in patients with SLE.

Vasospasm, especially associated with migraine, may also produce TVL without any of the visual phenomena typically seen during a migraine attack.[13,72,73,74,75,76] Vasospasm of the retinal vessels has been documented by ophthalmoscopy during some attacks of monocular TVL. Vasospastic TVL may be induced by exercise or sexual intercourse.[77,78] Exercise-induced TVL may last minutes to hours.[77] TVL in young individuals is often benign and related to migraine. Tippin et al reviewed 83 cases of TVL or ocular infarction before the age of 45 years; cerebral TIAs occurred in 9 patients but no case of stroke was found.[79] Forty-one percent of the patients had headaches or orbital pain accompanying their TVL spells and an additional 25.3% had severe headaches independent of the visual loss. Of the original 83 patients, 42 were reexamined after a mean period of 5.8 years. None of the patients in this group had a stroke. The clinical status at follow-up did not correlate with duration of visual loss (TVL or ocular infarction), frequency (single or recurrent episodes), gender, presence of headache or heart disease, cigarette smoking, use of oral contraceptives, or abnormal findings on echocardiogram or blood studies. The authors concluded that TVL and ocular infarction occurring in younger patients are associated with a more benign clinical course than seen in older persons, and that migraine is the most common cause for visual loss in this group. O'Sullivan et al described nine young adults (median age 19.5 years) who suffered from TVL.[75] The attacks of TVL were of short duration and associated with premonitory symptoms in five patients and migrainous headache in two. In five patients, visual loss progressed in a lacunar pattern (vision was lost in a series of blobs), unlike the "curtain" pattern characteristic of TVL in older patients. Investigation revealed no evidence of an embolic or atheromatous etiology. In two patients, a minor abnormality was found on echocardiography. The authors conclude that TVL in young adults has a different clinical pattern and may have a different etiology compared with that seen in older patients. The pattern of visual loss in some cases suggests that the choroidal rather than retinal circulation is primarily affected.

TVL lasting 15 to 20 minutes (occasionally up to 7 hours) may occur during episodes of spontaneous anterior chamber hemorrhage (hyphema).[16,80] In these patients, TVL may be associated with erythropsia (seeing red) and color desaturation. Such hemorrhages are most likely to occur after cataract extraction and are particularly apt to occur after placement of an iris-fixated lens implant. Other potential causes of spontaneous anterior chamber hemorrhages include vascular anomalies of the iris (e.g., in myotonic dystrophy or Sturge-Weber syndrome), microhemangiomas, diffuse hemangiomatosis of childhood, neoplasms (e.g., melanoma or retinoblastoma), diseases of blood or vessels (e.g., leukemia, hemophilia, scurvy, lymphoma), rubeosis iridis, severe iritis, fibrovascular membranes, juvenile xanthogranuloma, occult trauma or delayed bleeding after trauma, hydrophthalmos, malignant exophthalmos, histiocytosis X, and postsclerotomy with cautery.[80] Episodes of TVL lasting up to 24 hours have been described with recurrent hyphema after deep sclerotomy with collagen implant.[81] The uveitis-glaucoma-hyphema (UGH) syndrome is an unusual cause of monocular TVL following cataract extraction and intraocular lens implantation.[13,82] Patients may present with the full triad or with its individual elements, with symptoms often developing years after cataract surgery. ▶ Table 8.1 compares the symptoms of TVL in retinal emboli compared with the UGH syndrome.[82]

Table 8.1 Comparison between the classic symptoms of visual loss in patients with TVL due to retinal emboli and the UGH syndrome

	TVL due to retinal embolus	TVL due to UGH syndrome
Speed of onset	Sudden (seconds)	Gradual (minutes)
Recovery	Rapid (seconds to minutes)	Slow (hours to days)
Character	Dark curtain over vision	Gradual misting of vision Erythropsia (red vision)
Location	Sector loss	Diffuse
Pain	None	With or without ache in affected eye

Abbreviations: TVL, transient visual loss; UGH, uveitis–glaucoma–hyphema.

Intermittent angle closure glaucoma may also cause brief episodes of monocular TVL that are usually, though not always, associated with ipsilateral eye pain and occasionally simultaneous dilation of the pupil.[13,16] A 51-year-old man who experienced monocular TVL in his right eye 10 to 15 minutes following sexual intercourse was found to have narrow angles; his symptoms resolved following bilateral peripheral iridotomies.[83] Exercise-induced visual disturbances may also occur during attacks of pigmentary glaucoma.[77] Episodes of monocular TVL lasting 2 to 3 minutes induced by changes in posture have been described following scleral buckle placement, likely due to intermittent obstruction of the central retinal artery circulation by the encircling element.[84]

Finally, TVL may also be associated with congenital anomalies, such as peripapillary staphyloma and morning glory syndrome.[45,85,86] Episodes of TVL with these anomalies may last 15 to 20 seconds or up to 20 minutes, the latter duration mimicking TVL with thromboembolic disease. Episodes of TVL in peripapillary staphyloma may be associated with intermittent dilation of the retinal veins and may be orthostatic.

An uncommon cause of monocular TVL described as a "curtain being drawn" and lasting for 1 to 20 minutes occurred in a 61-year-old man with vasculopathic risk factors. Amaurosis fugax related to atherosclerotic disease was first considered but, a CT angiography (CTA) revealed a dislocated lens as the surprise cause of the TVL.[87]

Patients with monocular TVL lasting for minutes and associated with visible retinal emboli need to be evaluated for vascular (e.g., carotid or aortic disease) and cardiac thromboembolism. Stroke risk factors (e.g., smoking, hypertension, diabetes mellitus, and hyperlipidemia) should be evaluated and controlled. Studies to evaluate the carotid arteries include carotid Doppler, MR angiography (MRA), CTA, and conventional angiography. Cardiac investigations include transthoracic and transesophageal echocardiography and cardiac MRI. In a study of 18 patients with branch or central retinal artery occlusion, transesophageal echocardiography revealed a possible cardiac or thoracic source of embolus in 13 patients (72%), whereas a potential carotid source of embolus was present in three of 16 patients (19%).[88] In patients found to have a right-to-left shunt on echocardiography and a history of ocular ischemia associated with monocular TVL and/or retinal artery occlusion, consider evaluation for venous thromboses in the lower extremities and pelvis with ultrasonography (class III, level C).[71]

Hurwitz et al performed a prospective clinical and arteriographic study comparing patients with monocular TVL and patients with other transient hemispheric cerebral ischemic attacks.[89] In 93 patients with monocular TVL, a potentially operable atherosclerotic carotid lesion (defined as ≥ 50% stenosis or ulceration on the side of TVL) was found in 66% of the patients, and the 7-year cumulative rate of cerebral infarction in these patients was 14%. In 212 patients with other hemispheric TIAs, an operable carotid lesion was found in 51% of patients, with the 7-year cumulative rate of infarction of 27%. Therefore, in approximately two-thirds of patients with monocular TVL, a potentially operable carotid lesion may be found.

Volkers et al performed a prospective study of 341 patients to assess the risk of vascular complications associated with different characteristics of monocular TVL. The complications they found included outcome events of vascular death, stroke, myocardial infarction, or retinal infarction in 60 patients (17%). Characteristics of monocular TVL independently associated with complications included involvement of only the peripheral part of the visual field (hazard ratio [HR]: 6.5), constricting onset of vision loss (HR: 3.5), downward onset of vision loss (HR: 1.9), upward resolution of vision loss (HR: 2.0), and the occurrence of more than three attacks (HR: 1.7). In the study, peripheral vision loss was the most powerful predictor of impending vascular disease. Downward onset of visual field loss was attributed to emboli and upward resolution of vision loss was thought to occur with restoration of blood flow to the lower retina. This study showed that monocular TVL has a high rate of complications and characteristics of vision loss may help with prognosis assessment.[90]

In patients with monocular TVL (or other carotid distribution TIAs or nondisabling stroke) and ipsilateral carotid stenosis of 70 to 99%, carotid endarterectomy (CEA) may be indicated. Surgery may be recommended in this setting if the patient is a good surgical candidate and the perioperative complication rate of the surgery is less than 6%.[91] CEA in this group reduces the 2-year ipsilateral stroke rate from 26 to 9%, and decreases the major or fatal ipsilateral stroke rate from 13.1 to 2.5%. The benefit of surgery in the 70% or greater stenosis patients is greatest among men, in patients with a recent stroke as a qualifying event, and in patients with hemispheric (vs. visual) symptoms.[92] The benefit of surgery is twice as great for patients with 90 to 99% carotid stenosis versus 70 to 79% stenosis. The frequency of major functional impairment was much lower in the surgical group than in the medical group.[93]

However, it has been shown that patients with hemispheric TIA obtained a benefit from surgical endarterectomy (3-year stroke rate of 11% treated surgically vs. 18% treated medically), but patients with retinal TIA (monocular TVL) had worse outcomes with surgery (stroke rate of 9% surgical vs. 7.2% medical treatment). Additionally, studies have shown that individuals with retinal TIA had half the 3-year risk of ipsilateral stroke compared with those who had hemispheric TIA (7.2 vs. 18%). These studies suggest that although patients with hemispheric TIA and 70 to 99% carotid stenosis may benefit from surgical intervention, medical treatment may be preferred for patients with monocular TVL.[94]

In patients with monocular TVL (or other carotid distribution TIA or nondisabling stroke) and 50 to 69% ipsilateral carotid stenosis, the 5-year rate of any ipsilateral stroke was 15.7% in the surgical group and 22.2% in the medical group.[92] Therefore, CEA in patients with symptomatic carotid stenosis of 50 to 69% yields only moderate reduction in stroke risk, with the absolute risk reduction being about 10% at 5 years. Among patients with ICA stenosis, the prognosis is better for those presenting with TVL than for those presenting with hemispheric TIAs.[95] Decisions about treatment must take into account the patient's risk factors, and the surgical perioperative complication rates must be less than 6%. Additionally, indications for endovascular stenting approaches should be taken into consideration and patients who meet the following criteria may be considered: (1) recurrent symptoms despite medical therapy, (2) hemodynamic instability, (3) impending rupture of pseudoaneurysm, and (4) contraindications to anticoagulation.[96] Patient's age and cardiac risk factors should also be considered. While the Carotid Revascularization Endarterectomy vs. Stenting Trial (CREST) found there was no significant difference in the rates of the primary end point (any periprocedural stroke, myocardial infarction (MI), death, or postprocedural ipsilateral stroke) between endovascular stenting and CEA (7.2 and 6.8%, respectively), the lower incidence of periprocedural stroke in the CEA group was offset in the primary endpoint by the lower incidence of periprocedural MI in the stenting group. In addition, patients younger than 70 years had a slightly better outcome with stenting and patients older than 70 years had a better outcome with CEA.[97]

In patients with monocular TVL and less than 50% carotid stenosis, the stroke rate was not significantly lower in the surgery group (14.9%) than in the medical group (18.7%).[92] A cardiac or aortic embolic source should be sought and, if none is found, treatment should consist of aspirin and stroke risk factor reduction. In patients with a cardioembolic source, especially those with atrial fibrillation, anticoagulation may be warranted in the absence of contraindications. Patients older than 50 years with a history of monocular TVL lasting minutes without visible retinal emboli should have an evaluation for GCA (e.g., erythrocyte sedimentation rate, C-reactive protein, and consideration of temporal artery biopsy; class II, level C).

Patients with evidence of monocular TVL resulting from ocular hypoperfusion (e.g., venous stasis retinopathy and the ocular ischemic syndrome) might have decreased retinal artery pressure on ophthalmodynamometry (although not universally available). The patient should be investigated for carotid stenosis, but if the carotid imaging is hemodynamically insignificant, then ophthalmic artery stenosis or occlusion may also be an etiology. When carotid stenosis is severe, carotid endarterectomy may be used to reestablish flow[98,99]; when the ICA is totally occluded, a superficial temporal artery to middle cerebral artery bypass procedure may be considered if the external carotid artery is patent.[100] With early treatment, resolution of the hypoperfusion syndrome may occur; unfortunately, no therapy is clearly effective. In one study, carotid endarterectomy was effective for improving or preventing the progress of chronic ocular ischemia caused by internal carotid stenosis; visual acuity improved in 5 of 11 patients and had not worsened in the other 6 patients.[98] Reestablishment of flow in a previously stenotic ICA may actually produce further visual difficulties by increasing perfusion to the ciliary arteries and causing dramatic increase in intraocular pressure. Carotid endarterectomy and superficial temporal artery to middle cerebral artery bypass procedures have been combined with laser panretinal photocoagulation, peripheral retinal cryotherapy, or both. These latter procedures are thought to decrease the oxygen requirement of the eye and thus reduce the drive for neovascularization. Rarely, ocular ischemic syndrome may be improved by the calcium channel blocker, verapamil.[57] Intravitreal anti-vascular endothelial growth factor or triamcinolone therapy can be useful to treat macular edema complicating ocular ischemic syndrome.[48]

If no thromboembolic source for the episodes of TVL is found, further studies should be considered. These include MRI/MRA of the brain to investigate for possible brain ischemia or vascular malformations, and laboratory studies including sedimentation rate, complete blood count, antiphospholipid antibodies, antinuclear antibodies, collagen vascular disease profile, and studies to investigate the presence of dysproteinemia (class III–IV, level U). If all of these studies are negative, an echocardiography may be considered. A rare case of monocular TVL caused by a cardiac tumor (papillary fibroelastoma) found on echocardiography was reported in a 45-year-old man.[101] Newer implanted cardiac monitors may also detect occult atrial fibrillation or other cardiac arrhythmia that might be missed on routine electrocardiography.

Young patients (< 45 years old) with monocular TVL are unlikely to have significant carotid disease. A cardiac embolic source as well as a vasculitis or coagulopathy must be sought. As noted earlier, monocular TVL in younger patients has a more benign clinical course than that found in an older population, and migraine is a likely cause for many episodes. Calcium channel blockers (e.g., verapamil or nifedipine), if not otherwise contraindicated, may be considered in some of these patients to reduce the frequency of episodes of TVL.[76,78,102]

Finally, all patients with monocular TVL lasting minutes should have a complete ophthalmoscopic examination to investigate such conditions as intermittent angle closure glaucoma, morning glory syndrome, and peripapillary staphyloma. A case of intermittent branch retinal artery occlusion causing monocular TVL in a 15-year-old girl was diagnosed on fundus examination, which revealed intensive edema of the superior retina.[103] Spontaneous anterior chamber hemorrhage (hyphema) should also be considered, especially in patients with associated erythropsia and in those who have undergone cataract extraction.

Episodes of monocular TVL lasting hours are rare. However, such spells may occur with thromboembolic disease, as a postprandial phenomenon associated with critical carotid stenosis, and with migraine. One patient experienced monocular TVL lasting for 2 hours, as well as nocturnal sinus bradycardia of 40 beats per minute, following administration of topical latanoprost.[104] The patient had complete recovery after cessation of latanoprost. Monocular TVL lasting hours may be a symptom of impending central retinal vein occlusion.[105]

An approach to the evaluation of patients with monocular TVL is presented in ▶ Fig. 8.1.

8.7 Are the Episodes of TVL Binocular?

Episodes of bilateral simultaneous TVL are usually due to migraine, bilateral occipital lobe ischemia, or other occipital structural lesions, such as tumors and AVMs. However, TVO lasting seconds may occur in one or both eyes in patients with increased intracranial pressure and papilledema. Also, patients with bilateral severe carotid occlusive disease may have bilateral TVL on exposure to bright light.

The presence of a small area of visual loss or a mild disturbance of vision that progressively increases over 15 minutes or longer (i.e., march and buildup) is highly characteristic of migraine.[106] This visual abnormality is usually bilateral and homonymous. The patient need not have headaches for this diagnosis to be made. Most patients describe abnormal positive visual symptoms associated with the episodes. Most commonly, fortification spectra are described around an area of scotoma. These scintillations or distortions within the area of visual disturbance may resemble "heat waves" or "water running down a glass." The typical migraine visual aura starts as a flickering, uncolored zigzag in the center of the visual field that gradually progresses and expands toward the periphery of one hemifield and often leaves a temporary scotoma.[107] Migrainous visual may certainly occur in individuals older than 50 years and often occur in the absence of headache in this age group.[108] These episodes probably are not associated with an increased stroke risk. The spells are usually stereotyped, begin gradually, and progress, lasting several minutes to 1 hour, and usually include positive visual phenomena (bright images, colors, movement of images) affecting both eyes. In a study by Wijman et al, the migrainous visual auras were never accompanied by headache in 58% of patients, and 42% of individuals had no history of recurrent headache.[108] The risk of stroke in these patients was 11.5%, significantly less than the 33.3% noted in patients with TIAs but not significantly different from the rate of 13.6% in those with neither migrainous auras nor TIAs. Associated symptoms may include nausea, aphasia, eye pain, diplopia, dizziness, tinnitus, numbness, and paresthesias.

Rarely, the positive visual phenomena of migraine may persist for months to years, unassociated with electroencephalographic or MRI findings.[109] Patients with persistent migraine visual auras (migraine aura status) may demonstrate occipital hypoperfusion on brain single-photon emission computed tomography (SPECT).[110,111] This pathologic state may be responsive to lamotrigine.[110] In another form of persistent migraine aura, patients may experience a large number of consecutive (mostly) visual auras, very often without headache. Between the auras, the patient is without symptoms. Episodes can last for weeks, and within this period several migraine auras can occur on 1 day. Multiple treatments have been used with variable results. Beltramone and Donnet found success with lamotrigine for migraine aura, while Haan et al and Cupini and Stipa used acetazolamide effectively.[112,113,114] Rozen reported using furosemide effectively for two patients with persistent and prolonged migraine aura.[115] Afridi et al and Kaube et al used intranasal ketamine with success for prolonged aura.[116,117]

Visual disturbances similar to those that occur with migraine may rarely occur with cerebral structural lesions such as AVMs of the occipital lobe or tumors. These are often associated with headache and usually do not have the characteristic buildup and resolution of visual symptoms. Instead, these lesions usually produce symptoms that steadily increase in frequency and duration until they occur daily.

Occipital lobe tumors may rarely produce scintillating scotomas that mimic migraine.[16,118,119,120] In most of these cases, the tumors were diagnosed only after the patients developed papilledema or when a homonymous visual field defect was identified. Riaz et al described three patients with migraine with aura for many years of duration that preceded the diagnosis of meningioma.[120] In two patients, the tumors were occipital and in one patient frontotemporal. Visual symptoms in two of these patients were exceptional in their constant localization to the same hemianopic field, whereas in the third patient they involved either hemianopic field. The visual phenomena sometimes occurred independent of headache.

Occipital lobe AVMs may also produce visual symptoms and headache that may simulate migraine.[121,122,123,124,125] Visual symptoms with occipital AVMs are usually brief, episodic, unformed, and not associated with the angular, scintillating figures that occur with migraine. They also tend to occur consistently in the same visual field. However, the clinical symptoms classically noted with migraine may occasionally occur with occipital AVMs. Kupersmith et al described the clinical presentations of 70 patients with occipital AVMs.[123] At the time of presentation, headache was present in 39 (56%); the headache was throbbing in 19 cases (27%) with preceding homonymous positive visual phenomena with migraine-like features in the field contralateral to the AVM in 15 cases. A visual disturbance in the opposite field, not necessarily associated with headache, occurred in 39 patients (56%). Patients often described episodes of scintillating scotomas, jagged flickering fortification images, transient and permanent homonymous hemianopia, blurred vision in a hemifield, hemifield spots, tunnel vision, and diplopia. Three patients had transient field loss as a prodrome to grand mal seizures and two others had episodes of flickering vision associated with seizure activity on electroencephalography. Only 5 of the 23 patients with visual symptoms who had a homonymous field defect did not have recurrent headaches. Fifteen additional patients without visual symptoms, 8 of who had no recurrent headaches, had homonymous visual field defects. The authors concluded that, if "migraine" headache or visual symptoms are restricted to one side of the head (even if the visual field exam is normal), neuroimaging should be performed to investigate the possibility of an occipital AVM. Migraine in this setting is a diagnosis of exclusion. While some headache features and visual symptoms are similar between occipital AVMs and migraine, the two disorders are usually distinguishable. Kurita et al described a man with periodic right-sided throbbing headaches heralded by a visual prodrome of scintillating bright lights in the left visual field lasting several minutes.[124] The headaches decreased 18 months after radiosurgery for a right occipital AVM. Positive visual phenomena resembling migraine have also been described with cerebral venous sinus thrombosis.[126] Scintillating scotomas occasionally occur in patients with SLE, but it is not clear if they are a manifestation of a cerebrovascular disorder related to lupus or simply the coexistence of two separate disease processes.[16]

Although ictal and postictal TVL is unusual, the phenomenon is well recognized.[127,128,129] The visual deficits are almost always binocular and patients may complain of homonymous hemianopia or complete bilateral blindness. The duration may vary in length from seconds to months, and can be permanent following status epilepticus.[129,130]

Due to the cortical nature of the vision loss, patients may not recognize the visual deficit.[130]

In patients with no history of seizures, it can be difficult to clinically differentiate epileptic from migrainous visual loss. Panayiotopoulos described multiple cases of idiopathic occipital epilepsy and visual seizures (elementary visual hallucinations).[127,128] The visual symptoms typically lasted seconds and consisted of multiple, small, brightly colored, circular spots in a visual hemifield, often increasing in size or flashing. Patients reported transient loss of vision early in the episode. Symptoms often progressed to other sensory or motor manifestations, and secondary generalized convulsions. Although the visual symptoms were distinct from migraine visual aura in most patients, many patients with occipital lobe seizures developed an ictal or postictal migraine-like headache.

Misdiagnosis of occipital seizures as migraine and vice versa is not uncommon in clinical practice, especially since ictal and postictal migrainous headaches are common. A recent retrospective study by Hartl et al analyzed the characteristics of the auras in epilepsy and migraine of 27 patients. The duration of visual aura was typically seconds in epilepsy and minutes in migraine. Aura duration longer than 5 minutes was 100% sensitive and 92% specific for identifying migraine patients. The aura in epilepsy typically remained restricted to a visual hemifield, stereotypically affecting only one hemifield. Centrifugal or centripetal spread of the visual aura was seen only in migraine patients ($p = 0.0007$). Accompanying migraine symptoms of nausea/vomiting or photo-/phonophobia were common in migraine patients and not seen in any epilepsy patients. None of the patients exhibited visual migrainous aura that evolved into an epileptic seizure ("migralepsy").[131]

Dreier et al described two patients with migraine who experienced migrainous aura-like symptoms several minutes after the onset of acute headache induced by subarachnoid hemorrhage.[132] The cases suggest that subarachnoid hemorrhage is a trigger for migrainous aura.

Symptoms similar to the scintillating scotomas of migraine may also occur with acute vitreous or retinal detachment.[16] In these patients, the visual symptoms are clearly monocular, last longer than typical migrainous visual aura, and occur without any associated headache. Scintillating scotomas, as well as monocular TVLs, have also been described associated with ICA dissection.[42,133,134] The first of the three patients described by Ramadan et al developed sudden severe right occipital headache followed minutes later by nausea and bright dots in both visual fields that spread centrifugally during a 10-minute period and persisted for several hours.[133] The second perceived scintillating and nonmarching "snowflakes" in the entire visual field of the right eye that lasted 10 minutes, during which the right eye lost vision. This was followed by right frontotemporal sharp pain that lasted for another hour. The third patient noted the abrupt onset of seeing stationary, sharp-edged gray shapes (e.g., triangles, squares, and zigzag lines) outlined in bright red and blue and superimposed on a glaring background. These positive visual phenomena were perceived in the left eye and lasted for 3 days. She later developed another episode of visual phenomena in the left eye associated with left supraorbital and temporal throbbing headache. The first patient's episode was binocular but atypical for migraine aura in that the positive visual phenomena lasted for hours; in the other two patients, the symptoms were monocular, and in one of these the positive symptoms lasted for days, again atypical for migraine aura. Tomaschütz et al reported in a patient "jagged lines" followed by "circular vision loss," which was also monocular.[134] As noted earlier, in a study of 146 patients with extracranial carotid artery dissection, 23 of the 41 patients with transient monocular visual loss described it as "scintillations" or "flashing lights" (often related to postural changes suggesting choroidal hypoperfusion).[42]

Patients with restrictive thyroid eye disease may occasionally complain of flashing lights in the superior visual field on upgaze, possibly phosphenes as a result of either compression of the globe by a tight inferior rectus muscle or traction on the insertion of the inferior rectus muscle.[135] Twelve of 30 patients with thyroid eye disease experienced flashing lights on upward gaze and all had tight inferior rectus muscles.[135]

Binocular episodes of TVL may be due to bilateral occipital ischemia secondary to disease of the vertebrobasilar circulation (rarely bilateral retinal ischemia from systemic hypotension or bilateral carotid disease). Episodes of visual loss or blurring in patients with vertebrobasilar TIA usually occur in association with other symptoms of transient brainstem, cerebellar, or posterior cerebral ischemia, including vertigo, dysarthria, dysphagia, diplopia, weakness, sensory disturbances (especially perioral numbness), coordination difficulties, and gait instability. However, TVL symptoms may occur in isolation and may warn of an impending larger ischemic event, as has been reported in a patient with moyamoya disease.[136] Visual loss or blurring of vision in these patients is bilateral and symmetric, may be hemianopic or diffuse, and usually lasts several minutes or occasionally less than a minute (but not seconds, as noted with obscurations of vision noted with papilledema and increased intracranial pressure). The scintillating and expanding scotomas of migraine rarely occur with vertebrobasilar TIAs, and migrainous visual phenomena usually last 20 to 30 minutes, somewhat longer than visual loss noted with vertebrobasilar TIAs. Interestingly, Hilton-Jones et al described a patient with a large frontal lobe tumor who experienced frequent, stereotyped episodes of bilateral, simultaneous visual loss lasting 5 to 30 minutes.[137] This patient reportedly did not have papilledema.

Other unusual causes of bilateral TVL should be mentioned. Transient bilateral blindness lasting minutes to hours may rarely occur with GCA, vertebrobasilar insufficiency, or bilateral impending anterior ischemic optic neuropathy.[138] Bilateral TVL lasting minutes to several hours during sexual arousal may be associated with narrow-angle glaucoma.[139] Bilateral or unilateral TVL lasting days after LASIK has been associated with steroid-induced elevated IOP.[140] A case of bilateral TVL lasting for 2 minutes due to occipital lobe seizure was triggered by a solitary cysticercus granuloma in the occipital lobe.[141] As noted earlier, bilateral TVL may be the sole manifestation of occipital lobe epilepsy.[127] In fact, prolonged (48 hours) visual loss may occur with occipital seizures (status epilepticus amauroticus).[142] Transient vision loss has been described due to neurotoxicity (e.g., exposure to iodinated contrast or glycine). Transient cortical blindness lasting hours, days, or even weeks may occur after cerebral angiography (i.e., contrast-induced neurotoxicity).[143,144,145,146,147,148] A case has even been reported of transient cortical blindness lasting 9 days after placement of a peripherally inserted central venous catheter (PICC) for TPN.[149]

Temporary bilateral blindness (pupils normal or nonreactive) may occur with irritability, confusion, bradycardia, nausea, hypertension, dyspnea, and seizures during or after transurethral prostatic resection (TURP).[150] This TURP syndrome is thought to be caused by excessive absorption of nonelectrolyte irrigating fluid through the prostatic venous sinuses into the general circulation. Glycine toxicity on the optic nerves or cortex, caused by excessive glycine absorption, is the likely mechanism of visual loss. The symptoms and signs of the TURP syndrome resolve within 24 hours with intravenous pyridoxine and arginine hydrochloride. A case of a 6-year-old female child with newly diagnosed ornithine transcarbamylase deficiency developed binocular TVL lasting for 72 hours and had associated MRI findings of cortical hyperintensity and adjacent subcortical hypointensity on fluid-attenuated inversion recovery imaging of the right occipital lobe, leading to a diagnosis of acute reversible cortical blindness due to her metabolic disease.[151] Transient cortical blindness can also follow trauma due to occipital lobe contusion.[152]

Bilateral TVL lasting up to several weeks may occur with the posterior reversible encephalopathy syndrome (PRES), also known as reversible posterior leukoencephalopathy syndrome or reversible posterior cerebral edema syndrome. PRES is a clinicoradiologic diagnosis of varying severity that is frequently associated with acute hypertension (e.g., due to renal failure or preeclampsia/eclampsia), infection, sepsis, septic shock, autoimmune disease (e.g., SLE or polyarteritis nodosa), acute intermittent porphyria, organ transplantation, or exposure to chemotherapy or immunosuppressive therapy (e.g., cyclosporine, tacrolimus, or interleukin-2 therapy).[13,153,154,155,156,157,158,159,160,161] Disruption of the blood–brain barrier through increased pressure in the cerebral venous system is a potential etiology of PRES.[161]

8.8 What Is the Evaluation for Binocular TVL?

The evaluation of patients with bilateral TVL must include a thorough history, especially directed at the characteristics and temporal course of TVL episodes and any associated symptoms. A complete neuro-ophthalmologic examination, including visual field testing, should be performed. If episodes last seconds and papilledema is present, MRI and MR venogram of the head may be indicated (class III, level C). If imaging is negative, a spinal tap may be warranted (class III, level C). If episodes of bilateral visual loss occur only on exposure to bright light, evaluation of the carotid arteries is indicated. Patients with typical expanding migraine scintillations and positive phenomena lasting 20 to 30 minutes that have been noted to occur on different sides at different times and headaches that have been documented to occur on different sides at different times usually do not require further workup. Abnormalities on visual field examination suggesting a retrochiasmal lesion or atypical migraine-like phenomena should prompt neuroimaging (class III–IV, level C). Patients with visual symptoms that are brief, episodic, unformed, and not associated with the angular, scintillating figures might also require MRI or MR angiography (class III–IV, level U). When either migraine-like headache or visual symptoms are restricted to one side of the head (even if the visual field exam is normal), a neuroimaging study for occipital AVM is reasonable (class III–IV, level U). Patients with migraine and symptoms or signs of collagen vascular disease require a collagen vascular disease profile. Electroencephalography or a trial of anticonvulsant medication may be warranted if occipital epilepsy is likely (class III, level U).

The evaluation of patients with vertebrobasilar TIAs usually starts with brain MRI and MRA of the head and neck; cerebral angiography may also be considered. A cardiac embolic source should always be considered and, if warranted, transthoracic or transesophageal echocardiography may be performed (class III–IV, level C). Treatment includes control of stroke risk factors and antiplatelet drugs or anticoagulation.

If the presentation of TVL is within 72 hours, the American Heart Association recommends hospital admission if the patient meets the age, blood pressure, clinical features, and symptom duration (ABCD) score of 3. For presentation between 3 and 7 days, hospitalization is still recommended if the patient has a known untreated source of ischemia.[102] Additionally, the 2009 American Heart Association/American Stroke Association guidelines recommend that all patients with TIA undergo neuroimaging evaluation within 24 hours of symptom onset, followed by additional diagnostic studies.[71]

An approach to the evaluation of patients with bilateral TVL is presented in ▶ Fig. 8.2.

References

[1] Bremner FD, Sanders MD, Stanford MR. Gaze evoked amaurosis in dysthyroid orbitopathy. Br J Ophthalmol. 1999; 83(4):501

[2] Danesh-Meyer HV, Savino PJ, Bilyk JR, Sergott RC, Kubis K. Gaze-evoked amaurosis produced by intraorbital buckshot pellet. Ophthalmology. 2001; 108(1):201–206

[3] Knapp ME, Flaharty PM, Sergott RC, Savino PJ, Mazzoli RA, Flanagan JC. Gaze-induced amaurosis from central retinal artery compression. Ophthalmology. 1992; 99(2):238–240

[4] Kohmoto H, Oohira A. Gaze-evoked scotomata in metastatic orbital tumor. Neuro-ophthalmology. 1993; 13:223–226

[5] Mezer E, Gdal-On M, Miller B. Orbital metastasis of renal cell carcinoma masquerading as Amaurosis fugax. Eur J Ophthalmol. 1997; 7(3):301–304

[6] Smith L, Kriss A, Gregson R, Thompson D, Taylor D. Gaze evoked amaurosis in neurofibromatosis type II. Br J Ophthalmol. 1998; 82(5):584–585

[7] Sivak-Callcott J, Carpenter JS, Rosen CL, Ellis B, Hix C. Gaze-evoked amaurosis associated with an intracranial aneurysm. Arch Ophthalmol. 2004; 122(9):1404–1406

[8] Sibony P, Shindo M. Orbital osteoma with gaze-evoked amaurosis. Arch Ophthalmol. 2004; 122(5):788–789

[9] Otto CS, Coppit GL, Mazzoli RA, et al. Gaze-evoked amaurosis: a report of five cases. Ophthalmology. 2003; 110(2):322–326

[10] Patel MM, Lefebvre DR, Lee NG, Brachtel E, Rizzo J, Freitag SK. Gaze-evoked amaurosis from orbital breast carcinoma metastasis. Ophthal Plast Reconstr Surg. 2013; 29(4):e98–e101

[11] Koch MU, Houtman AC, de Keizer RJ. Gaze-evoked amaurosis with cavernous sinus meningioma. Eye (Lond). 2006; 20(7):840–843

[12] Segal S, Salyani A, DeAngelis DD. Gaze-evoked amaurosis secondary to an intraorbital foreign body. Can J Ophthalmol. 2007; 42(1):147–148

[13] Thurtell MJ, Rucker JC. Transient visual loss. Int Ophthalmol Clin. 2009; 49(3):147–166

[14] Sobottka Ventura AC, Remonda L, Mojon DS. Intermittent visual loss and exophthalmos due to the Blue rubber bleb nevus syndrome. Am J Ophthalmol. 2001; 132(1):132–135

[15] O'Duffy D, James B, Elston J. Idiopathic intracranial hypertension presenting with gaze-evoked amaurosis. Acta Ophthalmol Scand. 1998; 76(1):119–120

[16] Miller NR. Walsh and Hoyt's Clinical Neuro-ophthalmology. 4th ed. Baltimore, MD: Williams & Wilkins; 1991:2300–2307, 2526–2528

[17] Katz B, Hoyt WF. Gaze-evoked amaurosis from vitreopapillary traction. Am J Ophthalmol. 2005; 139(4):631–637

[18] Orlans HO, Bremner FD. Dysthyroid orbitopathy presenting with gaze-evoked amaurosis: case report and review of the literature. Orbit. 2015; 34(6):324–326

[19] Seery LS, Zaldívar RA, Garrity JA. Amaurosis and optic disc blanching during upgaze in graves ophthalmopathy. J Neuroophthalmol. 2009; 29(3):219–222

[20] Sheth HG, O'Sullivan EP, Graham EM, Plant GT. Gaze-evoked amaurosis in optic neuropathy due to probable sarcoidosis. Eye (Lond). 2006; 20(9):1078–1080

[21] Kumar R, Madge SN, Selva D, Pirgousis P, Goss AN. Gaze-evoked amaurosis-post reconstruction of orbital floor fracture with a bone graft: case report. J Oral Maxillofac Surg. 2010; 68(12):3053–3054

[22] Manor RS, Yassur Y, Hoyt WF. Reading-evoked visual dimming. Am J Ophthalmol. 1996; 121(2):212–214

[23] O'Sullivan E, Shaunak S, Matthews T, Wade J, Kennard C, Simcock P. Transient monocular blindness. J Neurol Neurosurg Psychiatry. 1995; 59(5):559

[24] Wall M, George D. Idiopathic intracranial hypertension. A prospective study of 50 patients. Brain. 1991; 114 Pt 1A:155–180

[25] Ammache Z, Graber M, Davis P. Idiopathic stabbing headache associated with monocular visual loss. Arch Neurol. 2000; 57(5):745–746

[26] Grigorian AP, Spaeth G. An explanation of transient visual loss associated with leaking filtering bleb. Am J Ophthalmol. 2004; 138(5):869–870

[27] Sunil M, Payne C, Panda M. Transient binocular visual loss: a rare presentation of ventriculoperitoneal shunt malfunction. BMJ Case Rep. 2011; 2011:bcr1020114929

[28] Awad AM, Estephan B, Warnack W, Stüve O. Optic neuritis presenting with amaurosis fugax. J Neurol. 2009; 256(12):2100–2103

[29] Romano JG, Babikian VL, Wijman CAC, Hedges TR, III. Retinal ischemia in aortic arch atheromatous disease. J Neuroophthalmol. 1998; 18(4):237–241

[30] Giltner JW, Thomas ER, Rundell WK. Amaurosis fugax associated with congenital vascular defect. Int Med Case Rep J. 2016; 9:169–172

[31] Bruno A, Corbett JJ, Biller J, Adams HP, Jr, Qualls C. Transient monocular visual loss patterns and associated vascular abnormalities. Stroke. 1990; 21(1):34–39

[32] Goodwin JA, Gorelick PB, Helgason CM. Symptoms of amaurosis fugax in atherosclerotic carotid artery disease. Neurology. 1987; 37(5):829–832

[33] Pessin MS, Duncan GW, Mohr JP, Poskanzer DC. Clinical and angiographic features of carotid transient ischemic attacks. N Engl J Med. 1977; 296(7):358–362

[34] Lavallée PC, Cabrejo L, Labreuche J, et al. Spectrum of transient visual symptoms in a transient ischemic attack cohort. Stroke. 2013; 44(12):3312–3317

[35] Marshall J, Meadows S. The natural history of amaurosis fugax. Brain. 1968; 91(3):419–434

[36] Sharma S, Brown GC, Pater JL, Cruess AF. Does a visible retinal embolus increase the likelihood of hemodynamically significant carotid artery stenosis in patients with acute retinal arterial occlusion? Arch Ophthalmol. 1998; 116(12):1602–1606

[37] Klein R, Klein BE, Jensen SC, Moss SE, Meuer SM. Retinal emboli and stroke: the Beaver Dam Eye Study. Arch Ophthalmol. 1999; 117(8):1063–1068

[38] Tanaka K, Uehara T, Kimura K, et al. Japan TIA Research Group 2009–2011. Features of patients with transient monocular blindness: a multicenter retrospective study in Japan. J Stroke Cerebrovasc Dis. 2014; 23(3):e151–e155

[39] Kaiboriboon K, Piriyawat P, Selhorst JB. Light-induced amaurosis fugax. Am J Ophthalmol. 2001; 131(5):674–676

[40] Galetta SL, Balcer LJ, Liu GT. Giant cell arteritis with unusual flow-related neuro-ophthalmologic manifestations. Neurology. 1997; 49(5):1463–1465

[41] Donders RC, Dutch TMB Study Group. Clinical features of transient monocular blindness and the likelihood of atherosclerotic lesions of the internal carotid artery. J Neurol Neurosurg Psychiatry. 2001; 71(2):247–249

[42] Biousse V, Touboul P-J, D'Anglejan-Chatillon J, Lévy C, Schaison M, Bousser MG. Ophthalmologic manifestations of internal carotid artery dissection. Am J Ophthalmol. 1998; 126(4):565–577

[43] Kerty E. The ophthalmology of internal carotid artery dissection. Acta Ophthalmol Scand. 1999; 77(4):418–421

[44] Levin LA, Mootha VV. Postprandial transient visual loss. A symptom of critical carotid stenosis. Ophthalmology. 1997; 104(3):397–401

[45] Gass JDM. Stereoscopic Atlas of Macular Disease. Diagnosis and Treatment. 4th ed. St. Louis, MO: Mosby; 1997:464–466, 984–985

[46] Malhotra R, Gregory-Evans K. Management of ocular ischaemic syndrome. Br J Ophthalmol. 2000; 84(12):1428–1431

[47] Cohen R, Padilla J, Light D, Diller R. Carotid artery occlusive disease and ocular manifestations: importance of identifying patients at risk. Optometry. 2010; 81(7):359–363

[48] Mendrinos E, Machinis TG, Pournaras CJ. Ocular ischemic syndrome. Surv Ophthalmol. 2010; 55(1):2–34

[49] Borruat F-X, Bogousslavsky J, Uffer S, Klainguti G, Schatz NJ. Orbital infarction syndrome. Ophthalmology. 1993; 100(4):562–568

[50] Casson RJ, Fleming FK, Shaikh A, James B. Bilateral ocular ischemic syndrome secondary to giant cell arteritis. Arch Ophthalmol. 2001; 119(2):306–307

[51] Gupta A, Jalali S, Bansal RK, Grewal SPS. Anterior ischemic optic neuropathy and branch retinal artery occlusion in cavernous sinus thrombosis. J Clin Neuroophthalmol. 1990; 10(3):193–196

[52] Hamed LM, Guy JR, Moster ML, Bosley T. Giant cell arteritis in the ocular ischemic syndrome. Am J Ophthalmol. 1992; 113(6):702–705

[53] Lamirel C, Newman NJ, Biousse V. Vascular neuro-ophthalmology. Handb Clin Neurol. 2009; 93:595–611

[54] Hwang J-M, Girkin CA, Perry JD, Lai JC, Miller NR, Hellmann DB. Bilateral ocular ischemic syndrome secondary to giant cell arteritis progressing despite corticosteroid treatment. Am J Ophthalmol. 1999; 127(1):102–104

[55] Lewis JR, Glaser JS, Schatz NJ, Hutson DG. Pulseless (Takayasu) disease with ophthalmic manifestations. J Clin Neuroophthalmol. 1993; 13(4):242–249

[56] Meire FM, De Laey JJ, Van Thienen MN, Schuddinck L. Retinal manifestations in fibromuscular dysplasia. Eur J Ophthalmol. 1991; 1(2):63–68

[57] Winterkorn JMS, Beckman RL. Recovery from ocular ischemic syndrome after treatment with verapamil. J Neuroophthalmol. 1995; 15(4):209–211

[58] Zimmerman CF, Van Patten PD, Golnik KC, Kopitnik TA, Jr, Anand R. Orbital infarction syndrome after surgery for intracranial aneurysms. Ophthalmology. 1995; 102(4):594–598

[59] Peredo R, Vilá S, Goñi M, Colón E, Ríos-Solá G. Reactive thrombocytosis: an early manifestation of Takayasu arteritis. J Clin Rheumatol. 2005; 11(5):270–273

[60] Hayreh SS. Ocular vascular occlusive disorders: natural history of visual outcome. Prog Retin Eye Res. 2014; 41:1–25

[61] Andracchi S, Kupersmith MJ, Nelson PK, Slakter JS, Setton A, Berenstein A. Visual loss from arterial steal in patients with maxillofacial arteriovenous malformation. Ophthalmology. 2000; 107(4):730–736

[62] Kearns TP, Siekert RG, Sundt TM. The ocular aspects of carotid artery bypass surgery. Trans Am Ophthalmol Soc. 1978; 76:247–265

[63] Hayreh SS, Podhajsky PA, Zimmerman B. Ocular manifestations of giant cell arteritis. Am J Ophthalmol. 1998; 125(4):509–520

[64] Hayreh SS, Podhajsky PA, Zimmerman B. Occult giant cell arteritis: ocular manifestations. Am J Ophthalmol. 1998; 125(4):521–526

[65] Wykes WN, Adams GGW, Cullen JF. Temporal arteritis: visual loss associated with posture. Neuro-ophthalmology. 1984; 4(2):107–109

[66] Finelli PF. Alternating amaurosis fugax and temporal arteritis. Am J Ophthalmol. 1997; 123(6):850–851

[67] Case Records of the Massachusetts General Hospital. Case records of the Massachusetts General Hospital. Weekly clinicopathological exercises. Case 3-1999. A 41-year-old woman with muscle weakness, painful paresthesias, and visual problems. N Engl J Med. 1999; 340(4):300–307

[68] Donders RC, Kappelle LJ, Derksen RH, et al. Transient monocular blindness and antiphospholipid antibodies in systemic lupus erythematosus. Neurology. 1998; 51(2):535–540

[69] Levine SR, Deegan MJ, Futrell N, Welch KM. Cerebrovascular and neurologic disease associated with antiphospholipid antibodies: 48 cases. Neurology. 1990; 40(8):1181–1189

[70] Muñoz-Negrete FJ, Casas-Lleras P, Pérez-López M, Rebolleda G. Hypercoagulable workup in ophthalmology. When and what [in Spanish]. Arch Soc Esp Oftalmol. 2009; 84(7):325–332

[71] Vodopivec I, Cestari DM, Rizzo JF, III. Management of transient monocular vision loss and retinal artery occlusions. Semin Ophthalmol. 2017; 32(1):125–133

[72] Bernard GA, Bennett JL. Vasospastic amaurosis fugax. Arch Ophthalmol. 1999; 117(11):1568–1569

[73] Booy R. Amaurosis fugax in a young woman. Lancet. 1990; 335(8704):1538

[74] Burger SK, Saul RF, Selhorst JB, Thurston SE. Transient monocular blindness caused by vasospasm. N Engl J Med. 1991; 325(12):870–873

[75] O'Sullivan F, Rossor M, Elston JS. Amaurosis fugax in young people. Br J Ophthalmol. 1992; 76(11):660–662

[76] Winterkorn JM, Kupersmith MJ, Wirtschafter JD, Forman S. Brief report: treatment of vasospastic amaurosis fugax with calcium-channel blockers. N Engl J Med. 1993; 329(6):396–398

[77] Jehn A, Frank Dettwiler B, Fleischhauer J, Sturzenegger M, Mojon DS. Exercise-induced vasospastic amaurosis fugax. Arch Ophthalmol. 2002; 120(2):220–222

[78] Teman AJ, Winterkorn JMS, Weiner D. Transient monocular blindness associated with sexual intercourse. N Engl J Med. 1995; 333(6):393

[79] Tippin J, Corbett JJ, Kerber RE, Schroeder E, Thompson HS. Amaurosis fugax and ocular infarction in adolescents and young adults. Ann Neurol. 1989; 26(1):69–77

[80] Kosmorsky GS, Rosenfeld SI, Burde RM. Transient monocular obscuration–? amaurosis fugax: a case report. Br J Ophthalmol. 1985; 69(9):688–690

[81] Ambresin A, Borruat F-X, Mermoud A. Recurrent transient visual loss after deep sclerectomy. Arch Ophthalmol. 2001; 119(8):1213–1215

[82] Cates CA, Newman DK. Transient monocular visual loss due to uveitis-glaucoma-hyphaema (UGH) syndrome. J Neurol Neurosurg Psychiatry. 1998; 65(1):131–132

[83] Lee MD, Odel JG, Rudich DS, Ritch R. Vision loss with sexual activity. J Glaucoma. 2016; 25(1):e46–e47

[84] Fineman MS, Regillo CD, Sergott RC, Spaeth G, Vander J. Transient visual loss and decreased ocular blood flow velocities following a scleral buckling procedure. Arch Ophthalmol. 1999; 117(12):1647–1648

[85] Ebner R. Morning glory syndrome, amaurosis fugax, and cortical laser tomography. Presented at the North American Neuro-Ophthalmology Society annual meeting, Tucson, Arizona, 1995

[86] Zarnegar SR, Chung S, Selhorst JB. An unusual cause of amaurosis fugax. Presented at the North American Neuro-Ophthalmology annual meeting, Tucson, Arizona, 1995

[87] Benninger F, Steiner I. Surprising cause of transient monocular vision loss. Pract Neurol. 2014; 14(6):448

[88] Kramer M, Goldenberg-Cohen N, Shapira Y, et al. Role of transesophageal echocardiography in the evaluation of patients with retinal artery occlusion. Ophthalmology. 2001; 108(8):1461–1464

[89] Hurwitz BJ, Heyman A, Wilkinson WE, Haynes CS, Utley CM. Comparison of amaurosis fugax and transient cerebral ischemia: a prospective clinical and arteriographic study. Ann Neurol. 1985; 18(6):698–704

[90] Volkers EJ, Donders RC, Koudstaal PJ, van Gijn J, Algra A, Jaap Kappelle L. Transient monocular blindness and the risk of vascular complications according to subtype: a prospective cohort study. J Neurol. 2016; 263(9):1771–1777

[91] Barnett HJM, Taylor DW, Haynes RB, et al. North American Symptomatic Carotid Endarterectomy Trial Collaborators. Beneficial effect of carotid endarterectomy in symptomatic patients with high-grade carotid stenosis. N Engl J Med. 1991; 325(7):445–453

[92] Barnett HJM, Taylor DW, Eliasziw M, et al. Benefit of carotid endarterectomy in patients with symptomatic moderate or severe stenosis. North American Symptomatic Carotid Endarterectomy Trial Collaborators. N Engl J Med. 1998; 339(20):1415–1425

[93] Haynes RB, Taylor DW, Sackett DL, Thorpe K, Ferguson GG, Barnett HJ. Prevention of functional impairment by endarterectomy for symptomatic high-grade carotid stenosis. North American Symptomatic Carotid Endarterectomy Trial Collaborators. JAMA. 1994; 271(16):1256–1259

[94] Lawlor M, Perry R, Hunt BJ, Plant GT. Strokes and vision: the management of ischemic arterial disease affecting the retina and occipital lobe. Surv Ophthalmol. 2015; 60(4):296–309

[95] Benavente O, Eliasziw M, Streifler JY, Fox AJ, Barnett HJ, Meldrum H, North American Symptomatic Carotid Endarterectomy Trial Collaborators. Prognosis after transient monocular blindness associated with carotid-artery stenosis. N Engl J Med. 2001; 345(15):1084–1090

[96] Kim KT, Baik SG, Park KP, Park MG. A case of complete recovery of fluctuating monocular blindness following endovascular treatment in internal carotid artery dissection. J Stroke Cerebrovasc Dis. 2015; 24(9):e283–e286

[97] Brott TG, Hobson RW, II, Howard G, et al. CREST Investigators. Stenting versus endarterectomy for treatment of carotid-artery stenosis. N Engl J Med. 2010; 363(1):11–23

[98] Kawaguchi S, Okuno S, Sakaki T, Nishikawa N. Effect of carotid endarterectomy on chronic ocular ischemic syndrome due to internal carotid artery stenosis. Neurosurgery. 2001; 48(2):328–332, discussion 322–323

[99] Rennie CA, Flanagan DW. Resolution of proliferative venous stasis retinopathy after carotid endarterectomy. Br J Ophthalmol. 2002; 86(1):117–118

[100] Kawaguchi S, Sakaki T, Morimoto T, Okuno S, Nishikawa N. Effects of bypass on ocular ischaemic syndrome caused by reversed flow in the ophthalmic artery. Lancet. 1999; 354(9195):2052–2053

[101] Mehrzad R, Bajaj R. A rare but important differential diagnosis in transient monocular blindness. BMJ Case Rep. 2014; 2014:bcr2014206812

[102] Pula JH, Kwan K, Yuen CA, Kattah JC. Update on the evaluation of transient vision loss. Clin Ophthalmol. 2016; 10:297–303

[103] Stepanov A, Hejsek L, Jiraskova N, Feuermannova A, Rencova E, Rozsival P. Transient branch retinal artery occlusion in a 15-year-old girl and review of the literature. Biomed Pap Med Fac Univ Palacky Olomouc Czech Repub. 2015; 159(3):508–511

[104] Luu ST, Lee AW, Chen CS. Transient monocular visual loss following administration of topical latanoprost: a case report. Can J Ophthalmol. 2009; 44(6):715

[105] Biousse V, Newman NJ, Sternberg P, Jr. Retinal vein occlusion and transient monocular visual loss associated with hyperhomocystinemia. Am J Ophthalmol. 1997; 124(2):257–260

[106] Russell MB, Olesen J. A nosographic analysis of the migraine aura in a general population. Brain. 1996; 119(Pt 2):355–361

[107] Fisher CM. Late-life (migrainous) scintillating zigzags without headache: one person's 27-year experience. Headache. 1999; 39(6):391–397

[108] Wijman CA, Wolf PA, Kase CS, Kelly-Hayes M, Beiser AS. Migrainous visual accompaniments are not rare in late life: the Framingham Study. Stroke. 1998; 29(8):1539–1543

[109] Liu GT, Schatz NJ, Galetta SL, Volpe NJ, Skobieranda F, Kosmorsky GS. Persistent positive visual phenomena in migraine. Neurology. 1995; 45(4): 664–668

[110] Chen W-T, Fuh J-L, Lu S-R, Wang S-J. Persistent migrainous visual phenomena might be responsive to lamotrigine. Headache. 2001; 41(8): 823–825

[111] Luda E, Bo E, Sicuro L, Comitangelo R, Campana M. Sustained visual aura: a totally new variation of migraine. Headache. 1991; 31(9):582–583

[112] Haan J, Sluis P, Sluis LH, Ferrari MD. Acetazolamide treatment for migraine aura status. Neurology. 2000; 55(10):1588–1589

[113] Beltramone M, Donnet A. Status migrainosus and migraine aura status in a French tertiary-care center: an 11-year retrospective analysis. Cephalalgia. 2014; 34(8):633–637

[114] Cupini LM, Stipa E. Migraine aura status and hyperhomocysteinaemia. Cephalalgia. 2007; 27(7):847–849

[115] Rozen TD. Treatment of a prolonged migrainous aura with intravenous furosemide. Neurology. 2000; 55(5):732–733

[116] Afridi SK, Giffin NJ, Kaube H, Goadsby PJ. A randomized controlled trial of intranasal ketamine in migraine with prolonged aura. Neurology. 2013; 80 (7):642–647

[117] Kaube H, Herzog J, Käufer T, Dichgans M, Diener HC. Aura in some patients with familial hemiplegic migraine can be stopped by intranasal ketamine. Neurology. 2000; 55(1):139–141

[118] Biousse V, Newman NJ, Lee AG, Eggenberger E, Patrinely JR, Kaufman D. Intracranial Ewing's sarcoma. J Neuroophthalmol. 1998; 18(3):187–191

[119] Pepin EP. Cerebral metastasis presenting as migraine with aura. Lancet. 1990; 336(8707):127–128

[120] Riaz G, Selhorst JB, Hennessey JJ. Meningeal lesions mimicking migraine. Neuro-ophthalmology. 1991; 11:41–48

[121] Haas DC. Arteriovenous malformations and migraine: case reports and an analysis of the relationship. Headache. 1991; 31(8):509–513

[122] Kupersmith MJ, Berenstein A, Nelson PK, ApSimon HT, Setton A. Visual symptoms with dural arteriovenous malformations draining into occipital veins. Neurology. 1999; 52(1):156–162

[123] Kupersmith MJ, Vargas ME, Yashar A, et al. Occipital arteriovenous malformations: visual disturbances and presentation. Neurology. 1996; 46 (4):953–957

[124] Kurita H, Shin M, Kirino T. Resolution of migraine with aura caused by an occipital arteriovenous malformation. Arch Neurol. 2000; 57(8): 1219–1220

[125] Spierings EL. Daily migraine with visual aura associated with an occipital arteriovenous malformation. Headache. 2001; 41(2):193–197

[126] Newman DS, Levine SR, Curtis VL, Welch KM. Migraine-like visual phenomena associated with cerebral venous thrombosis. Headache. 1989; 29(2):82–85

[127] Panayiotopoulos CP. Elementary visual hallucinations, blindness, and headache in idiopathic occipital epilepsy: differentiation from migraine. J Neurol Neurosurg Psychiatry. 1999; 66(4):536–540

[128] Panayiotopoulos CP. Visual phenomena and headache in occipital epilepsy: a review, a systematic study and differentiation from migraine. Epileptic Disord. 1999; 1(4):205–216

[129] Joseph JM, Louis S. Transient ictal cortical blindness during middle age. A case report and review of the literature. J Neuroophthalmol. 1995; 15(1):39–42

[130] Sadeh M, Goldhammer Y, Kuritsky A. Postictal blindness in adults. J Neurol Neurosurg Psychiatry. 1983; 46(6):566–569

[131] Hartl E, Angel J, Rémi J, Schankin CJ, Noachtar S. Visual auras in epilepsy and migraine – an analysis of clinical characteristics. Headache. 2017; 57(6): 908–916

[132] Dreier JP, Sakowitz OW, Unterberg AW, Benndorf G, Einhäupl KM, Valdueza JM. Migrainous aura starting several minutes after the onset of subarachnoid hemorrhage. Neurology. 2001; 57(7):1344–1345

[133] Ramadan NM, Tietjen GE, Levine SR, Welch KMA. Scintillating scotomata associated with internal carotid artery dissection: report of three cases. Neurology. 1991; 41(7):1084–1087

[134] Tomaschütz L, Dos Santos M, Schill J, Palm F, Grau A. Recurrent amaurosis fugax in a patient after Stanford type a dissection depending on blood pressure and haemoglobin level. Case Rep Vasc Med. 2012; 2012:254204

[135] Danks JJ, Harrad RA. Flashing lights in thyroid eye disease: a new symptom described and (possibly) explained. Br J Ophthalmol. 1998; 82(11):1309–1311

[136] Kim DS, Kang SG, Yoo DS, Huh PW, Cho KS, Kim MC. Sudden cortical blindness in an adult with moyamoya disease. Surg Neurol. 2007; 67(3): 303–307

[137] Hilton-Jones D, Ponsford JR, Graham N. Transient visual obscurations, without papilloedema. J Neurol Neurosurg Psychiatry. 1982; 45(9):832–834

[138] Diego M, Margo CE. Postural vision loss in giant cell arteritis. J Neuroophthalmol. 1998; 18(2):124–126

[139] Friedberg DN, Fox LE. Blurred vision during sexual arousal associated with narrow-angle glaucoma. Am J Ophthalmol. 1999; 128(5):647–648

[140] Frucht-Pery J, Landau D, Raiskup F, et al. Early transient visual acuity loss after LASIK due to steroid-induced elevation of intraocular pressure. J Refract Surg. 2007; 23(3):244–251

[141] Hussain S, Hussain K, Hussain S. Transient cortical blindness as a manifestation of solitary cysticercus granuloma. BMJ Case Rep. 2012; 2012. DOI: 10.1136/bcr-2012-007552

[142] Sawchuk KS, Churchill S, Feldman E, Drury I. Status epilepticus amauroticus. Neurology. 1997; 49(5):1467–1469

[143] Gibson JM, Cullen JF. Blindness and visual field defects following cerebral angiography. Neuro-ophthalmology. 1982; 2(4):297–303

[144] Tatli E, Buyuklu M, Altun A. An unusual but dramatic complication of coronary angiography: transient cortical blindness. Int J Cardiol. 2007; 121 (1):e4–e6

[145] Leong S, Fanning NF. Persistent neurological deficit from iodinated contrast encephalopathy following intracranial aneurysm coiling. A case report and review of the literature. Interv Neuroradiol. 2012; 18(1):33–41

[146] Shah PR, Yohendran J, Parker GD, McCluskey PJ. Contrast-induced transient cortical blindness. Clin Exp Optom. 2013; 96(3):333–335

[147] Mentzel HJ, Blume J, Malich A, Fitzek C, Reichenbach JR, Kaiser WA. Cortical blindness after contrast-enhanced CT: complication in a patient with diabetes insipidus. AJNR Am J Neuroradiol. 2003; 24(6):1114–1116

[148] Till V, Koprivsek K, Stojanovic S, Avramov P, Vulekovic P. Transient cortical blindness following vertebral angiography in a young adult with cerebellar haemangioblastoma. Pediatr Radiol. 2009; 39(11):1223–1226

[149] Yeh S, Bazzaz S, Foroozan R. Transient cortical blindness with leptomeningeal enhancement after attempted peripherally inserted central venous catheter placement. Arch Ophthalmol. 2005; 123(5):700–702

[150] Barletta JP, Fanous MM, Hamed LM. Temporary blindness in the TUR syndrome. J Neuroophthalmol. 1994; 14(1):6–8

[151] Prasun P, Altinok D, Misra VK. Ornithine transcarbamylase deficiency presenting with acute reversible cortical blindness. J Child Neurol. 2015; 30 (6):782–785

[152] Ng RH. Post-traumatic transient cortical blindness in a child with occipital bone fracture. J Clin Neurosci. 2016; 34:225–227

[153] Hinchey J, Chaves C, Appignani B, et al. A reversible posterior leukoencephalopathy syndrome. N Engl J Med. 1996; 334(8):494–500

[154] Karp BI, Yang JC, Khorsand M, Wood R, Merigan TC. Multiple cerebral lesions complicating therapy with interleukin-2. Neurology. 1996; 47(2):417–424

[155] Kesler A, Kaneti H, Kidron D. Transient cortical blindness in preeclampsia with indication of generalized vascular endothelial damage. J Neuroophthalmol. 1998; 18(3):163–165

[156] Kupferschmidt H, Bont A, Schnorf H, et al. Transient cortical blindness and bioccipital brain lesions in two patients with acute intermittent porphyria. Ann Intern Med. 1995; 123(8):598–600

[157] Baizabal-Carvallo JF, Barragán-Campos HM, Padilla-Aranda HJ, et al. Posterior reversible encephalopathy syndrome as a complication of acute lupus activity. Clin Neurol Neurosurg. 2009; 111(4):359–363

[158] Stanzani L, Fusi L, Gomitoni A, Roncoroni M, Villa P, Grampa G. A case of posterior reversible encephalopathy during polyarteritis nodosa vasculitis. Neurol Sci. 2008; 29(3):163–167

[159] Fabbian F, Pala M, Fallica E, et al. Posterior reversible encephalopathy syndrome in an 87-year-old woman with Escherichia coli bloodstream infection. Clin Exp Nephrol. 2010; 14(2):176–179

[160] Lateef A, Lim AY. Case reports of transient loss of vision and systemic lupus erythematosus. Ann Acad Med Singapore. 2007; 36(2):146–149

[161] Rao NM, Raychev R, Kim D, Liebeskind DS. Elucidating the mechanism of posterior reversible encephalopathy syndrome: a case of transient blindness after central venous catheterization. Neurologist. 2012; 18(6):391–394

9 Visual Field Defects

Beena M. Shah

Abstract

A visual field defect can topographically localize to specific lesions along the visual pathway. The laterality and pattern of the deficit help clinically localize the lesion and guide further evaluation (e.g., neuroimaging) of the underlying etiology. This chapter discusses the clinical pathways for the evaluation and differential diagnosis of a visual field defect, reviewing the literature in detail.

Keywords: visual field defect, arcuate defect, scotoma, homonymous hemianopia, bitemporal hemianopia

9.1 What Is the Topographical Diagnosis of Visual Field Defects?

The localization of visual field defects is outlined in ▸ Fig. 9.1.

9.2 Is the Visual Field Defect Unilateral?

Lesions affecting the retina, nerve fiber layer, or optic nerve produce visual field defects in the ipsilateral eye that correspond in position, shape, extent, and intensity to the lesion. The lesion may be inflammatory, ischemic, degenerative, or neoplastic. Because the nerve fiber layer arising from the peripheral retina arches over the fovea, superior or inferior nerve fiber layer damage results in arcuate-shaped visual field defects. Rarely, patients with a lesion of the anterior occipital lobe may have a unilateral, contralateral visual field defect (see discussion on monocular temporal crescent).

9.3 Is a Retinal Lesion Responsible for the Visual Field Defect?

Almost all retinal lesions resulting in visual field loss are visible ophthalmoscopically. Careful attention should be directed to the retina and retinal nerve fiber layer corresponding to the visual field defect. Patients with macular disease may also complain of metamorphopsia, micropsia, and positive photopsias (e.g., flashing lights) that are unusual in patients with optic neuropathies. Easily visible retinal lesions are not discussed in detail. In some cases, the retina may appear normal or near normal, and ancillary testing may be required to define the etiology as retinal (e.g., fluorescein angiography or focal, multifocal, or full field electroretinography). The following are some retinal disorders that may be difficult to visualize without careful attention to the macula with high magnification and stereoscopic viewing:
- Cystoid macular edema.
- Epiretinal membrane.
- Outer retinal inflammatory diseases.
- Multiple evanescent white dot syndrome (MEWDS).
- Acute macular neuroretinitis (AMN).
- Acute retinal pigment epitheliitis.
- Acute multifocal placoid pigment epitheliopathy (AMPPE).
- Acute zonal occult outer retinopathy (AZOOR).
- Serous detachment of the macula.
- Cone-rod dystrophy.
- Retinitis pigmentosa sine pigmento.
- Cancer-associated retinopathy (CAR).
- Melanoma-associated retinopathy (MAR).

Annular or ring scotomas may occur with retinopathies or optic neuropathies. Etiologies of annular or ring scotomas include pigmentary retinopathies, retinitis, choroiditis, blinding diffuse light, retinal migraine, myopia, CAR, open angle glaucoma (from coalescence of upper and lower arcuate scotomas), and optic neuropathies (e.g., anterior ischemic optic neuropathy). Bilateral annular or ring scotomas may be due to bilateral retinal or optic nerve disease but may also occur with bilateral occipital pole damage or occur on a functional (nonorganic) basis.

9.4 Is There Evidence for an Optic Neuropathy?

Central visual field defects (unilateral or bilateral) are the result of damage to the papillomacular bundle or optic nerve. Any visual field defect produced by a retinal lesion may be produced by a lesion of the optic nerve[1] and virtually any etiology may be responsible (e.g., glaucomatous, degenerative, ischemic, traumatic, inflammatory, infiltrative, compressive, or vascular optic neuropathy). Patients with a unilateral visual field defect and evidence for an optic neuropathy should undergo evaluation for an optic neuropathy (see Chapter 1). Patients with a unilateral hemianopic visual field defect (junctional scotoma of Traquair) may harbor a lesion of the optic nerve at the junction of the optic nerve and chiasm, such as a pituitary adenoma.[2]

In assessing optic nerve–related visual field defects, several anatomic points are worth remembering:
1. Fibers from peripheral ganglion cells occupy a more peripheral position of the optic disc, whereas fibers from ganglion cells located closer to the disc occupy a more central position.
2. Peripheral fibers course peripherally through the entire extent of the optic nerve.
3. The papillomacular bundle occupies a large sector-shaped region of the temporal disc. This bundle of fibers moves centrally in the more distal (posterior) portions of orbital optic nerve.
4. All retinal fibers retain their relative positions throughout the visual pathways except in the optic tract and at the lateral geniculate nucleus, where there is a rotation of 90 degrees that becomes "straightened out" in the optic radiations.

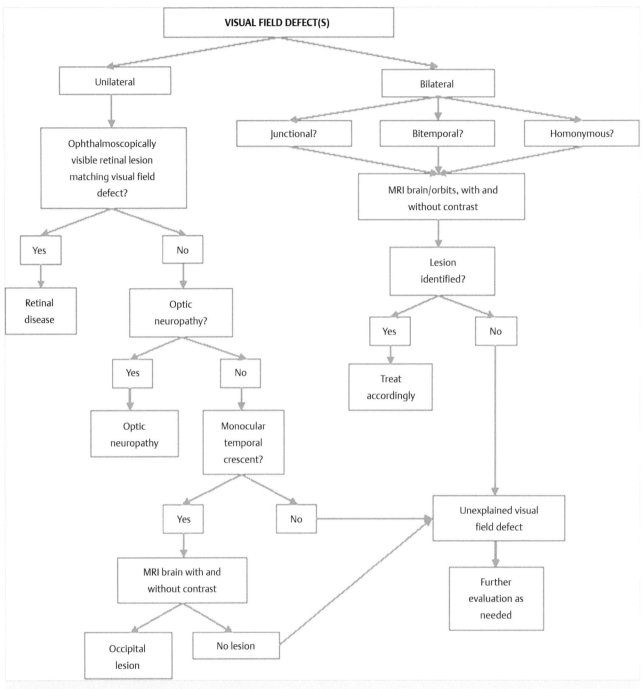

Fig. 9.1 Evaluation of visual field defects.

9.5 Is the Monocular Temporal Crescent Affected in Isolation?

Although monocular peripheral temporal visual field defects are most often the result of retinal or optic nerve disease, a lesion of the peripheral nasal fibers in the anterior occipital lobe may also produce a unilateral (monocular) temporal crescent-shaped visual field defect from 60 to 90 degrees ("half-moon syndrome").[3] Although retrochiasmal lesions in the visual pathway usually result in homonymous visual field loss, the monocular temporal crescent is the one exception. Homonymous visual field loss with sparing of this temporal crescent or selective involvement of this area localizes the lesion to the occipital lobe, and neuroimaging should be directed to the contralateral calcarine cortex.[4,5]

9.6 Is the Visual Field Defect Bilateral?

Bilateral lesions of the retina or optic nerve may result in bilateral visual field defects. In the absence of evidence for bilateral retinal disease or bilateral optic neuropathy, bilateral visual field loss results from disease affecting the optic chiasm or retrochiasmal pathways. The rest of this section reviews the clinical features of bilateral superior or inferior altitudinal defects and bilateral central or cecocentral scotomas.

Bilateral superior or inferior altitudinal defects are mostly caused by bilateral optic nerve or retinal disease. Rarely, large prechiasmal lesion compresses both nerves inferiorly to cause bilateral superior hemianopia. Compression of nerves from below may also elevate them against the dural shelves extending out from the intracranial end of the optic canals and cause bilateral inferior altitudinal defects. Bilateral symmetric damage to postchiasmal pathways may also cause bilateral altitudinal defects; bilateral lesions of medial aspect of lateral geniculate body may cause bilateral inferior hemianopias.

Bilateral cecocentral or central scotomas may be bilateral optic neuropathy of any cause (e.g., compressive). However, more common etiologies include toxic or nutritional amblyopia, bilateral demyelinating optic neuritis, syphilis, Leber hereditary optic neuropathy, bilateral macular disease, or bilateral occipital lesions involving macular projections.

9.7 Is the Visual Field Defect Junctional in Nature?

Nerve fibers originating in the retina follow a specific topographic arrangement in the optic nerve and chiasm. Compressive lesions at the junction of the intracranial optic nerve and optic chiasm may produce characteristic visual field defects. Optic nerve involvement at the junction of the optic chiasm results in unilateral visual field loss (optic neuropathy). If fibers from the inferonasal retina of the contralateral eye (Wilbrand's knee) are involved, there will also be a superotemporal visual field defect in the contralateral eye.

The intracranial optic nerves extend posteriorly from the optic foramen and join at the optic chiasm. Within the chiasm, fibers from the nasal retina of each eye cross into the contralateral optic tract, and fibers from the temporal retina pass uncrossed into the ipsilateral optic tract. Within the intracranial optic nerve, the crossed (nasal retinal) and uncrossed (temporal retinal) fibers are anatomically separated at the junction of the optic nerve and chiasm. In addition, inferior nasal crossing fibers may loop anteriorly for a short distance into the contralateral optic nerve. These fibers are often referred to as the anterior knee or Wilbrand's knee.

Lesions at the junction of the optic nerve and chiasm may produce specific types of visual field defects that allow topographic localization. Selective compression of the crossed or uncrossed visual fibers at the junction may result in a unilateral temporal or nasal hemianopic field defect, respectively. In addition, involvement of the inferonasal fibers of the anterior knee (Wilbrand's knee) results in a superotemporal visual field defect contralateral to the lesion.

In 1927, H. M. Traquair used the term *junctional scotoma* to refer to a unilateral temporal hemicentral field defect caused by compression of the nasal fibers crossing in the intracranial optic nerve at the junction of the optic nerve and chiasm. Miller and Newman emphasized that the *junctional scotoma* described by Traquair refers to a strictly unilateral temporal scotoma that is assumed to arise from a lesion at the junction of the optic nerve and chiasm.[1] Unfortunately, some confusion has arisen regarding the use of the term junctional scotoma. As opposed to the defect described by Traquair, some authors have used the term to refer to an ipsilateral optic neuropathy with a contralateral superotemporal visual field defect. This superotemporal defect is caused by compression of the inferonasal fibers from the contralateral eye traveling in Wilbrand's knee.

To clarify this distinction, Miller, citing J. Lawton Smith, recommended that the unilateral temporal visual field defect described by Traquair should be referred to as the "junctional scotoma of Traquair" to differentiate it from the contralateral superotemporal defect more commonly referred to as the "junctional scotoma."[1]

The existence of Wilbrand's knee has come into question. Wilbrand was restricted to examining human subjects who had undergone enucleation. In the enucleated eye, the nerve fibers atrophied and became distinct from the nerve fibers of the normal eye as seen on myelin staining. Horton, utilizing axon labeling techniques in nonenucleated monkeys, was unable to demonstrate crossing fibers looping into the contralateral optic nerve (Wilbrand's knee).[6] Lee et al also challenged the existence of the Wilbrand's knee. After the resection of the ON at the ON-chiasm in three different patients, junctional scotomas could not be detected by visual perimetry. Lee et al supported Horton's hypothesis that the Wilbrand's knee does not exist in humans with intact visual apparatus.[7]

Nevertheless, whether Wilbrand's knee exists anatomically, the localizing value of junctional visual field loss to the junction of the optic nerve and chiasm remains undiminished because chiasmal compression alone may result in the contralateral superotemporal visual field defect (junctional scotoma). Karanjia and Jacobson described a junctional scotoma due to a focal lesion (pituitary tumor) of the prechiasmatic segment of the distal optic nerve and stressed the "exquisite localizing value" of a junctional scotoma.[8]

Trobe and Glaser noted that junctional visual field loss was due to a mass lesion in 98 out of 100 cases.[9] The differential diagnosis of a junctional syndrome includes pituitary tumors, suprasellar meningiomas, supraclinoid aneurysms, craniopharyngiomas, and gliomas.[10] Chiasmal neuritis, pachymeningitis, and trauma are rare etiologies of the junctional syndrome. Junctional visual field abnormalities may also occur on a functional (nonorganic) basis.

Patients with the junctional scotoma of Traquair or the junctional scotoma should be considered to have a compressive lesion at the junction of the optic nerve and chiasm until proven otherwise. Neuroimaging studies, preferably magnetic resonance imaging (MRI), should be directed to this location. Patients with junctional scotoma may be unaware of a small superotemporal visual field defect, and patients presenting with strictly unilateral visual complaints may be misdiagnosed as having an optic neuritis or other unilateral optic neuropathy. Therefore, in any patient with presumed unilateral visual loss, careful visual field testing should be performed in the contralateral asymptomatic eye.

9.8 Is a Bitemporal Hemianopsia Present?

Bitemporal hemianopsia may be peripheral, paracentral, or central. The visual field defect may "split" or "spare" the macular central field. The bitemporal defect usually is the result of a compressive mass lesion at the level of the optic chiasm.[1] The following are lists of possible etiologies of a chiasmal lesion (Box 9.1).

Box 9.1 Etiologies of chiasmal lesions

Most common etiologies of a chiasmal lesion:
- Pituitary apoplexy.[11,12,13]
- Pituitary tumor (especially pituitary adenoma).[14,15,16,17,18,19,20]
- Optic chiasm diastasis from pituitary tumor.[21]
- Meningioma.[22]
- Craniopharyngioma.[23,24,25]
- Dysgerminoma.
- Suprasellar aneurysm.
- Chiasmal glioma.[26,27,28]

Less common etiologies of a chiasmal lesion:
- Abscess.
- Anaplastic astrocytoma.[27]
- Arachnoid cyst.
- Aspergillosis.
- Cavernous hemangioma.[29,30]
- Chiasmal hematoma (chiasmal apoplexy).[31]
- Chondroma.
- Chordoma.
- Choristomas.
- Colloid cyst.
  - Third ventricle cyst.
  - Pituitary gland cyst.[32]
- Dermoid.
- Dolichoectatic internal carotid arteries.[33,34]
- Enchondromatosis (Ollier disease).
- Ependymoma.
- Epidermoid.
- Esthesioneuroblastoma.
- Extramedullary hematopoiesis.[35]
- Fibrous dysplasia.
- Gangliocytoma.[36]
- Ganglioglioma.[37]
- Giant cell tumor of bone.
- Glioma.
- Granular cell myoblastoma.
- Hemangioblastoma.[38]
- Hemangioma.[39]
- Hemangiopericytoma.
- Histiocytosis X.
- Hydrocephalus and distention of the third ventricle.
- Intrasellar.
- Langerhans cell histiocytoma.[40]

- Leukemia and lymphoma.[41,42]
- Lipoma.
- Lymphocytic hypophysitis.[43,44,45,46,47,48,49,50,51,52,53,54]
- Lymphohistiocytosis.[55]
- Melanoma.[56]
- Meningeal carcinomatosis.
- Metastatic disease to brain or pituitary gland.[57,58]
- Mucocele or mucopyocele.
- Multiple myeloma.
- Nasopharyngeal cancer.
- Nonneoplastic pituitary gland enlargement.
- Paraganglioma.
- Plasmacytoma.
- Rathke cleft cyst.[59,60,61,62,63]
- Rhabdomyosarcoma.[64]
- Sarcoma.
- Schwannoma.
- Septum pellucidum cyst.
- Sinus histiocytosis with lymphadenopathy (Rosai-Dorfman disease).
- Sinus tumors.
- Sphenoid sinus.
- Syphilitic granuloma.
- Teratoma.
- Vascular malformation.
- Venous aneurysm arising from carotid-cavernous sinus fistula.[65]
- Venous angioma.

Other causes of chiasmal syndrome:
- Hydrocephalus.[66]
- Cobalamin deficiency.[67]
- Demyelinating disease.[67,68]
- Empty sella syndrome (primary or secondary).[69]
- Chiasmal ischemia.
- Optochiasmic arachnoiditis.
- Foreign body–induced granuloma (e.g., muslin).
- Idiopathic.
- Infection:
  - Chronic fungal infection.
  - Cryptococcus.
  - Cysticercosis.[70]
  - Encephalitis.
  - Epstein-Barr virus.[71]
  - Meningitis.
  - Mucormycosis.[72]
  - Nasopharyngeal and sinus infections.
  - Syphilis.
  - Tuberculosis.
- Inflammatory:
  - Collagen vascular disease (e.g., systemic lupus erythematosus).[73,74]
  - Rheumatoid pachymeningitis.
  - Sarcoidosis (e.g., granuloma).
  - Multiple sclerosis.
- Posthemorrhagic.
- Posttraumatic.
- Radiation necrosis.
- Shunt catheter.

- Toxic (see toxic optic neuropathies):
  - Tobacco–alcohol toxicity.[75]
  - Ethchlorvynol (Placidyl).
  - Pheniprazine (Catron).
- Trauma, including postsurgical.[76,77,78]
- Fat packing after transsphenoidal hypophysectomy.[79,80]
- Tethering scar tissue causing delayed visual deterioration after pituitary surgery.[81]
- Vascular occlusion.
- Vasculitis.[67]
- Hereditary (probably autosomal recessive) chiasmal optic neuropathy.[82]
- Nonorganic (functional).[83]

Pseudochiasmal visual field defects (i.e., bitemporal defects that do not respect the vertical midline) may be due to tilted discs, colobomas, bilateral nasal retinal disease (e.g., schisis), glaucoma, and bilateral optic neuropathies. Neuroimaging (preferably MRI) should be directed at the optic chiasm in all patients with bitemporal defects that respect the vertical midline.

Certain anatomic relationships are important in evaluating chiasmal visual field defects:
- The ratio of crossed-to-uncrossed fibers is 53:47.
- Uncrossed fibers, both dorsal and ventral, maintain their relative position at the lateral aspects of the chiasm and pass directly into the ipsilateral optic tract.
- Dorsal extramacular crossing fibers from each eye decussate posteriorly in the chiasm and then directly enter the dorsomedial aspect of contralateral optic tract.
- Macular fibers that cross do so in the central and posterior portions of chiasm.
- Some inferonasal retina fibers, primarily peripheral fibers, may loop in Wilbrand's loop (although anatomic existence of this structure is questioned).

9.9 Is a Binasal Hemianopsia Present?

Most organic nasal visual field defects are actually arcuate in nature. Bilateral irregular nasal defects may be associated with optic disc drusen, but such defects do not obey the vertical midline and in fact are generally arcuate in nature. Binasal defects are usually due to bilateral intraocular disease of the retina or optic nerve (e.g., chronic papilledema, ischemic optic neuropathy, glaucoma, optic nerve drusen, or retinal disease such as sector retinitis pigmentosa or retinoschisis). Rarely compression of the lateral chiasm may result in a binasal defect. Bilateral nasal defect may occur with hydrocephalus with third ventricle enlargement causing lateral displacement of optic nerves against the supraclinoid portion of the internal carotid arteries. Binasal defects have also been described in patients with primary empty sella syndrome and with other suprasellar lesions.[84]

An unusual binasal visual field impairment has been noted with spontaneous intracranial hypotension from a dural cerebrospinal fluid leak.[85] Some of these patients have a binasal defect with peripheral depressions most severe in the upper

nasal quadrants but also involving the lower nasal and upper temporal quadrants.

9.10 Is a Homonymous Hemianopsia Present?

Homonymous visual field impairments appear with lesions of the retrochiasmal pathways. Those affecting the optic tract and lateral geniculate body tend to be incongruous, but the more posteriorly the lesion is located in the optic radiation, the greater the congruity of the defects. In general, tumors produce sloping field defects, whereas vascular lesions produce sharp field defects. The localization of homonymous field defects depends on the nature of the field defect and associated neuro-ophthalmologic and neurologic findings. Homonymous field defects may be caused by lesions affecting the optic tract, lateral geniculate body, optic radiations, or occipital lobe. Rarely, an occipital lesion may cause a monocular field defect (see monocular crescent, above). In general, complete homonymous hemianopias are nonlocalizing and may be seen with any lesions of the retrochiasmal pathway, including lesions of the lateral geniculate body, optic radiations, and striate cortex.

9.11 Is the Homonymous Hemianopia Caused by an Optic Tract Lesion?

In the optic tract, macular fibers lie dorsolaterally, peripheral fibers from the upper retina are situated dorsomedially, and peripheral fibers from the lower retina run ventrolaterally. Complete unilateral optic tract lesions cause a complete macular splitting homonymous hemianopia, usually without impaired visual acuity, unless the lesion extends to involve the optic chiasm or nerve. Partial optic tract lesions are more common than complete lesions and result in an incongruous field defect that may be scotomatous. (The only other postchiasmatic location for a lesion causing a scotomatous hemianopic visual field defect is the occipital lobe.) Optic tract lesions are often associated with a relative afferent pupillary defect (RAPD) in the eye with the temporal field loss (contralateral to the side of the lesion). An afferent pupillary defect in the contralateral eye in a patient with normal visual acuity bilaterally and a complete homonymous hemianopia is usually indicative of optic tract involvement.[1] Wilhelm et al described a possible exception to this clinical rule. These authors described a RAPD contralateral to the lesions in 16 of 43 patients with congruous homonymous hemianopias (optic tract lesions excluded).[86] Responsible lesions were postgeniculate and closer than 10 mm to the lateral geniculate nucleus. A RAPD did not occur in lesions farther than 18 mm from the lateral geniculate nucleus. The authors postulated that the RAPD was probably not caused by a lesion of the visual pathway per se, but by a lesion of intercalated neurons between the visual pathways and the pupillomotor centers in the pretectal area of the midbrain. Another abnormality of the pupil that may occur with optic tract lesions is due to concurrent third nerve involvement by the pathologic process causing the tract damage. In these cases, the pupil ipsilateral to the lesion may be large and poorly reactive. Finally, many patients with chronic optic tract lesions develop bilateral optic atrophy with a characteristic "wedge," "band," or "bow-tie" pallor in the contralateral eye (identical to that seen in some patients with bitemporal visual field loss from chiasmal lesions), and a more generalized pallor in the ipsilateral optic nerve associated with loss of nerve fiber layer in the superior and inferior arcuate regions corresponding to the bulk of temporal fibers subserving the nasal visual fields (hemianopic optic atrophy).[1] Hemianopic optic atrophy indicates postchiasmal, preoptic radiation involvement (i.e., optic tract or lateral geniculate body damage), but has also been rarely described in congenital retrogeniculate lesions.[1]

Etiologies of optic tract lesions include space-occupying lesions (e.g., glioma, meningioma, craniopharyngioma, metastasis, pituitary adenoma, ectopic pinealoma, abscess, and sella arachnoidal cyst), aneurysms, arteriovenous malformations, dolichoectatic basilar arteries, demyelinating disease, and trauma, including neurosurgical procedures (e.g., temporal lobectomy, insertion of intraventricular shunt).[1,87,88,89,90,91,92,93,94,95] Patients undergoing posterior pallidotomy for parkinsonism may develop mild-to-moderate contralateral homonymous superior quadrantanopias associated with small paracentral scotomas likely due to optic tract damage.[96] A congenital optic tract syndrome has also been described.[97] A complete neurologic examination and MRI, with specific attention to the optic tract region, are warranted in all patients suspected of having an optic tract lesion. If MRI fails to reveal the responsible lesion, then MR angiography or cerebral angiography may be warranted in nontraumatic cases to investigate the presence of vascular lesions (e.g., aneurysm).

9.12 Is the Homonymous Hemianopia Caused by a Lesion of the Lateral Geniculate Body?

In the lateral geniculate body, axons from ganglion cells superior to fovea are located medially, axons originating from ganglion cells inferior to fovea are located laterally, and macular fibers terminate in a large central area. As axons leave the lateral geniculate body they re-rotate back to their original positions so that within the optic radiations and the striate cortex, fibers that have synapsed with axons from superior retinas are located in superior radiations and above the calcarine fissure in the striate cortex, whereas fibers that have synapsed with axons from the inferior retinas are located in the inferior optic radiations and below the calcarine fissure. Upper field fibers originate in the medial aspect of lateral geniculate nucleus and travel through the parietal lobes, whereas lower fields originate from the lateral aspect of the lateral geniculate body and make a loop in the temporal lobe (Meyer's loop or the Meyer-Archambault loop). Lateral geniculate body lesions may also cause a complete macular splitting homonymous hemianopia.[1] Partial lesions result in an incongruous homonymous field defect. Hemianopic optic atrophy may develop and no RAPD is usually evident. Although the study of Wilhelm et al suggested that a RAPD may occasionally be present with lateral geniculate body or parageniculate optic radiation lesions,[86] this observation has not been confirmed by other investigators.

Although lesions of the optic tract or lateral geniculate body often cause incongruous field defects, two relatively specific patterns of congruous homonymous field defects with abruptly sloping borders, associated with sectorial optic atrophy, have been attributed to focal lesions of the lateral geniculate body caused by infarction in the territory of specific arteries. Occlusion of the anterior choroidal artery may cause a homonymous defect in the upper and lower quadrants with sparing of a horizontal sector (quadruple sector anopia).[98] This defect occurs because the lateral geniculate body is organized in projection columns oriented vertically that represent sectors of the field parallel to the horizontal meridians, and the anterior choroidal artery supplies the hilum and anterolateral part of the nucleus. Bilateral lateral geniculate lesions may therefore cause bilateral hourglass-shaped visual field defects[99] or bilateral blindness. In three reported cases of isolated bilateral involvement of the lateral geniculate bodies, the pathogenesis included anterior choroidal syphilitic arteritis, methanol toxicity-producing coagulative necrosis of the lateral geniculate body, and geniculate myelinolysis associated with the rapid correction of hyponatremia, respectively.[100] Barton described another patient with bilateral sector anopia ("hourglass" pattern) due to probable osmotic demyelination.[101] Interruption of the posterior lateral choroidal artery that perfuses the central portion of the lateral geniculate causes a horizontal homonymous sector defect (wedge shaped).[98,102,103,104] In posterior lateral choroidal territory infarction, the homonymous quadrantanopia may be associated with hemisensory loss and neuropsychological dysfunction (transcortical aphasia, memory disturbances), and delayed contralateral abnormal movements.[103] A homonymous horizontal sector anopia is not diagnostic of a lateral geniculate body lesion, however, as a similar sector defect may occur with lesions affecting the optic radiations[105] or, rarely, the occipital cortex in the region of the calcarine fissure,[106] the temporooccipital junction, the parietotemporal region, or in the distribution of the superficial sylvian artery territory.[107] Finally, a patient has been described with bilateral lateral geniculate lesions with bilateral sector defects with preservation of the visual fields in an hourglass distribution.[108] The patient was a 28-year-old woman who developed incongruous binasal and bitemporal visual field defects 1 week after having a febrile gastroenteritis, characterized by severe diarrhea, while traveling in Mexico. MRI demonstrated bilaterally increased signal intensity within the lateral geniculate bodies. The severe diarrhea was thought to be associated with an aseptic bilateral lateral geniculitis resulting in the hourglass-shaped visual fields. There is also documentation of a 31-year-old primigravida woman with preeclampsia developing reversible vision loss with signs of posterior reversible encephalopathy syndrome (PRES) bilaterally in the lateral geniculate regions on MRI. There were no other abnormalities noted along other parts of the retrogeniculate pathway. This patient had a previous history of migraine with aura and presented to the hospital postrupture of amniotic membranes at 38 weeks of gestation. The evidence with this patient suggests that there was hypoperfusion of choroidal vessels as a complication of the preeclampsia. Several theories about the pathogenesis have been suggested, including one that suggests that placental hypoperfusion could lead to cytokine release that may promote endothelial dysfunction causing vasogenic cerebral edema and PRES. This case also supports the notion that vasoconstriction is the pathological basis for PRES along with presenting an example of PRES causing bilateral LGN lesions.[109]

Patients with lesions of the lateral geniculate body may have no other signs or symptoms of neurologic involvement or may have associated findings related to thalamic or corticospinal tract involvement. Etiologies for lateral geniculate damage include infarction, arteriovenous malformation, trauma, tumor, inflammatory disorders, demyelinating disease, and toxic exposure (e.g., methanol).[89,98,100,102,103,108,110] MRI, with attention to the lateral geniculate region, is indicated in all cases.[102,103,111]

9.13 Is the Lesion Causing the Homonymous Hemianopia Located in the Optic Radiations?

Lesions of the proximal portion of the optic radiations may result in a complete homonymous hemianopia with macular splitting. Superior homonymous quadrantic defects ("pie-in-the-sky" field defects) may result from a lesion in the temporal (Meyer's) loop of the optic radiations or in the inferior bank of the calcarine fissure. In a study of 30 patients with superior quadrantanopias, lesions were occipital in 83%, temporal in 13%, and parietal in 3%.[112] In temporal lobe lesions, the superior quadrantic defect is usually, but not always, incongruous,[1] and the inferior margins of the defects may have sloping borders and may cross beyond the horizontal midline. Also, the ipsilateral nasal field defect is often denser and comes closer to fixation than the defect in the contralateral eye. Macular vision may or may not be involved with the quadrantic defect.[1]

Although visual field defects often may occur in isolation with temporal lobe lesions,[112] other signs of neurologic impairment may be evident.[113] With dominant temporal lobe involvement, aphasic syndromes may occur, whereas nondominant lesions may be associated with impaired recognition of facial emotional expression, sensory amusia (inability to appreciate various characteristics of music), and aprosodias (impaired appreciation of emotional overtones of spoken language). Other abnormalities seen with temporal lobe dysfunction include memory impairment and seizures. Etiologies for temporal lobe dysfunction include space-occupying lesions (e.g., tumors, abscesses, hemorrhage), arteriovenous malformations, infarction, infections, congenital malformations, demyelinating disease, and trauma (e.g., temporal lobectomy).[34,114] MRI is required in all patients.

Hughes et al studied the visual field defects in 32 patients after temporal lobe resection.[114] Visual field defects were present in 31 of the 32 patients, but none of the patients were aware of the deficits. Points nearest fixation were relatively spared, and defects were greatest in the sector closest to the vertical meridian in the eye ipsilateral to the resection. Ipsilateral and contralateral field defects differed in topography and in depth. Thus, this study demonstrated that certain fibers from the ipsilateral eye travel more anteriorly and laterally in Meyer's loop and supports the hypothesis that visual field defects due to anterior retrogeniculate lesions are incongruous because of anatomic differences in the afferent pathway.[114] There might be a difference in the incidence of visual field defects produced by anterior temporal lobectomy (ATL) versus amygdalohippocampectomy (AH) which spares lateral temporal anatomy for patients with intractable epilepsy. A study in 2000 performed both procedures found that there was no significant difference in the incidence of visual field defects between the groups. A total of 29 patients were enrolled in this study, 14 receiving AH and 15 receiving ATL.[99] However, a retrospective study in 2009 looking at the differences between ATL and AH found that proportionately the visual field defects are significantly less pronounced after AH than with ATL. This study analyzed 55 patients, 18 had undergone AH and 33 underwent ATL.[115]

Involvement of the optic radiations in the depth of the parietal lobe gives rise to a congruous homonymous hemianopia, denser below than above ("pie-on-the-floor" defect). Such defects are usually more congruous than those produced by lesions of the temporal lobe, and because the entire optic radiation passes through the parietal lobe, large lesions may produce complete homonymous hemianopia with macular splitting.[1] Patients may often be unaware of their visual field defects. Patients do not have associated pupillary abnormalities, and optic atrophy does not occur unless the responsible lesion is congenital.

In a study of 41 patients with inferior quadrantanopias, 76% were due to occipital lesions, 22% due to parietal lesions, and 2% due to temporal lesions.[112] In patients with occipital lesions, the field defects often occurred in isolation, whereas other localizing signs of parietal involvement were evident in 89% of patients with parietal lesions. Thus, although visual field defects may occur in relative isolation with parietal lobe lesions, lesions in this location more often betray themselves by other signs of neurologic dysfunction.[113] Parietal lobe lesions may be associated with contralateral somatosensory impairment, including impaired object recognition, impaired position sense, impaired touch and pain sensation, and tactile extinction. Dominant parietal lesions may cause apraxia, finger agnosia, acalculia, right–left disorientation, alexia, and aphasic disturbances, whereas nondominant lesions may be associated with anosognosia (denial of neurologic impairment), autotopagnosia (failure to recognize hemiplegic limbs as belonging to self), spatial disorientation, hemispatial neglect, constructional apraxia (abnormal drawing and copying), and dressing apraxia. Pathologic processes associated with parietal dysfunction are essentially the same as those that may cause temporal lobe dysfunction and are best evaluated by MRI.

Lepore studied nine patients with alexia without agraphia and found that three had complete right homonymous hemianopia, two had complete right homonymous hemianopia with additional binocular or monocular left field loss, two had right superior quadrantanopia, and the last two had bilateral superior or inferior quadrantanopia.[116] Right superior quadrant vision was impaired in eight patients, and no patient demonstrated an isolated right inferior quadrantanopia or an isolated left homonymous field defect. No patient attained 20/20 visual acuity bilaterally. Lepore concluded that bilateral visual field loss and decreased visual acuity occur in many cases of alexia without agraphia. The frequent presence of a right superior quadrantic field defect implies a critical role in reading for the ventral outflow pathways of the dominant calcarine cortex. Although right homonymous hemianopia and a left occipital lobe and splenium lesions remain the paradigm for alexia without agraphia, bilateral field loss, decreased visual acuity, and bihemispheric disease are common and may adversely affect the integrity of neural reading mechanisms.

Most pure alexia (alexia without agraphia) is caused by a single lesion to the dominant visual cortex also involving the splenium. There is a report of a 56-year-old right-handed male patient with right homonymous hemianopia reported to have a pure alexia caused by separate lesions in the splenium and the optic radiation. Magnetic resonance angiography revealed mild stenosis at the origin of the right vertebral artery and there was also stenosis of the left distal posterior cerebral artery. This pattern of lesions also sheds light onto the mechanism for developing pure alexia.[117]

9.14 Is the Visual Field Defect Caused by an Occipital Lesion?

Homonymous quadrantic visual field defects may occur with unilateral occipital lesions.[118] Superior quadrantic defects may be seen with inferior calcarine lesions, and inferior quadrantic defects may occur with superior calcarine lesions. A patient with a neurologically isolated quadrantanopia is likely to have a lesion in the occipital lobe, although, in the case of a superior quadrantanopia, the possibility of a temporal lobe lesion cannot be excluded using clinical criteria only.[112] As noted earlier, quadrantanopias caused by lesions of the parietal lobe usually are associated with other localizing signs.[112] Often field defects due to calcarine lesions have a sharp horizontal edge that would not be caused by tumors or trauma because it is unlikely that they would injure only one bank of the calcarine fissure and leave the fellow calcarine bank untouched. Horton and Hoyt suggested that a lesion of the extrastriate cortex (areas V2 and V3) would be more likely to explain the sharp horizontal edge of the defect because areas V2 and V3 are divided along the horizontal meridian into separate halves flanking the striate (V1) cortex and, consequently, the upper and lower quadrants in extrastriate cortex are physically isolated on opposite sides of the striate cortex.[119] Although a lesion in this location (e.g., a tumor) may have irregular margins, if it crosses the representation of the horizontal meridian in extrastriate cortex it will produce a quadrantic visual field defect with a sharp horizontal border because of the split layout of the upper and lower quadrants of V2/V3. Thus, a homonymous quadrantanopia respecting the horizontal meridian is not a "pathognomonic" sign of extrastriate cortical disease but may occur with striate lesions.[120] A congruous inferior quadrantanopia with borders aligned on both the vertical and horizontal meridians has also been described with a lesion of the superior fibers of the optic radiations near the contralateral trigone where the fascicles of visual axons become compact as they approach the calcarine cortex.[121]

Gray et al reported two patients with unique homonymous hemianopias from occipital lesions.[122] One patient had vertical meridian sparing and the other displayed horizontal meridian sparing. MRI correlation with the defects confirmed that the vertical hemianopic meridian is represented along the border of the calcarine lip and the horizontal meridian lies at the base of the calcarine banks deep within the calcarine fissure. Galetta and Grossman reported two patients further demonstrating that the horizontal meridian is represented at the calcarine fissure base in the primary visual cortex.[123]

Medial occipital lesions cause highly congruous homonymous field defects.[85,124,125] When both the upper and the lower calcarine cortices are affected, a complete homonymous hemianopia, usually with macular sparing, develops. Sparing of the central 5 degrees of vision (macular sparing) is common with occipital lesions, probably due to a combination of a large macular representation and dual blood supply.[1] The central 10 to 15 degrees of vision fill a majority of the total surface area of the occipital cortex (as much as 50–60%).[85,126,127,128] The authors considers macular sparing to be present when at least 5 degrees of central visual field is spared; macular sparing of 3 degrees or less may be due to wandering fixation and may not be clinically meaningful. Patients with purely occipital lesions are often aware of the hemianopia, whereas patients with larger or more anterior lesions, affecting parietal regions or associative pathways to the primary or secondary visual association cortex, may be unaware of their deficit. Celesia et al, however, prospectively studied 32 consecutive patients with homonymous field defects caused by ischemic infarcts and found hemianopic anosognosia, defined as the unawareness of visual loss in the homonymous hemifield (or hemiquadrant) in 20 patients (63%).[129] Hemianopic anosognosia occurred predominantly in right-sided lesions (16 of 26 patients or 62%), but also was present in 4 of 6 patients (67%) with left-sided lesions. Hemianopic anosognosia was associated with somatic anosognosia in 9 patients and hemineglect in 17 patients. Eight patients had pure homonymous hemianopia without cognitive, motor, or somatosensory deficits; four of these patients had awareness of visual defect and three had hemianopic anosognosia. Patients in these two groups had similar anatomic lesions. Patients with phosphenes, photopsias, or visual hallucinations were usually aware of their visual field loss. The authors suggest that hemianopic anosognosia is most often related to failure of discovery of the deficits, occasionally with severe visual hemineglect, sometimes to generalized cognitive impairment, or to a combination of these factors. The authors further conclude (1) there is no specific cortical area for conscious visual perception; (2) visual awareness is processed by a distributed network including multiple visual cortices, parietal and frontal lobes, the pulvinar, and the lateral geniculate bodies (lesions localized at various nodes or centers in the network may produce similar phenomena); and (3) both hemispheres are involved in visual processing and conscious awareness.

Ogawa et al analyzed lesions between the occipital tip and the posterior portion of the medial area of the striate cortex. The study found that central homonymous hemianopia tended to be incomplete in patients with lesions in the posterior portion of the medial area of the striate. However, patients with occipital tip lesions suffered from complete central homonymous hemianopia and quadrantanopia. Ogawa et al suggested that fibers related to the central visual field are less dense in the posterior portion of the medial area compared to the occipital tip. The authors also concluded the concentration of fibers increases when approaching the occipital tip.[130]

Lesions of the striate cortex may be classified as anterior, intermediate, or posterior.[1,4,85,127] Anterior lesions lie adjacent to the parieto-occipital fissure and affect the monocular temporal crescent of the contralateral visual field (temporal crescent or half-moon syndrome). This area constitutes less than 10% of the total surface area of the striate cortex and the defect begins approximately 60 degrees from fixation. Both upper and lower temporal crescents may be scotomatous in the field of one eye, or only the upper or lower temporal crescent may be involved. Conversely, the temporal crescent may be spared with lesions that destroy the entire calcarine cortex except for the anterior tip.[4,5] Posterior lesions are located in the posterior 50 to 60% of the striate cortex, including the occipital pole and operculum, affect macular vision (i.e., the central 10 degrees in the contralateral hemifield), and therefore cause scotomatous defects. Intermediate lesions lie between the anterior and posterior confines and affect from 10 to 60 degrees in the contralateral hemifield. The most common cause of unilateral occipital disease is infarction in the distribution of the posterior cerebral artery.[124,125,131] Other etiologies include venous infarction, hemorrhage, arteriovenous malformation and fistulas, tumor, abscess, and trauma.[91,92,132,133,134] Thus, MRI is warranted in all patients.

Bilateral occipital lobe lesions may occur from a single or from consecutive events and may cause bilateral homonymous scotomas, usually with some macular sparing ("ring" scotomas) that respects the vertical midline.[1] In some cases, there may be "tunnel" or "keyhole" fields with bilateral complete homonymous hemianopias except for macular sparing. Careful testing in these cases reveals that the macular sparing respects the vertical midline. Bilateral lesions affecting the superior or inferior calcarine cortices may produce bilateral altitudinal defects that may mimic the visual field abnormalities seen with bilateral optic nerve or retinal disease.[135,136] Bilateral upper calcarine bank lesions may have associated neurologic findings including Balint syndrome (apraxia of gaze, optic ataxia, decreased visual attention, and simultanagnosia), abnormal depth perception, defective revisualization of spatial relations, topographic disorientation, and disorientation to place.[113,137] Bilateral lesions of the inferior banks of the calcarine fissure may be associated with prosopagnosia (inability to identify faces visually), cerebral dyschromatopsia, amnesia, and difficulty revisualizing the morphology and appearance of people and objects.[113,137] Bilateral lesions of the visual cortices, often due to large bilateral posterior cerebral artery infarcts involving both banks of the calcarine fissure and both temporal lobes, cause cortical blindness often associated with agitated delirium and amnesia.[113,137]

Cortical blindness implies visual impairment due to discrete involvement of the occipital cortices bilaterally, whereas cerebral blindness is a more general term indicating visual loss from any process affecting the retrogeniculate visual pathways. The essential features of cortical and cerebral blindness include complete loss of all visual sensation including all appreciation of light and dark; loss of reflex lid closure to bright illumination and to threatening gestures; retention of the reflex constriction of the pupils to illumination and to convergence movements; and integrity of the normal structure of the retina as verified by ophthalmoscopy.[1] There are many etiologies of cerebral and cortical blindness, including hypoxia, infarction, hemorrhage, eclampsia, hypertensive encephalopathy, tentorial herniation from cerebral mass, tumor, arteriovenous malformation, infection (e.g., progressive multifocal leukoencephalopathy, Creutzfeldt-Jakob disease (CJD), subacute sclerosing panencephalitis, HIV encephalitis, syphilis, encephalitis, abscess), inflammation (e.g., sarcoidosis), demyelinating disease, trauma, metabolic disorders (e.g., adrenoleukodystrophy, hypoglycemia, porphyria, mitochondrial encephalopathies), toxins (e.g., lead, mercury, ethanol, carbon monoxide), medications (e.g., cyclosporine, tacrolimus, interleukin-2), radiation encephalopathy, Alzheimer disease, postictal after seizures, and complications of cerebral angiography.[1,131,138,139,140,141,142,143,144] Occasionally, patients with cortical blindness deny their visual defect (Anton's syndrome).

9.15 What If a Homonymous Visual Field Defect Is Present But Neuroimaging Is Normal?

As noted earlier, MRI is indicated in all patients with a homonymous visual field defect, except in acute or traumatic cases, in which computed tomography (CT) imaging is usually adequate, or in patients in whom MRI is contraindicated (e.g., ferromagnetic aneurysmal clip, metallic fragments, and pacemakers). There are several clinical situations in which MRI may be normal in a patient with a homonymous hemianopia[145]:

1. Homonymous hemianopia or cortical blindness may be an early or initial finding in some patients with the Heidenhain variant of CJD, and in most of these patients routine MRI or CT is normal.[145,146,147,148,149,150] Some patients, however, will have symmetric hyperintensities in the basal ganglia and/or gray matter of the occipital cortex on T2-weighted and proton-weighted images,[151] and some will have abnormalities in the cortex, basal ganglia, and thalamus on diffusion-weighted MRI.[148,152,153,154,155,156,157] Bilateral symmetric, high signal intensities on T2-weighted images were present in the basal ganglia of 109 (67%) of 162 patients with CJD, and thus MRI was thought to be reasonably sensitive (67%) and highly specific (93%) in the diagnosis of this entity.[158] The electroencephalogram (EEG) is often initially normal in these patients, although it usually eventually shows characteristic periodic complexes in most patients. Patients soon also develop mentation impairment, myoclonus, and other signs of CJD, but initially the diagnosis may be quite difficult. Abnormalities in the cerebrospinal fluid, such as the presence of 14–3–3 protein or neuron-specific enolase, may assist in the diagnosis.[151,156,157,159,160,161,162,163,164,165] For example, the presence of the 14–3–3 brain protein in the cerebrospinal fluid has a positive predictive value for CJD of 94.7%, whereas its absence has a negative predictive value of 92.4%.[161,164] In other studies, the sensitivity was 94 to 97% and the specificity 74 to 87%.[156,157,162] False negatives have been documented[166] and false positives have been noted with herpes simplex encephalitis, meningoencephalitis, stroke, hypoxic brain injury, carcinomatous meningitis, vascular dementia, Hashimoto encephalopathy, intracerebral metastasis, frontotemporal dementia, dementia with Lewy bodies, and Alzheimer disease.[162,164,166,167,168] The 14–3–3 protein assay may be positive in paraneoplastic neurologic disorders that may mimic CJD, but the immunoblasting pattern of this protein distinguishes most patients with paraneoplastic disorders from those with CJD.[169]

2. Some patients with Alzheimer disease or Lewy body disease may develop a homonymous field defect.[145,170,171] MRI may be normal or show only diffuse atrophy, and the EEG is normal or shows only mild diffuse slowing. This diagnosis is suspected in patients with a slowly progressive dementia without other "focal" neurologic findings, and the dementia usually far outweighs the visual field impairment. However, some patients may present with visual changes prior to more significant decline in other cognitive areas. Dyslexia, incomplete homonymous hemianopia, preserved color identification with abnormal color vision on Ishihara, and simultanagnosia have been reported in patients with visual variant of Alzheimer disease (VVAD).[172]

3. Most patients with field defects from cerebral infarction or hypoxia demonstrate MRI changes compatible with ischemia. However, Moster et al described two patients, one with bilateral homonymous congruous hemianopic central scotomata after carbon monoxide poisoning and the other with bilateral congruous inferior visual scotomata after global hypoxia, who were initially diagnosed with "functional" visual loss.[173] Neither CT nor MRI adequately demonstrated the source of the visual dysfunction, but single photon emission computed tomography (SPECT) in one patient and positron emission tomography (PET) imaging in the other confirmed the organic substrate of the visual impairment. Wang et al also reported two patients with organophosphate intoxication associated with cortical visual loss who had normal MRI but abnormal hypometabolism of the visual cortex demonstrated on PET scanning.[174] Brazis et al also presented a patient with a homonymous visual field defect secondary to cerebral infarction with normal MRI.[145] Functional imaging techniques, such as SPECT or PET, should thus be considered in patients with suspected cortical visual loss and normal CT or MRI studies. Functional MRI is also a possible method for the objective detection of abnormalities in the afferent visual system.[175]

4. Transient homonymous hemianopia with normal CT imaging has rarely been reported with nonketotic hyperglycemia.[145,176] These patients had other positive visual phenomena associated with a homonymous hemianopia. Thus, nonketotic hyperglycemia may present with positive visual phenomena associated with a homonymous field defect and normal neuroimaging.

5. Functional (nonorganic) hemianopias are associated with normal imaging studies.[177,178,179] One method of determining if a field defect is nonorganic is to test saccadic eye movements into the supposedly absent portion of the field, with the patient assuming that eye movements and not visual fields are being tested. Demonstrating "hemianopic" defects with both eyes open is often useful.[177] Another method is to place a 30-diopter Fresnel prism into the upper quadrants of a trial frame.[180] After visual fields are obtained without the prism, the prism is placed first base-out and then base-in, and with each change the fields are repeated. Patients with pathologic hemianopsias shift their superior field 15 degrees to the right or to the left of the central vertical meridian with the prism base-in or -out, respectively, whereas patients with suspected functional hemifield defect do not shift their superior sectors in a similar fashion.

9.16 What Treatments Can Be Offered to Patients with Homonymous Hemianopias?

Treatment of processes causing visual field impairment is directed at the underlying etiology. Unfortunately, patients with homonymous hemianopias have a consistently poor rehabilitation outcome, with no more than 20% of patients undergoing spontaneous recovery within the first several months of brain injury.[181,182]

Smith suggested the use of Fresnel press-on prisms in patients with homonymous hemianopia.[183] The prism is placed on the outside half of the lens ipsilateral to the hemianopia with the base toward that side (e.g., for a patient with a right homonymous hemianopia, a 15- to 30-diopter prism is placed base-out on the right half of the right lens). The goal is to increase the patient's scanning skills. Although prisms may help some patients, and although patients with the prisms perform significantly better than controls on visual perception tasks, there is overall no difference in activities of daily living functioning.[184]

Moss et al used monocular sector prisms to get two patients with complete homonymous hemianopia to vision that meets qualifications to legally drive. Both patients were fitted with glasses and press-on 57-PD peripheral monocular sector prisms on the lens ipsilateral to the VF defect with prisms oriented obliquely above and below the visual axis. Kinetic perimetry was reassessed both monocularly and binocularly (with and without prisms). The patients were a 24-year-old male and a 31-year-old male, both suffered a stroke that damaged their visual fields. The patients had 95- and 82-degree angle of continuous, horizontal, binocular VF before using the prisms, and increased their binocular VF to 115- and 112-degree angles, respectively, after using the prisms.[185]

Reading problems are common in patients with homonymous field defects.[186] Patients with right hemianopias cannot see which letters or words follow those they have already read, and patients with left hemianopias often lose their place when reading, beginning again on an unrelated line. A right homonymous hemianopia also disrupts the motor preparation of reading saccades during text reading.[186] A ruler to guide the patient's vision is often useful, and some patients with hemianopias can improve their reading by turning the material 90 degrees and reading vertically in their intact hemifields. Hemianopic patients may also be trained to perform large saccades into the blind field and to search their entire field in various patterns, resulting in some visual improvement.[181,187]

Patients with cortical or cerebral blindness with some visual preservation may benefit by referral to low-vision specialists for instruction in various visual aids to assist reading and other daily activities. Restorative rehabilitation programs addressing neuronal plasticity have not shown to be effective as of yet. Studies suggest that neuronal cortical plasticity in adulthood have the potential to be the target for treatment and visual rehabilitation in the future. Currently, visual restoration and rehabilitation has not shown to be effective in clinical practice mainly because the physiological processes are not understood clearly.[188]

9.17 What Should Be Done with an Unexplained Visual Field Defect?

Patients with an unexplained unilateral or bilateral visual field defect should have careful attention paid to the corresponding areas of the retina and optic nerve on ophthalmoscopy. Some patients may have occult retinal and/or choroidal vascular disease that may be detected only by timed and directed (to the location predicted by the visual field defect) fluorescein angiography.[189] Visual defects respecting the vertical midline with a bitemporal or homonymous "flavor" should undergo a neuroimaging study. Rarely, patients with unilateral or bilateral nasal defects respecting the vertical midline may harbor an underlying compressive lesion.[1] In addition, apparently altitudinal (superior or inferior) bilateral visual field defects may actually represent bilateral lesions of the optic nerves or retrochiasmal pathway.

Constriction of the visual fields may occur in media opacities, miotic pupils, or uncorrected refractive error; as an artifact of testing; in occult retinal disease (e.g., retinitis pigmentosa, CAR, etc.); with any optic neuropathy (e.g., optic neuritis, ischemic optic neuropathy, and glaucoma); with bilateral retrochiasmal lesions (e.g., occipital stroke); or in nonorganic patients. In fact, any combination of these entities (e.g., an optic neuropathy and a retrochiasmal homonymous hemianopsia) may produce any number of combinations of associated visual field defects. The simple algorithm presented obviously cannot account for every one of these combinations. Electrophysiologic testing such as electroretinography, visual-evoked potentials, and other ancillary testing such as fluorescein angiography may disclose an abnormality in the retina or optic nerve even in the absence of an ophthalmoscopically visible lesion. Pattern visual-evoked potentials aid in the diagnosis of functional visual loss.[190] Testing confrontational visual fields at both 1 and 2 meter testing may disclose a nonorganic "tunnel" visual field compared with an organic "funnel" and physiologically expanded visual field.

References

[1] Miller NR, Newman NJ. Topical diagnosis of lesions in the visual sensory pathway. In: Miller NR, Newman NJ, eds. Walsh and Hoyt's Clinical Neuro-ophthalmology. 5th ed. Baltimore: Williams & Wilkins; 1998:237–386

[2] Mojon DS, Odel JG, Rios RJ, Hirano M. Pituitary adenoma revealed by paracentral junctional scotoma of Traquair. Ophthalmologica. 1997; 211(2): 104–108

[3] Chavis PS, al-Hazmi A, Clunie D, Hoyt WF. Temporal crescent syndrome with magnetic resonance correlation. J Neuroophthalmol. 1997; 17(3):151–155

[4] Landau K, Wichmann W, Valavanis A. The missing temporal crescent. Am J Ophthalmol. 1995; 119(3):345–349

[5] Lepore FE. The preserved temporal crescent: the clinical implications of an "endangered" finding. Neurology. 2001; 57(10):1918–1921

[6] Horton JC. Wilbrand's knee of the primate optic chiasm is an artefact of monocular enucleation. Trans Am Ophthalmol Soc. 1997; 95:579–609

[7] Lee JH, Tobias S, Kwon JT, Sade B, Kosmorsky G. Wilbrand's knee: does it exist? Surg Neurol. 2006; 66(1):11–17, discussion 17

[8] Karanjia N, Jacobson DM. Compression of the prechiasmatic optic nerve produces a junctional scotoma. Am J Ophthalmol. 1999; 128(2):256–258

[9] Trobe JD, Glaser JS. The Visual Fields Manual: A Practical Guide to Testing and Interpretation. Gainesville, FL: Triad; 1983:176

[10] Hershenfeld SA, Sharpe JA. Monocular temporal hemianopia. Br J Ophthalmol. 1993; 77(7):424–427

[11] Bills DC, Meyer FB, Laws ER, Jr, et al. A retrospective analysis of pituitary apoplexy. Neurosurgery. 1993; 33(4):602–608, discussion 608–609

[12] Biousse V, Newman NJ, Oyesiku NM. Precipitating factors in pituitary apoplexy. J Neurol Neurosurg Psychiatry. 2001; 71(4):542–545

[13] Embil JM, Kramer M, Kinnear S, Light RB. A blinding headache. Lancet. 1997; 350(9072):182

[14] Abe T, Matsumoto K, Kuwazawa J, Toyoda I, Sasaki K. Headache associated with pituitary adenomas. Headache. 1998; 38(10):782–786

[15] Ikeda H, Yoshimoto T. Visual disturbances in patients with pituitary adenoma. Acta Neurol Scand. 1995; 92(2):157–160

[16] Kerrison JB, Lynn MJ, Baer CA, Newman SA, Biousse V, Newman NJ. Stages of improvement in visual fields after pituitary tumor resection. Am J Ophthalmol. 2000; 130(6):813–820

[17] Kupersmith MJ, Rosenberg C, Kleinberg D. Visual loss in pregnant women with pituitary adenomas. Ann Intern Med. 1994; 121(7):473–477

[18] Lee AG, Sforza PD, Fard AK, Repka MX, Baskin DS, Dauser RC. Pituitary adenoma in children. J Neuroophthalmol. 1998; 18(2):102–105

[19] Peter M, De Tribolet N. Visual outcome after transsphenoidal surgery for pituitary adenomas. Br J Neurosurg. 1995; 9(2):151–157

[20] Petruson B, Jakobsson KE, Elfverson J, Bengtsson BA. Five-year follow-up of nonsecreting pituitary adenomas. Arch Otolaryngol Head Neck Surg. 1995; 121(3):317–322

[21] Duru S, Ceylan S, Ceylan S. Optic chiasm diastasis in a pituitary tumor. Case illustration. J Neurosurg. 1999; 90(2):363

[22] Kinjo T, al-Mefty O, Ciric I. Diaphragma sellae meningiomas. Neurosurgery. 1995; 36(6):1082–1092

[23] Fahlbusch R, Honegger J, Paulus W, Huk W, Buchfelder M. Surgical treatment of craniopharyngiomas: experience with 168 patients. J Neurosurg. 1999; 90(2):237–250

[24] Honegger J, Buchfelder M, Fahlbusch R. Surgical treatment of craniopharyngiomas: endocrinological results. J Neurosurg. 1999; 90(2): 251–257

[25] Mikelberg FS, Yidegiligne HM. Axonal loss in band atrophy of the optic nerve in craniopharyngioma: a quantitative analysis. Can J Ophthalmol. 1993; 28(2):69–71

[26] Cirak B, Unal O, Arslan H, Cinal A. Chiasmatic glioblastoma of childhood. A case report. Acta Radiol. 2000; 41(4):375–376

[27] Miyairi Y, Tada T, Tanaka Y, Hongo K, Kobayashi S. Anaplastic astrocytoma invading the optic chiasm through the optic pathway. J Neurosurg. 2000; 93 (4):716

[28] Rossi LN, Pastorino G, Scotti G, et al. Early diagnosis of optic glioma in children with neurofibromatosis type 1. Childs Nerv Syst. 1994; 10(7): 426–429

[29] Cobbs CS, Wilson CB. Intrasellar cavernous hemangioma. Case report. J Neurosurg. 2001; 94(3):520–522

[30] Hwang JF, Yau CW, Huang JK, Tsai CY. Apoplectic optochiasmal syndrome due to intrinsic cavernous hemangioma. Case report. J Clin Neuroophthalmol. 1993; 13(4):232–236

[31] Pakzaban P, Westmark K, Westmark R. Chiasmal apoplexy due to hemorrhage from a pituitary adenoma into the optic chiasm: case report. Neurosurgery. 2000; 46(6):1511–1513, discussion 1513–1514

[32] Bladowska J, Bednarek-Tupikowska G, Biel A, Sąsiadek M. Colloid cyst of the pituitary gland: case report and literature review. Pol J Radiol. 2010; 75(2): 88–93

[33] Jacobson DM. Symptomatic compression of the optic nerve by the carotid artery: clinical profile of 18 patients with 24 affected eyes identified by magnetic resonance imaging. Ophthalmology. 1999; 106(10):1994–2004

[34] Slavin ML. Bitemporal hemianopia associated with dolichoectasia of the intracranial carotid arteries. J Clin Neuroophthalmol. 1990; 10(1):80–81

[35] Aarabi B, Haghshenas M, Rakeii V. Visual failure caused by suprasellar extramedullary hematopoiesis in beta thalassemia: case report. Neurosurgery. 1998; 42(4):922–925, discussion 925–926

[36] McCowen KC, Glickman JN, Black PM, Zervas NT, Lidov HG, Garber JR. Gangliocytoma masquerading as a prolactinoma. Case report. J Neurosurg. 1999; 91(3):490–495

[37] Liu GT, Galetta SL, Rorke LB, et al. Gangliogliomas involving the optic chiasm. Neurology. 1996; 46(6):1669–1673

[38] Sawin PD, Follett KA, Wen BC, Laws ER, Jr. Symptomatic intrasellar hemangioblastoma in a child treated with subtotal resection and adjuvant radiosurgery. Case report. J Neurosurg. 1996; 84(6):1046–1050

[39] Bourekas EC, Tzalonikou M, Christoforidis GA. Case 1. Cavernous hemangioma of the optic chiasm. AJR Am J Roentgenol. 2000; 175(3): 888–891, 891

[40] Job OM, Schatz NJ, Glaser JS. Visual loss with Langerhans cell histiocytosis: multifocal central nervous system involvement. J Neuroophthalmol. 1999; 19(1):49–53

[41] Lee AG, Tang RA, Roberts D, Schiffman JS, Osborne A. Primary central nervous system lymphoma involving the optic chiasm in AIDS. J Neuroophthalmol. 2001; 21(2):95–98

[42] McFadzean RM, McIlwaine GG, McLellan D. Hodgkin's disease at the optic chiasm. J Clin Neuroophthalmol. 1990; 10(4):248–254

[43] Abe T, Matsumoto K, Sanno N, Osamura Y. Lymphocytic hypophysitis: case report. Neurosurgery. 1995; 36(5):1016–1019

[44] Beressi N, Cohen R, Beressi J-P, et al. Pseudotumoral lymphocytic hypophysitis successfully treated by corticosteroid alone: first case report. Neurosurgery. 1994; 35(3):505–508, discussion 508

[45] Honegger J, Fahlbusch R, Bornemann A, et al. Lymphocytic and granulomatous hypophysitis: experience with nine cases. Neurosurgery. 1997; 40(4):713–722, discussion 722–723

[46] Jabre A, Rosales R, Reed JE, Spatz EL. Lymphocytic hypophysitis. J Neurol Neurosurg Psychiatry. 1997; 63(5):672–673

[47] Kerrison JB, Lee AG, Weinstein JM. Acute loss of vision during pregnancy due to a suprasellar mass. Surv Ophthalmol. 1997; 41(5):402–408

[48] Kristof RA, Van Roost D, Klingmüller D, Springer W, Schramm J. Lymphocytic hypophysitis: non-invasive diagnosis and treatment by high dose methylprednisolone pulse therapy? J Neurol Neurosurg Psychiatry. 1999; 67(3):398–402

[49] Lee J-H, Laws ER, Jr, Guthrie BL, Dina TS, Nochomovitz LE. Lymphocytic hypophysitis: occurrence in two men. Neurosurgery. 1994; 34(1):159–162, discussion 162–163

[50] Naik RG, Ammini A, Shah P, Sarkar C, Mehta VS, Berry M. Lymphocytic hypophysitis. Case report. J Neurosurg. 1994; 80(5):925–927

[51] Nishioka H, Ito H, Fukushima C. Recurrent lymphocytic hypophysitis: case report. Neurosurgery. 1997; 41(3):684–686, discussion 686–687

[52] Stelmach M, O'Day J. Rapid change in visual fields associated with suprasellar lymphocytic hypophysitis. J Clin Neuroophthalmol. 1991; 11(1):19–24

[53] Thodou E, Asa SL, Kontogeorgos G, Kovacs K, Horvath E, Ezzat S. Clinical case seminar: lymphocytic hypophysitis: clinicopathological findings. J Clin Endocrinol Metab. 1995; 80(8):2302–2311

[54] Tubridy N, Molloy J, Saunders D, Belli A, Powell M, Plant GT. Postpartum pituitary hypophysitis. J Neuroophthalmol. 2001; 21(2):106–108

[55] Galetta SL, Stadtmauer EA, Hicks DG, Raps EC, Plock G, Oberholtzer JC. Reactive lymphohistiocytosis with recurrence in the optic chiasm. J Clin Neuroophthalmol. 1991; 11(1):25–30

[56] Aubin MJ, Hardy J, Comtois R. Primary sellar haemorrhagic melanoma: case report and review of the literature. Br J Neurosurg. 1997; 11(1):80–83

[57] Baeesa SS, Benoit BG. Solitary metastasis of breast carcinoma in the optic chiasm. Br J Neurosurg. 1999; 13(3):319–321

[58] Morita A, Meyer FB, Laws ER, Jr. Symptomatic pituitary metastases. J Neurosurg. 1998; 89(1):69–73

[59] el-Mahdy W, Powell M. Transsphenoidal management of 28 symptomatic Rathke's cleft cysts, with special reference to visual and hormonal recovery. Neurosurgery. 1998; 42(1):7–16, discussion 16–17

[60] Fischer EG, DeGirolami U, Suojanen JN. Reversible visual deficit following debulking of a Rathke's cleft cyst: a tethered chiasm? J Neurosurg. 1994; 81(3):459–462

[61] Rao GP, Blyth CP, Jeffreys RV. Ophthalmic manifestations of Rathke's cleft cysts. Am J Ophthalmol. 1995; 119(1):86–91

[62] Voelker JL, Campbell RL, Muller J. Clinical, radiographic, and pathological features of symptomatic Rathke's cleft cysts. J Neurosurg. 1991; 74(4):535–544

[63] Yamamoto M, Jimbo M, Ide M, Umebara Y, Hagiwara S, Kubo O. Recurrence of symptomatic Rathke's cleft cyst: a case report. Surg Neurol. 1993; 39(4):263–268

[64] Arita K, Sugiyama K, Tominaga A, Yamasaki F. Intrasellar rhabdomyosarcoma: case report. Neurosurgery. 2001; 48(3):677–680

[65] Wolansky LJ, Shaderowfsky PD, Sander R, Frohman LP, Kalnin AJ, Lee HJ. Optic chiasmal compression by venous aneurysm: magnetic resonance imaging diagnosis. J Neuroimaging. 1997; 7(1):46–47

[66] Bogdanovic MD, Plant GT. Chiasmal compression due to obstructive hydrocephalus. J Neuroophthalmol. 2000; 20(4):266–267

[67] Wilhelm H, Grodd W, Schiefer U, Zrenner E. Uncommon chiasmal lesions: demyelinating disease, vasculitis, and cobalamin deficiency. Ger J Ophthalmol. 1993; 2(4–5):234–240

[68] Newman NJ, Lessell S, Winterkorn JM. Optic chiasmal neuritis. Neurology. 1991; 41(8):1203–1210

[69] Kosmorsky GS, Straga JM. A descent thing to do for the chiasm. J Neuroophthalmol. 1997; 17(1):53–56

[70] Chang GY, Keane JR. Visual loss in cysticercosis: analysis of 23 patients. Neurology. 2001; 57(3):545–548

[71] Beiran I, Krasnitz I, Zimhoni-Eibsitz M, Gelfand YA, Miller B. Paediatric chiasmal neuritis-typical of post-Epstein-Barr virus infection? Acta Ophthalmol Scand. 2000; 78(2):226–227

[72] Lee BL, Holland GN, Glasgow BJO. Chiasmal infarction and sudden blindness caused by mucormycosis in AIDS and diabetes mellitus. Am J Ophthalmol. 1996; 122(6):895–896

[73] Frohman LP, Frieman BJ, Wolansky L. Reversible blindness resulting from optic chiasmitis secondary to systemic lupus erythematosus. J Neuroophthalmol. 2001; 21(1):18–21

[74] Siatkowski RM, Scott IU, Verm AM, et al. Optic neuropathy and chiasmopathy in the diagnosis of systemic lupus erythematosus. J Neuroophthalmol. 2001; 21(3):193–198

[75] Danesh-Meyer H, Kubis KC, Wolf MA, Lessell S. Chiasmopathy? Surv Ophthalmol. 2000; 44(4):329–335

[76] Carter K, Lee AG, Tang RA, et al. Neuro-ophthalmologic complications of sinus surgery. Neuroophthalmology. 1998; 19:75–82

[77] Domingo Z, de Villiers JC. Post-traumatic chiasmatic disruption. Br J Neurosurg. 1993; 7(2):141–147

[78] Heinz GW, Nunery WR, Grossman CB. Traumatic chiasmal syndrome associated with midline basilar skull fractures. Am J Ophthalmol. 1994; 117(1):90–96

[79] McHenry JG, Spoor TC. Chiasmal compression from fat packing after transsphenoidal resection of intrasellar tumor in two patients. Am J Ophthalmol. 1993; 116(2):253

[80] Slavin ML, Lam BL, Decker RE, Schatz NJ, Glaser JS, Reynolds MG. Chiasmal compression from fat packing after transsphenoidal resection of intrasellar tumor in two patients. Am J Ophthalmol. 1993; 115(3):368–371

[81] Czech T, Wolfsberger S, Reitner A, Görzer H. Delayed visual deterioration after surgery for pituitary adenoma. Acta Neurochir (Wien). 1999; 141(1):45–51

[82] Pomeranz HD, Lessell S. A hereditary chiasmal optic neuropathy. Arch Ophthalmol. 1999; 117(1):128–131

[83] Miele DL, Odel JG, Behrens MM, Zhang X, Hood DC. Functional bitemporal quadrantopia and the multifocal visual evoked potential. J Neuroophthalmol. 2000; 20(3):159–162

[84] Charteris DG, Cullen JF. Binasal field defects in primary empty sella syndrome. J Neuroophthalmol. 1996; 16(2):110–114

[85] Horton JC, Fishman RA. Neurovisual findings in the syndrome of spontaneous intracranial hypotension from dural cerebrospinal fluid leak. Ophthalmology. 1994; 101(2):244–251

[86] Wilhelm H, Wilhelm B, Petersen D, et al. Relative afferent pupillary defects in patients with geniculate and retrogeniculate lesions. Neuro-ophthalmology. 1996; 16(4):219–224

[87] Chun BB, Lee AG, Coughlin WF, Floyd DT, May EF. Unusual presentations of sellar arachnoid cyst. J Neuroophthalmol. 1998; 18(4):246–249

[88] Freitag SK, Miller NR, Kosmorsky G. Visual loss in a 42-year-old man. Surv Ophthalmol. 2000; 44(6):507–512

[89] Groom M, Kay MD, Vicinanza-Adami C, Santini R. Optic tract syndrome secondary to metastatic breast cancer. Am J Ophthalmol. 1998; 125(1):115–118

[90] Guirgis MF, Lam BL, Falcone SF. Optic tract compression from dolichoectatic basilar artery. Am J Ophthalmol. 2001; 132(2):283–286

[91] Liu GT, Galetta SL. Homonymous hemifield loss in childhood. Neurology. 1997; 49(6):1748–1749

[92] Molia L, Winterkorn JMS, Schneider SJ. Hemianopic visual field defects in children with intracranial shunts: report of two cases. Neurosurgery. 1996; 39(3):599–603

[93] Shults WT, Hamby S, Corbett JJ, Kardon R, Winterkorn JS, Odel JG. Neuro-ophthalmic complications of intracranial catheters. Neurosurgery. 1993; 33(1):135–138

[94] Slavin ML. Acute homonymous field loss: really a diagnostic dilemma. Surv Ophthalmol. 1990; 34(5):399–407

[95] Vargas ME, Kupersmith MJ, Setton A, Nelson K, Berenstein A. Endovascular treatment of giant aneurysms which cause visual loss. Ophthalmology. 1994; 101(6):1091–1098

[96] Biousse V, Newman NJ, Carroll C, et al. Visual fields in patients with posterior GPi pallidotomy. Neurology. 1998; 50(1):258–265

[97] Murphy MA, Grosof DH, Hart WM, Jr. Congenital optic tract syndrome: magnetic resonance imaging and scanning laser ophthalmoscopy findings. J Neuroophthalmol. 1997; 17(4):226–230

[98] Luco C, Hoppe A, Schweitzer M, Vicuña X, Fantin A. Visual field defects in vascular lesions of the lateral geniculate body. J Neurol Neurosurg Psychiatry. 1992; 55(1):12–15

[99] Egan RA, Shults WT, So N, Burchiel K, Kellogg JX, Salinsky M. Visual field deficits in conventional anterior temporal lobectomy versus amygdalohippocampectomy. Neurology. 2000; 55(12):1818–1822

[100] Donahue SP, Kardon RH, Thompson HS. Hourglass-shaped visual fields as a sign of bilateral lateral geniculate myelinolysis. Am J Ophthalmol. 1995; 119 (3):378–380

[101] Barton JJS. Bilateral sectoranopia from probable osmotic demyelination. Neurology. 2001; 57(12):2318–2319

[102] Borruat F-X, Maeder P. Sectoranopia after head trauma: evidence of lateral geniculate body lesion on MRI. Neurology. 1995; 45(3)(,)(Pt 1):590–592

[103] Neau J-P, Bogousslavsky J. The syndrome of posterior choroidal artery territory infarction. Ann Neurol. 1996; 39(6):779–788

[104] Wein F, Miller NR, Vaphiades MS. An unusual homonymous visual field defect. Surv Ophthalmol. 2000; 44(4):324–328

[105] Carter JE, O'Connor P, Shacklett D, Rosenberg M. Lesions of the optic radiations mimicking lateral geniculate nucleus visual field defects. J Neurol Neurosurg Psychiatry. 1985; 48(10):982–988

[106] Grossman M, Galetta SL, Nichols CW, Grossman RI. Horizontal homonymous sectoral field defect after ischemic infarction of the occipital cortex. Am J Ophthalmol. 1990; 109(2):234–236

[107] Grochowicki M, Vighetto A. Homonymous horizontal sectoranopia: report of four cases. Br J Ophthalmol. 1991; 75(10):624–628

[108] Greenfield DS, Siatkowski RM, Schatz NJ, Glaser JS. Bilateral lateral geniculitis associated with severe diarrhea. Am J Ophthalmol. 1996; 122(2): 280–281

[109] Stem MS, Fahim A, Trobe JD, Parmar HA, Ibrahim M. Lateral geniculate lesions causing reversible blindness in a pre-eclamptic patient with a variant of posterior reversible encephalopathy syndrome. J Neuroophthalmol. 2014; 34(4):372–376

[110] Kosmorsky G, Lancione RR, Jr. When fighting makes you see black holes instead of stars. J Neuroophthalmol. 1998; 18(4):255–257

[111] Horton JC, Landau K, Maeder P, Hoyt WF. Magnetic resonance imaging of the human lateral geniculate body. Arch Neurol. 1990; 47(11):1201–1206

[112] Jacobson DM. The localizing value of a quadrantanopia. Arch Neurol. 1997; 54(4):401–404

[113] Brazis PW, Masdeu JC, Biller J. Localization in Clinical Neurology. 4th ed. Philadelphia, PA: Lippincott Williams & Wilkins; 2001:453–521

[114] Hughes TS, Abou-Khalil B, Lavin PJM, Fakhoury T, Blumenkopf B, Donahue SP. Visual field defects after temporal lobe resection: a prospective quantitative analysis. Neurology. 1999; 53(1):167–172

[115] Mengesha T, Abu-Ata M, Haas KF, et al. Visual field defects after selective amygdalohippocampectomy and standard temporal lobectomy. J Neuroophthalmol. 2009; 29(3):208–213

[116] Lepore FE. Visual deficits in alexia without agraphia. Neuroophthalmology. 1998; 19:1–6

[117] Maeshima S, Osawa A, Sujino K, Fukuoka T, Deguchi I, Tanahashi N. Pure alexia caused by separate lesions of the splenium and optic radiation. J Neurol. 2011; 258(2):223–226

[118] Horton JC, Hoyt WF. Quadrantic visual field defects. A hallmark of lesions in extrastriate (V2/V3) cortex. Brain. 1991; 114(Pt 4):1703–1718

[119] Horton JC, Hoyt WF. The representation of the visual field in human striate cortex. A revision of the classic Holmes map. Arch Ophthalmol. 1991; 109 (6):816–824

[120] McFadzean RM, Hadley DM. Homonymous quadrantanopia respecting the horizontal meridian. A feature of striate and extrastriate cortical disease. Neurology. 1997; 49(6):1741–1746

[121] Borruat F-X, Siatkowski RM, Schatz NJ, Glaser JS. Congruous quadrantanopia and optic radiation lesion. Neurology. 1993; 43(7):1430–1432

[122] Gray LG, Galetta SL, Schatz NJ. Vertical and horizontal meridian sparing in occipital lobe homonymous hemianopias. Neurology. 1998; 50(4):1170–1173

[123] Galetta SL, Grossman RI. The representation of the horizontal meridian in the primary visual cortex. J Neuroophthalmol. 2000; 20(2):89–91

[124] Pessin MS, Kwan ES, DeWitt LD, Hedges TR, III, Gale D, Caplan LR. Posterior cerebral artery stenosis. Ann Neurol. 1987; 21(1):85–89

[125] Pessin MS, Lathi ES, Cohen MB, Kwan ES, Hedges TR, III, Caplan LR. Clinical features and mechanism of occipital infarction. Ann Neurol. 1987; 21(3): 290–299

[126] Gray LG, Galetta SL, Siegal T, Schatz NJ. The central visual field in homonymous hemianopia. Evidence for unilateral foveal representation. Arch Neurol. 1997; 54(3):312–317

[127] McFadzean R, Brosnahan D, Hadley D, Mutlukan E. Representation of the visual field in the occipital striate cortex. Br J Ophthalmol. 1994; 78(3):185–190

[128] Wong AMF, Sharpe JA. Representation of the visual field in the human occipital cortex: a magnetic resonance imaging and perimetric correlation. Arch Ophthalmol. 1999; 117(2):208–217

[129] Celesia GG, Brigell MG, Vaphiades MS. Hemianopic anosognosia. Neurology. 1997; 49(1):88–97

[130] Ogawa K, Ishikawa H, Suzuki Y, Oishi M, Kamei S. Clinical study of the visual field defects caused by occipital lobe lesions. Cerebrovasc Dis. 2014; 37(2): 102–108

[131] Belden JR, Caplan LR, Pessin MS, Kwan E. Mechanisms and clinical features of posterior border-zone infarcts. Neurology. 1999; 53(6):1312–1318

[132] Bartolomei J, Wecht DA, Chaloupka J, Fayad P, Awad IA. Occipital lobe vascular malformations: prevalence of visual field deficits and prognosis after therapeutic intervention. Neurosurgery. 1998; 43(3):415–421, discussion 421–423

[133] Kupersmith MJ, Berenstein A, Nelson PK, ApSimon HT, Setton A. Visual symptoms with dural arteriovenous malformations draining into occipital veins. Neurology. 1999; 52(1):156–162

[134] Kupersmith MJ, Vargas ME, Yashar A, et al. Occipital arteriovenous malformations: visual disturbances and presentation. Neurology. 1996; 46 (4):953–957

[135] Hansen HV. Bilateral inferior altitudinal hemianopia. Neuroophthalmology. 1993; 13:81

[136] Lakhanpal A, Selhorst JB. Bilateral altitudinal visual fields. Ann Ophthalmol. 1990; 22(3):112–117

[137] Caplan LR. Visual perception abnormalities. Presented at the 42nd annual meeting of the American Academy of Neurology, Miami, Florida; 1990

[138] Blake PY, Miller NR. Progressive bilateral homonymous visual field defects caused by a left hemisphere arteriovenous malformation: resolution after embolization. Neuro-ophthalmology. 1999; 21(1):17–23

[139] Hinchey J, Chaves C, Appignani B, et al. A reversible posterior leukoencephalopathy syndrome. N Engl J Med. 1996; 334(8):494–500

[140] Karp BI, Yang JC, Khorsand M, Wood R, Merigan TC. Multiple cerebral lesions complicating therapy with interleukin-2. Neurology. 1996; 47(2):417–424

[141] Kupferschmidt H, Bont A, Schnorf H, et al. Transient cortical blindness and biocoipital brain lesions in two patients with acute intermittent porphyria. Ann Intern Med. 1995; 123(8):598–600

[142] Ormerod LD, Rhodes RH, Gross SA, Crane LR, Houchin KW. Ophthalmologic manifestations of acquired immune deficiency syndrome-associated progressive multifocal leukoencephalopathy. Ophthalmology. 1996; 103(6): 899–906

[143] Pomeranz HD, Henson JW, Lessell S. Radiation-associated cerebral blindness. Am J Ophthalmol. 1998; 126(4):609–611

[144] Steg RE, Kessinger A, Wszolek ZK. Cortical blindness and seizures in a patient receiving FK506 after bone marrow transplantation. Bone Marrow Transplant. 1999; 23(9):959–962

[145] Brazis PW, Lee AG, Graff-Radford N, Desai NP, Eggenberger ER. Homonymous visual field defects in patients without corresponding structural lesions on neuroimaging. J Neuroophthalmol. 2000; 20(2):92–96

[146] Aguglia U, Gambarelli D, Farnarier G, Quattrone A. Different susceptibilities of the geniculate and extrageniculate visual pathways to human Creutzfeldt-Jakob disease (a combined neurophysiological-neuropathological study). Electroencephalogr Clin Neurophysiol. 1991; 78(6):413–423

[147] Felton WL. Presented at the 28th Annual Meeting of the Frank B. Walsh Meeting, Salt Lake City, Utah, February 10–11, 1996

[148] Jacobs DA, Lesser RL, Mourelatos Z, Galetta SL, Balcer LJ. The Heidenhain variant of Creutzfeldt-Jakob disease: clinical, pathologic, and neuroimaging findings. J Neuroophthalmol. 2001; 21(2):99–102

[149] Vargas ME, Kupersmith MJ, Savino PJ, Petito F, Frohman LP, Warren FA. Homonymous field defect as the first manifestation of Creutzfeldt-Jakob disease. Am J Ophthalmol. 1995; 119(4):497–504

[150] Warren FE, Vargas ME, Seidman I, Kupersmith MJ. Homonymous field defect in an HIV negative, at risk individual. Presented at the 24th Annual Frank B. Walsh Society meeting, Los Angeles, California, February 28–29, 1992

[151] Kropp S, Schulz-Schaeffer WJ, Finkenstaedt M, et al. The Heidenhain variant of Creutzfeldt-Jakob disease. Arch Neurol. 1999; 56(1):55–61

[152] Bahn MM, Kido DK, Lin W, Pearlman AL. Brain magnetic resonance diffusion abnormalities in Creutzfeldt-Jakob disease. Arch Neurol. 1997; 54(11): 1411–1415

[153] Bahn MM, Parchi P. Abnormal diffusion-weighted magnetic resonance images in Creutzfeldt-Jakob disease. Arch Neurol. 1999; 56(5):577–583

[154] Mittal S, Farmer P, Kalina P, Kingsley PB, Halperin J. Correlation of diffusion-weighted magnetic resonance imaging with neuropathology in Creutzfeldt-Jakob disease. Arch Neurol. 2002; 59(1):128–134

[155] Na DL, Suh CK, Choi SH, et al. Diffusion-weighted magnetic resonance imaging in probable Creutzfeldt-Jakob disease: a clinical-anatomic correlation. Arch Neurol. 1999; 56(8):951–957

[156] Zerr I, Pocchiari M, Collins S, et al. Analysis of EEG and CSF 14–3–3 proteins as aids to the diagnosis of Creutzfeldt-Jakob disease. Neurology. 2000; 55(6): 811–815

[157] Zerr I, Schulz-Schaeffer WJ, Giese A, et al. Current clinical diagnosis in Creutzfeldt-Jakob disease: identification of uncommon variants. Ann Neurol. 2000; 48(3):323–329

[158] Schröter A, Zerr I, Henkel K, Tschampa HJ, Finkenstaedt M, Poser S. Magnetic resonance imaging in the clinical diagnosis of Creutzfeldt-Jakob disease. Arch Neurol. 2000; 57(12):1751–1757

[159] Aksamit AJ, Jr, Preissner CM, Homburger HA. Quantitation of 14–3–3 and neuron-specific enolase proteins in CSF in Creutzfeldt-Jakob disease. Neurology. 2001; 57(4):728–730

[160] Green AJE, Thompson EJ, Stewart GE, et al. Use of 14–3–3 and other brain-specific proteins in CSF in the diagnosis of variant Creutzfeldt-Jakob disease. J Neurol Neurosurg Psychiatry. 2001; 70(6):744–748

[161] Hsich G, Kenney K, Gibbs CJ, Lee KH, Harrington MG. The 14–3–3 brain protein in cerebrospinal fluid as a marker for transmissible spongiform encephalopathies. N Engl J Med. 1996; 335(13):924–930

[162] Lemstra AW, van Meegen MT, Vreyling JP, et al. 14–3–3 testing in diagnosing Creutzfeldt-Jakob disease: a prospective study in 112 patients. Neurology. 2000; 55(4):514–516

[163] Poser S, Mollenhauer B, Kraubeta A, et al. How to improve the clinical diagnosis of Creutzfeldt-Jakob disease. Brain. 1999; 122(Pt 12):2345–2351

[164] Zerr I, Bodemer M, Gefeller O, et al. Detection of 14–3–3 protein in the cerebrospinal fluid supports the diagnosis of Creutzfeldt-Jakob disease. Ann Neurol. 1998; 43(1):32–40

[165] Zerr I, Bodemer M, Räcker S, et al. Cerebrospinal fluid concentration of neuron-specific enolase in diagnosis of Creutzfeldt-Jakob disease. Lancet. 1995; 345(8965):1609–1610

[166] Chapman T, McKeel DW, Jr, Morris JC. Misleading results with the 14–3–3 assay for the diagnosis of Creutzfeldt-Jakob disease. Neurology. 2000; 55(9): 1396–1397

[167] Burkhard PR, Sanchez J-C, Landis T, Hochstrasser DF. CSF detection of the 14–3–3 protein in unselected patients with dementia. Neurology. 2001; 56 (11):1528–1533

[168] Hernández Echebarría LE, Saiz A, Graus F, et al. Detection of 14–3–3 protein in the CSF of a patient with Hashimoto's encephalopathy. Neurology. 2000; 54(7):1539–1540

[169] Saiz A, Graus F, Dalmau J, et al. Detection of 14–3–3 brain protein in the cerebrospinal fluid of patients with paraneoplastic neurological disorders. Ann Neurol. 1999; 46:774–777

[170] Bashir K, Elble RJ, Ghobrial M, Struble RG. Hemianopsia in dementia with Lewy bodies. Arch Neurol. 1998; 55(8):1132–1135

[171] Trick GL, Trick LR, Morris P, Wolf M. Visual field loss in senile dementia of the Alzheimer's type. Neurology. 1995; 45(1):68–74

[172] Kaeser PF, Ghika J, Borruat FX. Visual signs and symptoms in patients with the visual variant of Alzheimer disease. BMC Ophthalmol. 2015; 15:65

[173] Moster ML, Galetta SL, Schatz NJ. Physiologic functional imaging in "functional" visual loss. Surv Ophthalmol. 1996; 40(5):395–399

[174] Wang A-G, Liu R-S, Liu J-H, Teng MM, Yen MY. Positron emission tomography scan in cortical visual loss in patients with organophosphate intoxication. Ophthalmology. 1999; 106(7):1287–1291

[175] Miki A, Nakajima T, Fujita M, Takagi M, Abe H. Functional magnetic resonance imaging in homonymous hemianopsia. Am J Ophthalmol. 1996; 121(3):258–266

[176] Harden CL, Rosenbaum DH, Daras M. Hyperglycemia presenting with occipital seizures. Epilepsia. 1991; 32(2):215–220

[177] Keane JR. Patterns of hysterical hemianopia. Neurology. 1998; 51(4): 1230–1231

[178] Martin TJ. Threshold perimetry of each eye with both eyes open in patients with monocular functional (nonorganic) and organic vision loss. Am J Ophthalmol. 1998; 125(6):857–864

[179] Thompson JC, Kosmorsky GS, Ellis BD. Field of dreamers and dreamed-up fields: functional and fake perimetry. Ophthalmology. 1996; 103(1): 117–125

[180] Carlow TJ. Functional hemianopsia: identified with Fresnel prisms and quantitative perimetry. Presented at the North American Neuro-Ophthalmology Society meeting, Tucson, Arizona, 1995

[181] Kerkhoff G, Münssinger U, Meier EK. Neurovisual rehabilitation in cerebral blindness. Arch Neurol. 1994; 51(5):474–481

[182] Kerkhoff G, Münßinger U, Haaf E, Eberle-Strauss G, Stögerer E. Rehabilitation of homonymous scotomata in patients with postgeniculate damage of the visual system: saccadic compensation training. Restor Neurol Neurosci. 1992; 4(4):245–254

[183] Smith JL. New pearls check list. J Clin Neuroophthalmol. 1981; 1:78

[184] Rossi PW, Kheyfets S, Reding MJ. Fresnel prisms improve visual perception in stroke patients with homonymous hemianopia or unilateral visual neglect. Neurology. 1990; 40(10):1597–1599

[185] Moss AM, Harrison AR, Lee MS. Patients with homonymous hemianopia become visually qualified to drive using novel monocular sector prisms. J Neuroophthalmol. 2014; 34(1):53–56

[186] Leff AP, Scott SK, Crewes H, et al. Impaired reading in patients with right hemianopia. Ann Neurol. 2000; 47(2):171–178

[187] Kerkhoff G. Neurovisual rehabilitation: recent developments and future directions. J Neurol Neurosurg Psychiatry. 2000; 68(6):691–706

[188] Grunda T, Marsalek P, Sykorova P. Homonymous hemianopia and related visual defects: Restoration of vision after a stroke. Acta Neurobiol Exp (Warsz). 2013; 73(2):237–249

[189] Rizzo JF, III. Occult retinal and choroidal vascular disease. The value of timed and directed fluorescein angiography. Ophthalmology. 1993; 100(9):1407–1416

[190] Xu S, Meyer D, Yoser S, Mathews D, Elfervig JL. Pattern visual evoked potential in the diagnosis of functional visual loss. Ophthalmology. 2001; 108(1):76–80, discussion 80–81

10 Diplopia

Murtaza M. Mandviwala and Alec L. Amram

Abstract

Diplopia can result from a variety of underlying ocular, neurologic, or neuro-ophthalmic disorders. A careful history and examination can help localize the diplopia and direct evaluation and management (e.g., monocular vs. binocular, vertical vs. horizontal, and transient vs. persistent). This chapter discusses the clinical pathway for evaluating and diagnosing diplopia, reviewing the literature in detail.

Keywords: diplopia, double vision, monocular diplopia, binocular diplopia, vertical diplopia, horizontal diplopia

10.1 Acknowledgment

The authors gratefully acknowledge the input of Joseph Hough, MD in reviewing this chapter.

10.2 Introduction

In this chapter, we divide diplopia into several categories: monocular versus binocular and horizontal versus vertical. The evaluation for diplopia is outlined in ▶ Fig. 10.1.

10.3 Is the Diplopia Monocular?

Monocular diplopia can usually be diagnosed by history alone. Diplopia that is monocular remains present while covering the uninvolved eye and resolves when the involved eye is occluded. Monocular diplopia may thus occur unilaterally or bilaterally and should be distinguished from binocular diplopia which occurs when using the two eyes together. The patient should be asked if the diplopia resolves with covering "either eye" to establish the binocular or monocular nature of the diplopia. The second image in monocular diplopia is often described as a less clear and partially superimposed "ghost image" or "halo" on the first image. A pinhole may dramatically reduce the patient's symptoms. Patients without a clear history of monocular diplopia can be asked to keep a diary of their symptoms with specific instructions to document the details for review at a future visit. A pinhole can be given to patients with suspected monocular diplopia to try at home. This "take-home" pinhole can be made in the office out of a business card or a note card using a pen or pencil to make a small-diameter hole. The patient can then try the pinhole at home during the episode of diplopia to test if it resolves the symptoms.

Monocular diplopia usually implies a problem within the eye itself and may respond to refraction, artificial tear trial, or contact lens trial. Box 10.1 lists the ocular causes of monocular diplopia. Monocular diplopia usually does not require any further neuro-ophthalmologic evaluation.

Box 10.1 Ocular causes of monocular diplopia

- Refractive error[1] including astigmatism.
- Poorly fitting contact lens.
- Corneal abnormalities:
  - Keratoconus.
  - Corneal surface abnormality.
  - Tear film disorders including dry eye.
  - Refractive surgery.
  - Corneal transplant.
- Lid abnormalities:
  - Chalazion.
  - Lid position abnormalities.
- Iris abnormalities:
  - Iridotomy/iridectomy.
  - Miotic pupils.
- Lens abnormalities:
  - Cataract.
  - Subluxation or dislocation.
  - Intraocular lens (e.g., positioning holes, decentered lens).
- Retinal abnormalities:
  - Epiretinal membrane or scar.

Another less common form of bilateral but monocular diplopia is cerebral polyopia.[2] The images in cerebral polyopia, unlike those of monocular diplopia secondary to ocular disease, are seen with equal clarity, do not improve with pinhole use, and are unchanged in appearance whether the patient is viewing binocularly or monocularly. Some patients see only two images; others may see many or even hundreds of images occurring in a grid-like pattern ("entomopia" or "insect eye").[3] Some patients experience polyopia only in certain positions of gaze. Patients with cerebral polyopia often have associated signs of occipital or parieto-occipital region damage, such as homonymous visual field defects, difficulty with visually guided reaching, cerebral achromatopsia or dyschromatopsia, object agnosia, and abnormal visual afterimages. These patients require neuroimaging (e.g., magnetic resonance imaging, MRI), to investigate the etiology of the polyopia. Cerebral infarction is the most common etiology, although cerebral polyopia may also occur with tumors, multiple sclerosis, encephalitis, seizures, and with migraine.[2]

Detection of higher order aberrations by wavefront analysis has also been helpful in the evaluation of monocular diplopia. Chalita et al reported that horizontal coma is associated with monocular diplopia at all pupil sizes and total coma is associated with monocular diplopia at 5 and 7 mm pupil sizes in patients who have recently undergone laser in situ keratomileusis (LASIK).[4,5] Post-LASIK coma may be corrected by wavefront-guided surface ablation with topical mitomycin C.[6] Similarly, Melamud et al reported two patients with monocular diplopia and comatic aberration who underwent wavefront-guided LASIK

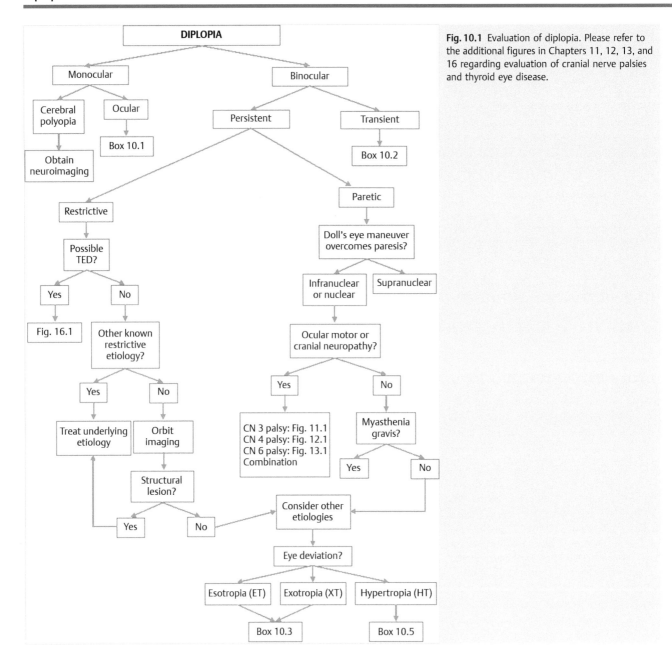

Fig. 10.1 Evaluation of diplopia. Please refer to the additional figures in Chapters 11, 12, 13, and 16 regarding evaluation of cranial nerve palsies and thyroid eye disease.

surgery to have their vision significantly improved when compared with preoperative vision.[7] Spherical aberration and secondary astigmatism detected by wavefront analysis in a patient with monocular diplopia and cortical cataract has also been reported.[8] Another patient presented with monocular diplopia in both eyes with bilateral cataracts who had irregularities on her simulated retinal images of a point source (point spread function) detected by wavefront analysis.[9] The diplopia in both of these patients resolved after cataract removal.[8,9]

10.4 Is the Diplopia Binocular?

A history of binocular diplopia is associated with ocular misalignment. Identification of specific clinical signs and symptoms may allow identification of specific etiologies for the diplopia.

10.5 Is the Deviation Vertical or Horizontal?

If there are no distinctive or obvious signs to indicate diagnosis of a specific etiology for the diplopia, then the vertical or horizontal nature of the deviation may allow further classification of the problem.

10.6 Is the Diplopia Transient or Persistent?

Diplopia may be noted only in certain fields of gaze (e.g., only on looking down in some patients with fourth nerve palsies) and may fluctuate during the day (e.g., diplopia in thyroid ophthalmopathy may be more apparent in the early morning, or worse in the evening with myasthenia gravis). Patients with truly intermittent diplopia may be asymptomatic at examination and eye misalignment may be subtle or not demonstrated. Box 10.2 lists the causes of transient diplopia. These etiologies are discussed in more detail in subsequent sections on horizontal and vertical diplopia.

Box 10.2 Causes of transient diplopia

- Transient ischemia:
  - Transient ocular muscle ischemia (e.g., giant cell arteritis).
  - Vertebrobasilar artery ischemia.
- Decompensation of preexisting phoria.
- Retinal hemifield slide phenomena.
- Myasthenia gravis.
- Muscle or mechanical.
  - Thyroid ophthalmopathy.
  - Brown syndrome.
  - Silent sinus syndrome.
- Intermittent phenomena.
  - Migraine.
  - Neuromyotonia.
  - Intermittent or paroxysmal skew deviation.
  - Superior oblique myokymia.
  - Paroxysmal superior rectus and levator palpebrae spasm.
  - Increased intracranial pressure.
  - Multiple sclerosis (days to weeks).

10.7 Is This an Ocular Motor Cranial Neuropathy?

Ocular motor cranial nerve palsies are discussed in the chapters on third nerve palsies (Chapter 11), fourth nerve palsies (Chapter 12), and sixth nerve palsies (Chapter 13).

10.8 Is There Evidence for a Restrictive Ophthalmoplegia Due to Orbital Disease?

Orbital signs, such as proptosis, chemosis, and injection, should be looked for in patients with diplopia. Forced ductions may reveal a restrictive component to the diplopia. Orbital wall fracture, orbital tumors, silent sinus syndrome, orbital inflammatory disease, or trauma may result in a restrictive strabismus. Orbital imaging is indicated when concern for these conditions exists.

10.9 Is This Myasthenia Gravis?

The evaluation and management of myasthenia gravis is discussed in Chapter 15. For any patient with painless, pupil-sparing, nonproptotic ophthalmoplegia or diplopia, consider a diagnosis of myasthenia gravis as part of the differential.

10.10 Is This Thyroid Eye Disease?

Although transient or persistent diplopia and ophthalmoplegia may occur without other signs of thyroid eye disease, identification of the distinctive signs of thyroid disease as described in Chapter 16 is essential in the evaluation of any patient with diplopia.

10.11 Is This a Supranuclear Process?

The doll's eye (or doll's head) maneuver involves rapid forced horizontal and vertical head movements to activate the vestibulo-ocular reflex. In a patient with negative forced ductions and no evidence for restrictive ophthalmoplegia, this maneuver may overcome a supranuclear ophthalmoplegia (see Chapter 14). Failure of the maneuver to overcome the ophthalmoplegia suggests an infranuclear etiology.

10.12 What Are Phorias and Tropias? How Does the Examiner Assess Horizontal Eye Muscle Function?

A phoria is a latent ocular misalignment that is overcome by fusion. Fusion is the merging of images from each eye into a single perception. Sensory fusion is the cortical integration of two images, whereas motor fusion represents the corrective movements of the eyes required to maintain eye alignment on a single target. Breakdown of fusion due to fatigue, stress, or illness may allow a preexisting phoria to become an intermittent or manifest tropia. The degree of eye deviation may be approximately equal in all directions of gaze (comitant) or may vary in different positions of gaze (incomitant). Horizontal deviations from decompensation of prior childhood strabismus are typically comitant. Breakdown of acquired deviations, such as an old fourth nerve palsy, may be incomitant.

Ductions (each eye moving separately) and versions (the eyes moving conjugately) should be assessed. In assessing normal eye excursion, an imaginary vertical line through the lower lacrimal punctum should coincide with a boundary line between the inner third and outer two-thirds of cornea. If more cornea is hidden, adduction is excessive; if more cornea is visible and if some sclera is visible, adduction is limited. If abduction is normal, the corneal limbus should touch the outer canthus. If the limbus passes that point and some of the cornea is hidden, abduction is excessive; if some of the sclera remains visible, abduction is limited.[10]

10.13 What Are the Causes of Binocular Horizontal Diplopia (Esotropia and Exotropia)?

Horizontal binocular diplopia is usually due to disease processes affecting the medial and/or lateral rectus muscles, the innervation of these muscles (including ocular motor cranial nerves and neuromuscular junction), or processes affecting fusion or convergence and divergence mechanisms.[11] By definition, patients with horizontal diplopia experience two images side by side. The separation of images may vary or remain unchanged at far or near fixation. For example, the image separation from a left abducens nerve palsy is typically worse at a distance than at close range and worse on left gaze.

Box 10.3 categorizes the causes of binocular horizontal diplopia as either disorders causing esotropia (ET) or exotropia (XT). Congenital and childhood strabismus syndromes (Box 10.3) are mentioned but not discussed in depth. For a thorough discussion of childhood strabismus syndromes, the reader is referred to the excellent text of von Noorden.[10] Disorders of vergence, such as convergence insufficiency, convergence spasm, and divergence insufficiency, are also in the differential diagnosis of binocular horizontal diplopia.

Box 10.3 Etiologies of esotropia/exotropia and acquired horizontal diplopia

- Esotropia:
  - Age-related distant esotropia.[12,13,14,15,16,17]
  - Childhood strabismus syndromes.
  - Change of angle of preexisting childhood strabismus or loss of suppression scotoma.
  - Decompensation of a long-standing esophoria.
  - Consecutive esotropia (after strabismus surgery).
  - Optical causes (e.g., optical center change in glasses, over-minus in accommodative esophoria).
  - Sensory esotropia (usually not associated with diplopia).
  - Disorders of muscle and restrictive syndromes:
    – Orbital myositis (orbital pseudotumor).
    – Thyroid eye disease.
    – Medial orbital wall fracture.
    – Postsurgical esotropia.
    – Isolated lateral rectus weakness.
    – Muscle trauma.
    – Progressive external ophthalmoplegia syndromes.
    – Anomalous orbital structures (e.g., extraocular muscles inserting into an abnormal location, fibrous bands, and discrete anomalous muscles).[18]
    – Other orbital disease processes.
  - Disorders of the neuromuscular junction (e.g., myasthenia gravis).
  - Disorders of cranial nerves:
    – Sixth nerve palsy.
    – Ocular neuromyotonia.
  - Central disorders:
    – Cyclic esotropia.
    – Periodic alternating esotropia.
    – Divergence insufficiency or paralysis.
    – Acute acquired comitant esotropia.
    – Spasm of the near reflex.
    – Midbrain pseudo–sixth nerve palsy.
    – Thalamic esotropia.
    – Acquired motor fusion deficiency.
    – Hemifield slide phenomena.
- Exotropia:
  - Childhood strabismus syndromes.
  - Change of angle of preexisting childhood strabismus or loss of suppression scotoma.
  - Decompensation of a long-standing exophoria.
  - Consecutive exotropia (after strabismus surgery).
  - Exotropia secondary to vitreous hemorrhage.
  - Optical causes.
  - Sensory exotropia (often not associated with diplopia).
  - Disorders of the muscle.
    – Orbital myositis (orbital pseudotumor).
    – Thyroid eye disease (uncommon).
    – Postsurgical exotropia.
    – Isolated medial rectus weakness.
    – Muscle trauma.
    – Progressive external ophthalmoplegia syndromes.
    – Other orbital disease processes.
  - Disorders of the neuromuscular junction (e.g., myasthenia gravis).
  - Disorders of cranial nerves:
    – Third nerve palsy.
    – Ocular neuromyotonia.
  - Central disorders.
  - Acquired motor fusion deficiency.
  - Internuclear ophthalmoplegia (WEMINO syndrome and WEBINO syndrome) and the one-and-a-half syndrome (paralytic pontine exotropia).
  - Vitamin E deficiency (e.g., abetalipoproteinemia).
  - Convergence insufficiency and paralysis.
  - Hemifield slide phenomena.

10.14 What Are the Childhood Strabismus Syndromes Causing Esotropia and Exotropia?

Childhood strabismus syndromes may be confused with acquired causes of ET and XT in adulthood. Most childhood ETs are comitant and present at an early age with "crossed-eyes" or amblyopia. Childhood comitant ETs may be due to hyperopia or impaired accommodation or convergence.[19] Incomitant childhood ETs include A-pattern and V-pattern esodeviations, in which the esodeviation is worse on upward and downward gaze, respectively, retraction syndromes (see below), and mechanical-restrictive esodeviation due to congenital fibrosis of the medial rectus muscle. Some patients with congenital nystagmus are able to decrease the amplitude or frequency of their nystagmus by convergence (nystagmus blockage syndrome) and thus an esotropia develops.

Occasionally, adults with a long-standing asymptomatic esophoria may present with diplopia due to "decompensation."[20] This decompensation of a long-standing esophoria may occur following head trauma, refractive changes, medication or drug use causing central nervous system depression (e.g., alcohol or sedatives), systemic illness, or for other unclear reasons. History and examination often reveal evidence of long-standing strabismus, including a history of childhood strabismus or patching, the presence of past head turn, or horizontal comitance.

Childhood XT is less frequent than childhood ET. The XT may be intermittent or persistent, and sometimes adults with exophoria or intermittent XT may present with diplopia due to the inability to adequately compensate for the ocular misalignment (decompensation of exophoria).

Duane retraction syndrome is characterized by a narrowing of the palpebral fissure and globe retraction on adduction.[21] Three forms have been described.[22] In Duane type I, abduction is limited, but adduction is normal or only slightly limited. In type II, adduction is impaired, but abduction is normal or slightly limited. In type III, both adduction and abduction are impaired. Eye deviation may or may not be present in primary position but if it is present, then ET is usually present in type I and III patients, whereas XT is more frequent in type II patients. Type I presents more often in females and the early teenage years, whereas types II and III present more often in the early 20 s.[23] Although many patients adopt a head turn to maintain single binocular vision, these patients rarely complain of spontaneous diplopia. They often acknowledge their own diplopia, if specifically asked, and state that they do recognize two images when their eyes are misaligned. In all types, there may be a vertical deviation of the adducting eye with "up-shoots" and "down-shoots" that may be decreased with lateral rectus recession and Y splitting.[24,25,26,27] Duane retraction syndrome is predominantly congenital. Several genetic variants of Duane syndrome have been identified.[28] Such genetic abnormalities presumably affect either the creation or survival of cranial nerve VI neurons (HOXA1 gene) or guidance of growing cranial nerve VI axons to the lateral rectus (CHN1 and SALL4 genes). High-resolution imaging of Duane syndrome shows two consistent features: (1) the absence of abducens nerve or abducens nerve nucleus (2) muscle abnormalities (atrophy or hypertrophy) of the lateral rectus muscle.[29,30,31,32,33,34] However, in patients with the type II variant, the abducens nerve and an aberrant branch of the oculomotor nerve may dually innervate the lateral rectus muscle.[22,34,35,36] An acquired Duane-like syndrome has been described in patients with pontine glioma, rheumatoid arthritis, following trigeminal rhizotomy, Wildervanck syndrome,[37] and after removal of an orbital cavernous hemangioma by lateral orbitotomy.

Consecutive esotropia refers to esodeviation that occurs iatrogenically after surgical overcorrection of an exodeviation. Consecutive exotropia similarly results from surgical overcorrection of ET or may arise spontaneously in a previously esotropic patient, especially in association with poor vision in the deviating eye (sensory exotropia). Lee et al reported that the esodeviation of consecutive ET can be decreased by prism glasses.[38]

10.15 What Are Sensory Esotropia and Sensory Exotropia?

Sensory deviations including ET or XT result from reduced visual acuity in one eye. These patients do not complain of diplopia because of the visual loss. Loss of fusion in cases of visual loss may allow a preexisting phoria to become manifest. Sidikaro and von Noorden reported on 121 patients with sensory heterotropias and noted that ET and XT occurred with almost equal frequency when the onset of visual impairment occurred at birth or between birth and age 5.[39] Sensory XT, however, predominates in older children and adults.

10.16 What Disorders of the Extraocular Muscles Are Associated with Horizontal Diplopia?

Idiopathic orbital inflammatory syndrome (IOIS) is characterized by the following features: (1) typically unilateral (but may be bilateral); (2) clinical symptoms and signs of orbital involvement (e.g., proptosis, chemosis, pain, injection, ophthalmoplegia); (3) orbital imaging shows focal or diffuse inflammatory lesion; (4) histopathology reveals a fibroinflammatory lesion; and (5) oftentimes, no other identifiable local or systemic causes.[40,41] In our own experience, only about 10 to 20% of patients present with local or systemic causes. The most common of these nonidiopathic causes are sarcoidosis and IgG4-related systemic disease.[42,43]

When the inflammatory process is confined to one or multiple extraocular muscles, the process is referred to as orbital myositis, although some authors feel that orbital pseudotumor and orbital myositis may be distinct entities.[44] Patients present with acute or subacute orbital pain and diplopia. Findings include conjunctival chemosis and injection, ptosis, and proptosis. Angle-closure glaucoma may rarely occur.[45] The process may be unilateral or bilateral and usually resolves with corticosteroid therapy,[44] antitumor necrosis factor agents, anti-CD20 agents,[46] mycophenolate mofetil,[47,48] or radiation therapy.[49] The illness is often monophasic, but recurrent episodes may occur. Characteristics associated with recurrences include male gender, lack of proptosis, eyelid retraction, horizontal extraocular muscle involvement, multiple or bilateral extraocular muscle involvement, muscle tendon sparing on neuroimaging, and lack of response to steroids or nonsteroidal anti-inflammatory agents.[50] Orbital myositis may be associated with systemic diseases such as Crohn disease,[51,52] celiac disease, eosinophilic granulomatosis with polyangiitis,[53] systemic lupus erythematosus,[40,54] Whipple disease,[55] relapsing polychondritis,[56] rheumatoid arthritis, Behçet disease,[57] Lyme disease,[58] linear scleroderma,[54,59,60] IgG4-related systemic disease,[43] and granulomatosis with polyangiitis, relapsing polychondritis.[61] Recurrent orbital myositis may occasionally be familial[62] and orbital myositis may rarely be paraneoplastic.[63]

Neuroimaging reveals enlarged and often extraocular muscles, usually with tendinous insertion involvement (as opposed to tendon sparing in thyroid ophthalmopathy). Extraorbital extension of the inflammatory process to the cavernous sinus, middle cranial fossa, supraorbital and infraorbital nerves, lacrimal glands, or nasal sinuses may occur.[64,65] The differential diagnosis of orbital pseudotumor is outlined in Box 10.4.

Box 10.4 Differential diagnosis of orbital pseudotumor

- Thyroid eye disease (see ▶ Table 10.1).
- Orbital cellulitis (e.g., orbital apex syndrome).
  - Bacterial.
  - Fungal.
    - Aspergillosis.[66,67,68,69,70]
    - Mucormycosis.[71,72,73]
    - Bipolaris hawaiiensis.[74]
    - Actinomycosis.[75]
  - Cysticercosis.[40]
  - Trichinosis.[76]
- Low-flow dural-cavernous sinus fistula.
- Neoplastic.
  - Metastatic.
    - Breast cancer (false "orbital pseudotumor" presentation).[40,77,78,79]
    - Lymphoid hyperplasia.
    - Non-Hodgkin lymphoma and Hodgkin disease.
    - Seminoma (bilateral nonspecific inflammatory or Graves-like orbitopathy not due to direct orbital metastasis).
- Infiltrative.
  - Erdheim-Chester disease (idiopathic infiltration of the heart, lungs, retroperitoneum, bones, and other tissues by xanthomatous histiocytes and Touton giant cells).[80,81,82]
  - Orbital amyloidosis.[40,83,84]
  - Sinus histiocytosis with massive lymphadenopathy (Rosai-Dorfman disease).[85]
- Inflammatory.
  - Sarcoidosis.[40,86,87,88,89]
  - Giant cell arteritis.[90]
  - Orbital polymyositis and giant cell myocarditis.
  - Systemic inflammatory diseases (granulomatosis with polyangiitis,[61] systemic lupus erythematosus).[91]
  - IgG4-related disease.[42,43]

Table 10.1 Clinical differential diagnosis of orbital myositis and thyroid eye disease

Orbital myositis	Thyroid eye disease
Males and females equally affected	Females predominate
Acute or subacute onset	Gradual onset
Often severe orbital pain	Painless or "foreign body" sensation
Motility problems early	Motility problems late
May have limited ductions	Restrictive ductions
No lid lag or retraction	Lid lag and retraction
Neuroimaging of orbit	
Enlarged muscles irregular	Enlarged muscles often smooth
Tendon spared	Tendon may be involved
Often unilateral	Often bilateral

Orbital polymyositis or giant cell myocarditis is a rare, distinct nosologic entity characterized by progressive, often painful bilateral ophthalmoplegia with thickened extraocular muscles and cardiac arrhythmia often leading to death.[92,93,94] Pathologically, the extraocular and cardiac muscles showed diffuse mononuclear and giant cell inflammation. Cardiac transplantation may be lifesaving.[93]

Orbital biopsy may be required to confirm the diagnosis and rule out alternative etiologies. Biopsy is generally not recommended in typical cases of IOIS and pure myositis presentation, in which surgical biopsy may damage the muscle. Likewise, orbital apex and very posterior lesions may not be accessible safely for biopsy and may damage the optic nerve at risk.[41] Pathologic studies in typical orbital myositis reveal inflammatory infiltrates composed mainly of small well-differentiated mature lymphocytes admixed with plasma cells in a diffuse or multifocal pattern. The muscle fibers are swollen and separated by edema and fibrosis with loss of normal striations and degeneration of muscle fibers.[41] Other atypical histopathologic patterns including extensive sclerosis, true vasculitis, granulomatous inflammation, toll-like receptor staining,[95] and tissue eosinophilia can be used for subclassification of orbital pseudotumor.[41] There

is no definite correlation between clinicotherapeutic outcome and these atypical findings. However, special staining for IgG4 disease is indicated in IOIS.

Thyroid eye disease (thyroid orbitopathy, thyroid ophthalmopathy, or Graves disease) is a disorder characterized clinically by lid retraction, lid lag in downward gaze, exophthalmos, diplopia (due to extraocular muscle inflammation or fibrosis), potential visual loss due to compressive optic neuropathy or corneal damage, and signs and symptoms of orbital congestion.[96,97,98,99,100] The restrictive extraocular muscle involvement may be confirmed by impaired ocular motility during forced duction testing. The extraocular muscles predominantly affected include the inferior, medial, and superior rectus muscles, and as muscle tightness or restriction increases, the diplopia worsens in the direction of gaze opposite that of the involved muscle(s). Thus, hypertropia and esotropia are quite common deviations in thyroid eye disease, but exotropia is uncommon due to less frequent involvement of the lateral rectus muscle. In fact, if a patient with thyroid eye disease is noted to be exotropic, superimposed myasthenia gravis should be considered, as there is an increased risk of myasthenia gravis in patients with thyroid eye disease.[101,102] Thyroid eye disease is further discussed in Chapter 16. Thyroid eye disease and orbital myositis may resemble each other clinically. Differential features are outlined in ▶ Table 10.1.

The diagnosis of myasthenia gravis should be considered in all patients with painless ptosis and/or ocular motor weakness without pupillary involvement or proptosis. Weakness and fatigue confined to the extraocular muscles or lids combined with orbicularis oculi paresis is especially suggestive of this diagnosis. Myasthenia gravis may cause hypertropia, esotropia, or exotropia, and can mimic many neurogenic conditions including abducens nerve palsies, gaze abnormalities, divergence paresis, and internuclear ophthalmoplegia. Therefore, in any patient with an abnormality of horizontal gaze, myasthenia gravis should at least be considered. Myasthenia gravis is discussed further in Chapter 15.

Orbital trauma may result in horizontal diplopia due to orbital wall, floor, or other orbital bone fractures.[10,103,104] Medial rectus muscle incarceration accompanying medial orbital wall fracture may lead to ET with impaired abduction or XT with impaired adduction. Medial orbital wall injury may occur iatrogenically during endoscopic transnasal sinus surgery.[10,103] Also, medial or lateral orbital surgery (e.g., optic nerve sheath fenestration) may directly injure the medial or lateral rectus muscles resulting in muscle paresis occasionally followed by scarring and restrictive ET or XT, respectively. Other ocular surgeries (e.g., pterygium surgery, scleral buckle, and glaucoma Setons) may also result in horizontal diplopia.

Isolated medial rectus paresis is rare and results in XT due to unopposed action of the lateral rectus muscle. The XT increases on gaze opposite the involved muscle and is associated with impaired ipsilateral adduction. Impaired monocular adduction is more often noted with internuclear ophthalmoplegia (INO) than with isolated medial rectus palsy due to a partial third nerve palsy. Isolated medial rectus muscle paresis may occur with myasthenia gravis, orbital myositis, muscle trauma, or orbital disease. Lesions of the oculomotor nerve cause medial rectus paresis but not in isolation. Because the neurons controlling the medial rectus muscle probably lie at three different locations within the oculomotor nucleus, it is unlikely that a medial rectus paralysis would be the sole manifestation of a brainstem oculomotor nuclear lesion.

Although isolated lateral rectus paresis is most often due to lesions of the sixth cranial nerve, other processes, including myasthenia gravis, orbital myositis, muscle trauma, and orbital lesions, may impair the muscle directly.

10.17 What Disorders of the Cranial Nerves Cause Horizontal Diplopia?

Unilateral sixth cranial nerve injury results in an incomitant esodeviation that is worsened with gaze into the field of the weak lateral rectus muscle. Patients may employ a compensatory face turn in the direction of the paralyzed lateral rectus muscle to limit diplopia. Abduction is often limited on the side of the lesion. With bilateral paralysis, both eyes may be in a position of adduction causing an esotropia that increases with any horizontal deviation from primary gaze. Myasthenia gravis may mimic an isolated sixth nerve palsy, so in some patients with isolated abduction paresis, further evaluation with anti-acetylcholine receptor antibody testing and possibly electromyography with repetitive stimulation testing may be the next step, especially if there are signs of fatigability of the muscle paresis or associated ptosis. Sixth cranial nerve palsies are further discussed in Chapter 13 and ocular myasthenia gravis is discussed in Chapter 15.

Lesions of the third cranial nerve may cause an XT (with or without a hyperdeviation) because of weakness of the medial rectus muscle with the eye deviating toward the side of the preserved lateral rectus muscle. This XT is usually associated with other signs of third nerve affection, including paresis of eye elevation and depression, ptosis, and pupillary involvement. Third cranial nerve palsies are further discussed in Chapter 11.

Ocular neuromyotonia (ONM) is a rare disorder characterized by episodic (lasting seconds to minutes) horizontal or vertical diplopia, occurring either spontaneously or following sustained (10–20 seconds) eccentric gaze.[105,106,107,108,109,110,111,112,113,114,115] Most patients have had prior radiation therapy to the sellar or parasellar region (months to years before onset of the ONM) for tumors including chordoma, pituitary tumors,[116,117,118] craniopharyngioma, chondrosarcoma, rhabdomyosarcoma, thalamic glioma, sinonasal carcinoma, and medulloblastoma. There are rare cases of ONM following surgery and radiation therapy for nonsellar or parasellar tumors such as nasopharyngeal carcinoma,[119] cerebellar medulloblastoma,[120] and ethmoidal sinonasal carcinoma.[120] One report documented the occurrence of ONM in a patient postradiation and surgical treatment for a posterior fossa medulloblastoma with parasellar metastasis.[121] In some cases, however, no responsible structural lesion or history of radiation therapy is noted.[122] Rarely, ONM may be due to a compressive lesion,[123] such as an aneurysm,[105,108,124,125] dolichoectatic basilar artery,[126] thyroid eye disease,[107,127,128] Paget disease of bone,[129] cavernous sinus trigeminal schwannoma,[130] cavernous sinus meningioma,[131,132] or after cavernous sinus thrombosis secondary to mucormycosis.[133] One patient had fourth nerve involvement where spasms of the superior oblique muscle were induced only by alcohol intake,[108] whereas another developed ONM several years after myelography with thorium dioxide (Thorotrast).[115] Intramedullary stroke[134] and brainstem demyelination[135] have also been reported to cause ONM.

ONM is thought to reflect impaired muscle relaxation due to inappropriate discharges from oculomotor, trochlear, or abducens neurons or axons with unstable cellular membrane potassium channels.[136] Patients with ONM often benefit from membrane stabilizing agents such as carbamazepine[127,128] and gabapentin.[128] One patient noted that she could terminate episodes of ocular depression instantly by forcefully directing her gaze upward, and thus stretching the affected muscle might also prove to be an effective way of ending attacks.[137] A second patient discovered that by wearing goggles and consciously restricting her lateral vision, episodes of diplopia resolved.[138] Another patient's ONM resolved after microvascular decompression of the oculomotor nerve.[139] When evaluating a patient with diplopia exclusively occurring in eccentric gaze, even without ptosis, myasthenia gravis should be considered.[140] Patients with unexplained transient episodic diplopia should thus be specifically tested for diplopia and ocular misalignment following sustained eccentric gaze.

10.18 What Other Central Disorders Cause Horizontal Diplopia?

Other central disorders causing horizontal diplopia include cyclic esotropia, periodic alternating esotropia, divergence insufficiency and paralysis, convergence spasm, convergence insufficiency and paralysis, acquired motor fusion deficiency, INO and the one-and-a-half syndrome, vitamin E deficiency, and the hemifield slip phenomenon. Exotropia due to vitreous hemorrhage is included here, as the diplopia may be due to impaired fusional mechanisms. INO, the one-and-a-half syndrome, and the motility disorder associated with vitamin E deficiency (abetalipoproteinemia) may all cause horizontal diplopia (and occasionally vertical diplopia when associated with skew deviation) and are discussed in Chapter 17.

10.19 What Is Cyclic Esotropia?

Cyclic esotropia is a rare condition characterized by a regularly recurring ET that often occurs with regular 48-hour cycles.[141,142] There is often a 24-hour period of normal binocular vision followed by a 24-hour period of manifest ET; 72 and 96-hour cycles have also been reported. The ET may eventually become constant. Cyclic ET usually appears in young children but may also occur in adults.[141,142] The condition usually starts without precipitant but has been described after strabismus following intermittent XT,[143] cataract surgery, traumatic aphakia, surgical removal of a third ventricular astrocytoma, and in association with optic atrophy or retinal detachment.[141] Rare cases have been described with overlapping symptoms of ONM and cyclic ET which occasionally resolved with carbamazepine or ocular muscle recession.[144,145,146] The etiology of this condition is unknown with possible links to ONM,[144,145,146] oculomotor nerve hyperactivity (although there are no associated abnormalities of the pupil or lid), abducens nerve dysfunction, strabismus interrupted by periodic intervals of fusion, or, most likely, a disorder of central mechanisms. Cyclic ET is usually managed by surgical correction of the affected ocular muscle, but surgeons have also used botulinum toxin injection[147,148] and prisms[149] to alleviate the condition.

10.20 What Is Periodic Alternating Esotropia?

Periodic alternating esotropia is a rare cyclic disorder typically associated with periodic alternating nystagmus (PAN) or periodic alternating gaze (PAG).[150] While one eye maintains fixation, the other eye undergoes a phase of waxing then waning inward deviation. The cycle is completed by a phase of varying inward deviation in the eye that was initially fixating after a transition period of orthotropia during which fixation changes. This condition is invariably associated with severe brain dysfunction and is especially noted in young children with ataxia or hydrocephalus.

10.21 What Constitutes Divergence Insufficiency and Divergence Paralysis?

Weakness of divergence is characterized by intermittent or constant ET at distance with fusion and near.[10,151,152,153,154,155,156,157] Duction and version testing is relatively full bilaterally. The angle of strabismus remains unchanged (comitant) or may be decreased on gaze to either side. Fusional divergence is reduced or absent. Fusional divergence is measured by placing prisms of progressively larger strength base-in over one eye while the subject is fixating at distance and near and noting when the fixation image appears double (break point). Patients with divergence weakness should also demonstrate normal speed and amplitude of horizontal saccades.[158]

When ET at distance due to divergence impairment occurs in an otherwise healthy individual, it is referred to as "divergence insufficiency" or "primary divergence insufficiency," whereas when it occurs in association with neurologic disease it is called "divergence paralysis" or "secondary divergence insufficiency." Primary divergence insufficiency is usually observed in young adults, is self-limited, and may be treated with base-out prisms or occasionally surgery.[10,151,152,153,154,156,157] Recent data suggest that divergence insufficiency in adults is mostly associated with some benign neurological process.[159] That said, neuro-ophthalmologists must be on the lookout for convergence excess, basic esotropia or esophoria, divergence paralysis, or sixth nerve palsy.

In one study, 95% of patients with primary divergence insufficiency were older than 50 years and symptoms resolved in 40% of patients after a median of 5 months.[154] The more recent term for primary divergence insufficiency among seniors is "age-related distant esotropia."[12,13,14,160] This diagnosis is made if the exam demonstrates orthophoria or asymptomatic esophoria of no more than 10 prism diopters (PD) at 33 cm, with symptomatic distance esotropia measuring at least twice the near esophoria.[15] MRI studies of age-related divergence insufficiency show sagging eyes with peripheral displacement of all rectus muscle pulleys (especially lateral and superior rectus pulleys) resulting in horizontal or vertical strabismus.[16,161]

Divergence paralysis (secondary divergence insufficiency) is usually noted with brainstem disease. It has been reported with multiple sclerosis, intracranial masses (e.g., pontomedullary glioma), brainstem hemorrhage or infarction, head trauma, increased intracranial pressure (e.g., pseudotumor cerebri, neurobrucellosis, frontal lobe glioblastoma), spontaneous intracranial hypotension syndrome, cerebellar lesions, cranio-cervical junction abnormalities (e.g., Chiari malformation), hydrocephalus, meningitis, encephalitis, syphilis, clivus lymphoma, acute lymphoblastic leukemia, chronic lymphocytic leukemia, diazepam ingestion, giant cell arteritis, Miller Fisher syndrome, Wernicke encephalopathy, Parkinson disease, Machado-Joseph disease, progressive supranuclear palsy, and after lumbar puncture or epidural block.[151,152,153,154,155,156,157,162,163,164,165,166,167,168,169] Abducens nerve palsy may also cause esotropia that is worse at a distance than near, and indeed some authors believe that divergence paralysis does not exist and that all such cases actually represent bilateral abducens nerve palsies. However, three findings occur with divergence paralysis but not with bilateral sixth nerve palsies: (1) fusional divergence is reduced or absent, (2) the esotropia not only remains unchanged during horizontal gaze but may even decrease, and (3) saccadic velocities are normal.

In a study of 17 adults with divergence weakness, none of the patients were found to have concurrent neurologic disease.[170] Thirteen patients remained stable, three improved, and one progressed. Sixteen patients were treated successfully: 12 with prisms and 4 with strabismus surgery. One patient was not treated. The authors concluded that divergence weakness is usually an isolated condition that tends to remain stable and respond to treatment with prisms or strabismus surgery. In another study of 15 patients with divergence paresis, three cases were idiopathic and the rest were associated with diverse central nervous system diseases.[155] Although six of these patients had posterior fossa disease, neuroimaging showed no common circumscribed lesion site or evidence of increased intracranial pressure, and thus divergence paresis was considered a nonlocalizing cause of horizontal diplopia. Divergence paresis may be mimicked by myasthenia gravis.[155]

As noted earlier, unilateral or bilateral abducens nerve paresis may cause an acute ET with the deviation greater at distance than near. This deviation may eventually become comitant ("spread of comitance"), in which case it will be difficult to recognize the paretic element. Acute acquired comitant ET may occur in childhood and may be benign.[10] For example, it may develop after artificial interruption of fusion by occlusion of one eye. A previous esophoria may decompensate and become manifest after fusion has been disrupted. Acquired comitant ET in childhood may also occur with central nervous system tumors, especially brainstem and cerebellar tumors and tumors of the corpus callosum, and with Chiari I malformation. Thus, these patients should undergo neuroimaging.[156,159,171,172,173,174] It has also been described after head trauma in a child on carbamazepine.[175] The mechanism of acute acquired comitant ET is unknown.

10.22 What Is Convergence Spasm?

Convergence spasm usually occurs on a functional basis. Patients exhibit intermittent episodes of sustained maximal convergence associated with accommodative spasm (induced myopia) and miosis.[10,176,177] The spasm may be triggered by asking the patient to fixate an object held closely before the eyes; after the fixation object has been removed, the eyes will remain in a convergent position.[10] Quick saccades back and forth in the horizontal plane may also induce the spasm.

Patients with spasm of the near reflex often complain of headache, diplopia, photophobia, and blurred vision and often have tunnel visual fields. Patients may initially be thought to have unilateral or bilateral abducens nerve paresis or myasthenia gravis. Observation of miosis during the spasm in a patient with apparent unilateral or bilateral limitation of abduction and severe myopia (8–10 diopters) indicates the correct diagnosis.[176,177,178,179] This miosis generally resolves as soon as either eye is occluded.[178] Also, despite apparent weakness of abduction, patients have full abduction when one eye is patched or during duction testing. Convergence spasm may occasionally be confused with divergence paralysis in that in both instances there is ET at distance fixation. With convergence spasm, however, fusional divergence is normal and visual acuity at distance is decreased.

Spasm of the near reflex may rarely be associated with organic disease of the central and ocular motor system. Increased or sustained convergence may be seen with lesions of the diencephalic–mesencephalic junction. For example, a pseudo–sixth nerve palsy may occur from midbrain lesions (midbrain pseudo–sixth nerve palsy), perhaps due to an excess of convergence tone.[180] In a study of patients with pseudo-abducens palsy and "top-of-the-basilar" infarcts, the smallest infarcts producing an ipsilateral pseudo-abducens palsy were located just rostral to the oculomotor nucleus, near the midbrain–diencephalic junction.[180] Two patients with only contralateral pseudo-abducens palsy had subthalamic and thalamic infarction, and four patients with bilateral pseudo-abducens palsy had larger infarcts involving the midbrain. All patients with pseudo-abducens palsy had upgaze palsy. The authors concluded that lesions near the midbrain–diencephalic junction are important for the development of pseudo-abducens palsy and that this abnormality and convergence-retraction nystagmus are both manifestations of abnormal vergence activity. Inhibitory descending pathways for convergence may pass through the thalamus and decussate in the subthalamic region.[180] A case of pseudo–sixth nerve palsy has been ascribed to brainstem infarction due to deep cerebral venous thrombosis.[181] Acute esotropia has been described with contralateral thalamic infarction in the territory of the mesencephalic artery (acute thalamic esotropia). Tonic activation of the medial rectus muscle in these cases could result from damage to direct inhibitory projections from the thalamus or impairments of inputs to midbrain neurons involved in vergence control. Acute thalamic hemorrhage may cause bilateral asymmetric esotropia with the contralateral eye more affected than the ipsilateral eye.[182] Bilateral pseudo–sixth nerve palsies have been described with symmetric bilateral paramedian thalamic lesions without midbrain involvement.[183] Other etiologies of increased or sustained spasm of the near reflex include Wernicke–Korsakoff syndrome, Arnold–Chiari malformation, encephalitis, hepatic encephalopathy, neurosyphilis, vertebrobasilar ischemia, multiple sclerosis, labyrinthine fistula, trauma, posterior fossa tumor, pituitary adenoma, phenytoin intoxication, cyclic oculomotor palsy, Raeder paratrigeminal syndrome, ocular inflammation, conversion disorders, thalamic glioblastoma, cerebral aneurysm, Miller Fisher syndrome, and ocular myasthenia gravis.[10,176,177,179,182,184,185,186,187]

10.23 What Constitutes Convergence Insufficiency and Convergence Paralysis?

Patients with an exodeviation greater at close range than at a distance have convergence insufficiency type XT. Adduction is usually normal, there is a remote near point of convergence, and fusional convergence is decreased at near fixation.[10] This condition is common among teenagers and college students, especially those with an increased visual work load, but may also be seen in the elderly. It often develops at times of stress or fatigue, but also may be noted during systemic infection or after head trauma. Acquired cerebral lesions, especially affecting the nondominant parietal lobe, may rarely be responsible.[188] Patients with convergence insufficiency typically complain of eyestrain and ache. After brief periods of reading, the letters will blur and run together and often diplopia occurs during near work. Typically, the patient will close or cover one eye while reading to obtain relief from visual fatigue.

Patients with convergence paralysis, as opposed to convergence insufficiency, often harbor a lesion of the midbrain. Diplopia exists only at near fixation, adduction is normal, and the patient is unable to converge. Preservation of accommodation or pupillary miosis at close range confirms an organic etiology. Other signs of midbrain damage usually are present including impaired vertical gaze, upbeat or downbeat nystagmus, convergence-retraction nystagmus, and eyelid retraction. Many conditions are associated with convergence paralysis, including Parkinson disease, progressive supranuclear palsy, dorsal midbrain tumors, midbrain hemorrhage or infarction, multiple sclerosis, polyarteritis nodosa, encephalitis, metabolic causes, trauma, subdural hematoma, and drugs.[189,190,191] Dissociated unilateral convergence paralysis has been described with thalamotectal hemorrhage.[192] Selective convergence loss with light-near dissociation has been described with bilateral paramedian thalamic infarction.[183]

10.24 What Is Acquired Motor Fusion Deficiency?

Motor fusion is a function of the extrafoveal retinal periphery.[10] Acquired motor fusional deficiency is a rare condition that represents loss of both fusional convergence and divergence that may occur after head trauma, stroke, brain tumor, or neurosurgery.[10] It is assumed to be due to midbrain damage. Patients complain of eyestrain and are unable to maintain single vision for any length of time. Despite apparent ocular alignment, patients complain of transient or permanent diplopia. Fusional amplitudes are absent, but stereopsis and sensory fusion are intact during brief episodes of fusion. There is no effective therapy.

10.25 Why Is Vitreous Hemorrhage Sometimes Associated with a Secondary Exotropia?

Fujikado et al described eight patients with exotropia and binocular diplopia after recovery from vitreous hemorrhage.[193] Vitreous hemorrhages were bilateral in three patients and unilateral in five patients. Diplopia occurred in all patients after vitrectomy. Exotropia was present in all of the patients, and seven of the eight also had vertical strabismus with an average deviation of six prism diopters. The authors concluded that diplopia after vitrectomy for long-standing vitreous hemorrhage may occur due to fusion impairment (i.e., sensory XT) comparable to that occasionally seen after surgery for traumatic cataract.

10.26 What Is the Hemifield Slide Phenomenon?

The retinal hemifield slide or slip phenomenon is a rare cause of intermittent binocular diplopia noted in some patients with lesions of the optic chiasm. This phenomenon typically occurs with complete or nearly complete bitemporal hemianopic visual field defects (but can occur in any pattern of nonoverlapping residual visual fields) with disruption of ocular fusion and decompensation of a previous phoria. The underlying pathophysiology is loss of binocularity due to lack of cortical representation of corresponding points in the visual field from each eye (i.e., transection of the chiasm creates two independent, free-floating hemifields, with each eye projecting only to the ipsilateral visual cortex). Patients complain of intermittent diplopia and difficulty with near work. On examination, no ocular motor palsy is noted despite the subjective complaint of diplopia. If the eyes intermittently converge (esotropia), a blank

space is produced between the vertical meridians as the eyes "slip" inward and the remaining hemifields drift apart horizontally. Ocular divergence (exotropia) causes overlapping of the vertical meridians, resulting in superimposition of images from noncorresponding retinal areas. Hemifield slide diplopia may also occur from altitudinal visual field defects.[194] Two cases have been described in which heteronymous altitudinal field defects resulted in loss of fusion and transient overlap of preserved hemifields. This phenomenon resulted in complaints of diplopia similar to that described with bitemporal hemianopia. The patients had superior altitudinal field defects in one eye and inferior defects in the other. One complained of vertical diplopia and the other had vertical and horizontal diplopia.

10.27 How Does One Examine a Patient with the Complaint of Vertical Diplopia?

Patients with vertical diplopia complain of seeing two images, one atop or diagonally displaced from the other. The evaluation of these patients starts with a careful history, including queries concerning previous eye muscle surgeries, childhood strabismus, and history of patching or orthoptic exercises. The examiner must question whether the diplopia is monocular, and thus likely secondary to abnormalities of the ocular media/surface (including refractive error), or binocular due to impaired ocular motility. By asking pertinent questions and observing the posture of the patient's head, a likely diagnosis can usually be reached even before physical examination begins.[10,195] If the patient complains of vertical diplopia in primary gaze, often one of the vertically acting extraocular muscles is underacting: the right and/or left inferior rectus, superior rectus, inferior oblique, or superior oblique. The examiner should then ask if the vertical separation between images is worse on gaze to the left or right. If, for example, vertical separation of images is worse on gaze to the right, then four of the eight extraocular muscles may be underacting (the right superior or inferior rectus or the left inferior or superior oblique). If the separation is worse on gaze to the right and down, the right inferior rectus or left superior oblique must be underacting; if the image separation worsens or improves with left or right head tilt, torsional abnormalities, especially due to oblique muscle involvement, should be suspected.

Patients with binocular vertical diplopia may adopt a compensatory head, face, or chin position to move their eyes into a gaze angle that achieves binocular single vision. Underaction of the superior or inferior rectus muscles is compensated by neck flexion or extension (chin down or chin up), which seeks to avoid the eye position of maximum image separation. Torsional diplopia is usually caused by underaction of the superior or inferior oblique muscles and may be associated with an angular head tilt. This head tilt is assumed to avoid the vertical and torsional image separation.

The Parks-Bielschowsky three-step test is important in the evaluation of vertical diplopia:
1. Determine whether there is a right or left hypertropia or hyperphoria in primary position. For example, if there is a right hypertropia in primary position and the lesion is

paretic then there is a paresis of one of the right eye depressors (right inferior rectus or superior oblique) or left eye elevators (left superior rectus or inferior oblique).

2. Compare the amount of vertical deviation in right and left gaze. For example, if the right hypertropia increases in left gaze, either the right superior oblique or the left superior rectus is underacting.

3. Compare the vertical deviation in right head tilt and left head tilt (Bielschowsky head-tilt test). For example, if the vertical deviation increases with right head tilt, the right superior oblique must be weak; if the hyperdeviation increases on left head tilt, the left superior rectus is weak.

4. Ocular torsion ("fourth step" of the "three-step test") may be measured with the double Maddox rod test, which utilizes a red Maddox rod over the right eye and a white Maddox rod over the left eye in a trial frame. A thin base-down prism may be placed before one eye to separate the horizontal lines induced. The tilt of the retinal image is opposite the tilt of the horizontal line, as seen by the patient. Therefore, when the line is seen slanted toward the nose, an excyclodeviation is present, whereas if the tilt is toward the temple, an incyclodeviation is present. The line is always tilted in the direction in which the offending muscle would rotate the eye if it were acting alone.[10] For example, a patient with right superior oblique muscle palsy will describe the red line to be lower than the white line and relatively intorted or slanted toward the nose. The Maddox rod is then turned until the two lines are parallel and the magnitude of the cyclotropia can be read off the trial frame. Cyclodeviation may also be noted with indirect ophthalmoscopy.[10] Normally, the average location of the fovea in relation to the optic nerve head is 0.3 disc diameters below a horizontal line extending through the geometric center of the optic disc. From this position, an imaginary horizontal line will cross the optic nerve head just below the halfway point between its geometric center and lower pole. Incyclotorsion is present when the fovea appears above a line extending horizontally from the center of the optic nerve head, and excyclotorsion is present when the fovea is below a line extending horizontally from just below the lower pole of the optic disc.

5. Tilt the exam chair back and reexamine the ocular deviation with the patient in supine position ("fifth step" of the "three-step test"). Skew deviation is the only condition that should result in a positive upright-supine test. According to Wong et al, patients with skew deviation have at least a 50% decrease in vertical misalignment during supine positioning.[196] As such, a positive upright-supine test warrants neuroimaging.

Finally, if restrictive ophthalmopathy is thought to be responsible for vertical misalignment, the forced duction test can be used to differentiate whether limitation of ocular movement is due to extraocular muscle paresis or antagonist extraocular muscle tethering.

10.28 What Are the Etiologies of Vertical Diplopia?

Binocular vertical diplopia may be due to supranuclear processes, ocular motor nerve dysfunction, neuromuscular junction disease, diseases of eye muscle, mechanical processes causing vertical eye misalignment, and even retinal disease.[197] Etiologies responsible for vertical binocular diplopia and hypertropia/hyperphoria are outlined in Box 10.5.

Box 10.5 Etiologies of binocular vertical diplopia and hypertropia/hyperphoria

- Supranuclear causes.
  - Supranuclear monocular elevation paresis (congenital or acquired).
  - Skew deviation.
  - Vertical one-and-a-half syndrome.
  - Wernicke encephalopathy.
  - Paroxysmal superior rectus and levator palpebrae spasm with multiple sclerosis.
  - Vitreous hemorrhage.
- Ocular motor nerve dysfunction.
  - Third nerve palsy.
  - Fourth nerve palsy.
  - Hypertropia (small) accompanying sixth nerve palsy.
  - Superior oblique myokymia.
  - Ocular neuromyotonia.
  - Ophthalmoplegic migraine.
  - Wernicke encephalopathy.
  - Miller Fisher syndrome.
  - Guillain–Barré syndrome.
  - Decompensation of a long-standing phoria.
  - Increased intracranial pressure.
- Neuromuscular junction disease.
  - Myasthenia gravis.
  - Botulism.
- Diseases of the eye muscle.
  - Isolated paresis of a vertical-acting extraocular muscle (e.g., due to congenital causes, myasthenia gravis, Graves disease, botulism, trauma, postsurgery, trochleitis, orbital metastasis, orbital pseudotumor, and muscle ischemia form giant cell arteritis).
    - Superior oblique muscle.
    - Inferior oblique muscle.
    - Superior rectus muscle.
    - Inferior rectus muscle.
  - Decompensation of a long-standing phoria.
  - Graves disease.
  - Chronic progressive external ophthalmoplegia (CPEO) syndromes.
  - After surgery (e.g., cataract operation).
  - Congenital strabismus syndromes.
  - Dissociated vertical deviation (DVD).
  - Congenital "double elevator" palsy (monocular elevation deficiency).
  - Double depressor paralysis (unilateral paralysis of the inferior rectus and superior oblique; may be congenital or acquired).
  - n Physiologic hyperdeviation on lateral gaze (asymptomatic).
- Mechanical processes causing vertical eye misalignment.
  - Graves disease.
  - Brown superior oblique tendon sheath syndrome.
    - Congenital.

- Acquired (e.g., superomedial orbital trauma, tenosynovitis or myositis, adhesions, metastasis to the superior oblique muscle, frontal sinus osteoma, pansinusitis, psoriasis, peribulbar anesthesia, blepharoplasty, maxillofacial or sinus surgery, and superior oblique tuck).
  - Superior oblique click syndrome (e.g., due to schwannoma or giant cell tumor of sheath of superior oblique tendon).
- Acquired Brown syndrome associated with underaction of the ipsilateral superior oblique muscle ("canine tooth syndrome").
- Orbital floor blowout fracture.
- Maxillary sinusitis (silent sinus syndrome).
- Direct trauma to the extraocular muscles (e.g., intramuscular hematoma).
- Congenital inferior rectus fibrosis.
- Anomalous orbital structures, such as extraocular muscles inserting into an abnormal location, fibrous bands, and discrete anomalous muscles.[18]
- Strabismus fixus (generalized fibrosis of extraocular muscles).
- Postoperative sequelae (including retinal detachment surgery, orbital surgery, strabismus surgery, and cataract surgery).
- Orbital inflammation (myositis) and pseudotumor.
- Metastatic infiltration of extraocular muscles.
- Orbital tumors.
- Fallen eye syndrome (long-standing superior oblique muscle paresis in patients who habitually fixate with the paretic eye may develop hypodeviation of the uninvolved eye caused by contracture of the contralateral inferior rectus muscle).
- Rising eye syndrome (long-standing inferior oblique muscle palsy may result in contracture and fibrosis of the contralateral superior rectus.
- Miscellaneous.
  - Hemifield slide phenomenon from dense bitemporal hemianopia or heteronymous altitudinal field defects.
  - Foveal displacement syndrome (e.g., due to subretinal or epiretinal neovascular membranes).

10.29 What Supranuclear Processes May Cause Vertical Diplopia?

Monocular elevation paresis ("double elevator palsy") may occur on a peripheral basis (e.g., due to primary inferior rectus restriction, primary superior rectus palsy, myasthenia gravis, or a fascicular third nerve lesion) or with pretectal supranuclear lesions. Supranuclear monocular elevation paresis may be congenital[198,199] or acquired, with the latter due to a lesion contralateral to the paretic eye or ipsilateral to the paretic eye that interrupts efferents from the rostral interstitial nucleus of the medial longitudinal fasciculus to the superior rectus and inferior oblique subnuclei.[200,201] Double elevator palsy may simply be an asymmetric upgaze palsy that clinically presents as monocular elevation paresis in the more severely affected eye.[201] Patients do not have subjective diplopia in primary position and demonstrate limitation of monocular elevation that is the same from primary position, adduction, or abduction, confirming a supranuclear basis for the elevation impairment. Patients may have associated pupillary abnormalities, convergence impairment, and other neurologic signs of brainstem involvement but do not have ptosis, lid retraction, proptosis, and positive forced ductions. A vertical one-and-a-half syndrome, with vertical upgaze palsy and monocular paresis of downgaze on the side of the lesion or contralateral to the lesion, and skew deviation, a vertical misalignment resulting from supranuclear derangement, may also cause vertical diplopia. These and the ocular tilt reaction (OTR), discussed in Chapter 14, may also be associated with vertical diplopia. A tonic OTR may simulate superior oblique palsy.[202] Five patients with OTR had a three-step test suggesting superior oblique palsy (bilateral in one patient), but no patient had the expected excyclotorsion of the hypertropic eye. Two patients had conjugate ocular torsion (intorsion of the hypertropic eye and extorsion of the hypotropic eye) and two patients had only intorsion of the hypotropic eye. All had neurologic deficits consistent with more widespread brainstem disease. The authors concluded that vertical ocular deviations that localize to superior oblique palsy on three-step testing are not always caused by fourth nerve weakness. When a patient with an apparent fourth nerve palsy has ocular torsion inconsistent with a superior oblique (SO) palsy, OTR should be suspected, especially if posterior fossa or vestibular dysfunction coexist. Because results of the Bielschowsky head tilt test may be positive in patients with the OTR, the feature distinguishing OTR from SO palsy is the direction of torsion. The authors advocate a fourth step—evaluation of ocular torsion—in addition to the standard three steps.

Wernicke encephalopathy is due to thiamine deficiency and is especially seen in the context of chronic alcohol abuse. Patients with Wernicke encephalopathy may endorse vertical diplopia due to a supranuclear or nuclear lesion. This is associated with other signs of brainstem and cerebellar dysfunction (e.g., nystagmus, gaze palsies, gait ataxia), confusion, memory impairment, and peripheral polyneuropathy.

Paroxysmal superior rectus and levator palpebrae spasm is a rare and unique disorder described in a single patient with multiple sclerosis.[203] Paroxysms of vertical diplopia and lid retraction in this patient lasted 3 to 4 seconds and examination revealed intermittent right hypertropia, lid retraction, and restriction of downgaze. MRI revealed multiple lesions consistent with multiple sclerosis, including a midbrain lesion involving the third nerve fascicle. Carbamazepine relieved all symptoms caused by spontaneous spasm of the superior rectus/levator complex.

10.30 What Cranial Nerve Impairments Cause Vertical Diplopia?

Third nerve palsies may cause vertical and horizontal binocular diplopia and are discussed in Chapter 11. Fourth cranial nerve palsies are a common cause of acquired binocular vertical diplopia[10,204] and are discussed in Chapter 12.

Increased intracranial pressure may rarely cause transient diplopia.[205] A patient has been described with recurrent attacks of a right third nerve palsy causing diplopia in addition to headaches, papilledema, periodic urinary incontinence, and other neurologic findings. The transient third nerve palsy lasted about 5 minutes and eventually the patient developed persistent third nerve palsy. At autopsy, the patient had right frontal and temporal brain metastases with herniation of the hippocampal gyrus that stretched the right third nerve.

Superior oblique myokymia is a rare disorder of unknown etiology characterized symptomatically by oscillopsia and episodic vertical and/or torsional diplopia. This disorder is discussed in Chapter 17. ONM may also cause vertical diplopia and is discussed earlier.

Ophthalmoplegic migraine usually starts in the first decade of life and usually affects the oculomotor nerve, although rare trochlear nerve or multiple ocular motor nerve involvement has been described.[206] Clinical criteria essential for the diagnosis of ophthalmoplegic migraine include (1) a history of typical migraine headache (severe, throbbing, unilateral but occasionally bilateral or alternating) lasting hours to days; (2) ophthalmoplegia that may include one or more nerves and may alternate sides with attacks (extraocular muscle paralysis may occur with the first attack of headache or, rarely, precede it; usually, however, the paralysis appears subsequent to an established migraine pattern); and (3) exclusion of other causes by neuroimaging, surgery, or autopsy. Friedman et al studied 5,000 patients with migraine and found eight examples (0.16%) of ophthalmoplegic migraine.[207] All eight patients had recurrent attacks of headache (usually orbital), usually accompanied by nausea and vomiting, and an ipsilateral third nerve palsy. The third nerve paresis reached a maximum as the headache began to resolve and persisted for 1 to 4 weeks. Third nerve paralysis during an attack is often complete or nearly so, but partial third nerve paresis, including isolated superior division third nerve paresis, may occur.[208] Most patients have normal neuro-ophthalmologic examinations between attacks, but some patients may demonstrate partial third nerve paresis or even signs of aberrant regeneration. The differential diagnosis of ophthalmoplegic migraine is that of painful ophthalmoplegia in general; during the initial attack, structural lesions, especially aneurysms, should be suspected, and the evaluation should proceed as described for third nerve palsies (Chapter 11). The diagnosis should thus be made with caution, especially if the first attack occurs in adulthood, and only after other causes of painful ophthalmoplegia have been excluded by appropriate laboratory and neuroimaging studies.[205]

Miller Fisher syndrome (ophthalmoplegia associated with ataxia and areflexia) or Guillain–Barré syndrome (associated with diffuse muscle paresis, areflexia, etc.) may also be associated with vertical diplopia.[195] Miller Fisher syndrome, Guillain–Barré syndrome with ophthalmoplegia, Bickerstaff brainstem encephalitis, and acute ophthalmoparesis without ataxia are all associated with the anti-GQ1b IgG autoantibody.[209,210]

Although patients with sixth cranial nerve palsies mainly complain of horizontal binocular diplopia with esotropia or esophoria on examination, some patients endorse vertical as well as horizontal diplopia.[211] Hyperdeviation with sixth nerve palsies may occur in primary gaze but is usually most prominent to the side of the palsy with the hyperdeviation measuring

4 to 16 prism diopters. Patients with isolated sixth nerve palsies with hyperdeviation have normal vertical ductions, no torsional abnormality on double Maddox rod testing, and negative head tilt test. Rarely, up- or down-shooting of the paretic eye may be noted on attempted abduction. The hyperdeviation may be due to mechanical factors (decreased vertical stabilization of globe due to weak lateral rectus) or vertical substitution movement in the face of one paretic muscle.[211] Although hyperdeviation may occur with isolated sixth nerve palsies, one must always be concerned that the hyperdeviation in a patient with a sixth nerve palsy reflects concomitant involvement of the third or fourth cranial nerve (e.g., with cavernous sinus pathology), associated skew deviation, or myasthenia gravis. Conditions suggesting additional causes for a hyperdeviation with a sixth nerve palsy include a positive head tilt test, cyclotropia on double Maddox rod testing, concomitant nystagmus or other signs of brainstem dysfunction, associated ptosis, or decreased vertical muscle ductions.

10.31 What Disease Processes Affecting the Neuromuscular Junction Cause Vertical Diplopia?

A common cause of intermittent diplopia is myasthenia gravis. Myasthenia gravis may masquerade as a fourth nerve palsy with vertical duction limitations, cyclotropia, and a positive head tilt test. Increased vertical deviation with sustained upgaze and improvement of the deviation after eye closure are suggestive of myasthenia gravis. Ocular myasthenia gravis is discussed in detail in Chapter 15. Botulism may also be associated with vertical diplopia but typically has systemic weakness and pupil involvement bilaterally.

10.32 What Disease Processes Affecting the Extraocular Muscles Cause Vertical Diplopia?

Isolated paresis of a vertical-acting extraocular muscle may cause vertical binocular diplopia. Myasthenia gravis should be considered in all such cases. Other etiologies of isolated vertical-acting extraocular muscle palsy include local trauma (e.g., cataract surgery), vascular disease (especially muscle ischemia with giant cell arteritis), thyroid ophthalmopathy, congenital causes, and the etiologies of restrictive ophthalmopathy noted below.[10,212] Isolated superior rectus palsy causes ipsilateral hypotropia in primary position, impaired ocular elevation in abduction, trace excyclotorsion, and absent Bell's phenomenon. Head tilt is usually toward the sound side but may be toward the side of palsy. Superior rectus palsy may be associated with ipsilateral ptosis, especially in congenital cases. Also, a pseudoptosis may be noted on the side of hypotropia when the nonparetic eye fixates. Isolated inferior rectus palsy is often congenital and results in hypertropia in primary gaze, incyclotorsion, impaired depression of the eye in abduction, pseudoptosis of the sound eye when the paretic eye fixates, and a head tilt to either side. Isolated inferior oblique muscle paresis is rare and results in hypotropia in primary gaze, impaired elevation in adduction, incyclotorsion, and a head tilt, most often toward the paralyzed side. The head tilt test is positive on tilting the head toward the normal side. Although superior oblique muscle paresis is most often due to fourth nerve palsies, this muscle may also be affected by myasthenia gravis, botulism, trochleitis, orbital metastasis, orbital inflammatory pseudotumor (myositis), and trauma to the trochlea.[195,204,213] Occasionally, damage to the trochlea (e.g., due to dog bite or frontal sinus surgery) may cause acquired Brown syndrome (see below) associated with underaction of the ipsilateral superior oblique muscle referred to as the "canine tooth syndrome." Isolated superior oblique myositis may cause mild limitation of elevation of the eye in adduction.[214]

Rarely, vertical binocular diplopia may occur from chronic progressive external ophthalmoplegia (often associated with ptosis, orbicularis oculi paresis, and occasionally pigmentary retinopathy). These patients rarely experience diplopia despite prominent external ophthalmoplegia.

Decompensation of a long-standing phoria may cause hypertropia and vertical diplopia.[215] A phoria will become manifest and break down into a tropia if fusion is broken. This occurs transiently by occluding or blurring vision in one eye, when a patient is tired, when a patient has taken a central nervous system depressant such as alcohol or sedative medications, or during a febrile illness. More persistent decompensation may occur following head trauma, with changing refractive needs, often for unclear reasons. Neuro-ophthalmologic history and examination often reveal supportive evidence of long-standing strabismus including a history of childhood strabismus or patching, the presence of a head tilt or turn (demonstrated on old photos), and large vertical fusional amplitude (6–20 prism diopters). Vertical fusional amplitudes are measured by presenting vertically oriented prisms of gradually increasing strength in front of one eye after first neutralizing any manifest tropia. The amount of prism needed to produce diplopia over that needed to neutralize the tropia (if present) represents the fusional amplitude (normal vertical fusional amplitudes are two to four prism diopters).

A number of congenital conditions may be associated with vertical deviation of the eyes without vertical diplopia. These conditions include congenital strabismus syndromes, DVD, congenital double elevator or double depressor palsy, and asymptomatic physiologic hyperdeviation on lateral gaze. Congenital strabismus syndromes may be associated with overaction of the inferior or superior oblique muscles, causing V-pattern exotropia or esotropia and A-pattern exotropia or esotropia, respectively. Patients with these patterns of congenital strabismus do not have hyperdeviation in primary gaze, do not have a positive head tilt test, do not have ductional limitation, and do not have cyclodeviation. DVD, characterized by upward turn of the nonfixating eye, may also accompany congenital strabismus, especially esotropia. Monocular occlusion of either eye produces elevation of the occluded eye without corresponding depression of the uncovered eye (i.e., DVD does not follow Hering's law). The eye under cover "floats" up and out and may also excyclotort. After removal of the cover, the eye makes a slow downward movement to reach midline accompanied by incyclotorsion. The deviation is often variable, bilateral, and asymmetric. There is no ductional limitation, head tilt test is negative, and the deviation is not gaze dependent. Congenital

"double elevator" palsy (monocular elevation deficiency) may be due to inferior rectus restriction (with positive forced ductions to elevation, no muscle paralysis, and normal saccades of the superior rectus), elevator weakness (with negative forced ductions, evidence of paralysis of vertical muscles, and reduced saccadic velocities in upgaze of the affected eye), or a combination of inferior rectus restriction and weak elevators (with positive forced ductions in elevation, reduced upward vertical saccadic velocities in involved eye, and variable muscle paresis). Von Noorden noted that one must consider the possibility that double elevator paralysis is a misnomer and that generalized weakness of elevation is caused by long-standing superior rectus palsy, the deviation having spread throughout the entire upward field of gaze and the inferior rectus having become contracted.[10] Double depressor paralysis (unilateral paralysis of the inferior rectus and superior oblique) is rare and may be congenital or acquired.[10] Again, von Noorden suspects that the so-called double depressor paralyses are caused by long-standing inferior rectus muscle paralysis and secondary superior rectus contracture.[10]

It should be noted that many patients may have asymptomatic physiologic hyperdeviation on lateral gaze. Slavin et al noted a physiologic hyperdeviation of greater than two prism diopters that simulates overaction of the inferior oblique muscle in 77% of normal subjects.[216] The hyperdeviation occurred in any field of gaze and never measured greater than 10 prism diopters. Forty-seven percent of the patients showed an isolated left hyperdeviation in right upgaze and right hyperdeviation in left upgaze, 32% had either a right hyperdeviation in left upgaze or a left hyperdeviation in right upgaze, and 85% of patients had a V pattern of less than 15 prism diopters. No patient had hyperdeviation in primary gaze or hyperdeviation induced by head tilt, and no patients complained of vertical diplopia. Thus, physiologic hyperdeviation should not be considered with hyperdeviation in primary gaze, hyperdeviation induced by head tilt in primary gaze, significant downgaze hyperdeviation, duction limitation, or uncrossed hyperdeviation in peripheral gaze (e.g., a left hyperdeviation on gaze to the left and up).

10.33 What Mechanical Processes Cause Vertical Eye Misalignment?

Restrictive ophthalmopathy may result in vertical binocular diplopia. Restrictive ophthalmopathy is defined as limitation of eye movement associated with a positive forced duction test. An increase in intraocular pressure (>5 mm) in the direction against the restriction is indirect evidence of restriction (differential intraocular pressure). Normal saccadic velocities favor a restrictive ophthalmopathy as a cause for diplopia rather than an ocular motor nerve palsy.[10,195]

Thyroid eye disease is a common cause of horizontal or vertical diplopia. "Tightness" and restriction of the extraocular muscles preferentially affect the inferior rectus, medial rectus, and superior rectus, in that order. Limitation of elevation in one or both eyes is by far the most common defect of ocular motility. Vertical misalignment with thyroid eye disease is usually associated with other characteristic signs such as lid lag, lid retraction, and proptosis. Patients often have ductional limitation in the vertical plane and may also have cyclodeviation and a positive head tilt test. The forced duction test is often positive and the diagnosis is aided by demonstrating appropriate extraocular muscle enlargement with orbital ultrasound, computed tomography (CT), or MRI.

Thyroid eye disease may present as an apparent superior oblique muscle paresis on the three-step test and may thus be mistaken for fourth nerve palsy.[213,216] This clinical picture is caused by the restrictive process affecting the opposite inferior rectus muscle (hypotropic eye) with the hypotropia greatest in the field of superior rectus. Clues to the diagnosis of thyroid eye disease rather than superior oblique weakness, in a patient with hyperdeviation, include the following:

1. Increased vertical deviation in upgaze.
2. Increased intraocular tension (> 5 mm) in upgaze.
3. When a "subacute" or "chronic" superior oblique palsy is diagnosed (i.e., when the hyperdeviation is greater on upgaze), consider that a restrictive process may be operative; if ductions are normal, differential intraocular pressure should be evaluated.
4. If a patient with acute diplopia is found to have a hypertropia greater on upgaze than downgaze, a diagnosis of superior oblique palsy should be withheld.

Thyroid eye disease is discussed in detail in Chapter 16.

With the Brown superior oblique tendon sheath syndrome, there is an inability to elevate the adducted eye above the midhorizontal plane.[10] This condition may be bilateral in about 10% of patients. A mechanical restriction to free movement of the superior oblique tendon at the pulley may prevent the upward and inward movement of the globe, thus mimicking paresis of the inferior oblique muscle. Episodic vertical diplopia results from entrapment of the eye on gaze downward and inward or in the field of action of the superior oblique. The eye may then release suddenly, occasionally associated with the sensation or actual hearing of a click. Some minimal restriction of elevation may persist even in full abduction and there may be slight down-shoot of the adducted eye mimicking superior oblique overaction. Hypotropia in primary gaze, a compensatory head posture (chin up due to hypotropia with a head turn toward the involved side), and a V-pattern exotropia may be noted in addition to positive forced duction testing. This syndrome is often congenital but may be acquired due to superomedial orbital trauma, tenosynovitis or myositis, adhesions, metastasis to the superior oblique muscle, frontal sinus osteoma, pansinusitis, psoriasis, peribulbar anesthesia, blepharoplasty, implantation of a glaucoma tube shunt, maxillofacial or sinus surgery, and superior oblique tuck.[10,217,218,219,220,221,222] In congenital cases, MRI may show enlargement of the tendon–trochlea complex with this complex being of irregular shape and of intermediate signal intensity.[223,224]

The superior oblique click syndrome is a form of intermittent acquired Brown' syndrome with a clinical picture that alternates between a Brown-type syndrome and a superior oblique muscle palsy.[225] The clinical features depend on the direction in which the muscle is impeded. The click, often audible to the patient and/or the examiner, may signal the release of the restriction. The click is palpable in the superonasal orbit. Lesions are located within the sheath of the anterior superior oblique tendon, and include schwannoma and giant cell tumor of the tendon.

Some reports suggest that Brown syndrome and superior oblique palsy have the same origin.[226,227] Coussens and Ellis reported a case in which a male patient had Brown syndrome and his father had congenital superior oblique palsy.[226] The authors proposed that both syndromes arise from a developmental defect in the superior oblique muscle–tendon–trochlea complex. If the tendon is lax or absent, it is superior oblique palsy; if the tendon is strained, it manifests as Brown syndrome.

The differential of Brown syndrome includes, primarily, paralysis of the inferior oblique muscle. Forced ductions distinguish these syndromes. Other restrictions of elevation (such as thyroid eye disease, the inferior rectus muscle fibrosis, double elevator palsy, and orbital floor fractures) usually cause elevation restriction from any gaze position and are not limited to elevation restriction in adduction.[10] However, orbital floor fracture and thyroid ophthalmopathy may simulate Brown syndrome.[10,228,229]

Orbital blowout fractures frequently incarcerate the inferior rectus muscle and its surrounding tissue. Characteristic findings may include any of the following[218,230]:

1. Edema and ecchymosis of the involved eye.
2. Diplopia often presents in all positions of gaze immediately posttrauma that may persist in upgaze or downgaze.
3. Paresthesia of the infraorbital area due to damage to the infraorbital nerve.
4. Enophthalmos, either early or late.
5. Entrapment of the inferior rectus, inferior oblique, and/or surrounding tissue resulting in restriction of upward gaze with positive forced duction testing. Inferior rectus paresis, resulting in hypertropia in primary position in the involved eye, may also occur due to direct nerve or muscle trauma.
6. Hypotropia in primary position that increases in upgaze.
7. Frequent intraocular damage.

Other causes of restrictive ophthalmopathy include direct trauma to the extraocular muscles (e.g., intramuscular hematoma), congenital inferior rectus fibrosis (often with ipsilateral ptosis), strabismus fixus (generalized fibrosis of extraocular muscles), postoperative sequelae (including retinal detachment surgery, orbital surgery, strabismus surgery, sinus surgery, and cataract surgery), orbital inflammation (myositis), metastatic infiltration of extraocular muscles, and other orbital tumors.[195,231,232,233] Orbital lesions are usually associated with pain, proptosis, chemosis, or other findings that betray their location. Also, with long-standing muscle paralysis, the antagonist muscle may become contracted and fibrotic. Thus, patients with long-standing superior oblique muscle paresis who habitually fixate with the paretic eye may develop the fallen eye syndrome.[195] This syndrome manifests as a unilateral superior oblique muscle paresis presenting with hypodeviation of the uninvolved eye that worsens in abduction caused by contracture of the contralateral inferior rectus muscle. Conversely, long-standing inferior oblique muscle palsy may result in the rising eye syndrome due to contracture and fibrosis of the contralateral superior rectus muscle (the contralateral eye rises during attempted abduction).[195] Transient recurrent vertical diplopia, likely due to intermittent transient fusion impairment, has been described with maxillary sinusitis associated with lowering of the orbital floor (silent sinus syndrome).[234,235,236] The spectrum of silent sinus syndrome includes enophthalmos, hypoglobus, transient vertical diplopia, lid retraction, lagophthalmos, and blurred vision.[235,236]

The congenital inferior rectus fibrosis syndrome is a rare familial or sporadic syndrome manifested by downward fixation of one or both eyes associated with marked ptosis, restricted elevation (of equal magnitude from adduction, primary position, and abduction), positive forced ductions, and a backward (chin-up) head tilt.[10,232] CT imaging may show atrophy of the involved inferior rectus muscle.[233] In some cases, pathologic studies have shown absence of the superior division of the oculomotor nerve and its corresponding alpha motor neurons, and abnormalities of the levator palpebrae superioris and superior rectus (the muscles innervated by the superior division of the oculomotor nerve). Thus, congenital fibrosis of the extraocular muscles likely results from an abnormality in the development of the extraocular muscle lower motor neuron system.[232]

Vertical diplopia after cataract surgery requires some comment. Three categories of strabismus or diplopia have been noted after cataract surgery[237]:

1. Preexisting condition (e.g., thyroid eye disease) in which misalignment was masked by a dense cataract.
2. Conditions secondary to prolonged occlusion by the cataract (e.g., sensory deprivation). Disruption of binocularity may be caused by long-term occlusion. Also, fusional amplitude can be reduced by the occluding cataract. Improved vision following surgery renders the preexisting ocular conditions symptomatic.
3. Surgical trauma to extraocular muscles or orbital soft tissue (injury to inferior rectus muscle causing paresis or contracture is most common).

Capó and Guyton studied 19 patients with vertical strabismus after cataract surgery and noted that the vertical deviation was greater in the field of action of the presumed tight muscle in 16 of the 19 patients.[238] An ipsilateral hypertropia with superior rectus muscle overaction subsequently developed in two patients with an initial hypotropia. The authors noted that myotoxicity from direct injection of local anesthetics into an extraocular muscle probably causes transient paresis followed by segmental contracture of the involved muscle. Mild contractures result in strabismus with a motility pattern of an overactive muscle, whereas larger amounts of contracture lead to restrictive strabismus. In another prospective study of 20 consecutive patients with acquired vertical diplopia after cataract surgery, Capó et al noted that 50% of involved muscles were overactive, 39% were restricted, and 11% were paretic.[239] In overactive strabismus, versions showed overaction of the affected muscle with no significant underaction of its antagonist, the deviation increased in the field of action of the affected muscle, and forced ductions were negative or mildly positive. In restrictive cases, the affected muscle was tight by forced duction testing and the deviation was either comitant or worse in the field of action of the antagonist muscle. In paretic cases, the diagnosis was reached by limited ductions in the field of action of the affected muscle, accompanied by negative forced-duction testing. The inferior rectus was involved in 17 patients (61%) and superior rectus muscle in 11 (39%). The odds of damaging the inferior rectus, as opposed to superior rectus, with peribulbar anesthesia was 4.8 times higher than with retrobulbar blocks. The authors drew the following conclusions concerning

motility disturbances causing acquired strabismus after cataract surgery:

1. Myotoxic effects of local anesthesia could result in temporary or permanent muscle weakness.
2. Superior rectus overaction may occur from superior rectus contracture secondary to temporary paresis of the inferior rectus muscle caused by local anesthetic.
3. Inferior rectus muscle contracture may result from direct penetration by needle, with elevated tissue pressure due to hematoma or a large amount of anesthetic within the muscle, followed by secondary vascular compromise and ensuing muscle fibrosis.
4. In the series, restrictive and overactive motility disorders predominate, suggesting that most cases with persistent vertical strabismus after cataract surgery result from muscle contracture rather than from permanent muscle paresis.

The authors concluded that in this patient population, permanent vertical strabismus following cataract surgery results more often from muscle overaction or restriction as opposed to paresis. Both the superior and inferior recti can be injured with retrobulbar anesthesia; peribulbar injections affect the inferior rectus muscle more frequently.[239] Occasionally, a permanent extraocular muscle paresis occurs, possibly secondary to nerve damage, but this mechanism is unclear. Corboy and Jiang reported 31 cases of postoperative hypotropia following 2,143 cataract operations and noted that myotoxicity or perimuscular inflammation from anesthesia likely produced contracture hypotropia and restricted elevation of the globe.[240]

Koide et al reported 18 eyes of 17 patients with diplopia after retrobulbar anesthesia for cataract surgery.[241] Several cases showed superior or inferior deviations, but most patients had nonuniform disturbances of ocular motility. In another study, orthoptic evaluations were carried out in 118 cataract surgery patients (all of who underwent retrobulbar anesthetic injections) at 1 month before, 1 day after, 1 week after, and 1 month after surgery.[242] Preoperatively, 16 patients had ocular misalignment; 10 were phoric, 4 were intermittently tropic, and 2 were tropic. Follow-up evaluation was obtained for 101 patients (86%) at 1 day, 91 (77%) at 1 week, and 88 (75%) at 1 month. A change in ocular alignment occurred in 22 of 101 patients (22%) at 1 day, 9 of 91 (10%) at 1 week, and 6 of 88 (7%) at 1 month. Only one patient who had a change in alignment at 1 month was symptomatic. The authors concluded that change in ocular alignment after uneventful cataract surgery occurred in 7% of patients, but symptomatic diplopia was uncommon (1 in 118) in this small series. Johnson noted persistent vertical diplopia after cataract surgery in 0.23% of patients in whom retrobulbar anesthesia was performed.[243] No cases were found after topical anesthesia.

Vertical strabismus after cataract surgery may also result from inferior oblique muscle injury from local anesthesia. Hunter et al described four patients without preexisting strabismus who developed diplopia following cataract surgery.[237] Three had delayed-onset hypertropia with fundus extorsion in the eye that underwent surgery, consistent with inferior oblique muscle overaction secondary to presumed contracture. The fourth patient had an intermediate-onset hypotropia with fundus intorsion in the eye that underwent surgery, consistent with inferior oblique paresis. The inferior oblique muscle contracture observed in three patients may have been caused by local anesthetic myotoxicity, whereas the early paresis observed in one patient may have been due to mechanical trauma or anesthetic toxicity directly to the nerve innervating the muscle. Inferior oblique muscle or nerve injury should be considered as another possible cause of postoperative vertical strabismus, especially when significant fundus torsion accompanies a vertical deviation. As noted earlier, a Brown syndrome may also occur after cataract surgery. The number of cases of diplopia after cataract surgery seems to be declining with the increasing use of topical rather than retrobulbar anesthesia.

10.34 What Is the Foveal Displacement Syndrome?

Binocular diplopia may occasionally occur with retinal disease. In one study, 52% of causes responsible for foveal displacement syndrome was due to epiretinal membrane, whereas 31% of these causes was due to ocular surgery.[244] Burgess et al described 11 patients with subretinal neovascular membranes in one eye who developed binocular diplopia before and after effective photocoagulation therapy (the foveal displacement syndrome).[245] The diplopia was thought to be due to a rivalry between central and peripheral fusional mechanisms. The subretinal neovascular membrane produced a shift of the foveal photoreceptor array toward the proliferating neovascular complex. If the unaffected eye is covered, the affected eye will have to realign, mimicking a true tropia. For example, an inferior foveal lesion will mimic a hypertropia in the affected eye. All patients demonstrated the following:

1. The affected eye deviated (measured tropia) away from the position of the retinal lesion (e.g., a lesion inferior to the fovea produces a superior scotoma).
2. The affected eye deviated upward (toward the scotoma).
3. The distal diplopic image was downward (toward the retinal image).

The diplopia in this condition responds only transiently to prisms. Surgical removal of the subretinal neovascular membrane may correct the diplopia, at least transiently.[246] Foveal displacement syndrome may also occur in patients with epiretinal membranes.[247,248] Benegas et al described seven patients with binocular diplopia concurrent with macular disease, including epiretinal membranes (six patients) and vitreomacular traction (one patient).[247] All seven patients had aniseikonia and all had concomitant small-angle strabismus. The response to treatment with prisms was variable. The authors concluded that aniseikonia, caused by separation or compression of photoreceptors, is likely a contributing factor to the existence of diplopia and the inability to fuse in patients with macular disease. Silverberg et al presented seven patients with binocular diplopia due to macular disease, including subretinal neovascularization, epiretinal membrane, and central serous retinopathy.[248] All except one had a small-angle, comitant hyperdeviation with no muscle paresis. Neither prism correction nor manipulation of the refractive errors corrected the diplopia. However, a partially occlusive foil (Bangerter) of density ranging from 0.4 to 1.0 placed in front of the affected eye provided an effective treatment, allowing peripheral fusion to be maintained.

The retinal hemifield slide or slip phenomenon, a rare cause of intermittent binocular diplopia noted in some patients with lesions of the optic chiasm, can cause vertical diplopia and is discussed earlier. Finally, subjective symptoms of vertical or horizontal diplopia may also occur on a nonorganic basis (fictitious diplopia).

References

[1] Woods RL, Bradley A, Atchison DA. Monocular diplopia caused by ocular aberrations and hyperopic defocus. Vision Res. 1996; 36(22):3597–3606

[2] Jones MR, Waggoner R, Hoyt WF. Cerebral polyopia with extrastriate quadrantanopia: report of a case with magnetic resonance documentation of V2/V3 cortical infarction. J Neuroophthalmol. 1999; 19(1):1–6

[3] Lopez JR, Adornato BT, Hoyt WF. 'Entomopia': a remarkable case of cerebral polyopia. Neurology. 1993; 43(10):2145–2146

[4] Chalita MR, Xu M, Krueger RR. Correlation of aberrations with visual symptoms using wavefront analysis in eyes after laser in situ keratomileusis. J Refract Surg. 2003; 19(6):S682–S686

[5] Chalita MR, Chavala S, Xu M, Krueger RR. Wavefront analysis in post-LASIK eyes and its correlation with visual symptoms, refraction, and topography. Ophthalmology. 2004; 111(3):447–453

[6] Chalita MR, Roth AS, Krueger RR. Wavefront-guided surface ablation with prophylactic use of mitomycin C after a buttonhole laser in situ keratomileusis flap. J Refract Surg. 2004; 20(2):176–181

[7] Melamud A, Chalita MR, Krueger RR, Lee MS. Comatic aberration as a cause of monocular diplopia. J Cataract Refract Surg. 2006; 32(3):529–532

[8] Fujikado T, Shimojyo H, Hosohata J, et al. Wavefront analysis of eye with monocular diplopia and cortical cataract. Am J Ophthalmol. 2006; 141(6): 1138–1140

[9] Pérez GM, Abenza S, De Casas A, Marín JM, Artal P. Cause of monocular diplopia diagnosed by combining double-pass retinal image assessment and Hartmann-Shack aberrometry. J Refract Surg. 2010; 26(4):301–304

[10] von Noorden GK. Binocular Vision and Ocular Motility. 5th ed. St Louis, MO: Mosby; 1996

[11] Brazis PW, Lee AG. Acquired binocular horizontal diplopia. Mayo Clin Proc. 1999; 74(9):907–916

[12] Mittelman D. Age-related distance esotropia. J AAPOS. 2006; 10(3):212–213

[13] Mittelman D. Surgical management of adult onset age-related distance esotropia. J Pediatr Ophthalmol Strabismus. 2011; 48(4):214–216, quiz 217

[14] Godts D, Mathysen DG. Distance esotropia in the elderly. Br J Ophthalmol. 2013; 97(11):1415–1419

[15] Chaudhuri Z, Demer JL. Characteristics and surgical results in patients with age-related divergence insufficiency esotropia. J AAPOS. 2015; 19(1): 98–99

[16] Chaudhuri Z, Demer JL. Sagging eye syndrome: connective tissue involution as a cause of horizontal and vertical strabismus in older patients. JAMA Ophthalmol. 2013; 131(5):619–625

[17] Chaudhuri Z, Demer JL. Divergence insufficiency esotropia is a misnomer-reply. JAMA Ophthalmol. 2013; 131(4):547–548

[18] Lueder GT. Anomalous orbital structures resulting in unusual strabismus. Surv Ophthalmol. 2002; 47(1):27–35

[19] Mohney BG. Common forms of childhood esotropia. Ophthalmology. 2001; 108(4):805–809

[20] Kushner BJ. Recently acquired diplopia in adults with long-standing strabismus. Arch Ophthalmol. 2001; 119(12):1795–1801

[21] Chung M, Stout JT, Borchert MS. Clinical diversity of hereditary Duane's retraction syndrome. Ophthalmology. 2000; 107(3):500–503

[22] DeRespinis PA, Caputo AR, Wagner RS, Guo S. Duane's retraction syndrome. Surv Ophthalmol. 1993; 38(3):257–288

[23] Kekunnaya R, Gupta A, Sachdeva V, et al. Duane retraction syndrome: series of 441 cases. J Pediatr Ophthalmol Strabismus. 2012; 49(3):164–169

[24] Sarfraz S, Zafar SN, Khan A. Duane's syndrome: surgical outcome and non ophthalmologic associations. J Ayub Med Coll Abbottabad. 2014; 26(3): 328–330

[25] Ganesh SC, Narendran K, Pandey J. Surgical outcome of graded Y split in patients with Duane's retraction syndrome. J Pediatr Ophthalmol Strabismus. 2014; 51(5):262

[26] Sukhija J, Kaur S. Isolated Y splitting and recession of the lateral rectus muscle in patients with exo-Duane syndrome. Strabismus. 2013; 21(1):1–2

[27] Altintas AG, Arifoglu HB, Arikan M, Simsek S. Clinical findings and surgical results of Duane retraction syndrome. J Pediatr Ophthalmol Strabismus. 2010; 47(4):220–226

[28] Bosley TM, Abu-Amero KK, Oystreck DT. Congenital cranial dysinnervation disorders: a concept in evolution. Curr Opin Ophthalmol. 2013; 24(5): 398–406

[29] Denis D, Cousin M, Zanin E, Toesca E, Girard N. MRI in Duane retraction syndrome: preliminary results [in French]. J Fr Ophtalmol. 2011; 34(7): 476–481

[30] Denis D, Dauletbekov D, Alessi G, Chapon F, Girard N. Duane retraction syndrome: MRI features in two cases. J Neuroradiol. 2007; 34(2):137–140

[31] Kang NY, Demer JL. Comparison of orbital magnetic resonance imaging in Duane syndrome and abducens palsy. Am J Ophthalmol. 2006; 142(5): 827–834

[32] Kim JH, Hwang JM. Does infantile abduction deficit indicate Duane retraction syndrome until disproven? J Child Neurol. 2014; 29(11):NP151–NP153

[33] Tuzcu EA, Bayarogullari H, Atci N, et al. Magnetic resonance imaging findings of the abducens nerves in type 1 Duane's retraction syndrome. Semin Ophthalmol. 2014; 29(3):142–145

[34] Xia S, Li RL, Li YP, Qian XH, Chong V, Qi J. MRI findings in Duane's ocular retraction syndrome. Clin Radiol. 2014; 69(5):e191–e198

[35] Parsa CF. Abducens nerve is present in type 2 Duane's retraction syndrome. Ophthalmology. 2013; 120(2):436–437

[36] Kim JH, Hwang JM. Presence of the abducens nerve according to the type of Duane's retraction syndrome. Ophthalmology. 2005; 112(1):109–113

[37] Taylan Sekeroglu H, Ozlem Sımsek-Kıper P, Eda Utıne G, Boduroglu K, Sefik Sanac A, Cumhur Sener E. Wildervanck syndrome: an uncommon cause of Duane syndrome. J Fr Ophtalmol. 2014; 37(8):e123–e124

[38] Lee EK, Yang HK, Hwang JM. Long-term outcome of prismatic correction in children with consecutive esotropia after bilateral lateral rectus recession. Br J Ophthalmol. 2015; 99(3):342–345

[39] Sidikaro Y, von Noorden GK. Observations in sensory heterotropia. J Pediatr Ophthalmol Strabismus. 1982; 19(1):12–19

[40] Lacey B, Chang W, Rootman J. Nonthyroid causes of extraocular muscle disease. Surv Ophthalmol. 1999; 44(3):187–213

[41] Mombaerts I, Goldschmeding R, Schlingemann RO, Koornneef L. What is orbital pseudotumor? Surv Ophthalmol. 1996; 41(1):66–78

[42] Goto H, Takahira M, Azumi A, Japanese Study Group for IgG4-Related Ophthalmic Disease. Diagnostic criteria for IgG4-related ophthalmic disease. Jpn J Ophthalmol. 2015; 59(1):1–7

[43] Wallace ZS, Khosroshahi A, Jakobiec FA, et al. IgG4-related systemic disease as a cause of "idiopathic" orbital inflammation, including orbital myositis, and trigeminal nerve involvement. Surv Ophthalmol. 2012; 57(1):26–33

[44] Mombaerts I, Koornneef L. Current status in the treatment of orbital myositis. Ophthalmology. 1997; 104(3):402–408

[45] Bernardino CR, Davidson RS, Maus M, Spaeth GL. Angle-closure glaucoma in association with orbital pseudotumor. Ophthalmology. 2001; 108(9): 1603–1606

[46] Suhler EB, Lim LL, Beardsley RM, et al. Rituximab therapy for refractory orbital inflammation: results of a phase 1/2, dose-ranging, randomized clinical trial. JAMA Ophthalmol. 2014; 132(5):572–578

[47] Hatton MP, Rubin PA, Foster CS. Successful treatment of idiopathic orbital inflammation with mycophenolate mofetil. Am J Ophthalmol. 2005; 140(5): 916–918

[48] Thorne JE, Jabs DA, Qazi FA, Nguyen QD, Kempen JH, Dunn JP. Mycophenolate mofetil therapy for inflammatory eye disease. Ophthalmology. 2005; 112(8):1472–1477

[49] Prabhu RS, Kandula S, Liebman L, et al. Association of clinical response and long-term outcome among patients with biopsied orbital pseudotumor receiving modern radiation therapy. Int J Radiat Oncol Biol Phys. 2013; 85 (3):643–649

[50] Mannor GE, Rose GE, Moseley IF, Wright JE. Outcome of orbital myositis. Clinical features associated with recurrence. Ophthalmology. 1997; 104(3): 409–413, discussion, 414

[51] Durno CA, Ehrlich R, Taylor R, Buncic JR, Hughes P, Griffiths AM. Keeping an eye on Crohn's disease: orbital myositis as the presenting symptom. Can J Gastroenterol. 1997; 11(6):497–500

[52] Squires RH, Jr, Zwiener RJ, Kennedy RH. Orbital myositis and Crohn's disease. J Pediatr Gastroenterol Nutr. 1992; 15(4):448–451

[53] Takanashi T, Uchida S, Arita M, Okada M, Kashii S. Orbital inflammatory pseudotumor and ischemic vasculitis in Churg-Strauss syndrome: report of two cases and review of the literature. Ophthalmology. 2001; 108(6): 1129–1133

[54] Serop S, Vianna RN, Claeys M, De Laey JJ. Orbital myositis secondary to systemic lupus erythematosus. Acta Ophthalmol (Copenh). 1994; 72(4): 520–523

[55] Orssaud C, Poisson M, Gardeur D. Orbital myositis, recurrence of Whipple's disease [in French]. J Fr Ophtalmol. 1992; 15(3):205–208

[56] Mariani AF, Malik AI, Chevez-Barrios P, et al. Idiopathic orbital inflammation associated with relapsing polychondritis. Ophthal Plast Reconstr Surg. 2017; 33(3S) Sup pl 1:S167–S168

[57] Roh JH, Koh SB, Kim JH. Orbital myositis in Behçet's disease: a case report with MRI findings. Eur Neurol. 2006; 56(1):44–45

[58] Carvounis PE, Mehta AP, Geist CE. Orbital myositis associated with Borrelia burgdorferi (Lyme disease) infection. Ophthalmology. 2004; 111(5):1023–1028

[59] Ramboer K, Demaerel P, Baert AL, Casteels I, Dralands G. Linear scleroderma with orbital involvement: follow up and magnetic resonance imaging. Br J Ophthalmol. 1997; 81(1):90–91

[60] Suttorp-Schulten MS, Koornneef L. Linear scleroderma associated with ptosis and motility disorders. Br J Ophthalmol. 1990; 74(11):694–695

[61] Perry SR, Rootman J, White VA. The clinical and pathologic constellation of Wegener granulomatosis of the orbit. Ophthalmology. 1997; 104(4): 683–694

[62] Maurer I, Zierz S. Recurrent orbital myositis: report of a familial incidence. Arch Neurol. 1999; 56(11):1407–1409

[63] Harris GJ, Murphy ML, Schmidt EW, Hanson GA, Dotson RM. Orbital myositis as a paraneoplastic syndrome. Arch Ophthalmol. 1994; 112(3): 380–386

[64] de Jesús O, Inserni JA, Gonzalez A, Colón LE. Idiopathic orbital inflammation with intracranial extension. Case report. J Neurosurg. 1996; 85(3):510–513

[65] Song YS, Choung HK, Park SW, Kim JH, Khwarg SI, Jeon YK. Ocular adnexal IgG4-related disease: CT and MRI findings. Br J Ophthalmol. 2013; 97(4): 412–418

[66] Hutnik CML, Nicolle DA, Munoz DG. Orbital aspergillosis. A fatal masquerader. J Neuroophthalmol. 1997; 17(4):257–261

[67] Johnson TE, Casiano RR, Kronish JW, Tse DT, Meldrum M, Chang W. Sino-orbital aspergillosis in acquired immunodeficiency syndrome. Arch Ophthalmol. 1999; 117(1):57–64

[68] Levin LA, Avery R, Shore JW, Woog JJ, Baker AS. The spectrum of orbital aspergillosis: a clinicopathological review. Surv Ophthalmol. 1996; 41(2): 142–154

[69] Massry GG, Hornblass A, Harrison W. Itraconazole in the treatment of orbital aspergillosis. Ophthalmology. 1996; 103(9):1467–1470

[70] Slavin ML. Primary aspergillosis of the orbital apex. Arch Ophthalmol. 1991; 109(11):1502–1503

[71] Balch K, Phillips PH, Newman NJ. Painless orbital apex syndrome from mucormycosis. J Neuroophthalmol. 1997; 17(3):178–182

[72] Dooley DP, Hollsten DA, Grimes SR, Moss J, Jr. Indolent orbital apex syndrome caused by occult mucormycosis. J Clin Neuroophthalmol. 1992; 12(4):245–249

[73] Downie JA, Francis IC, Arnold JJ, Bott LM, Kos S. Sudden blindness and total ophthalmoplegia in mucormycosis. A clinicopathological correlation. J Clin Neuroophthalmol. 1993; 13(1):27–34

[74] Maskin SL, Fetchick RJ, Leone CR, Jr, Sharkey PK, Rinaldi MG. Bipolaris hawaiiensis-caused phaeohyphomycotic orbitopathy. A devastating fungal sinusitis in an apparently immunocompetent host. Ophthalmology. 1989; 96(2):175–179

[75] Sullivan TJ, Aylward GW, Wright JE. Actinomycosis of the orbit. Br J Ophthalmol. 1992; 76(8):505–506

[76] Behrens-Baumann W, Freissler G. Computed tomographic appearance of extraocular muscle calcification in a patient with seropositive trichinosis. Am J Ophthalmol. 1990; 110(6):709–710

[77] Goldberg RA, Rootman J. Clinical characteristics of metastatic orbital tumors. Ophthalmology. 1990; 97(5):620–624

[78] Goldberg RA, Rootman J, Cline RA. Tumors metastatic to the orbit: a changing picture. Surv Ophthalmol. 1990; 35(1):1–24

[79] Toller KK, Gigantelli JW, Spalding MJ. Bilateral orbital metastases from breast carcinoma. A case of false pseudotumor. Ophthalmology. 1998; 105 (10):1897–1901

[80] Esmaeli B, Ahmadi A, Tang R, Schiffman J, Kurzrock R. Interferon therapy for orbital infiltration secondary to Erdheim-Chester disease. Am J Ophthalmol. 2001; 132(6):945–947

[81] Shields JA, Karcioglu ZA, Shields CL, Eagle RC, Wong S. Orbital and eyelid involvement with Erdheim-Chester disease. A report of two cases. Arch Ophthalmol. 1991; 109(6):850–854

[82] Valmaggia C, Neuweiler J, Fretz C, Gottlob I. A case of Erdheim-Chester disease with orbital involvement. Arch Ophthalmol. 1997; 115(11): 1467–1468

[83] Çeviker N, Baykaner K, Akata F, et al. Primary amyloidosis of an extraocular muscle. Neuroophthalmology. 1997; 18:147–148

[84] Murdoch IE, Sullivan TJ, Moseley I, et al. Primary localised amyloidosis of the orbit. Br J Ophthalmol. 1996; 80(12):1083–1086

[85] Nemir J, Trninic I, Duric KS, Jakovcevic A, Mrak G, Paladino J. Extranodal right-optic nerve Rosai-Dorfman disease: a rare localization case report. Surg Neurol Int. 2016; 7 Suppl 44:S1158–S1162

[86] Cornblath WT, Elner V, Rolfe M. Extraocular muscle involvement in sarcoidosis. Ophthalmology. 1993; 100(4):501–505

[87] Patel AS, Kelman SE, Duncan GW, Rismondo V. Painless diplopia caused by extraocular muscle sarcoid. Arch Ophthalmol. 1994; 112(7):879–880

[88] Segal EI, Tang RA, Lee AG, Roberts DL, Campbell GA. Orbital apex lesion as the presenting manifestation of sarcoidosis. J Neuroophthalmol. 2000; 20 (3):156–158

[89] Takahashi T, Fujita N, Takeda K, Tanaka K, Nagai H. A case of sarcoid myopathy with external ocular muscle involvement–diagnosis and follow-up study with 99mTc pyrophosphate scintigraphy [in Japanese]. Rinsho Shinkeigaku. 2000; 40(2):145–148

[90] de Heide LJ, Talsma MA. Giant-cell arteritis presenting as an orbital pseudotumor. Neth J Med. 1999; 55(4):196–198

[91] Woo TL, Francis IC, Wilcsek GA, Coroneo MT, McNab AA, Sullivan TJ, Australasian Orbital and Adnexal Wagener's Study Group. Australasian orbital and adnexal Wegener's granulomatosis. Ophthalmology. 2001; 108 (9):1535–1543

[92] Kattah JC, Zimmerman LE, Kolsky MP, et al. Bilateral orbital involvement in fatal giant cell polymyositis. Ophthalmology. 1990; 97(4):520–525

[93] Leib ML, Odel JG, Cooney MJ. Orbital polymyositis and giant cell myocarditis. Ophthalmology. 1994; 101(5):950–954

[94] Stevens AW, Grossman ME, Barr ML. Orbital myositis, vitiligo, and giant cell myocarditis. J Am Acad Dermatol. 1996; 35(2, Pt 2):310–312

[95] Wladis EJ, Iglesias BV, Adam AP, Nazeer T, Gosselin EJ. Toll-like receptors in idiopathic orbital inflammation. Ophthal Plast Reconstr Surg. 2012; 28(4): 273–276

[96] Bartley GB. The epidemiologic characteristics and clinical course of ophthalmopathy associated with autoimmune thyroid disease in Olmsted County, Minnesota. Trans Am Ophthalmol Soc. 1994; 92:477–588

[97] Bartley GB, Fatourechi V, Kadrmas EF, et al. The incidence of Graves' ophthalmopathy in Olmsted County, Minnesota. Am J Ophthalmol. 1995; 120(4):511–517

[98] Bartley GB, Fatourechi V, Kadrmas EF, et al. Clinical features of Graves' ophthalmopathy in an incidence cohort. Am J Ophthalmol. 1996; 121(3): 284–290

[99] Bartley GB, Fatourechi V, Kadrmas EF, et al. Chronology of Graves' ophthalmopathy in an incidence cohort. Am J Ophthalmol. 1996; 121(4): 426–434

[100] Bartley GB, Gorman CA. Diagnostic criteria for Graves' ophthalmopathy. Am J Ophthalmol. 1995; 119(6):792–795

[101] Lee AG, Brazis PW. Therapeutic neuro-ophthalmology. In: Appel SH, ed. Current Neurology. Vol 17. Amsterdam: IOS Press; 1997:265–292

[102] Vargas ME, Warren FA, Kupersmith MJ. Exotropia as a sign of myasthenia gravis in dysthyroid ophthalmopathy. Br J Ophthalmol. 1993; 77(12): 822–823

[103] Eitzen JP, Elsas FJ. Strabismus following endoscopic intranasal sinus surgery. J Pediatr Ophthalmol Strabismus. 1991; 28(3):168–170

[104] Merle H, Gerard M, Raynaud M. Isolated medial orbital blow-out fracture with medial rectus entrapment. Acta Ophthalmol Scand. 1998; 76(3): 378–379

[105] Abdulla N, Eustace P. A case of ocular neuromyotonia with tonic pupil. J Neuroophthalmol. 1999; 19(2):125–127

[106] Barroso L, Hoyt WF. Episodic exotropia from lateral rectus neuromyotonia–appearance and remission after radiation therapy for a thalamic glioma. J Pediatr Ophthalmol Strabismus. 1993; 30(1):56–57

[107] Chung SM, Lee AG, Holds JB, Roper-Hall G, Cruz OA. Ocular neuromyotonia in Graves dysthyroid orbitopathy. Arch Ophthalmol. 1997; 115(3):365–370

[108] Ezra E, Spalton D, Sanders MD, Graham EM, Plant GT. Ocular neuromyotonia. Br J Ophthalmol. 1996; 80(4):350–355

[109] Frohman EM, Zee DS. Ocular neuromyotonia: clinical features, physiological mechanisms, and response to therapy. Ann Neurol. 1995; 37(5):620–626

[110] Fu ER. Ocular neuromyotonia–an unusual ocular motility complication after radiation therapy for nasopharyngeal carcinoma. Ann Acad Med Singapore. 1995; 24(6):895–897

[111] Haupert CL, Newman NJ. Ocular neuromyotonia 18 years after radiation therapy. Arch Ophthalmol. 1997; 115(10):1331–1332

[112] Helmchen C, Dieterich M, Straube A, Büttner U. "Abducens neuromyotonia" with partial oculomotor paralysis [in German]. Nervenarzt. 1992; 63(10): 625–629

[113] Morrow MJ, Kao GW, Arnold AC. Bilateral ocular neuromyotonia: oculographic correlations. Neurology. 1996; 46(1):264–266

[114] Newman SA. Gaze-induced strabismus. Surv Ophthalmol. 1993; 38(3): 303–309

[115] Yee RD, Purvin VA. Ocular neuromyotonia: three case reports with eye movement recordings. J Neuroophthalmol. 1998; 18(1):1–8

[116] Fricke J, Neugebauer A, Kirsch A, Rüssmann W. Ocular neuromyotonia: a case report. Strabismus. 2002; 10(2):119–124

[117] Kim SB, Oh SY, Chang MH, Kyung SE. Oculomotor neuromyotonia with lid ptosis on abduction. J AAPOS. 2013; 17(1):97–99

[118] Much JW, Weber ED, Newman SA. Ocular neuromyotonia after gamma knife stereotactic radiation therapy. J Neuroophthalmol. 2009; 29(2):136–139

[119] Kau HC, Tsai CC. Abducens ocular neuromyotonia in a patient with nasopharyngeal carcinoma following concurrent chemoradiotherapy. J Neuroophthalmol. 2010; 30(3):266–267

[120] Ela-Dalman N, Arnold AC, Chang LK, Velez FG, Lasky JL, III. Abducens nerve ocular neuromyotonia following non-sellar or parasellar tumors. Strabismus. 2007; 15(3):149–151

[121] de Saint Sardos A, Vincent A, Aroichane M, Ospina LH. Ocular neuromyotonia in a 15-year-old girl after radiation therapy. J AAPOS. 2008; 12(6):616–617– Epub2008Aug15

[122] Yürüten B, Ilhan S. Ocular neuromyotonia: a case report. Clin Neurol Neurosurg. 2003; 105(2):140–142

[123] Versino M, Colnaghi S, Todeschini A, et al. Ocular neuromyotonia with both tonic and paroxysmal components due to vascular compression. J Neurol. 2005; 252(2):227–229

[124] Cruz FM, Blitz AM, Subramanian PS. Partial third nerve palsy and ocular neuromyotonia from displacement of posterior communicating artery detected by high-resolution MRI. J Neuroophthalmol. 2013; 33(3):263–265

[125] Park HY, Hwang JM, Kim JS. Abducens neuromyotonia due to internal carotid artery aneurysm. J Neurol Sci. 2008; 270(1–2):205–208

[126] Tilikete C, Vial C, Niederlaender M, Bonnier PL, Vighetto A. Idiopathic ocular neuromyotonia: a neurovascular compression syndrome? J Neurol Neurosurg Psychiatry. 2000; 69(5):642–644

[127] Giardina AS, Slagle WS, Greene AM, Musick AN, Eckermann DR. Novel case of ocular neuromyotonia associated with thyroid-related orbitopathy and literature review. Optom Vis Sci. 2012; 89(12):e124–e134

[128] Roper-Hall G, Chung SM, Cruz OA. Ocular neuromyotonia: differential diagnosis and treatment. Strabismus. 2013; 21(2):131–136

[129] Boschi A, Spiritus M, Cioffi M, et al. Ocular neuromyotonia in a case of Paget's disease of bone. Neuro-ophthalmology. 1997; 18(2):67–71

[130] Oohira A, Furuya T. Ocular neuromyotonia with spastic lid closure. J Neuroophthalmol. 2006; 26(4):244–247

[131] Jacob M, Vighetto A, Bernard M, Tilikete C. Ocular neuromyotonia secondary to a cavernous sinus meningioma. Neurology. 2006; 66(10):1598–1599

[132] Salchow DJ, Wermund TK. Abducens neuromyotonia as the presenting sign of an intracranial tumor. J Neuroophthalmol. 2011; 31(1):34–37

[133] Harrison AR, Wirtschafter JD. Ocular neuromyotonia in a patient with cavernous sinus thrombosis secondary to mucormycosis. Am J Ophthalmol. 1997; 124(1):122–123

[134] Banks MC, Caruso PA, Lessell S. Midbrain-thalamic ocular neuromyotonia. Arch Ophthalmol. 2005; 123(1):118–119

[135] Menon D, Sreedharan SE, Gupta M, Nair MD. A novel association of ocular neuromyotonia with brainstem demyelination: two case reports. Mult Scler. 2014; 20(10):1409–1412

[136] Plant GT. Putting ocular neuromyotonia in context. J Neuroophthalmol. 2006; 26(4):241–243

[137] Safran AB, Magistris M. Terminating attacks of ocular neuromyotonia. J Neuroophthalmol. 1998; 18(1):47–48

[138] Weston K, Bush K, Afshar F, Rowley S. Can he fix it? Yes, he can! BMJ. 2010; 341:c6645

[139] Inoue T, Hirai H, Shimizu T, et al. Ocular neuromyotonia treated by microvascular decompression: usefulness of preoperative 3D imaging: case report. J Neurosurg. 2012; 117(6):1166–1169

[140] Jang J, Chang M, Kyung S. Ocular neuromyotonia and myasthenia gravis. J Pediatr Ophthalmol Strabismus. 2015; 52(3):190–191

[141] Riordan-Eva P, Vickers SF, McCarry B, Lee JP. Cyclic strabismus without binocular function. J Pediatr Ophthalmol Strabismus. 1993; 30(2):106–108

[142] Tapiero B, Pedespan JM, Rougier MB, Huslin V, Massicault B, Le Rebeller MJ. Cyclic strabismus. Presentation of two new cases and critical review of the literature [in French]. J Fr Ophtalmol. 1995; 18(6–7):411–420

[143] Ma L, Kong D, Fan Z, Zhao J. Consecutive cyclic esotropia after surgery for intermittent exotropia. Can J Ophthalmol. 2014; 49(5):e107–e108

[144] Roper-Hall G, Cruz OA, Espinoza GM, Chung SM. Cyclic (alternate day) vertical deviation–possible forme fruste of ocular neuromyotonia. J AAPOS. 2013; 17(3):248–252

[145] Miller NR, Lee AG. Adult-onset acquired oculomotor nerve paresis with cyclic spasms: relationship to ocular neuromyotonia. Am J Ophthalmol. 2004; 137(1):70–76

[146] Gadoth A, Kipervasser S, Korczyn AD, Neufeld MY, Kesler A. Acquired oculomotor nerve paresis with cyclic spasms in a young woman, a rare subtype of neuromyotonia. J Neuroophthalmol. 2013; 33(3):247–248

[147] Jones A, Jain S. Botulinum toxin: a novel treatment for pediatric cyclic esotropia. J AAPOS. 2014; 18(6):614–615

[148] Lai YH, Fredrick DR. Alteration of cyclic frequency by botulinum toxin injection in adult onset cyclic esotropia. Br J Ophthalmol. 2005; 89(11):1540–1541

[149] Voide N, Presset C, Klainguti G, Kaeser PF. Nonsurgical treatment of cyclic esotropia. J AAPOS. 2015; 19(2):196–198

[150] Hamed LM, Silbiger J. Periodic alternating esotropia. J Pediatr Ophthalmol Strabismus. 1992; 29(4):240–242

[151] Akman A, Dayanir V, Sefik Sanaç A, Kansu T. Acquired esotropia as presenting sign of cranio-cervical junction anomalies. Neuroophthalmology. 1995; 15(6):311–314

[152] Arai M, Fujii S. Divergence paralysis associated with the ingestion of diazepam. J Neurol. 1990; 237(1):45–46

[153] Friling R, Yassur Y, Merkin L, et al. Divergence paralysis versus bilateral sixth nerve palsy in an incomplete Miller-Fisher syndrome. Neuro-ophthalmology. 1993; 13(4):215–217

[154] Jacobson DM. Divergence insufficiency revisited: natural history of idiopathic cases and neurologic associations. Arch Ophthalmol. 2000; 118(9):1237–1241

[155] Lepore FE. Divergence paresis: a nonlocalizing cause of diplopia. J Neuroophthalmol. 1999; 19(4):242–245

[156] Lewis AR, Kline LB, Sharpe JA. Acquired esotropia due to Arnold-Chiari I malformation. J Neuroophthalmol. 1996; 16(1):49–54

[157] Schanzer B, Bordaberry M, Jeffery AR, McNeil DE, Phillips PC. The child with divergence paresis. Surv Ophthalmol. 1998; 42(6):571–576

[158] Leigh RJ, Zee DS. The Neurology of Eye Movements. 3rd ed. New York: Oxford University Press; 1999

[159] Herlihy EP, Phillips JO, Weiss AH. Esotropia greater at distance: children vs adults. JAMA Ophthalmol. 2013; 131(3):370–375

[160] Yadav S, Young J, Voas-Clarke C, Marsh IB, Durnian JM. Treatment of age-related distance esotropia with unilateral lateral rectus resection. J AAPOS. 2014; 18(5):446–448

[161] Demer JL. The Apt Lecture. Connective tissues reflect different mechanisms of strabismus over the life span. J AAPOS. 2014; 18(4):309–315

[162] Brown SM, Iacuone JJ. Intact sensory fusion in a child with divergence paresis caused by a pontine glioma. Am J Ophthalmol. 1999; 128(4):528–530

[163] Horton JC, Fishman RA. Neurovisual findings in the syndrome of spontaneous intracranial hypotension from dural cerebrospinal fluid leak. Ophthalmology. 1994; 101(2):244–251

[164] Mokri B, Piepgras DG, Miller GM. Syndrome of orthostatic headaches and diffuse pachymeningeal gadolinium enhancement. Mayo Clin Proc. 1997; 72(5):400–413

[165] Ohyagi Y, Yamada T, Okayama A, et al. Vergence disorders in patients with spinocerebellar ataxia 3/Machado-Joseph disease: a synoptophore study. J Neurol Sci. 2000; 173(2):120–123

[166] Tekeli O, Tomaç S, Gürsel E, Hasiripi H. Divergence paralysis & intracranial hypertension due to neurobrucellosis. A case report. Binocul Vis Strabismus Q. 1999; 14(2):117–118

[167] Versino M, Hurko O, Zee DS. Disorders of binocular control of eye movements in patients with cerebellar dysfunction. Brain. 1996; 119(Pt 6):1933–1950

[168] Bakker SL, Gan IM. Temporary divergence paralysis in viral meningitis. J Neuroophthalmol. 2008; 28(2):111–113

[169] Tsuda H, Sekiya R, Tanaka K, Kishida S. Isolated divergence paralysis due to midbrain tegmentum infarction. Intern Med. 2011; 50(10):1131

[170] Wiggins RE, Jr, Baumgartner S. Diagnosis and management of divergence weakness in adults. Ophthalmology. 1999; 106(7):1353–1356

[171] Biousse V, Newman NJ, Petermann SH, Lambert SR. Isolated comitant esotropia and Chiari I malformation. Am J Ophthalmol. 2000; 130(2):216–220

[172] Hoyt CS, Good WV. Acute onset concomitant esotropia: when is it a sign of serious neurological disease? Br J Ophthalmol. 1995; 79(5):498–501

[173] Weeks CL, Hamed LM. Treatment of acute comitant esotropia in Chiari I malformation. Ophthalmology. 1999; 106(12):2368–2371

[174] Simon JW, Waldman JB, Couture KC. Cerebellar astrocytoma manifesting as isolated, comitant esotropia in childhood. Am J Ophthalmol. 1996; 121(5):584–586

[175] Fukuo Y, Abe T, Hayasaka S. Acute comitant esotropia in a boy with head trauma and convulsions receiving carbamazepine. Ophthalmologica. 1998; 212(1):61–62

[176] al-Din SN, Anderson M, Eeg-Olofsson O, Trontelj JV. Neuro-ophthalmic manifestations of the syndrome of ophthalmoplegia, ataxia and areflexia: a review. Acta Neurol Scand. 1994; 89(3):157–163

[177] Goldstein JH, Schneekloth BB. Spasm of the near reflex: a spectrum of anomalies. Surv Ophthalmol. 1996; 40(4):269–278

[178] Newman NJ, Lessell S. Pupillary dilatation with monocular occlusion as a sign of nonorganic oculomotor dysfunction. Am J Ophthalmol. 1989; 108(4):461–462

[179] Postert T, Büttner T, McMonagle U, Przuntek H. Spasm of the near reflex: case report and review of the literature. Neuro-ophthalmology. 1997; 17(3):149–152

[180] Pullicino P, Lincoff N, Truax BT. Abnormal vergence with upper brainstem infarcts: pseudoabducens palsy. Neurology. 2000; 55(3):352–358

[181] Bernstein R, Bernardini GL. Abnormal vergence with upper brainstem infarcts: pseudoabducens palsy. Neurology. 2001; 56(3):424–425

[182] Hertle RW, Bienfang DC. Oculographic analysis of acute esotropia secondary to a thalamic hemorrhage. J Clin Neuroophthalmol. 1990; 10(1):21–26

[183] Wiest G, Mallek R, Baumgartner C. Selective loss of vergence control secondary to bilateral paramedian thalamic infarction. Neurology. 2000; 54(10):1997–1999

[184] Thompson SH, Miller NR. Disorders of pupillary function, accommodation, and lacrimation. In: Miller NR, Newman NJ, eds. Walsh and Hoyt's Clinical Neuro-Ophthalmology. 5th ed. Baltimore, MD: Williams & Wilkins; 1998:1016–1018

[185] Fekete R, Baizabal-Carvallo JF, Ha AD, Davidson A, Jankovic J. Convergence spasm in conversion disorders: prevalence in psychogenic and other movement disorders compared with controls. J Neurol Neurosurg Psychiatry. 2012; 83(2):202–204

[186] Jeong SH, Oh YM, Kim CY, Kim JS. Bimedial rectus hypermetabolism in convergence spasm as observed on positron emission tomography. J Neuroophthalmol. 2008; 28(3):217–218

[187] Weber KP, Thurtell MJ, Halmagyi GM. Teaching NeuroImage: Convergence spasm associated with midbrain compression by cerebral aneurysm. Neurology. 2008; 70(15):e49–e50

[188] Ohtsuka K, Maekawa H, Takeda M, Uede N, Chiba S. Accommodation and convergence insufficiency with left middle cerebral artery occlusion. Am J Ophthalmol. 1988; 106(1):60–64

[189] Racette BA, Gokden MS, Tychsen LS, Perlmutter JS. Convergence insufficiency in idiopathic Parkinson's disease responsive to levodopa. Strabismus. 1999; 7(3):169–174

[190] Spierer A, Huna R, Rechtman C, Lapidot D. Convergence insufficiency secondary to subdural hematoma. Am J Ophthalmol. 1995; 120(2):258–260

[191] Wylie J, Campbell C, Pope J, Akikusa J, Laxer RM, Nicolle D. Convergence paralysis as a manifestation of polyarteritis nodosa. Can J Neurol Sci. 2006; 33(4):423–425

[192] Lindner K, Hitzenberger P, Drlicek M, Grisold W. Dissociated unilateral convergence paralysis in a patient with thalamotectal haemorrhage. J Neurol Neurosurg Psychiatry. 1992; 55(8):731–733

[193] Fujikado T, Ohmi G, Ikeda T, Lewis JM, Tano Y. Exotropia secondary to vitreous hemorrhage. Graefes Arch Clin Exp Ophthalmol. 1997; 235(3):143–148

[194] Borchert MS, Lessell S, Hoyt WF. Hemifield slide diplopia from altitudinal visual field defects. J Neuroophthalmol. 1996; 16(2):107–109

[195] Spector RH. Vertical diplopia. Surv Ophthalmol. 1993; 38(1):31–62

[196] Wong AM, Colpa L, Chandrakumar M. Ability of an upright-supine test to differentiate skew deviation from other vertical strabismus causes. Arch Ophthalmol. 2011; 129(12):1570–1575

[197] Brazis PW, Lee AG. Binocular vertical diplopia. Mayo Clin Proc. 1998; 73(1):55–66

[198] Bell JA, Fielder AR, Viney S. Congenital double elevator palsy in identical twins. J Clin Neuroophthalmol. 1990; 10(1):32–34

[199] Ziffer AJ, Rosenbaum AL, Demer JL, Yee RD. Congenital double elevator palsy: vertical saccadic velocity utilizing the scleral search coil technique. J Pediatr Ophthalmol Strabismus. 1992; 29(3):142–149

[200] Hommel M, Bogousslavsky J. The spectrum of vertical gaze palsy following unilateral brainstem stroke. Neurology. 1991; 41(8):1229–1234

[201] Thömke F, Hopf HC. Acquired monocular elevation paresis. An asymmetric upgaze palsy. Brain. 1992; 115(Pt 6):1901–1910

[202] Donahue SP, Lavin PJ, Hamed LM. Tonic ocular tilt reaction simulating a superior oblique palsy: diagnostic confusion with the 3-step test. Arch Ophthalmol. 1999; 117(3):347–352

[203] Ezra E, Plant GT. Paroxysmal superior rectus and levator palpebrae spasm: a unique presentation of multiple sclerosis. Br J Ophthalmol. 1996; 80(2):187–188

[204] von Noorden GK, Murray E, Wong SY. Superior oblique paralysis. A review of 270 cases. Arch Ophthalmol. 1986; 104(12):1771–1776

[205] Harrington DO, Flocks M. Ophthalmoplegic migraine; pathogenesis; report of pathological findings in a case of recurrent oculomotor paralysis. AMA Arch Opthalmol. 1953; 49(6):643–655

[206] Miller NR. Walsh and Hoyt's Clinical Neuro-ophthalmology. 4th ed. Baltimore, MD: Williams & Wilkins; 1991:2533–2538

[207] Friedman AP, Harter DH, Merritt HH. Ophthalmoplegic migraine. Arch Neurol. 1962; 7:320–327

[208] Katz B, Rimmer S. Ophthalmoplegic migraine with superior ramus oculomotor paresis. J Clin Neuroophthalmol. 1989; 9(3):181–183

[209] Odaka M, Yuki N, Hirata K. Anti-GQ1b IgG antibody syndrome: clinical and immunological range. J Neurol Neurosurg Psychiatry. 2001; 70(1):50–55

[210] Yuki N, Odaka M, Hirata K. Acute ophthalmoparesis (without ataxia) associated with anti-GQ1b IgG antibody: clinical features. Ophthalmology. 2001; 108(1):196–200

[211] Slavin ML. Hyperdeviation associated with isolated unilateral abducens palsy. Ophthalmology. 1989; 96(4):512–516

[212] von Noorden GK, Hansell R. Clinical characteristics and treatment of isolated inferior rectus paralysis. Ophthalmology. 1991; 98(2):253–257

[213] Moster ML, Bosley TM, Slavin ML, Rubin SE. Thyroid ophthalmopathy presenting as superior oblique paresis. J Clin Neuroophthalmol. 1992; 12(2):94–97

[214] Stidham DB, Sondhi N, Plager D, Helveston E. Presumed isolated inflammation of the superior oblique muscle in idiopathic orbital myositis. Ophthalmology. 1998; 105(12):2216–2219

[215] Burde RM, Savino PJ, Trobe JD. Clinical Decisions in Neuro-ophthalmology. 2nd ed. St Louis, MO: Mosby Yearbook; 1991:227

[216] Slavin ML, Potash SD, Rubin SE. Asymptomatic physiologic hyperdeviation in peripheral gaze. Ophthalmology. 1988; 95(6):778–781

[217] Alonso-Valdivielso JL, Alvarez Lario B, Alegre López J, Sedano Tous MJ, Buitrago Gómez A. Acquired Brown's syndrome in a patient with systemic lupus erythematosus. Ann Rheum Dis. 1993; 52(1):63–64

[218] Baker RS, Epstein AD. Ocular motor abnormalities from head trauma. Surv Ophthalmol. 1991; 35(4):245–267

[219] Coats DK, Paysse EA, Orenga-Nania S. Acquired Pseudo-Brown's syndrome immediately following Ahmed valve glaucoma implant. Ophthalmic Surg Lasers. 1999; 30(5):396–397

[220] Erie JC. Acquired Brown's syndrome after peribulbar anesthesia. Am J Ophthalmol. 1990; 109(3):349–350

[221] Saunders RA, Stratas BA, Gordon RA, Holgate RC. Acute-onset Brown's syndrome associated with pansinusitis. Arch Ophthalmol. 1990; 108(1):58–60

[222] Thorne JE, Volpe NJ, Liu GT. Magnetic resonance imaging of acquired Brown syndrome in a patient with psoriasis. Am J Ophthalmol. 1999; 127(2):233–235

[223] Sener EC, Özkan SB, Aribal ME, Sanac AS, Aslan B. Evaluation of congenital Brown's syndrome with magnetic resonance imaging. Eye (Lond). 1996; 10 (Pt 4):492–496

[224] Cousin M, Girard N, Denis D. MRI in congenital Brown's syndrome: report of 16 cases [in French]. J Fr Ophtalmol. 2013; 36(3):202–209

[225] White VA, Cline RA. Pathologic causes of the superior oblique click syndrome. Ophthalmology. 1999; 106(7):1292–1295

[226] Coussens T, Ellis FJ. Considerations on the etiology of congenital Brown syndrome. Curr Opin Ophthalmol. 2015; 26(5):357–361

[227] Suh SY, Le A, Demer JL. Size of the oblique extraocular muscles and superior oblique muscle contractility in Brown syndrome. Invest Ophthalmol Vis Sci. 2015; 56(10):6114–6120

[228] Hudson HL, Feldon SE. Late overcorrection of hypotropia in Graves ophthalmopathy. Predictive factors. Ophthalmology. 1992; 99(3):356–360

[229] Hughes DS, Beck L, Hill R, Plenty J. Dysthyroid eye disease presenting as Brown's syndrome. Acta Ophthalmol (Copenh). 1993; 71(2):262–265

[230] Egbert JE, May K, Kersten RC, Kulwin DR. Pediatric orbital floor fracture: direct extraocular muscle involvement. Ophthalmology. 2000; 107(10):1875–1879

[231] Carter K, Lee AG, Tang RA, et al. Neuro-ophthalmologic complications of sinus surgery. Neuro-ophthalmology. 1998; 19(2):75–82

[232] Engle EC, Goumnerov BC, McKeown CA, et al. Oculomotor nerve and muscle abnormalities in congenital fibrosis of the extraocular muscles. Ann Neurol. 1997; 41(3):314–325

[233] Hupp SL, Williams JP, Curran JE. Computerized tomography in the diagnosis of the congenital fibrosis syndrome. J Clin Neuroophthalmol. 1990; 10(2):135–139

[234] Borruat F-X, Jaques B, Dürig J. Transient vertical diplopia and silent sinus disorder. J Neuroophthalmol. 1999; 19(3):173–175

[235] Kubis KC, Danesh-Meyer H, Bilyk JR. Unilateral lid retraction during pregnancy. Surv Ophthalmol. 2000; 45(1):69–76

[236] Wan MK, Francis IC, Carter PR, Griffits R, van Rooijen ML, Coroneo MT. The spectrum of presentation of silent sinus syndrome. J Neuroophthalmol. 2000; 20(3):207–212

[237] Hunter DG, Lam GC, Guyton DL. Inferior oblique muscle injury from local anesthesia for cataract surgery. Ophthalmology. 1995; 102(3):501–509

[238] Capó H, Guyton DL. Ipsilateral hypertropia after cataract surgery. Ophthalmology. 1996; 103(5):721–730

[239] Capó H, Roth E, Johnson T, Muñoz M, Siatkowski RM. Vertical strabismus after cataract surgery. Ophthalmology. 1996; 103(6):918–921

[240] Corboy JM, Jiang X. Postanesthetic hypotropia: a unique syndrome in left eyes. J Cataract Refract Surg. 1997; 23(9):1394–1398

[241] Koide R, Honda M, Kora Y, Ozawa T. Diplopia after cataract surgery. J Cataract Refract Surg. 2000; 26(8):1198–1204

[242] Golnik KC, West CE, Kaye E, Corcoran KT, Cionni RJ. Incidence of ocular misalignment and diplopia after uneventful cataract surgery. J Cataract Refract Surg. 2000; 26(8):1205–1209

[243] Johnson DA. Persistent vertical binocular diplopia after cataract surgery. Am J Ophthalmol. 2001; 132(6):831–835

[244] De Pool ME, Campbell JP, Broome SO, Guyton DL. The dragged-fovea diplopia syndrome: clinical characteristics, diagnosis, and treatment. Ophthalmology. 2005; 112(8):1455–1462

[245] Burgess D, Roper-Hall G, Burde RM. Binocular diplopia associated with subretinal neovascular membranes. Arch Ophthalmol. 1980; 98(2):311–317

[246] Brazis PW, Lee AG, Bolling JP. Binocular vertical diplopia due to subretinal neovascular membrane. Strabismus. 1998; 6(3):127–131

[247] Benegas NM, Egbert J, Engel WK, Kushner BJ. Diplopia secondary to aniseikonia associated with macular disease. Arch Ophthalmol. 1999; 117(7):896–899

[248] Silverberg M, Schuler E, Veronneau-Troutman S, Wald K, Schlossman A, Medow N. Nonsurgical management of binocular diplopia induced by macular pathology. Arch Ophthalmol. 1999; 117(7):900–903

11 Third Nerve Palsies

William J. Hertzing and Alec L. Amram

Abstract

A third nerve palsy results from an injury to the oculomotor nerve. The palsy may be partial or complete, may cause partial or complete ptosis, and may spare or involve the pupil (e.g., fixed and dilated). Typically, there is paresis of adduction, elevation, depression, or any combination of these motility findings. The third nerve palsy may occur in isolation or with additional neurological features that may help to topographically localize the lesion. This chapter discusses the clinical pathways in localizing and diagnosing third nerve palsies, reviewing the literature in detail.

Keywords: third nerve palsy, oculomotor nerve, diplopia, ptosis, aneurysm

11.1 Acknowledgment

The authors gratefully acknowledge the input of Joseph Hough, MD in reviewing this chapter.

11.2 What Are the Clinical Features of a Third Cranial Nerve Palsy?

The oculomotor nerve (third cranial nerve) innervates the medial rectus, superior rectus, inferior rectus, and inferior oblique muscle, as well as the levator of the lid. It also contains parasympathetic fibers that supply the sphincter of the pupil and the ciliary body. A complete peripheral third nerve palsy (TNP) thus causes ptosis, a fixed and dilated pupil, and a down (hypotropic) and out (exotropic) resting eye position. Partial TNPs may cause (in combination or isolation) variable ptosis, mydriasis, and paresis of adduction, elevation, and depression. In this section, we discuss the localization of TNPs associated with other neurologic signs (nonisolated TNPs) and TNPs without other associated neurologic or neuro-ophthalmologic deficits (isolated TNPs).[1]

11.3 Localization

11.3.1 Is the TNP Isolated or Nonisolated? Can the TNP Be Localized?

We classify TNPs as either nonisolated or isolated. The isolated TNPs were defined as TNPs without associated neurologic findings (e.g., headache, other cranial neuropathies). Patients with

evidence for myasthenia gravis (e.g., variability, fatigue, Cogan lid twitch sign, enhancement of ptosis) are not included in the isolated TNP group. We define six types of TNP in Box 11.1. The localization of TNP is outlined in Box 11.2. Etiologies of TNP by localization are outlined in Box 11.3.

Box 11.1 Definitions of the Six Types of Third Nerve Palsy (TNP)

- Type 1: Nonisolated.
  - TNP is considered nonisolated if it has the following features:
    – Orbital disease (e.g., chemosis, proptosis, lid swelling, injection, and positive forced ductions).
    – Evidence to suggest myasthenia gravis (e.g., fatigability of the motility defect, Cogan lid twitch sign, orbicularis oculi weakness).
    – Multiple cranial nerve palsies (including bilateral TNP) or radiculopathy.
    – Brainstem signs (e.g., hemiplegia, cerebellar signs, other cranial nerve deficits).
    – Systemic, infectious, or inflammatory risk factors for TNP (e.g., history of previous malignancy, giant cell arteritis, collagen vascular disease).
    – Severe headache.
- Type 2: Traumatic.
  - Isolated unilateral TNP, which has a clearly established temporal relationship to significant previous head trauma and does not progress; patients with minor head trauma are not included.
- Type 3: Congenital.
  - Patient born with an isolated TNP.
- Type 4: Acquired, nontraumatic isolated.
  - Type 4A: TNP with a normal pupillary sphincter with completely palsied extraocular muscles.
  - Type 4B: TNP with normal pupillary sphincter and incomplete palsied extraocular muscles.
  - Type 4C: TNP with abnormal pupillary sphincter dysfunction and partial or complete extraocular muscle palsies.
- Type 5: Progressive or unresolved.
  - Patients with TNP that worsens after the acute stage (more than 2 weeks) or who develop new neurologic findings are considered to have *progressive TNP*.
  - Patients without resolution of TNP after 12 to 16 weeks are considered to have *unresolved TNP*.
- Type 6: Signs of aberrant regeneration.

- Lesions affecting the third nerve nucleus.
  - Oculomotor nucleus: ipsilateral complete cranial nerve (CN) III palsy; contralateral ptosis and superior rectus paresis.
  - Oculomotor subnucleus: isolated muscle palsy (e.g., inferior rectus).
  - Isolated levator subnucleus: isolated bilateral ptosis.
- Lesions affecting the third nerve fasciculus.
  - Isolated fascicle: partial or complete isolated CN III palsy with or without pupil involvement.
  - Paramedian mesencephalon: plus–minus syndrome (ipsilateral ptosis and contralateral eyelid retraction).
  - Fascicle, red nucleus/cerebellar peduncle: ipsilateral CN III palsy with contralateral ataxia and tremor (Claude).
  - Fascicle and cerebral peduncle: ipsilateral CN III palsy with contralateral hemiparesis (Weber).
  - Fascicle and red nucleus/substantia nigra: ipsilateral CN III palsy with contralateral choreiform movements (Benedikt).
- Lesions affecting the third nerve in the subarachnoid space.
  - Complete CN III palsy with or without other CN involvement.
  - Superior or inferior division palsy.
- Lesions affecting the third nerve in the cavernous sinus.
  - Painful or painless CN III palsy, with or without palsies of CN IV, VI, and V1.
  - CN III palsy with small pupil (Horner syndrome).
  - Primary aberrant CN III regeneration.
- Lesions affecting the third nerve in the superior orbital fissure.
  - CN III palsy with or without palsies of CN IV, VI, and V1; often with proptosis.
- Lesion affecting the third nerve in the orbit.
  - Superior and/or inferior CN III branch palsy.
  - CN III with involvement of optic nerve and/or other orbital structures: visual loss, proptosis, swelling of lids, and chemosis.

Source: Modified from Brazis et al[2] with permission from Lippincott Williams & Wilkins.

11.3.2 Is the TNP Due to a Nuclear Lesion?

Lesions of the third nerve nucleus are rare and often associated with other signs of mesencephalic involvement, especially vertical gaze impairment.[3,4,5,6,7,8] Nuclear lesions may be due to infarction, hemorrhage, tumor, infection, or trauma, and, thus, should be investigated by magnetic resonance imaging (MRI). Paresis of an isolated muscle innervated by the oculomotor nerve almost always results from an orbital lesion or from disease of the involved muscle or neuromuscular junction. For example, isolated inferior rectus paresis may occur secondary to trauma, myasthenia gravis, or vascular disease and may also occur on a congenital or idiopathic basis.[9] However, lesions of the inferior rectus subnucleus may also give rise to isolated weakness of the inferior rectus muscle.[10,11,12] Isolated inferior rectus paresis may also occur on a supranuclear basis with a lesion selectively interrupting fibers descending from the medial longitudinal fasciculus (MLF) to the inferior rectus subnucleus.[12] The levator palpebrae superioris muscles, the superior recti, and the constrictors of the pupils are affected bilaterally with nuclear lesions. Because medial rectus neurons probably lie at three different locations within the oculomotor nucleus, it is unlikely that a medial rectus paralysis (unilateral or bilateral) would be the sole manifestation of a nuclear lesion.[13] Most characteristic of oculomotor nuclear involvement is unilateral TNP, weakness of the ipsilateral and contralateral superior rectus, and bilateral incomplete ptosis.[14] On rare occasions, the ipsilateral superior rectus is spared while the contralateral superior rectus is paretic. Bilateral TNPs with sparing of the lid levators may also be caused by nuclear lesions (with sparing of the central caudal levator subnucleus).[15] Isolated bilateral ptosis with sparing of the extraocular muscles and pupils may occur with lesions involving the levator subnucleus and sparing more rostral oculomotor subnuclei.[16] After surgery for a fourth ventricle ependymoma, bilateral nuclear oculomotor palsies affecting only the levator and superior recti subnuclei have been described, resulting in third nerve paresis affecting only the levators and superior recti bilaterally.[17] Bilateral total ophthalmoplegia, bilateral complete ptosis, and large, unreactive pupils have been described with midbrain hematoma.[18] This constellation of findings was thought due to bilateral third nerve nuclear or fascicular damage or both, bilateral involvement of the interstitial nucleus of Cajal and the rostral nucleus of the MLF, and involvement of bilateral horizontal saccadic and smooth pursuit pathways.

11.3.3 Is the TNP Due to a Fascicular Lesion?

Lesions of the third nerve fascicle often accompany nuclear lesions because infarction is a common cause of a nuclear TNP, and the paramedian branches near the top of the basilar artery often feed both structures. For example, infarction of the dorsal paramedian midbrain may cause bilateral ptosis associated with unilateral paresis of all other muscles innervated by the oculomotor nerve (pupil spared) with sparing or involvement of the contralateral superior rectus muscle.[19] These unique findings suggest a lesion of the proximal third nerve fascicles and the central caudal subnucleus. Third nerve fascicular lesions are often caused by infarction, hemorrhage, or demyelination. Pure fascicular lesions cause a unilateral peripheral type of oculomotor palsy. Involvement of brainstem structures other than the fascicle of the third nerve identifies the mesencephalic location of the lesion.[20] Concomitant damage of the red nucleus and superior cerebellar peduncle causes contralateral ataxia and outflow tract cerebellar tremor (Claude syndrome), whereas a more anterior lesion, affecting the peduncle, gives rise to oculomotor palsy with contralateral hemiparesis (Weber syndrome). The TNP with Weber syndrome may affect or spare the pupillary fibers.[21] Larger lesions that affect the oculomotor fascicle and the red nucleus/substantia nigra region may produce TNP with contralateral choreiform movements or tremor (Benedikt syndrome),[22] sometimes associated with contralateral hemiparesis if the cerebellar peduncle is also involved. A pupil-sparing TNP associated with binocular cyclotorsion to the contralateral side—thereby indicating a left-sided midbrain lesion that included the fascicle of the third nerve and the supranuclear integration centers for torsional eye movements, the interstitial nucleus of Cajal, and the rostral interstitial nucleus of the MLF—has been described with a paramedian rostral midbrain infarction in a diabetic with giant cell arteritis.[23] Ipsilateral TNP and contralateral downbeat nystagmus may be caused by unilateral paramedian thalamopeduncular infarction.[24]

Rarely, a unilateral or bilateral fascicular third nerve lesion may occur in isolation without other ocular motor or neurologic signs or symptoms (see below).[25,26,27,28,29,30] Fascicular lesions, even when bilateral, may occasionally spare the pupil(s). Bilateral preganglionic internal ophthalmoplegia has been described with bilateral partial oculomotor fascicular lesions.[31] Because of the intra-axial topographic arrangement of fibers, fascicular lesions may cause TNP limited to specific oculomotor-innervated muscles.[32] Fascicular lesions have resulted in the following:

1. Isolated inferior oblique paresis.[33]
2. Unilateral fixed, dilated pupil unassociated with other neurologic dysfunction.[34]
3. Paresis of the superior rectus and inferior oblique without other evidence of oculomotor nerve involvement.[35]
4. Paresis of the superior rectus and medial rectus.[36]
5. Paresis of the levator, superior rectus, and medial rectus.[37]
6. Paresis of the inferior oblique, superior rectus, medial rectus, and levator with sparing of the inferior rectus muscle and pupil.[38,39,40]
7. Paresis of the inferior oblique, superior rectus, medial rectus, levator, and inferior rectus with pupillary sparing.[38,41]
8. Paresis of the left inferior rectus, left pupil, right superior rectus, convergence, and left medial rectus.[13]

Based on these clinical studies, it has been proposed that individual third nerve fascicles in the ventral mesencephalon are arranged topographically from lateral to medial as follows: inferior oblique, superior rectus, medial rectus and levator palpebrae, inferior rectus, and pupillary fibers.[33] A rostral-caudal topographic arrangement has also been suggested with pupillary fibers most superior, followed by fibers to the inferior rectus, inferior oblique, medial rectus, superior rectus, and levator, in that order.[36,39] This model also accounts for the description of superior and inferior division oculomotor palsies. The superior division paresis involves the superior rectus and levator muscles without involvement of other groups.[42,43,44] The inferior division oculomotor palsies cause paresis of inferior rectus, inferior oblique, medial rectus, and pupillary fibers with sparing of the superior rectus and levator.[44,45,46] Both divisional palsies may be associated with intra-axial midbrain lesions. Thus, although superior and inferior divisional TNP have classically been localized to anterior cavernous sinus or posterior orbital lesions, a divisional TNP may occur from damage at any location along the course of the oculomotor nerve, from the fascicle to the orbit.[44]

Fascicular TNP may occasionally be associated with ipsilateral ptosis and contralateral eyelid retraction (plus–minus lid syndrome).[47,48] This syndrome occurs with a small lesion located in the paramedian mesencephalon. There is involvement of the ipsilateral levator palpebrae fascicles as they emerge from the central caudal nucleus (the central caudal nucleus is spared) and the inhibitory pathways projecting to the levator palpebrae motor neurons immediately before their entrance in the central caudal nucleus. The plus–minus syndrome has been described with bilateral glioma extending to the paramedian midbrain and in thalamic-mesencephalic infarction; it also may occur with peripheral processes such as peripheral TNP, myasthenia gravis, orbital myositis, congenital ptosis, or orbital trauma.

11.3.4 Is the TNP Due to a Subarachnoid Lesion?

An isolated pupil-sparing peripheral TNP is most often related to an ischemic neuropathy or a lesion affecting its subarachnoid portion. Subarachnoid lesions may distort or injure the brainstem, and diffuse processes will show signs of meningeal irritation. Etiologies of TNPs due to a subarachnoid lesion are outlined in Box 11.3.

Box 11.3 Etiologies of third nerve palsy (TNP) by topographical localization

- Nuclear TNP.
  - Infarction or hemorrhage.[3,4,5,6,12,15,18,36]
  - Tumor.[7,10,17]
  - Infection (e.g., tuberculoma[49]).
  - Trauma.
  - Multiple sclerosis.[11]
  - Parinaud syndrome.[50]
- Fascicular TNP.
  - Infarction or hemorrhage.[6,8,13,19,21,24,27,28,30,32,33,36,37,41,42,51,52,53,54]
  - Tumor.[25,26,46,48,55,56,57]
  - Multiple sclerosis.[29,37,58]
  - Stereotactic surgery.[22]
  - Midbrain cavernous malformation.[59]
- Subarachnoid space.
  - Aneurysms of the internal carotid–posterior communicating, superior cerebellar, basilar, or posterior cerebral arteries.[60,61,62,63,64,65,66,67,68,69,70,71,72,73,74,75,76,77,78,79,80,81,82,83]
  - Cavernous malformation of the oculomotor nerve.[84]
  - Ectatic vessels.[85,86,87,88]
  - Basilar vasospasm (following perimesencephalic subarachnoid hemorrhage [SAH]).[89]
  - Tumors, especially meningiomas, chordomas, metastases, or primary tumors of the third nerve.[55,88,90,91,92,93,94,95,96,97,98,99,100,101,102,103,104,105,106,107,108,109,110,111]
  - Infectious or inflammatory processes of the meninges (e.g., sarcoidosis and granulomatosis with polyangiitis, tuberculosis meningitis[112]) and carcinomatous or lymphomatous meningitis.[55,70,74,94,113,114,115,116,117,118,119,120,121,122,123]
  - Ophthalmoplegic migraine.[124]
  - SAH (perimesencephalic,[125,126] with leukemia[127]).
  - Pseudotumor cerebri.
  - Spontaneous intracranial hypotension.[128]

- ○ Trauma, especially during neurosurgical procedures.[68,129,130,131,132]
- ○ Nerve infarction from diabetes, atherosclerosis, giant cell arteritis, or systemic lupus erythematosus (nerve infarction may also occur in the cavernous sinus or anywhere along the course of nerve).[74,75,94,133,134,135,136,137,138,139,140,141]
- ○ Uncal herniation.
- ○ Hydrocephalus.[142]
- • Cavernous sinus/superior orbital fissure.
  - ○ Aneurysm of the internal carotid or posterior communicating artery.[69,94,143,144,145,146,147,148]
  - ○ Dural carotid cavernous sinus fistula.[69,149,150,151,152,153,154,155,156]
  - ○ Internal carotid artery occlusion,[157] including iatrogenic (balloon test occlusion[158]).
  - ○ Cavernous sinus thrombosis or infection (e.g., tuberculoma[159]); superior ophthalmic vein thrombosis.[159,160,161,162]
  - ○ Tumors, including pituitary adenoma, meningioma, esthesioneuroblastoma, arachnoid cyst, neurinoma, schwannoma, nasopharyngeal carcinoma, myeloma, lymphoma, Hodgkin disease, teratoid rhabdoid tumor, and metastases.[69,90,163,164,165,166,167,168,169,170,171,172,173,174,175,176,177,178,179,180]
  - ○ Pituitary infarction or hemorrhage (pituitary apoplexy).[168,181,182,183,184]
  - ○ Gammopathy.
  - ○ Intraneural hemorrhage.[185]
  - ○ Mucocele of the sphenoid sinus.[186,187]
  - ○ Sphenoid sinusitis.[188]
  - ○ Tolosa–Hunt syndrome, Wegener granulomatosis with polyangiitis, or other granulomatous diseases.[69,92,94,189]
- • Orbit.
  - ○ Infections, inflammations, and granulomatous processes (e.g., orbital pseudotumor, Heerfordt syndrome).[190,191,192,193]
  - ○ Sphenoid sinus mucocele.[194]
  - ○ Tumors.[195,196]
  - ○ Dural arteriovenous malformation.[197]
  - ○ Trauma (including inferior division injury during surgical procedures[198]).
  - ○ Intraorbital oculomotor schwannoma.[199,200,201]
- • Unknown or varied localization.
  - ○ Congenital.[14,71,164,202,203,204,205,206,207,208]
  - ○ Migraine.[209,210,211,212]
  - ○ Viral infections (including herpes zoster ophthalmicus or Ramsay Hunt syndrome) and immunizations.[213,214,215,216,217,218,219]
  - ○ Lyme disease.[220,221]
  - ○ Neurobrucellosis.[222]
  - ○ Tuberculosis.[112]
  - ○ Diffuse neuropathic processes (e.g., Miller Fisher syndrome and chronic inflammatory demyelinating polyneuropathy [CIDP]).[223,224]
  - ○ Partial TNP associated with elevated antigalactocerebroside and anti-GM1 antibodies.[225]
  - ○ Cervical carotid artery dissection, stenosis, or occlusion.[226,227,228,229,230]
  - ○ Subdural hematomas.[231,232,233,234]

- ○ Glioblastoma multiforme.[235]
- ○ Unintentional subdural catheter.[236]
- ○ Submucosal diathermy to the inferior turbinates to improve the nasal airway.[237]
- ○ Toxic effects of drugs.[238,239]
  - – Cocaine.[240]
  - – Sildenafil citrate (Viagra).[241]
  - – Internal carotid cisplatin infusion (inferolateral trunk carotid artery neurovascular toxicity).[242,243]
  - – Dental anesthesia.
- ○ Radiation therapy.[244]

Third nerve schwannoma may cause a painful relapsing-remitting TNP mimicking the clinical syndrome of ophthalmoplegic migraine,[97] with development of hydrocephalus and impaired consciousness in severe cases.[245] Options for treatment include clinical observation, stereotactic radiation, or surgical resection. As TNP can be worsened during surgical management, stereotactic radiation may be a safer alternative.[246,247] Monocular elevator paresis from isolated superior rectus and/or inferior oblique dysfunction may occur in neurofibromatosis type 2-related schwannoma.[91] The third nerve is also susceptible to trauma in the subarachnoid space, especially during neurosurgical procedures.[68,130,131,247] Closed head trauma may cause TNP due to shearing injury resulting in distal fascicular damage or partial root avulsion.[129] A number of patients have presented with TNP precipitated by minor head trauma, found to have no abnormalities on cranial computed tomography (CT) scans, and subsequently discovered to have ipsilateral posterior communicating artery aneurysms.[72,80,248] Zhang et al noted that ptosis and pupillary involvement of a posttraumatic incomplete TNP improved after hematoma elimination.[249]

Compression of the third nerve by an aneurysm characteristically causes dilatation and unresponsiveness of the pupil. This can occur as the first and only symptom, as the pupillomotor fibers travel superficially in the dorsal portion of the nerve.[148] Compressive subarachnoid lesions may occasionally spare the pupil, however. Two explanations have been proposed: (1) compression may be evenly distributed and the relatively pressure-resistant, smaller-caliber pupillomotor fibers escape injury; or (2) the lesion compresses only the inferior portion of the nerve and spares the dorsally situated pupillomotor fibers. Aneurysmal TNP may be incomplete with at least one element of nerve dysfunction (i.e., ptosis, mydriasis, or extraocular muscle weakness) being absent. Ptosis has been described in isolation as the sole manifestation of third nerve compression by a posterior communicating artery (PComm) aneurysm.[65] Rarely, aneurysmal TNP may be transient and clear spontaneously.[66] Although TNP-causing aneurysms most often occur in the posterior communicating arteries, aneurysm of other arteries can impact third nerve function as well. A TNP was described in the setting of a SAH secondary to anterior cerebral A2 segment aneurysm. This is uncommon but should be taken into consideration when evaluating vascular neuroimaging studies.[250]

Treatment of TNP secondary to aneurysm may require surgical clipping and/or endovascular coiling.[251] However, caution must be taken while performing endovascular PComm coiling as it can cause perforation of the oculomotor nerve.[252] Use of papaverine after surgical clipping to reverse arterial spasm may also induce another transient TNP.[253,254] This can be avoided by diluting the normal 3% papaverine solution to 0.3% with normal saline while still maintaining a satisfactory result.[253]

A normal pupil in the setting of a complete somatic oculomotor paresis essentially excludes a diagnosis of aneurysm (see below). There are reports of patients in whom a painless, pupil-sparing but otherwise complete oculomotor paresis was the only sign of an aneurysm arising from the basilar artery.[255,256,257,258] Conversely, an isolated pupillary paralysis without ptosis or ophthalmoparesis is rarely caused by an aneurysm or other subarachnoid lesion.[99,259] Koennecke and Seyfert reported a patient with a common carotid artery dissection from intraoperative trauma whose mydriasis preceded a complete TNP by 12 hours.[228] Although rare, pupil-sparing TNP can be caused by upward compression of a large PComm aneurysm, demonstrating that unusual compressive lesions must be considered in addition to ischemic causes.[260]

11.3.5 Is the TNP Due to a Cavernous Sinus Lesion?

Cavernous sinus lesions affecting the third nerve often involve additional extraocular motor nerves, the ophthalmic branch of the trigeminal nerve, or sympathetic fibers. Sensory fibers from the ophthalmic division of the fifth CN join the oculomotor nerve within the lateral wall of the cavernous sinus. The frontal/orbital pain experienced by patients with enlarging aneurysms could thus be caused by direct irritation of the third nerve.[145] Compressive cavernous sinus lesions may also spare the pupil due to preferential involvement of the superior division of the oculomotor nerve, which carries no pupillomotor fibers.[146] Of note, apparent pupillary "sparing" of anterior cavernous sinus lesions may result from simultaneous nerve fiber injury to the pupillary sphincter and dilator, causing a mid-position fixed pupil, or may result from aberrant regeneration (see below). Ikeda et al described a patient with a painful, "severe" TNP with normal pupils due to a cavernous sinus aneurysm.[144] Lesions in the vicinity of the posterior clinoid process may for some time affect only the third nerve as it pierces the dura (e.g., breast and prostatic carcinoma).[90] Medial lesions in the cavernous sinus, such as carotid artery aneurysm, may affect only the ocular motor nerves but spare the more laterally located ophthalmic branch of the trigeminal nerve, resulting in painless ophthalmoplegia. Lesions that begin laterally present with retro-orbital pain first, and only later does ophthalmoparesis supervene. Lesions located in the cavernous sinus causing TNP are outlined in Box 11.3. The clinical findings and etiologies for processes located in the superior orbital fissure are similar to those of the cavernous sinus syndrome.

11.3.6 Is the TNP Due to an Orbital Lesion?

Lesions within the orbit that produce third nerve dysfunction usually produce other ocular motor dysfunction as well as optic neuropathy and proptosis.[195,196] Lesions may extend from the cavernous sinus to the orbital apex and vice versa, making clinical distinction between the two syndromes impossible. Isolated involvement of the muscles innervated by either the superior or the inferior oculomotor branch has classically been localized to an orbital process: often trauma, tumor, infection, or a sphenocavernous lesion.[192] However, as noted, the functional division of the third nerve is present probably even at the fascicular level, and a divisional pattern may occur from damage anywhere along the course of the nerve. Superior division or inferior division third nerve paresis may occur with subarachnoid lesions,[261] and isolated superior division paresis has been described with a superior cerebellar–posterior cerebral artery junction aneurysm that compressed and flattened the interpeduncular third nerve from below.[262] Superior branch palsy has also been described with basilar artery aneurysm, intracavernous carotid aneurysm, migraine, diabetes, lymphoma, sphenoidal abscess, sphenoid sinusitis, frontal sinus mucocele, viral illness, meningitis, and after craniotomy.[146,170,188,192,210,216,262,263,264] Even ophthalmoplegic migraine may cause recurrent paroxysmal superior division oculomotor palsy.[265] Isolated superior division-like paresis may be mimicked by myasthenia gravis.[266] Isolated inferior division involvement has occurred with trauma, mesencephalic infarction and tumor,[44,45,46] basilar artery aneurysm,[267] parasellar tumors (e.g., meningioma, schwannoma),[268] viral illness, orbital dural arteriovenous malformation,[197] as part of a more generalized vasculitic or demyelinating neuropathy,[269] and in association with elevated antigalactocerebroside and anti-GM1 antibodies.[225] Inferior division involvement from tumors may be pupil-sparing, perhaps due to insidious tumor growth sparing pressure-resistant pupillomotor fibers.

Partial or complete TNP may rarely follow dental anesthesia, presumably due to inadvertent injection of an anesthetic agent into the inferior dental artery or superior alveolar artery with subsequent retrograde flow into the maxillary artery, middle meningeal artery, and lacrimal branch of the ophthalmic artery.

11.4 Evaluation

11.4.1 What Is the Evaluation of Nonisolated TNP?

Appropriate investigations and neuroimaging studies in nonisolated TNP are directed at the precise area of interest, and this area is determined by associated localizing features.[1,270] In general, MRI with and without gadolinium enhancement is the neuroimaging modality of choice.[74] However, CT with CT angiography (CTA) is typically the best initial evaluation for TNP in the emergency room setting followed by gadolinium-enhanced cranial MRI with MR angiography (MRA). CT scanning is also the appropriate first-choice neuroimaging study in patients being evaluated for acute head trauma or acute vascular events (infarction or hemorrhage). Contrast-enhanced CT scanning with narrow (2-mm) collimation should also be considered for patients who cannot tolerate MRI or in whom MRI is contraindicated (e.g., pacemaker, claustrophobia, metallic clips in head, etc.).[74,77] If there are clinical signs of a meningeal process, lumbar puncture (LP) should be performed. The evaluation of a patient with TNP is summarized in ► Fig. 11.1.

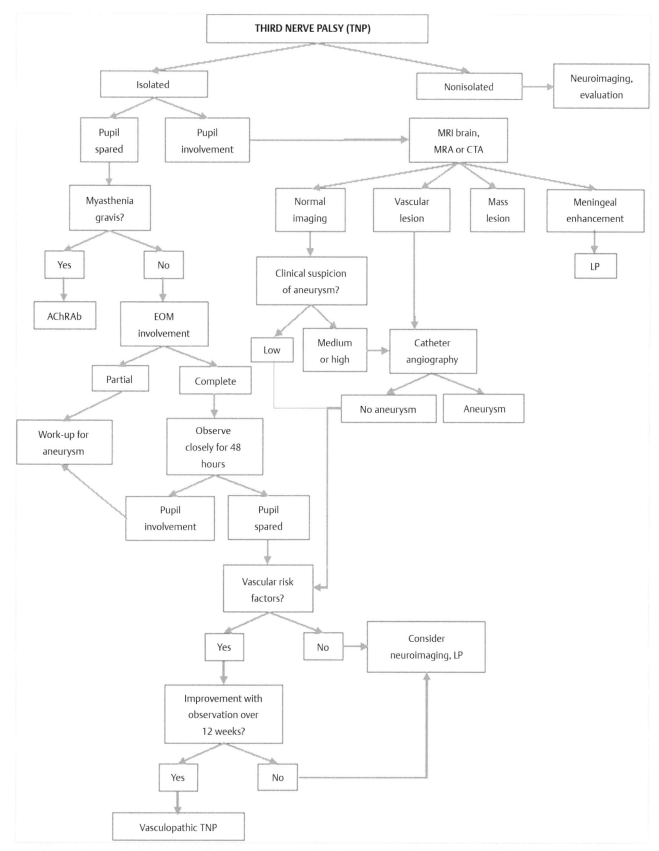

Fig. 11.1 Evaluation of third nerve palsy (TNP).

11.4.2 Is the TNP Due to Trauma?

Traumatic isolated TNP (type 2) should undergo CT scanning to evaluate associated central nervous system damage (e.g., subdural or intracerebral hematoma) as indicated by associated neurologic signs and symptoms.[129,130,131,132,232] TNP after mild head trauma has been observed in association with otherwise asymptomatic lesions (e.g., cerebral aneurysm).[72,80,271] Although uncommon, neuroimaging may be warranted in patients with TNP after minimal or trivial trauma to exclude mass lesions or cerebral aneurysms (class III–IV, level C).

11.4.3 Is the TNP Congenital?

Congenital isolated TNP (type 3) is rare, usually unilateral, and may occur in isolation or in association with other neurologic and systemic abnormalities, including congenital facial nerve palsies or other cranial neuropathies, facial capillary hemangioma, cerebellar hypoplasia, gaze palsy, ipsilateral nevus sebaceous of Jadassohn, mental retardation, and digital anomalies.[14,116,202,203,204,205,206,208] All patients have some degree of ptosis and ophthalmoplegia, and nearly all have pupillary involvement. In most cases, the pupil is miotic rather than dilated, likely secondary to aberrant third nerve regeneration, and is usually minimally reactive or nonreactive to light. Rarely, the pupil may be spared. Amblyopia is common.[206]

Occlusion therapy for amblyopia can be of significant benefit in patients with 20/40 or better visual acuity.[272] Stereopsis is uncommon in children who developed oculomotor palsy during the amblyogenic period but may be preserved if the patient experiences rapid recovery or develops a compensatory head tilt.[272] Most cases are spontaneous, but familial cases have been described. We recommend MRI in all patients with congenital TNPs, mainly to evaluate for associated intracranial structural abnormalities (class III–IV, level C).

11.4.4 Is the Isolated TNP Acquired and Nontraumatic?

Acquired, nontraumatic isolated TNP (type 4) may occur with lesions localized anywhere along the course of the third nerve from the fascicle to the orbit.[74] For clinical purposes, isolated TNP may be divided into three types (types 4A–4C) (Box 11.1).[1,273,274]

11.4.5 Does the Patient Have an Acquired Isolated TNP with a Normal Pupillary Sphincter with Completely Palsied Extraocular Muscles (Type 4A TNP)?

TNP with a normal pupillary sphincter and completely palsied extraocular muscles is almost never due to an intracranial aneurysm. However, one patient has been described in whom a painless, pupil-sparing, but otherwise complete TNP was the only sign of an aneurysm arising from the basilar artery.[255] A similar painful TNP has been described due to an aneurysm in the cavernous sinus,[144] and pupillary sparing may rarely occur

with pituitary adenoma. This type of TNP is most commonly caused by ischemia, especially associated with diabetes mellitus. In a retrospective review of 34 consecutive cases of isolated atraumatic TNP, diabetes mellitus was the most common etiology, accounting for 46% of cases.[74] Ischemic TNP may also occur with giant cell arteritis[74,75,133,134,137] and systemic lupus erythematosus. Pupil-sparing TNP has also been reported with sildenafil citrate[241] and cocaine use.[240] Ocular ischemia and ischemic TNP have been reported after administration of injectable calcium hydroxylapatite filler secondary to embolization.[275] Significant risk factors for ischemic oculomotor nerve palsies include diabetes, left ventricular hypertrophy, and elevated hematocrit.[140] Obesity, hypertension, and smoking are also probable risk factors. Ischemic damage to the trigeminal fibers in the oculomotor nerve may be the source of pain in ischemic-diabetic TNPs.[276] Ischemic TNP typically resolves over several weeks to months.[92,277,278,279]

Ischemic lesions of the oculomotor nerve often spare the pupil because the lesion is confined to the core of the nerve and does not affect peripherally situated pupillomotor fibers. However, the pupil is involved in about 25% of diabetic oculomotor palsies,[141,280] and diabetes may even cause a superior branch palsy of the oculomotor nerve. Pupil sparing has been documented in 62 to 86% of TNPs due to ischemia.[138] In differentiating a diabetic from an aneurysmal ischemic TNP, it is useful to note that ophthalmoplegia resolves more quickly in diabetic TNPs.[280] In a prospective study of 26 consecutive patients with diabetes-associated TNP, internal ophthalmoplegia occurred in 10 patients (38%).[138] The magnitude of anisocoria was 1 mm or less in most patients. Only two patients had anisocoria greater than 2.0 mm, and none had greater than 2.5 mm. No patient had a fully dilated, unreactive pupil. The authors concluded that pupil involvement in patients with diabetes-associated TNP occurs more often than has previously been recognized (14–32% in other studies), although the degree of anisocoria in any patient is usually 1 mm or less. When commenting on this study, Trobe stated, "we can presume that all patients who have oculomotor nerve palsies with anisocoria of greater than 2.0 mm are outliers for the diagnosis of ischemia."[281]

Postmortem examinations in three diabetic patients have demonstrated pathologic changes in the subarachnoid or cavernous sinus portion of the nerve. Ischemic TNP with pupillary sparing, however, has also been reported due to fascicular damage with mesencephalic infarcts documented on MRI.[23,30,41,52,282] Keane and Ahmadi, however, noted that most diabetic TNPs are peripheral.[283] In their MRI study of 49 diabetic patients with isolated, unilateral TNPs, only one was found to have a brainstem infarct. Of eight diabetics with midbrain infarcts and TNPs, seven had other central nervous system findings and five had bilateral TNPs.

In a prospective study of 16 patients with ischemic TNPs, 11 (69%) had progression of ophthalmoplegia with a median time between reported onset and peak severity of ophthalmoplegia of 10 days.[139] Almost all patients with an ischemic TNP will improve within 4 to 12 weeks of onset of symptoms.[135]

Sanders et al retrospectively reviewed 55 patients with vasculopathic TNP.[284] Of these, 42 (76%) had normal pupillary function. Of these 42 patients, 23 (55%) demonstrated an incomplete extraocular muscle palsy, defined as partially reduced ductions affecting all third nerve innervated extraocular muscles and levator (diffuse pattern) or partially reduced ductions that involved only some third nerve innervated muscles and levator (focal pattern). Twenty (87%) of these 23 patients showed a diffuse pattern of paresis and only three (13%) showed a focal pattern of paresis, affecting only the superior rectus and levator muscles (superior division weakness). Based on their series, the authors noted that most patients with extraocular muscle and levator involvement in pupil-sparing, incomplete TNPs of vasculopathic origin have a diffuse pattern of paresis, whereas pupil-sparing TNPs of aneurysmal origin often have a focal pattern of paresis.

Adults who develop type 4A TNP do not require angiography.[273,285] Although some authors recommend that neuroimaging need not be performed initially in presumed ischemic, neurologically isolated, complete, pupil-spared TNP, this is controversial in the modern neuroimaging era. The yield for detecting a compressive lesion is low but the risk of missing a treatable lesion has to be weighed against the cost of the study and the comfort level of the clinician and the patient. If the TNP resolves over time, then imaging may not be needed at all (class III–IV, level C). Neuroimaging should be performed in patients with no vasculopathic risk factors or in patients who do not improve by 12 weeks of follow-up (class III–IV, level B). Patients with type 4A TNP should be observed closely for the first week, as some patients with aneurysms may develop delayed pupil involvement, usually within the first 24 to 48 hours. Patients who develop pupil involvement should be reevaluated (see below). Vasculopathic risk factors, especially diabetes mellitus, hypertension, and increased cholesterol, should be sought and controlled. Patients over the age of 55 years, especially those with other symptoms suggestive of giant cell arteritis (e.g., headache, jaw or tongue claudication, polymyalgia rheumatica symptoms), should have a sedimentation rate determination.[134,137] Temporal artery biopsy should be performed if the sedimentation rate is elevated or other systemic symptoms are present (class III–IV, level C). Myasthenia gravis may rarely mimic this type of TNP, so an evaluation (e.g., Tensilon or Prostigmin test, anti-acetylcholine antibodies, etc.) should be considered, primarily in patients with fluctuating or fatiguing ptosis or ophthalmoplegia (class III–IV, level C). If the complete, pupil-spared TNP improves following a period of observation, no neuroimaging is required (class III–IV, level C). Some authors recommend noninvasive vascular studies (MRI with MRA or CTA) in all patients with TNP, regardless of whether or not they have diabetes or any other systemic vasculopathy, with the one exception being patients with an otherwise complete TNP (i.e., complete ptosis, no adduction, no depression, no elevation) but normally reactive, isocoric pupils.[285] See below for a further discussion about this topic.

11.4.6 Does the Patient Have an Acquired Isolated TNP with a Normal Pupillary Sphincter and Incomplete Palsied Extraocular Muscles (Type 4B TNP)?

Patients with an incomplete motor TNP with pupillary sparing require an MRI to rule out a mass lesion. If the MRI is normal,

cerebral vascular imaging should be considered to investigate the presence of an aneurysm, dural-cavernous sinus fistula, or high-grade carotid stenosis. Three-dimensional time-of-flight MRA or CTA may well reveal an aneurysm or other vascular malformation.[70,78,81,273,286] Catheter cerebral angiography remains the "gold standard" for the diagnosis of cerebral aneurysms.[281,287] Although MRA may be able to detect up to 95% of cerebral aneurysms that will bleed, it cannot completely exclude aneurysm as the etiology of a pupil-involved TNP. Jacobson and Trobe addressed whether or not MRA was adequate for evaluating for aneurysms in patients with TNP.[273] They noted that in 46 well-documented aneurysms of the posterior communicating artery causing TNP, the aneurysm diameters ranged from 3 to 17 mm (median 8 mm); 42 of these (91.3%) measured 5 mm or more, and 4 (8.7%) measured less than 5 mm.[77] They then investigated how sensitive MRA is in detecting aneurysms and found that MRA detected 64 (97%) of 66 aneurysms 5 mm or greater in diameter but only 15 (53.6%) of 28 aneurysms less than 5 mm in diameter. The relationship between aneurysm size and risk of rupture was then assessed. Among the 115 aneurysms 5 mm or greater, 15 (13.0%) ruptured. None of the 40 aneurysms with a diameter of less than 5 mm ruptured. Combining these data, the authors estimated that properly performed MRA will overlook only 1.5% of aneurysms that cause TNP and that will go on to rupture during the subsequent 8 years if untreated. Two small series also showed CTA is reliable for detecting up to 100% of aneurysms causing isolated TNP.[70,288] In another study comparing CTA to conventional angiography for ruptured aneurysms, the authors found CTA still missed some unruptured aneurysms smaller than 4 mm.[289] The sensitivity of CTA in combination with MRI/MRA is almost 100%.[278] The false positive rate for noninvasive imaging (MRA or CTA) compared to catheter angiography was 15% in a retrospective review of 286 patients with unruptured intracranial aneurysms, and was significantly higher for aneurysms < 4 mm in size ($p < 0.01$).[290]

MRA and CTA play an important role in the initial evaluation of patients with any isolated TNP due to their high sensitivity, especially for aneurysms 5 mm or larger. Although some sensitivity and specificity is lost for smaller aneurysms (< 4 mm), these lesions are less likely to cause a compressive lesion. When MRA and/or CTA is properly performed and interpreted, the risk of overlooking an aneurysm likely to rupture is nearly equal to the aggregate risk of stroke, myocardial infarction, or death associated with catheter angiography. However, because of the potentially drastic consequences of overlooking an aneurysm, MRA or CTA should be considered the definitive test only in patients with a relatively low likelihood of harboring an aneurysm or relatively high likelihood of suffering a complication during catheter angiography (e.g., age greater than 70, symptomatic atherosclerotic cardiovascular disease, significant cardiovascular or renal disease, Ehlers–Danlos syndrome). In patients with type 4B TNP (plus patient age greater than or equal to 40 years and vasculopathic factors present), these authors recommend MRI with an MRA or CTA. Catheter angiography is recommended if (1) worsening of extraocular muscle or iris sphincter impairment continues beyond 14 days; (2) iris sphincter impairment progresses to anisocoria > 1 mm[138]; (3) no recovery of function occurs within 12 weeks; or (4) signs of aberrant regeneration develop (class IV, level U).[273]

Pupil involvement is not diagnostic of aneurysmal compression, and up to 38% of presumed ischemic TNPs involve the pupil.[138] Thus, a certain number of negative cerebral angiograms are expected in the evaluation of pupil-involved TNP. The potential risks and complications of catheter angiography, however, must be considered in the decision for angiography. MRI and MRA are especially warranted for superior division TNP. Myasthenia gravis may rarely mimic a superior division TNP, so acetylcholine receptor antibody testing and electromyography with repetitive stimulation should be considered as part of the evaluation. If a patient with a partial TNP has signs of meningeal irritation, other CN palsies, or signs of more diffuse meningeal involvement (e.g., radiculopathies), then a spinal tap to investigate infectious, inflammatory, or neoplastic meningitis should be performed (class IV, level C). In cases of presumed or suspected SAH, CT may be the preferred initial imaging study followed by CTA and cerebral angiography as needed.

11.4.7 Does the Patient Have an Isolated Acquired TNP with Subnormal Pupillary Sphincter Dysfunction and Partial or Complete Extraocular Muscle Palsies (Type 4C TNP)?

Patients with a "relative pupil-sparing" TNP should have MRI to rule out the possibility of a compressive lesion. Such patients should also have a CT scan if a SAH is suspected and a subsequent cerebral angiogram if MRI is negative because of the possibility of a cerebral aneurysm. Cullom et al published a small prospective study of 10 patients with "relative pupillary-sparing" TNP and none of the patients demonstrated aneurysms.[136] These authors suggested that the prevalence of aneurysm in patients with palsies of this type may be low enough to preclude routine angiography in this group. This report and subsequent recommendation, however, was based on an insufficient patient sample (class IV, level U). Jacobson reported 24 patients with relative pupil-sparing TNP and found that 10 had nerve infarction, 8 had parasellar tumors, 2 had intracavernous carotid aneurysms, 1 had leptomeningeal carcinomatosis, 1 had Tolosa–Hunt syndrome, 1 had oculomotor neurilemmoma, and 1 had primary ocular neuromyotonia.[94] Also, others have reported internal carotid, posterior communicating, and basilar artery aneurysms in isolated TNP with relative pupillary sparing. Thus, cerebral angiography may still be warranted if MRI is negative (class IV, level C). Because 10 to 38% of patients with ischemic TNPs have pupillary dysfunction,[135,138] using these guidelines there will be a certain percentage of normal angiograms.

In the Jacobson and Trobe study discussed above, patients with partially impaired iris sphincters but completely impaired extraocular muscle function (relative pupil-sparing complete TNP) plus patient age greater than or equal to 40 years and vascular risk factors present, the authors recommended MRI followed by MRA (or CTA) if MRI does not show a nonaneurysmal cause.[273] Catheter angiography may still be required in these patients (class IV, level U).

In evaluating these patients, one must be cautious to avoid mistaking "pseudo"-pupil-sparing, due to aberrant regeneration

(below) or coexistent Horner syndrome, from true relative pupil sparing. In both of these conditions, a compressive lesion is likely localized in the cavernous sinus. Thus, pupil-sparing or pseudo-pupil-sparing TNPs may occur not only with extra-axial ischemic lesions but also in intra-axial (midbrain) lesions, a small proportion of subarachnoid compressive lesions, and a large proportion of cavernous sinus compressive lesions.[38]

Complete external and internal TNPs occurring in isolation are often due to compressive lesions or meningeal infiltration; thus, an MRI is warranted as a first step. If this study is negative, a cerebral angiogram is necessary to investigate aneurysm or dural-cavernous sinus fistula. If meningeal signs are present, spinal fluid evaluation is warranted. A noncontrast head CT scan should be performed for suspected SAH followed by a CTA. In patients with totally impaired iris sphincter function and impairment of extraocular muscle function ("pupil-blown TNP"), Jacobson and Trobe recommend MRI followed by catheter angiography if MRI does not disclose a nonaneurysmal cause.[273] A fully dilated and nonreactive pupil occurs in up to 71% of patients with aneurysmal compression and TNP. Aneurysms impair the pupil in 96% of TNP, and the remaining 4% in which the pupil is spared have only partial TNP.

11.4.8 What Neuroimaging Procedures Should Be Considered in a Patient with an Isolated TNP?

Lee et al reviewed the literature on MRI, MRA, CT, CTA, and catheter angiography in the management of the isolated TNP, and proposed the following guidelines[277]:

1. Isolated complete or partial internal dysfunction (pupil dilated) with completely normal external function of the third nerve and no ptosis: The risk for aneurysm in this setting is minimal and neuroimaging for aneurysm is probably not required. The papers that were reviewed in this manuscript, however, did not explicitly include or exclude isolated dilated pupils in their complete or incomplete TNPs. The clinician should look for other etiologies for isolated pupil dysfunction (e.g., tonic pupil, pharmacologic, sphincter damage).[291] Performing CT/CTA or MRI/MRA in this setting is low risk, however. This represents a practice guideline of moderate certainty based on class III–IV evidence (level B).

2. Partial external dysfunction TNP without internal dysfunction: The risk for aneurysm in patients with partial TNP is moderate (up to 30% of cases). Unfortunately, the risk for an individual patient is not well defined because other etiologies may cause partial external dysfunction with a normal pupil. For example, patients who have clear myasthenia gravis do not require additional aneurysm evaluation. Other nonaneurysmal etiologies including neoplastic, demyelinating, infiltrative, and ischemic etiologies may also cause a partial TNP without pupil involvement and may require neuroimaging. If the TNP is due to aneurysm, the TNP usually progresses over time to a complete TNP including pupil involvement. Although there may not be internal dysfunction (pupil involvement) in a partial external dysfunction TNP, the term pupil-sparing is probably not appropriate in this setting. That is, pupil involvement may occur over time in patients with partial

TNP due to aneurysm with initially no internal dysfunction. Absence of pupil involvement early in the course of a partial TNP may be due to incomplete compression of the pupil fibers by the aneurysm. Note: MRI with MRA or CTA in the acute setting is a reasonable screen in these cases. The patient should be followed clinically for progression or pupil involvement in the first week. If the cranial MRI with MRA or CTA is negative and if the risk of angiography (e.g., elderly, severe cardiovascular disease, abnormal serum creatinine) is high, then observation alone is reasonable and the clinician should look for alternative etiologies for a partial external dysfunction TNP (e.g., myasthenia gravis). The clinician should still consider catheter angiography in these cases if the risk of aneurysm is higher than the risk of angiography (technically inadequate MRA, progression to complete TNP, pupil involvement). The practice option for cranial MRI with MRA or CTA alone in this setting is of low certainty (level C) and is based on class III–IV evidence.

3. Complete external dysfunction with completely normal internal function TNP: This clinical situation indicates a very low risk for aneurysm, and the vasculopathic patient may be observed for improvement.* The pupil should be reexamined within the first week. Patients who develop pupil involvement should be evaluated using the recommendations outlined in the pupil-involving TNP sections of this chapter. If the patient has no vasculopathic risk factors, or if there is no improvement after 4 to 12 weeks, or if signs of aberrant regeneration develop, then cranial MRI with MRA or CTA should be performed. This practice guideline is of moderate certainty based on the available evidence (level B). Evaluation for myasthenia gravis should be considered in painless, nonproptotic, pupil-spared ophthalmoplegia depending on the clinical situation. *Note: Since Lee et al's review, many authors have since advocated for imaging all TNP patients regardless of pupil involvement and vasculopathic risk factors. There is never "zero risk" of missing a treatable lesion, and over time these less-invasive imaging modalities have become more accessible and affordable to patients.*

4. Partial external dysfunction with partial internal dysfunction TNP: An initial cranial MRI with MRA or CTA is reasonable. If these studies are of excellent quality and negative, then the clinician should follow the patient for progression or complete internal dysfunction. The risk for aneurysm in this setting, however (even with a negative MRI/MRA), is uncertain. Clinicians should still consider catheter angiography if the risk of aneurysm in an individual patient is higher than the risk of angiography. This practice option is of low to moderate certainty in patients with low clinical risk for aneurysm based on class III–IV evidence (level C) and there is some disagreement among experts (level U).

5. Complete external dysfunction with partial internal dysfunction TNP: The risk of aneurysm for complete external dysfunction with partial internal dysfunction (partial pupil or "relative pupil sparing") is also unknown but probably lower than that for partial external dysfunction with or without partial internal dysfunction. The risk for aneurysm in this setting (even with a negative MRI/MRA or CTA) is uncertain. The clinician should consider catheter angiography if the risk of aneurysm is deemed higher than risk of angiography. This practice option is of low to moderate certainty in patients with low clinical risk for aneurysm based on class III–IV evidence (level C) and there is significant disagreement among experts (level U).

6. Isolated complete internal dysfunction with partial or complete external dysfunction TNP: This clinical situation has the highest risk for aneurysm (86–100% of aneurysmal TNPs have pupil involvement). MRI with MRA or CTA of the head should be performed, but even with negative neuroimaging there should be a strong consideration for catheter angiography. This practice guideline is of moderate certainty based on class III evidence and consensus expert opinion (level B). There are insufficient data to make a recommendation on whether a catheter angiogram must be performed in these cases (level U).

7. Any patient with TNP and signs of SAH: The presence of SAH (on unenhanced CT scan or LP) essentially makes the issue of complete or incomplete TNP as well as application of the "rule of the pupil" moot. Unfortunately, most of the papers in the literature on aneurysm and TNP have included nonneurologically isolated cases including SAH. In general, an initial noncontrast CT scan (with consideration for LP) should be performed in patients with TNP and signs of SAH. The clinical picture of SAH (e.g., severe headache, meningismus, altered consciousness) can be mimicked by other intracranial etiologies such as pituitary apoplexy, and most clinicians would consider a CT scan as an initial neuroimaging study prior to consideration of angiography. Patients with SAH on CT scan should probably undergo catheter angiography. Patients who cannot undergo a catheter angiogram (e.g., morbidly obese and unable to be placed on the angiography table) may have to undergo cranial CT and CTA alone prior to intervention. In other cases of SAH, special MRI parameters including fluid attenuation inversion recovery (FLAIR) MRI and MRA may be useful. Catheter angiography should be strongly considered even if the evaluations for SAH (e.g., CT, LP) are negative. This practice guideline is of strong certainty based on class II–III evidence and consensus expert opinion (level B). More recent studies have analyzed the usefulness of CTA versus MRA for diagnosing SAH.

8. Patients who cannot undergo MRI or MRA: CT and CTA could be considered in selected cases, especially in acute settings, if MRA is not available, or if MRI is contraindicated (e.g., obesity, pacemaker). Although CTA has some advantages over MRA (especially if the location of the aneurysm is known), the superior quality of MRI compared to CT in evaluating the entire course of the third nerve makes the combination of MRI/MRA superior to CT/CTA as the screening study for TNP. It has been found that the combination of CT–CTA and MRI–MRA has a sensitivity approaching 95 to 100% and can identify almost every lesion.[278] If there is a high clinical suspicion of an aneurysm, standard catheter angiography should be considered as a follow-up to detect very small aneurysms,[89] but caution should be taken as it is very invasive and there is a small risk of neurologic morbidity and mortality (1–2%). Standard catheter angiography remains the gold standard for diagnosis.[89,273,278,290]

When selecting between noninvasive imaging modalities, consider patient and facility factors. A CTA may be the preferred method over MRA if the patient cannot lie still for an extended period, is morbidly obese beyond the weight and girth limitations of the MRI scanner, or has implanted devices that are not compatible with an MRI scanner (e.g., many pacemakers, pain pumps, and shunts). CTA is slightly more sensitive than MRA overall, but MRA does not have the complication of bony artifact that can obscure some vascular lesions that is seen with CTA. MRA does not require contrast, but results can be limited due to the reliance on blood flow to generate the images. MRA can usually be performed at the same time as the MRI, whereas a CTA might require transport to another imaging area. The facility's ability to quickly perform and study with high quality and the availability of a specialist to interpret the images may also impact the decision between CTA and MRA. In many cases, patients may undergo both a CTA and MRA. A catheter angiogram is often not necessary in low-risk patients if neither detects a lesion. However, if one or both shows a vascular lesion, the next step is catheter angiogram for further characterization and possible intervention.[277,292]

11.5 Is the TNP Progressive or Unresolved (Type 5 TNP)?

Patients with TNP that worsens after the acute stage (greater than 2 weeks) or who develop new neurologic findings are considered to have progressive TNP. Patients without resolution of TNP after 12 to 16 weeks are considered unresolved. These patients require MRI and MRA and consideration of standard angiography. If signs of meningeal irritation or multiple CN palsies are present, LP is indicated. Recurrent, transient, unilateral oculomotor nerve palsies may occur spontaneously in healthy individuals with no underlying disease at all.[293] This may be a useful consideration after all other causes have been ruled out.

11.6 Is the TNP Associated with Signs of Aberrant Regeneration (Type 6)?

Months to years after the occurrence of a TNP, clinical findings of aberrant regeneration of the third nerve may be noted. They include elevation of the lid on downward gaze (pseudo-von Graefe phenomenon) or adduction but lid depression during abduction. Other findings include limitation of elevation and depression of the eye with occasional eyeball retraction on attempted vertical gaze, adduction of the eye on attempted elevation or depression, and suppression of the vertical phase of the optokinetic response. The pupil may be in a miotic or mid-dilated position; it may be fixed to light but may respond to near (near-light dissociation) or constrict on adduction or down-gaze. Lagophthalmos, presumably caused by cocontraction of the levator and superior rectus muscles during Bell's phenomenon, has also been described.[294]

Aberrant regeneration may be seen after TNP due to congenital causes, trauma, aneurysm, migraine, and syphilis, but is very rarely, if ever, caused by ischemic neuropathy.[294,295] A single case of aberrant regeneration has been described after an ischemic stroke affecting the third nerve fascicle in the cerebral peduncle.[53] Misdirection of regenerating nerve fibers is likely the cause, but it has been postulated that the syndrome may be due to ephaptic neuron transmission of impulses or from chromatolysis-induced reorganization of third nerve nuclear synapses. Ephaptic transmission would explain the transient third nerve misdirection described with ophthalmoplegic migraine, temporal arteritis, pituitary apoplexy, and non-Hodgkin lymphoma.[296] Long-standing lesions, such as meningiomas of the cavernous sinus, trigeminal neuromas, large aneurysms, and pituitary tumors, may present as primary aberrant regeneration of the third nerve without a history of previous TNP.[297,298] Primary aberrant regeneration may rarely occur with extracavernous lesions, such as neurilemmoma, meningioma, asymmetric mammillary body, or intradural aneurysm.[299] Bilateral primary aberrant regeneration may also occur with abetalipoproteinemia (Bassen-Kornzweig syndrome).[300] On rare occasions, the pseudo-von Graefe phenomenon may develop contralateral to a regenerating paretic third nerve.[262]

All patients with nontraumatic TNP with aberrant regeneration (type 5) require MRI and MRA (and possibly angiography) to investigate the possibility of a compressive lesion. This is especially true if signs of aberrance develop in a patient with presumed "ischemic" TNP or in patients with primary aberrant regeneration.

References

[1] Lee AG, Onan HW, Brazis PW, Prager TC. An imaging guide to the evaluation of third cranial nerve palsies. Strabismus. 1999; 7(3):153–168

[2] Brazis PW, Masdeu JC, Biller J. Localization in Clinical Neurology. 4th ed. Philadelphia: Lippincott Williams & Wilkins; 2001

[3] Bengel D, Huffmann G. Oculomotor nuclear complex syndrome as a single sign of midbrain hemorrhage. Neuroophthalmology. 1994; 5:279–282

[4] Bogousslavsky J, Maeder P, Regli F, Meuli R. Pure midbrain infarction: clinical syndromes, MRI, and etiologic patterns. Neurology. 1994; 44(11):2032–2040

[5] Chee MW, Tan CB, Tjia HT. Nuclear third nerve palsy and somnolence due to stroke–a case report. Ann Acad Med Singapore. 1990; 19(3):382–384

[6] Gaymard B, Larmande P, de Toffol B, Autret A. Reversible nuclear oculomotor nerve paralysis. Caused by a primary mesencephalic hemorrhage. Eur Neurol. 1990; 30(3):128–131

[7] Nakao H, Ohtsuka K, Hashimoto M. Nuclear oculomotor nerve palsy caused by metastatic tumor. Neuroophthalmology. 1998; 20:36

[8] Saeki N, Yamaura A, Sunami K. Bilateral ptosis with pupil sparing because of a discrete midbrain lesion: magnetic resonance imaging evidence of topographic arrangement within the oculomotor nerve. J Neuroophthalmol. 2000; 20(2):130–134

[9] von Noorden GK, Hansell R. Clinical characteristics and treatment of isolated inferior rectus paralysis. Ophthalmology. 1991; 98(2):253–257

[10] Chou TM, Demer JL. Isolated inferior rectus palsy caused by a metastasis to the oculomotor nucleus. Am J Ophthalmol. 1998; 126(5):737–740

[11] Lee AG, Tang RA, Wong GG, Schiffman JS, Singh S. Isolated inferior rectus muscle palsy resulting from a nuclear third nerve lesion as the initial manifestation of multiple sclerosis. J Neuroophthalmol. 2000; 20(4):246–247

[12] Tezer I, Dogulu CF, Kansu T. Isolated inferior rectus palsy as a result of paramedian thalamopeduncular infarction. J Neuroophthalmol. 2000; 20(3):154–155

[13] Umapathi T, Koon SW, Mukkam RP, et al. Insights into the three-dimensional structure of the oculomotor nuclear complex and fascicles. J Neuroophthalmol. 2000; 20(2):138–144

[14] Pratt DV, Orenga-Nania S, Horowitz BL, Oram O. Magnetic resonance imaging findings in a patient with nuclear oculomotor palsy. Arch Ophthalmol. 1995; 113(2):141–142

[15] Bryan JS, Hamed LM. Levator-sparing nuclear oculomotor palsy. Clinical and magnetic resonance imaging findings. J Clin Neuroophthalmol. 1992; 12(1): 26–30

[16] Martin TJ, Corbett JJ, Babikian PV, Crawford SC, Currier RD. Bilateral ptosis due to mesencephalic lesions with relative preservation of ocular motility. J Neuroophthalmol. 1996; 16(4):258–263

[17] Sanli M, Altinurs N, Bavbek M. Partial bilateral oculomotor nucleus lesion following surgery of a fourth ventricle ependymoma. Neuroophthalmology. 1995; 15:103–105

[18] Worthington JM, Halmagyi GM. Bilateral total ophthalmoplegia due to midbrain hematoma. Neurology. 1996; 46(4):1176–1177

[19] Liu GT, Carrazana EJ, Charness ME. Unilateral oculomotor palsy and bilateral ptosis from paramedian midbrain infarction. Arch Neurol. 1991; 48(9): 983–986

[20] Liu GT, Crenner CW, Logigian EL, Charness ME, Samuels MA. Midbrain syndromes of Benedikt, Claude, and Nothnagel: setting the record straight. Neurology. 1992; 42(9):1820–1822

[21] Saeki N, Murai N, Sunami K. Midbrain tegmental lesions affecting or sparing the pupillary fibres. J Neurol Neurosurg Psychiatry. 1996; 61(4):401–402

[22] Borrás JM, Salazar FG, Grandas F. Oculomotor palsy and contralateral tremor (Benedikt's syndrome) following a stereotactic procedure. J Neurol. 1997; 244(4):272–274

[23] Dichgans M, Dieterich M. Third nerve palsy with contralateral ocular torsion and binocular tilt of visual vertical, indicating a midbrain lesion. Neuroophthalmology. 1995; 15:315–320

[24] Oishi M, Mochizuki Y. Ipsilateral oculomotor nerve palsy and contralateral downbeat nystagmus: a syndrome caused by unilateral paramedian thalamopeduncular infarction. J Neurol. 1997; 244(2):132–133

[25] Andreo LK, Gardner TA, Enzenauer RW. Third nerve palsy in an AIDS patient. Presented at the North American Neuro-Ophthalmology Society meeting, Durango, Colorado, February 27–March 3, 1994

[26] Barbas NR, Hedges TR, Schwenn M. Isolated oculomotor nerve palsy due to neoplasm in infancy. Neuro-ophthalmol. 1995; 15(3):157–160

[27] Getenet JC, Vighetto A, Nighoghossian N, Trouillas P. Isolated bilateral third nerve palsy caused by a mesencephalic hematoma. Neurology. 1994; 44(5): 981–982

[28] Kim JS, Kang JK, Lee SA, Lee MC. Isolated or predominant ocular motor nerve palsy as a manifestation of brain stem stroke. Stroke. 1993; 24(4):581–586

[29] Newman NJ, Lessell S. Isolated pupil-sparing third-nerve palsy as the presenting sign of multiple sclerosis. Arch Neurol. 1990; 47(7):817–818

[30] Thömke F, Tettenborn B, Hopf HC. Third nerve palsy as the sole manifestation of midbrain ischemia. Neuro-ophthalmology. 1995; 15(6): 327–335

[31] Hashimoto M, Ohtsuka K. Bilateral internal ophthalmoplegia as a feature of oculomotor fascicular syndrome disclosed by magnetic resonance imaging. Am J Ophthalmol. 1998; 125(1):121–123

[32] Ksiazek SM, Slamovits TL, Rosen CE, Burde RM, Parisi F. Fascicular arrangement in partial oculomotor paresis. Am J Ophthalmol. 1994; 118(1): 97–103

[33] Castro O, Johnson LN, Mamourian AC. Isolated inferior oblique paresis from brain-stem infarction. Perspective on oculomotor fascicular organization in the ventral midbrain tegmentum. Arch Neurol. 1990; 47(2):235–237

[34] Shuaib A, Israelian G, Lee MA. Mesencephalic hemorrhage and unilateral pupillary deficit. J Clin Neuroophthalmol. 1989; 9(1):47–49

[35] Gauntt CD, Kashii S, Nagata I. Monocular elevation paresis caused by an oculomotor fascicular impairment. J Neuroophthalmol. 1995; 15(1):11–14

[36] Saeki N, Murai H, Mine S, Yamaura A. Fascicular arrangement within the oculomotor nerve MRI analysis of a midbrain infarct. J Clin Neurosci. 2000; 7 (3):268–270

[37] Onozu H, Yamamoto S, Takou K, Hasyasaka S. Blepharoptosis in association with ipsilateral adduction and elevation palsy. A form of fascicular oculomotor palsy. Neuro-ophthalmology. 1998; 19(3):145–150

[38] Nadeau SE, Trobe JD. Pupil sparing in oculomotor palsy: a brief review. Ann Neurol. 1983; 13(2):143–148

[39] Schwartz TH, Lycette CA, Yoon SS, Kargman DE. Clinicoradiographic evidence for oculomotor fascicular anatomy. J Neurol Neurosurg Psychiatry. 1995; 59(3):338

[40] Shuaib A, Murphy W. Mesencephalic hemorrhage and third nerve palsy. J Comput Tomogr. 1987; 11(4):385–388

[41] Breen LA, Hopf HC, Farris BK, Gutmann L. Pupil-sparing oculomotor nerve palsy due to midbrain infarction. Arch Neurol. 1991; 48(1):105–106

[42] Guy JR, Day AL. Intracranial aneurysms with superior division paresis of the oculomotor nerve. Ophthalmology. 1989; 96(7):1071–1076

[43] Hriso E, Miller A, Masdeu JC. Monocular elevation weakness and ptosis. Neurology. 1990; 47 Suppl 1:309

[44] Ksiazek SM, Repka MX, Maguire A, et al. Divisional oculomotor nerve paresis caused by intrinsic brainstem disease. Ann Neurol. 1989; 26(6):714–718

[45] Abdollah A, Francis GS. Intraaxial divisional oculomotor nerve paresis suggests intraaxial fascicular organization. Ann Neurol. 1990; 28(4): 589–590

[46] Eggenberger ER, Miller NR, Hoffman PN, Nauta HJ, Green WR. Mesencephalic ependymal cyst causing an inferior divisional paresis of the oculomotor nerve: case report. Neurology. 1993; 43(11):2419–2420

[47] Gaymard B, Lafitte C, Gelot A, de Toffol B. Plus-minus lid syndrome. J Neurol Neurosurg Psychiatry. 1992; 55(9):846–848

[48] Vetrugno R, Mascalchi M, Marulli D, et al. Plus minus lid syndrome due to cerebral glioma. A case report. Neuroophthalmology. 1997; 18(3):149–151

[49] Gottlieb M, Kogan A, Kimball D. Intracranial tuberculoma presenting as an isolated oculomotor nerve paresis. J Emerg Med. 2015; 48(1):e1–e4

[50] Kumar Y, Hooda K, Sapire J. A case report of isolated oculomotor nerve nucleus infarct: a rare cause of Parinaud's syndrome. Conn Med. 2016; 80 (3):167–168

[51] Gaymard B, Huynh C, Laffont I. Unilateral eyelid retraction. J Neurol Neurosurg Psychiatry. 2000; 68(3):390–392

[52] Hopf HC, Gutmann L. Diabetic 3rd nerve palsy: evidence for a mesencephalic lesion. Neurology. 1990; 40(7):1041–1045

[53] Messé SR, Shin RK, Liu GT, Galetta SL, Volpe NJ. Oculomotor synkinesis following a midbrain stroke. Neurology. 2001; 57(6):1106–1107

[54] Chen L, Maclaurin W, Gerraty RP. Isolated unilateral ptosis and mydriasis from ventral midbrain infarction. J Neurol. 2009; 256(7):1164–1165

[55] Hart AJ, Allibone J, Casey AT, Thomas DG. Malignant meningioma of the oculomotor nerve without dural attachment. Case report and review of the literature. J Neurosurg. 1998; 88(6):1104–1106

[56] Ishikawa H, Satoh H, Fujiwara M, et al. Oculomotor nerve palsy caused by lung cancer metastasis. Intern Med. 1997; 36(4):301–303

[57] Landolfi JC, Thaler HT, DeAngelis LM. Adult brainstem gliomas. Neurology. 1998; 51(4):1136–1139

[58] Thömke F, Lensch E, Ringel K, Hopf HC. Isolated cranial nerve palsies in multiple sclerosis. J Neurol Neurosurg Psychiatry. 1997; 63(5):682–685

[59] Man BL, Fu YP. Isolated bilateral oculomotor nerve palsies due to a midbrain cavernous malformation. BMJ Case Rep. 2013; 2013:bcr2013201063

[60] Birchall D, Khangure MS, McAuliffe W. Resolution of third nerve paresis after endovascular management of aneurysms of the posterior communicating artery. AJNR Am J Neuroradiol. 1999; 20(3):411–413

[61] Branley MG, Wright KW, Borchert MS. Third nerve palsy due to cerebral artery aneurysm in a child. Aust N Z J Ophthalmol. 1992; 20(2):137–140

[62] DiMario FJ, Jr, Rorke LB. Transient oculomotor nerve paresis in congenital distal basilar artery aneurysm. Pediatr Neurol. 1992; 8(4):303–306

[63] Friedman JA, Piepgras DG, Pichelmann MA, Hansen KK, Brown RD, Jr, Wiebers DO. Small cerebral aneurysms presenting with symptoms other than rupture. Neurology. 2001; 57(7):1212–1216

[64] Giombini S, Ferraresi S, Pluchino F. Reversal of oculomotor disorders after intracranial aneurysm surgery. Acta Neurochir (Wien). 1991; 112(1–2): 19–24

[65] Good EF. Ptosis as the sole manifestation of compression of the oculomotor nerve by an aneurysm of the posterior communicating artery. J Clin Neuroophthalmol. 1990; 10(1):59–61

[66] Greenspan BN, Reeves AG. Transient partial oculomotor nerve paresis with posterior communicating artery aneurysm. A case report. J Clin Neuroophthalmol. 1990; 10(1):56–58

[67] Griffiths PD, Gholkar A, Sengupta RP. Oculomotor nerve palsy due to thrombosis of a posterior communicating artery aneurysm following diagnostic angiography. Neuroradiology. 1994; 36(8):614–615

[68] Horikoshi T, Nukui H, Yagishita T, Nishigaya K, Fukasawa I, Sasaki H. Oculomotor nerve palsy after surgery for upper basilar artery aneurysms. Neurosurgery. 1999; 44(4):705–710, discussion 710–711

[69] Keane JR. Cavernous sinus syndrome. Analysis of 151 cases. Arch Neurol. 1996; 53(10):967–971

[70] McFadzean RM, Teasdale EM. Computerized tomography angiography in isolated third nerve palsies. J Neurosurg. 1998; 88(4):679–684

[71] Mudgil AV, Repka MX. Ophthalmologic outcome after third cranial nerve palsy or paresis in childhood. J AAPOS. 1999; 3(1):2–8

[72] Park-Matsumoto YC, Tazawa T. Internal carotid-posterior communi-cating artery aneurysm manifesting as an unusual ocular motor paresis after minor head trauma–case report. Neurol Med Chir (Tokyo). 1997; 37(2):181–183

[73] Ranganadham P, Dinakar I, Mohandas S, Singh AK. A rare presentation of posterior communicating artery aneurysm. Clin Neurol Neurosurg. 1992; 94 (3):225–227

[74] Renowden SA, Harris KM, Hourihan MD. Isolated atraumatic third nerve palsy: clinical features and imaging techniques. Br J Radiol. 1993; 66(792): 1111–1117

[75] Richards BW, Jones FR, Jr, Younge BR. Causes and prognosis in 4,278 cases of paralysis of the oculomotor, trochlear, and abducens cranial nerves. Am J Ophthalmol. 1992; 113(5):489–496

[76] Striph GG. Consecutive oculomotor nerve palsy from a de novo cerebral aneurysm. J Clin Neuroophthalmol. 1993; 13(3):181–187

[77] Teasdale E, Statham P, Straiton J, Macpherson P. Non-invasive radiological investigation for oculomotor palsy. J Neurol Neurosurg Psychiatry. 1990; 53 (7):549–553

[78] Tomsak RL, Masaryk TJ, Bates JH. Magnetic resonance angiography (MRA) of isolated aneurysmal third nerve palsy. J Clin Neuroophthalmol. 1991; 11(1): 16–18

[79] Tummala RP, Harrison A, Madison MT, Nussbaum ES. Pseudomyasthenia resulting from a posterior carotid artery wall aneurysm: a novel presentation: case report. Neurosurgery. 2001; 49(6):1466–1468, discussion 1468–1469

[80] Walter KA, Newman NJ, Lessell S. Oculomotor palsy from minor head trauma: initial sign of intracranial aneurysm. Neurology. 1994; 44(1): 148–150

[81] Weinberg DA, Kaufman DI, Siebert JD, Pernicone JR. Negative MRI versus real disease. Surv Ophthalmol. 1996; 40(4):312–319

[82] Wolin MJ, Saunders RA. Aneurysmal oculomotor nerve palsy in an 11-year-old boy. J Clin Neuroophthalmol. 1992; 12(3):178–180

[83] Zimmer DV. Oculomotor nerve palsy from posterior communicating artery aneurysm. J La State Med Soc. 1991; 143(8):22–25

[84] Wolfe SQ, Manzano G, Langer DJ, Morcos JJ. Cavernous malformation of the oculomotor nerve mimicking a partially thrombosed posterior communicating artery aneurysm: report of two cases. Neurosurgery. 2011; 69(2):E470–E474

[85] Hashimoto M, Ohtsuka K, Akiba H, Harada K. Vascular compression of the oculomotor nerve disclosed by thin-slice magnetic resonance imaging. Am J Ophthalmol. 1998; 125(6):881–882

[86] Nakagawa H, Nakajima S, Nakajima Y, Furuta Y, Nishi O, Nishi K. Bilateral oculomotor nerve palsies due to posterior cerebral arterial compression relieved by microvascular decompression–case report. Neurol Med Chir (Tokyo). 1991; 31(1):45–48

[87] Zingale A, Chiaramonte I, Mancuso P, Consoli V, Albanese V. Craniofacial pain and incomplete oculomotor palsy associated with ipsilateral primitive trigeminal artery. Case report. J Neurosurg Sci. 1993; 37(4):251–255

[88] Babbitz JD, Harsh GR, IV. Concomitant ectatic posterior communicating artery and tentorial meningioma as a source of oculomotor palsy: case report. Neurosurgery. 2005; 57(6):E1316–, discussion E1316

[89] Jeong HW, Seo JH, Kim ST, Jung CK, Suh SI. Clinical practice guideline for the management of intracranial aneurysms. Neurointervention. 2014; 9(2): 63–71

[90] Cullom ME, Savino PJ. Adenocarcinoma of the prostate presenting as a third nerve palsy. Neurology. 1993; 43(10):2146–2147

[91] Egan RA, Thompson CR, MacCollin M, Lessell S. Monocular elevator paresis in neurofibromatosis type 2. Neurology. 2001; 56(9):1222–1224

[92] Hardenack M, Völker A, Schröder JM, Gilsbach JM, Harders AG. Primary eosinophilic granuloma of the oculomotor nerve. Case report. J Neurosurg. 1994; 81(5):784–787

[93] Ide C, De Coene B, Gilliard C, et al. Hemorrhagic arachnoid cyst with third nerve paresis: CT and MR findings. AJNR Am J Neuroradiol. 1997; 18(8): 1407–1410

[94] Jacobson DM. Relative pupil-sparing third nerve palsy: etiology and clinical variables predictive of a mass. Neurology. 2001; 56(6):797–798

[95] Kadota T, Miyawaki Y, Nakagawa H, Ishiguro S, Kuroda C. MR imaging of oculomotor nerve neurilemmoma. Magn Reson Imaging. 1993; 11(7): 1071–1075

[96] Kajiya Y, Nakajo M, Kajiya Y, Miyaji N. Oculomotor nerve invasion by lymphoma demonstrated by MRI. J Comput Assist Tomogr. 1995; 19(3): 502–504

[97] Kawasaki A. Oculomotor nerve schwannoma associated with ophthalmoplegic migraine. Am J Ophthalmol. 1999; 128(5):658–660

[98] Kawase T, Shiobara R, Ohira T, Toya S. Developmental patterns and characteristic symptoms of petroclival meningiomas. Neurol Med Chir (Tokyo). 1996; 36(1):1–6

[99] Kaye-Wilson LG, Gibson R, Bell JE, Steers AJW, Cullen JF. Oculomotor nerve neurinoma: early detection by magnetic resonance imaging. Neuro-ophthalmol. 1994; 14(1):37–41

[100] Kodsi SR, Younge BR. Acquired oculomotor, trochlear, and abducent cranial nerve palsies in pediatric patients. Am J Ophthalmol. 1992; 114(5):568–574

[101] Mehta VS, Singh RV, Misra NK, Choudhary C. Schwannoma of the oculomotor nerve. Br J Neurosurg. 1990; 4(1):69–72

[102] Norman AA, Farris BK, Siatkowski RM. Neuroma as a cause of oculomotor palsy in infancy and early childhood. J AAPOS. 2001; 5(1):9–12

[103] Ogilvy CS, Pakzaban P, Lee JM. Oculomotor nerve cavernous angioma in a patient with Roberts syndrome. Surg Neurol. 1993; 40(1):39–42

[104] Reifenberger G, Boström J, Bettag M, Bock WJ, Wechsler W, Kepes JJ. Primary glioblastoma multiforme of the oculomotor nerve. Case report. J Neurosurg. 1996; 84(6):1062–1066

[105] Robertson PL, Pavkovic I, Donovan C, Blaivas M. Immature teratoma of the leptomeninges in an 8-year-old child: unusual presentation with recurrent transient oculomotor nerve palsies and rapid progression to diffuse brain infarction. J Child Neurol. 1998; 13(3):143–145

[106] Sanchez Dalmau BF, Abdul-Rahim AS, Zimmerman RA. Young boy with progressive double vision. Surv Ophthalmol. 1998; 43(1):47–52

[107] Schultheiss R, Kristof R, Schramm J. Complete removal of an oculomotor nerve neurinoma without permanent functional deficit. Case report. Ger J Ophthalmol. 1993; 2(4–5):228–233

[108] Takano S, Endo M, Miyasaka Y, Yada K, Ohwada T, Takagi H. Neurinoma of the oculomotor nerve–case report. Neurol Med Chir (Tokyo). 1990; 30(2): 132–136

[109] Winterkorn JMS, Bruno M. Relative pupil-sparing oculomotor nerve palsy as the presenting sign of posterior fossa meningioma. J Neuroophthalmol. 2001; 21(3):207–209

[110] Iijima K, Tosaka M, Nagano T, et al. Oculomotor nerve schwannoma associated with acute hydrocephalus: case report. Neurol Med Chir (Tokyo). 2014; 54(8):654–658

[111] Werner M, Bhatti MT, Vaishnav H, Pincus DW, Eskin T, Yachnis AT. Isolated anisocoria from an endodermal cyst of the third cranial nerve mimicking an Adie's tonic pupil. J Pediatr Ophthalmol Strabismus. 2005; 42(3):176–179

[112] Huang P, Tai CT. Tuberculous meningitis with initial manifestation of isolated oculomotor nerve palsy. Acta Neurol Taiwan. 2005; 14(1):21–23

[113] Balm M, Hammack J. Leptomeningeal carcinomatosis. Presenting features and prognostic factors. Arch Neurol. 1996; 53(7):626–632

[114] Galetta SL, Sergott RC, Wells GB, Atlas SW, Bird SJ. Spontaneous remission of a third-nerve palsy in meningeal lymphoma. Ann Neurol. 1992; 32(1): 100–102

[115] Guarino M, Stracciari A, Cirignotta F, D'Alessandro R, Pazzaglia P. Neoplastic meningitis presenting with ophthalmoplegia, ataxia, and areflexia (Miller-Fisher syndrome). Arch Neurol. 1995; 52(5):443–444

[116] Ing EB, Sullivan TJ, Clarke MP, Buncic JR. Oculomotor nerve palsies in children. J Pediatr Ophthalmol Strabismus. 1992; 29(6):331–336

[117] Ishibashi A, Sueyoshi K, You M, Yokokura Y. MR findings in isolated oculomotor nerve palsy associated with infectious mononucleosis caused by Epstein-Barr virus infection. J Comput Assist Tomogr. 1998; 22(6):995–997

[118] Keane JR. Intermittent third nerve palsy with cryptococcal meningitis. J Clin Neuroophthalmol. 1993; 13(2):124–126

[119] Mark AS, Blake P, Atlas SW, Ross M, Brown D, Kolsky M. Gd-DTPA enhancement of the cisternal portion of the oculomotor nerve on MR imaging. AJNR Am J Neuroradiol. 1992; 13(5):1463–1470

[120] Newman NJ, Slamovits TL, Friedland S, Wilson WB. Neuro-ophthalmic manifestations of meningocerebral inflammation from the limited form of Wegener's granulomatosis. Am J Ophthalmol. 1995; 120(5):613–621

[121] Straube A, Bandmann O, Büttner U, Schmidt H. A contrast enhanced lesion of the III nerve on MR of a patient with ophthalmoplegic migraine as evidence for a Tolosa-Hunt syndrome. Headache. 1993; 33(8):446–448

[122] Ueyama H, Kumamoto T, Fukuda S, Fujimoto S, Sannomiya K, Tsuda T. Isolated third nerve palsy due to sarcoidosis. Sarcoidosis Vasc Diffuse Lung Dis. 1997; 14(2):169–170

[123] Nardone R, Herz M, Egarter-Vigl E, Tezzon F. Isolated oculomotor nerve palsy as the presenting clinical manifestation of a meningeal carcinomatosis: a case report. Neurol Sci. 2006; 27(4):288–290

[124] O'Hara MA, Anderson RT, Brown D. Magnetic resonance imaging in ophthalmoplegic migraine of children. J AAPOS. 2001; 5(5):307–310

[125] Reynolds MR, Vega RA, Murphy RK, Miller-Thomas MM, Zipfel GJ. Perimesencephalic subarachnoid hemorrhage associated with a painless, pupillary-involving third cranial nerve palsy: case report and literature review. Clin Neurol Neurosurg. 2012; 114(8):1168–1171

[126] Kamat AA, Tizzard S, Mathew B. Painful third nerve palsy in a patient with perimesencephalic subarachnoid haemorrhage. Br J Neurosurg. 2005; 19(3): 247–250

[127] Papke K, Masur H, Martinez-Rubio A, Ostermann H, Schuierer G. Complete bilateral oculomotor palsy: the only clinical sign of subarachnoid hemorrhage in leukemia. Acta Neurol Scand. 1993; 88(2):153–156

[128] Ferrante E, Savino A, Brioschi A, Marazzi R, Donato MF, Riva M. Transient oculomotor cranial nerves palsy in spontaneous intracranial hypotension. J Neurosurg Sci. 1998; 42(3):177–179, discussion 180

[129] Balcer LJ, Galetta SL, Bagley LJ, Pakola SJ. Localization of traumatic oculomotor nerve palsy to the midbrain exit site by magnetic resonance imaging. Am J Ophthalmol. 1996; 122(3):437–439

[130] Hedges TR, Hirsh LF. Bilateral third nerve palsy from "minor" head trauma. Neuroophthalmology. 1993; 13:219

[131] Kudo T. An operative complication in a patient with a true posterior communicating artery aneurysm: case report and review of the literature. Neurosurgery. 1990; 27(4):650–653

[132] Lepore FE. Disorders of ocular motility following head trauma. Arch Neurol. 1995; 52(9):924–926

[133] Berlit P. Isolated and combined pareses of cranial nerves III, IV and VI. A retrospective study of 412 patients. J Neurol Sci. 1991; 103(1):10–15

[134] Bondeson J, Asman P. Giant cell arteritis presenting with oculomotor nerve palsy. Scand J Rheumatol. 1997; 26(4):327–328

[135] Capó H, Warren F, Kupersmith MJ. Evolution of oculomotor nerve palsies. J Clin Neuroophthalmol. 1992; 12(1):21–25

[136] Cullom ME, Savino PJ, Sergott RC, Bosley TM. Relative pupillary sparing third nerve palsies. To arteriogram or not? J Neuroophthalmol. 1995; 15(3): 136–140, discussion 140–141

[137] Davies GE, Shakir RA. Giant cell arteritis presenting as oculomotor nerve palsy with pupillary dilatation. Postgrad Med J. 1994; 70(822):298–299

[138] Jacobson DM. Pupil involvement in patients with diabetes-associated oculomotor nerve palsy. Arch Ophthalmol. 1998; 116(6):723–727

[139] Jacobson DM, Broste SK. Early progression of ophthalmoplegia in patients with ischemic oculomotor nerve palsies. Arch Ophthalmol. 1995; 113(12): 1535–1537

[140] Jacobson DM, McCanna TD, Layde PM. Risk factors for ischemic ocular motor nerve palsies. Arch Ophthalmol. 1994; 112(7):961–966

[141] Naghmi R, Subuhi R. Diabetic oculomotor mononeuropathy: involvement of pupillomotor fibres with slow resolution. Horm Metab Res. 1990; 22(1): 38–40

[142] Cultrera F, D'Andrea M, Battaglia R, Chieregato A. Unilateral oculomotor nerve palsy: unusual sign of hydrocephalus. J Neurosurg Sci. 2009; 53(2): 67–70

[143] Hahn CD, Nicolle DA, Lownie SP, Drake CG. Giant cavernous carotid aneurysms: clinical presentation in fifty-seven cases. J Neuroophthalmol. 2000; 20(4):253–258

[144] Ikeda K, Tamura M, Iwasaki Y, Kinoshita M. Relative pupil-sparing third nerve palsy: etiology and clinical variables predictive of a mass. Neurology. 2001; 57(9):1741–1742

[145] Lanzino G, Andreoli A, Tognetti F, et al. Orbital pain and unruptured carotid-posterior communicating artery aneurysms: the role of sensory fibers in the third cranial nerve. Acta Neurochir (Wien). 1993; 120(1–2):7–11

[146] Silva MN, Saeki N, Hirai S, Yamaura A. Unusual cranial nerve palsy caused by cavernous sinus aneurysms. Clinical and anatomical considerations reviewed. Surg Neurol. 1999; 52(2):143–148, discussion 148–149

[147] Zingale A, Albanese V, Giuffrida A, Pappalardo P, Barbagallo G. Painful ophthalmoplegia syndrome (spheno-cavernous syndrome) caused by a ruptured posterior communicating artery aneurysm. A brief report. J Neurosurg Sci. 1997; 41(3):299–301

[148] Albayram S, Ozer H, Sarici A, Murphy K, Miller N. Unilateral mydriasis without ophthalmoplegia–a sign of neurovascular compression? Case report. Neurosurgery. 2006; 58(3):E582–E583, discussion E582–E583

[149] Acierno MD, Trobe JD, Cornblath WT, Gebarski SS. Painful oculomotor palsy caused by posterior-draining dural carotid cavernous fistulas. Arch Ophthalmol. 1995; 113(8):1045–1049

[150] Brazis PW, Capobianco DJ, Chang F-LF, McLeish WM, Earnest F, IV. Low flow dural arteriovenous shunt: another cause of "sinister" Tolosa-Hunt syndrome. Headache. 1994; 34(9):523–525

[151] Lee AG. Third nerve palsy due to a carotid cavernous fistula without external eye signs. Neuroophthalmology. 1996; 16:183–187

[152] Miyachi S, Negoro M, Handa T, Sugita K. Dural carotid cavernous sinus fistula presenting as isolated oculomotor nerve palsy. Surg Neurol. 1993; 39 (2):105–109

[153] Pérez Sempere A, Martinez Menéndez B, Cabeza Alvarez C, Calandre Hoenigsfeld L. Isolated oculomotor nerve palsy due to dural cavernous sinus fistula. Eur Neurol. 1991; 31(4):186–187

[154] Uehara T, Tabuchi M, Kawaguchi T, Mori E. Spontaneous dural carotid cavernous sinus fistula presenting isolated ophthalmoplegia: evaluation with MR angiography. Neurology. 1998; 50(3):814–816

[155] Yen M-Y, Mu-Huo M, Wang A-G, Liu J-H. Isolated oculomotor palsy caused by dural carotid cavernous sinus fistula. Neuroophthalmology. 1998; 20:38

[156] Masaya-Anon P. Isolated oculomotor nerve palsy in a white-eyed patient with dural carotid-cavernous sinus fistulas: a case report. J Med Assoc Thai. 2012; 95 Suppl 4:S143–S146

[157] Watanabe A, Horikoshi T, Uchida M, Kinouchi H. Internal carotid artery occlusion manifesting only as oculomotor nerve palsy. J Stroke Cerebrovasc Dis. 2008; 17(6):433–435

[158] Lopes DK, Mericle RA, Wakhloo AK, Guterman LR, Hopkins LN. Cavernous sinus syndrome during balloon test occlusion of the cervical internal carotid artery. Report of two cases. J Neurosurg. 1998; 89(4):667–670

[159] Grayeli AB, Redondo A, Salama J, Rey A. Tuberculoma of the cavernous sinus: case report. Neurosurgery. 1998; 42(1):179–181, discussion 181–182

[160] Bikhazi NB, Sloan SH. Superior orbital fissure syndrome caused by indolent Aspergillus sphenoid sinusitis. Otolaryngol Head Neck Surg. 1998; 118(1): 102–104

[161] Holland NR, Deibert E. CNS actinomycosis presenting with bilateral cavernous sinus syndrome. J Neurol Neurosurg Psychiatry. 1998; 64(1):4

[162] Polito E, Leccisotti A. Painful ophthalmoplegia caused by superior ophthalmic vein thrombosis. Neuro-ophthalmology. 1996; 16(3):189–192

[163] Barr D, Kupersmith MJ, Pinto R, Turbin R. Arachnoid cyst of the cavernous sinus resulting in third nerve palsy. J Neuroophthalmol. 1999; 19(4):249–251

[164] Ing EB, Purvin V. Progressive visual loss and motility deficit. Surv Ophthalmol. 1997; 41(6):488–492

[165] Kasner SE, Galetta SL, Vaughn DJ. Cavernous sinus syndrome in Hodgkin's disease. J Neuroophthalmol. 1996; 16(3):204–207

[166] Kurokawa Y, Uede T, Honda O, Honmou O. Successful removal of intracavernous neurinoma originating from the oculomotor nerve–case report. Neurol Med Chir (Tokyo). 1992; 32(4):225–228

[167] Lee AG, Tang RA. Third nerve palsy as the presenting manifestation of esthesioneuroblastoma. J Neuroophthalmol. 2000; 20(1):20–21

[168] Lee CC, Cho AS, Carter WA. Emergency department presentation of pituitary apoplexy. Am J Emerg Med. 2000; 18(3):328–331

[169] Liu GT, Kay MD, Byrne GE, Glaser JS, Schatz N. Ophthalmoparesis due to Burkitt's lymphoma following cardiac transplantation. Neurology. 1993; 43 (10):2147–2149

[170] Manabe Y, Kurokawa K, Kashihara K, Abe K. Isolated oculomotor nerve palsy in lymphoma. Neurol Res. 2000; 22(4):347–348

[171] Moster ML, Scimeca GH, Romayananda N, et al. Mandibular ameloblastoma metastatic to the cavernous sinus. Neuroophthalmology. 1996; 16:47–50

[172] North KN, Antony JH, Johnston IH. Dermoid of cavernous sinus resulting in isolated oculomotor nerve palsy. Pediatr Neurol. 1993; 9(3):221–223

[173] Shen WC, Yang DY, Ho WL, Ho YJ, Lee SK. Neurilemmoma of the oculomotor nerve presenting as an orbital mass: MR findings. AJNR Am J Neuroradiol. 1993; 14(5):1253–1254

[174] Tao ZD. Oculomotor neuropathy syndrome. A diagnostic challenge in nasopharyngeal carcinoma. Chin Med J (Engl). 1992; 105(7):567–571

[175] Wake A, Kakinuma A, Mori N, et al. Angiotropic lymphoma of paranasal sinuses with initial symptoms of oculomotor nerve palsy. Intern Med. 1993; 32(3):237–242

[176] Hustler A, Joy H, Hodgkins P. Isolated unilateral mydriasis with delayed oculomotor nerve palsy secondary to intracranial arachnoid cyst. J AAPOS. 2009; 13(3):308–309

[177] Kumar LP, Monica I, Uppin MS, Kotiyala VJ. Large oculomotor nerve schwannoma–rare entity: a case report with review of literature. J Cancer Res Ther. 2014; 10(4):1098–1100

[178] Inoue N, Watanabe H, Okamura K, et al. Atypical teratoid rhabdoid tumor in the cavernous sinus of a toddler presenting with oculomotor nerve palsy. Childs Nerv Syst. 2014; 30(8):1463–1466

[179] Park YM, Cho JH, Cho JY, Huh JS, Ahn JY. Non-Hodgkin's lymphoma of the sphenoid sinus presenting as isolated oculomotor nerve palsy. World J Surg Oncol. 2007; 5:86

[180] Ashker L, Weinstein JM, Dias M, Kanev P, Nguyen D, Bonsall DJ. Arachnoid cyst causing third cranial nerve palsy manifesting as isolated internal ophthalmoplegia and iris cholinergic supersensitivity. J Neuroophthalmol. 2008; 28(3):192–197

[181] Robinson R, Toland J, Eustace P. Pituitary apoplexy: a cause for painful third nerve palsy. Neuroophthalmology. 1990; 10:257–260

[182] Rossitch E, Jr, Carrazana EJ, Black PM. Isolated oculomotor nerve palsy following apoplexy of a pituitary adenoma. J Neurosurg Sci. 1992; 36(2):103–105

[183] Seyer H, Kompf D, Fahlbusch R. Optomotor palsies in pituitary apoplexy. Neuroophthalmology. 1992; 12:217–224

[184] Kobayashi H, Kawabori M, Terasaka S, Murata J, Houkin K. A possible mechanism of isolated oculomotor nerve palsy by apoplexy of pituitary adenoma without cavernous sinus invasion: a report of two cases. Acta Neurochir (Wien). 2011; 153(12):2453–2456, discussion 2456

[185] Miyao S, Takano A, Teramoto J, Fujitake S, Hashizume Y. Oculomotor nerve palsy due to intraneural hemorrhage in idiopathic thrombocytopenic purpura: a case report. Eur Neurol. 1993; 33(1):20–22

[186] Ashwin PT, Mahmood S, Pollock WS. Sphenoid sinus mucocoele mimicking aneurysmal oculomotor nerve palsy. Eye (Lond). 2001; 15(Pt 1):108–110

[187] Mohebbi A, Jahandideh H, Harandi AA. Sphenoid sinus mucocele as a cause of isolated pupil-sparing oculomotor nerve palsy mimicking diabetic ophthalmoplegia. Ear Nose Throat J. 2013; 92(12):563–565

[188] Chotmongkol V, Chainunsamit S. Superior branch palsy of the oculomotor nerve caused by acute sphenoid sinusitis. J Med Assoc Thai. 1999; 82(4):410–413

[189] Hermann M, Bobek-Billewicz B, Bullo B, Hermann A, Rutkowski B. Wegener's granulomatosis with unusual cavernous sinus and sella turcica extension. Eur Radiol. 1999; 9(9):1859–1861

[190] Kondoh K, Ohtsuka K, Hashimoto M, Nakamura Y. Inferior branch palsy of the oculomotor nerve caused by EB virus infection. Neuroophthalmology. 1998; 20:36

[191] Ohtsuka K, Hashimoto M, Nakamura Y. Enhanced magnetic resonance imaging in a patient with acute paralysis of the inferior division of the oculomotor nerve. Am J Ophthalmol. 1997; 124(3):406–409

[192] Stefanis L, Przedborski S. Isolated palsy of the superior branch of the oculomotor nerve due to chronic erosive sphenoid sinusitis. J Clin Neuroophthalmol. 1993; 13(4):229–231

[193] Blair MP, Rizen M. Heerfordt syndrome with internal ophthalmoplegia. Arch Ophthalmol. 2005; 123(7):1017

[194] Sethi DS, Lau DP, Chan C. Sphenoid sinus mucocoele presenting with isolated oculomotor nerve palsy. J Laryngol Otol. 1997; 111(5):471–473

[195] Goldberg RA, Rootman J. Clinical characteristics of metastatic orbital tumors. Ophthalmology. 1990; 97(5):620–624

[196] Goldberg RA, Rootman J, Cline RA. Tumors metastatic to the orbit: a changing picture. Surv Ophthalmol. 1990; 35(1):1–24

[197] Gray LG, Galetta SL, Hershey B, Winkelman AC, Wulc A. Inferior division third nerve paresis from an orbital dural arteriovenous malformation. J Neuroophthalmol. 1999; 19(1):46–48

[198] Bayramlar H, Miman MC, Demirel S. Inferior oblique paresis, mydriasis, and accommodative palsy as temporary complications of sinus surgery. J Neuroophthalmol. 2004; 24(3):225–227

[199] Nagashima H, Yamamoto K, Kawamura A, Nagashima T, Nomura K, Yoshida M. Pediatric orbital schwannoma originating from the oculomotor nerve. J Neurosurg Pediatr. 2012; 9(2):165–168

[200] Shamim MS, Bari ME, Chisti KN, Abbas A. A child with intra-orbital oculomotor nerve schwannoma without neurofibromatosis. Can J Neurol Sci. 2008; 35(4):528–530

[201] Scheller C, Rachinger JC, Prell J, et al. Intraorbital oculomotor nerve schwannoma affecting only the parasympathetic fibers. J Neurol Surg A Cent Eur Neurosurg. 2013; 74(2):120–123

[202] Good WV, Barkovich AJ, Nickel BL, Hoyt CS. Bilateral congenital oculomotor nerve palsy in a child with brain anomalies. Am J Ophthalmol. 1991; 111(5):555–558

[203] Hamed LM. Associated neurologic and ophthalmologic findings in congenital oculomotor nerve palsy. Ophthalmology. 1991; 98(5):708–714

[204] Parmeggiani A, Posar A, Leonardi M, Rossi PG. Neurological impairment in congenital bilateral ptosis with ophthalmoplegia. Brain Dev. 1992; 14(2):107–109

[205] Patel CK, Taylor DS, Russell-Eggitt IM, Kriss A, Demaerel P. Congenital third nerve palsy associated with mid-trimester amniocentesis. Br J Ophthalmol. 1993; 77(8):530–533

[206] Schumacher-Feero LA, Yoo KW, Solari FM, Biglan AW. Third cranial nerve palsy in children. Am J Ophthalmol. 1999; 128(2):216–221

[207] Tsaloumas MD, Willshaw HE. Congenital oculomotor palsy: associated neurological and ophthalmological findings. Eye (Lond). 1997; 11(Pt 4):500–503

[208] White WL, Mumma JV, Tomasovic JJ. Congenital oculomotor nerve palsy, cerebellar hypoplasia, and facial capillary hemangioma. Am J Ophthalmol. 1992; 113(5):497–500

[209] Mark AS, Casselman J, Brown D, et al. Ophthalmoplegic migraine: reversible enhancement and thickening of the cisternal segment of the oculomotor nerve on contrast-enhanced MR images. AJNR Am J Neuroradiol. 1998; 19(10):1887–1891

[210] O'Halloran HS, Lee WB, Baker RS, Pearson PA. Ophthalmoplegic migraine with unusual features. Headache. 1999; 39(9):670–673

[211] Prats JM, Mateos B, Garaizar C. Resolution of MRI abnormalities of the oculomotor nerve in childhood ophthalmoplegic migraine. Cephalalgia. 1999; 19(7):655–659

[212] Tocco P, Fenzi F, Cerini R, Monaco S. Adult-onset migraine-related ophthalmoplegia and omolateral fetal-type posterior cerebral artery. BMJ Case Rep. 2011; 2011:bcr1020114930

[213] Capoferri C, Martorina M, Menga M. Herpes Zoster ophthalmoplegia in two hemodialysis patients. Neuro-ophthalmology. 1997; 17(1):49–51

[214] Chang-Godinich A, Lee AG, Brazis PW, Liesegang TJ, Jones DB. Complete ophthalmoplegia after zoster ophthalmicus. J Neuroophthalmol. 1997; 17(4):262–265

[215] Mansour AM, Bailey BJ. Ocular findings in Ramsay Hunt syndrome. J Neuroophthalmol. 1997; 17(3):199–201

[216] Saeki N, Yotsukura J, Adachi E, Yamaura A. Isolated superior division oculomotor palsy in a child with spontaneous recovery. J Clin Neurosci. 2000; 7(1):62–64

[217] Sood A, Midha V, Sood N, Gupta D. Hepatitis B and pupil-sparing oculomotor nerve paresis. Clin Infect Dis. 1999; 29(5):1330–1331

[218] Zurevinsky J. Ocular palsies in ophthalmic zoster. Am Orthopt J. 1993; 43:130–134

[219] Lee CY, Tsai HC, Lee SS, Chen YS. Orbital apex syndrome: an unusual complication of herpes zoster ophthalmicus. BMC Infect Dis. 2015; 15:33

[220] Savas R, Sommer A, Gueckel F, Georgi M. Isolated oculomotor nerve paralysis in Lyme disease: MRI. Neuroradiology. 1997; 39(2):139–141

[221] Drenckhahn A, Spors B, Knierim E. Acute isolated partial oculomotor nerve palsy due to Lyme neuroborreliosis in a 5 year old girl. Eur J Paediatr Neurol. 2016; 20(6):977–979

[222] Işıkay S, Yılmaz K, Ölmez A. Neurobrucellosis developing unilateral oculomotor nerve paralysis. Am J Emerg Med. 2012; 30(9):2085.e5–2085.e7

[223] Arroyo JG, Horton JC. Acute, painful, pupil-involving third nerve palsy in chronic inflammatory demyelinating polyneuropathy. Neurology. 1995; 45(4):846–847

[224] Nagaoka U, Kato T, Kurita K, et al. Cranial nerve enhancement on three-dimensional MRI in Miller Fisher syndrome. Neurology. 1996; 47(6):1601–1602

[225] Go T. Partial oculomotor nerve palsy associated with elevated anti-galactocerebroside and anti-GM1 antibodies. J Pediatr. 2000; 137(3):425–426

[226] Balcer LJ, Galetta SL, Yousem DM, Golden MA, Asbury AK. Pupil-involving third-nerve palsy and carotid stenosis: rapid recovery following endarterectomy. Ann Neurol. 1997; 41(2):273–276

[227] Höllinger P, Sturzenegger M. Painful oculomotor nerve palsy - a presenting sign of internal carotid artery stenosis. Cerebrovasc Dis. 1999; 9(3):178–181

[228] Koennecke H, Seyfert S. Mydriatic pupil as the presenting sign of common carotid artery dissection. Stroke. 1998; 29(12):2653–2655

[229] Mokri B, Silbert PL, Schievink WI, Piepgras DG. Cranial nerve palsy in spontaneous dissection of the extracranial internal carotid artery. Neurology. 1996; 46(2):356–359

[230] Schievink WI, Mokri B, Garrity JA, Nichols DA, Piepgras DG. Ocular motor nerve palsies in spontaneous dissections of the cervical internal carotid artery. Neurology. 1993; 43(10):1938–1941

[231] Okuchi K, Fujioka M, Maeda Y, Kagoshima T, Sakaki T. Bilateral chronic subdural hematomas resulting in unilateral oculomotor nerve paresis and brain stem symptoms after operation–case report. Neurol Med Chir (Tokyo). 1999; 39(5):367–371

[232] Phookan G, Cameron M. Bilateral chronic subdural haematoma: an unusual presentation with isolated oculomotor nerve palsy. J Neurol Neurosurg Psychiatry. 1994; 57(9):1146

[233] Corrivetti F, Moschettoni L, Lunardi P. Isolated oculomotor nerve palsy as presenting symptom of bilateral chronic subdural hematomas: two consecutive case report and review of the literature. World Neurosurg. 2016; 88:686.e9–686.e12

[234] Matsuda R, Hironaka Y, Kawai H, Park YS, Taoka T, Nakase H. Unilateral oculomotor nerve palsy as an initial presentation of bilateral chronic

subdural hematoma: case report. Neurol Med Chir (Tokyo). 2013; 53(9): 616–619

[235] al-Yamany M, al-Shayji A, Bernstein M. Isolated oculomotor nerve palsy: an unusual presentation of glioblastoma multiforme. Case report and review of the literature. J Neurooncol. 1999; 41(1):77–80

[236] Haughton AJ, Chalkiadis GA. Unintentional paediatric subdural catheter with oculomotor and abducens nerve palsies. Paediatr Anaesth. 1999; 9(6): 543–548

[237] Green KM, Board T, O'Keeffe LJ. Oculomotor nerve palsy following submucosal diathermy to the inferior turbinates. J Laryngol Otol. 2000; 114 (4):285–286

[238] Pacifici L, Passarelli F, Papa G, Cannone L, Rossini PM. Acute third cranial nerve ophthalmoplegia: possible pathogenesis from alpha-II-interferon treatment. Ital J Neurol Sci. 1993; 14(7):579–580

[239] Soysal T, Ferhanoğlu B, Bilir M, Akman N. Oculomotor nerve palsy associated with vincristine treatment. Acta Haematol. 1993; 90(4):209–210

[240] Migita DS, Devereaux MW, Tomsak RL. Cocaine and pupillary-sparing oculomotor nerve paresis. Neurology. 1997; 49(5):1466–1467

[241] Donahue SP, Taylor RJ. Pupil-sparing third nerve palsy associated with sildenafil citrate (Viagra). Am J Ophthalmol. 1998; 126(3):476–477

[242] Alderson LM, Noonan PT, Choi IS, Henson JW. Regional subacute cranial neuropathies following internal carotid cisplatin infusion. Neurology. 1996; 47(4):1088–1090

[243] Wu HM, Lee AG, Lehane DE, Chi TL, Lewis RA. Ocular and orbital complications of intraarterial cisplatin. A case report. J Neuroophthalmol. 1997; 17(3):195–198

[244] Ebner R, Slamovits TL, Friedland S, Pearlman JL, Fowble B. Visual loss following treatment of sphenoid sinus carcinoma. Surv Ophthalmol. 1995; 40(1):62–68

[245] Wang QJ, Guo Y, Zhang Y, et al. 3D MRI of oculomotor nerve schwannoma in the prepontine cistern: a case report. Clin Imaging. 2013; 37(5):947–949

[246] Saetia K, Larbcharoensub N, Wetchagama N. Oculomotor nerve schwannoma: a case report and review of the literature. J Med Assoc Thai. 2011; 94(8):1002–1007

[247] Nonaka Y, Fukushima T, Friedman AH, Kolb LE, Bulsara KR. Surgical management of nonvascular lesions around the oculomotor nerve. World Neurosurg. 2014; 81(5–6):798–809

[248] Chen CC, Pai YM, Wang RF, Wang TL, Chong CF. Isolated oculomotor nerve palsy from minor head trauma. Br J Sports Med. 2005; 39(8):e34

[249] Zhang Y, Chen K, Liu B, Chen L. Incomplete oculomotor nerve palsy in the subarachnoid space caused by traumatic brain injury. Neurosciences (Riyadh). 2012; 17(2):159–160

[250] Fairbanks C, White JB. Oculomotor nerve palsy in the setting of an anterior cerebral A2 segment aneurysm. J Neurointerv Surg. 2011; 3(1):74–76

[251] Saito R, Sugawara T, Mikawa S, Fukuda T, Kohama M, Seki H. Pupil-sparing oculomotor nerve paresis as an early symptom of unruptured internal carotid-posterior communicating artery aneurysms: three case reports. Neurol Med Chir (Tokyo). 2008; 48(7):304–306

[252] Menovsky T, van der Zijden T, Voormolen M, et al. Perforated oculomotor nerve after endovascular coiling: complete regeneration after microsurgical repair. case report. J Neurol Surg A Cent Eur Neurosurg. 2013; 74 Suppl 1: e248–e254

[253] Chittiboina P, Willet O, Nanda A, Guthikonda B. Transient oculomotor nerve palsy after topical administration of intracisternal papaverine. Acta Neurochir (Wien). 2011; 153(2):431–433

[254] Menon G, Baldawa SS, Nair S. Transient oculomotor nerve palsy after topical administration of intracisternal papaverine. Acta Neurochir (Wien). 2011; 153(6):1357–1358

[255] Lustbader JM, Miller NR. Painless, pupil-sparing but otherwise complete oculomotor nerve paresis caused by basilar artery aneurysm. Case report. Arch Ophthalmol. 1988; 106(5):583–584

[256] Lynch JM, Hennessy MJ. Third nerve palsy: harbinger of basilar artery thrombosis and locked-in syndrome? J Stroke Cerebrovasc Dis. 2005; 14(1): 42–43

[257] Soria E, Camell H, Dang H. Pupil-sparing oculomotor palsy caused by fusiform arteriosclerotic aneurysm of the basilar artery–a case report. Angiology. 1989; 40(10):921–927

[258] Trobe JD. Third nerve palsy and the pupil. Footnotes to the rule. Arch Ophthalmol. 1988; 106(5):601–602

[259] Wilhelm H, Klier R, Tûth B, Wilhelm B. Oculomotor nerve paresis starting as isolated internal ophthalmoplegia. Neuro-ophthalmology. 1995; 15(4): 211–215

[260] Motoyama Y, Nonaka J, Hironaka Y, Park YS, Nakase H. Pupil-sparing oculomotor nerve palsy caused by upward compression of a large posterior communicating artery aneurysm. Case report. Neurol Med Chir (Tokyo). 2012; 52(4):202–205

[261] Guy J, Savino PJ, Schatz NJ, Cobbs WH, Day AL. Superior division paresis of the oculomotor nerve. Ophthalmology. 1985; 92(6):777–784

[262] Guy J, Engel HM, Lessner AM. Acquired contralateral oculomotor synkinesis. Arch Neurol. 1989; 46(9):1021–1023

[263] Chotmongkol V, Techasuknirun A. Superior division paresis of the oculomotor nerve caused by cryptococcal meningitis. J Med Assoc Thai. 1992; 75(9):548–550

[264] Ehrenpreis SJ, Biedlingmaier JF. Isolated third-nerve palsy associated with frontal sinus mucocele. J Neuroophthalmol. 1995; 15(2):105–108

[265] Riadh H, Mohamed G, Salah Y, Fehmi T, Fafani BH. Pediatric case of ophthalmoplegic migraine with recurrent oculomotor nerve palsy. Can J Ophthalmol. 2010; 45(6):643

[266] Dehaene I, Van Zandijcke M. Isolated paralysis of the superior division of the ocular motor nerve mimicked by myasthenia gravis. Neuro-ophthalmology. 1995; 15(5):257–258

[267] Kardon RH, Traynelis VC, Biller J. Inferior division paresis of the oculomotor nerve caused by basilar artery aneurysm. Cerebrovasc Dis. 1991; 1:171–176

[268] Carlow TJ, Johnson JK. Parasellar tumors: isolated pupil-sparing third nerve palsy. Neurology. 1990; 40 Suppl 1:309

[269] Cunningham ET, Jr, Good WV. Inferior branch oculomotor nerve palsy. A case report. J Neuroophthalmol. 1994; 14(1):21–23

[270] Brazis PW. Localization of lesions of the oculomotor nerve: recent concepts. Mayo Clin Proc. 1991; 66(10):1029–1035

[271] Levy RL, Geist CE, Miller NR. Isolated oculomotor palsy following minor head trauma. Neurology. 2005; 65(1):169

[272] Ng YS, Lyons CJ. Oculomotor nerve palsy in childhood. Can J Ophthalmol. 2005; 40(5):645–653

[273] Jacobson DM, Trobe JD. The emerging role of magnetic resonance angiography in the management of patients with third cranial nerve palsy. Am J Ophthalmol. 1999; 128(1):94–96

[274] Trobe JD. Isolated pupil-sparing third nerve palsy. Ophthalmology. 1985; 92 (1):58–61

[275] Sung MS, Kim HG, Woo KI, Kim YD. Ocular ischemia and ischemic oculomotor nerve palsy after vascular embolization of injectable calcium hydroxylapatite filler. Ophthal Plast Reconstr Surg. 2010; 26(4):289–291

[276] Bortolami R, D'Alessandro R, Manni E. The origin of pain in 'ischemic-diabetic' third-nerve palsy. Arch Neurol. 1993; 50(8):795

[277] Lee AG, Hayman LA, Brazis PW. The evaluation of isolated third nerve palsy revisited: an update on the evolving role of magnetic resonance, computed tomography, and catheter angiography. Surv Ophthalmol. 2002; 47(2): 137–157

[278] Bruce BB, Biousse V, Newman NJ. Third nerve palsies. Semin Neurol. 2007; 27(3):257–268

[279] Murchison AP, Gilbert ME, Savino PJ. Neuroimaging and acute ocular motor mononeuropathies: a prospective study. Arch Ophthalmol. 2011; 129(3): 301–305

[280] Dhume KU, Paul KE. Incidence of pupillary involvement, course of anisocoria and ophthalmoplegia in diabetic oculomotor nerve palsy. Indian J Ophthalmol. 2013; 61(1):13–17

[281] Trobe JD. Managing oculomotor nerve palsy. Arch Ophthalmol. 1998; 116 (6):798

[282] Murakami M, Kitano I, Hitoshi Y, Ushio Y. Isolated oculomotor nerve palsy following midbrain infarction. Clin Neurol Neurosurg. 1994; 96(2):188–190

[283] Keane JR, Ahmadi J. Most diabetic third nerve palsies are peripheral. Neurology. 1998; 51(5):1510

[284] Sanders S, Kawasaki A, Purvin VA. Patterns of extraocular muscle weakness in vasculopathic pupil-sparing, incomplete third nerve palsy. J Neuroophthalmol. 2001; 21(4):256–259

[285] Miller NR. Unequal pupils can be seen in diabetic 3rd nerve palsy. Evidence-Based Eye Care. 1999; 1:40–41

[286] Kaufman DI. Recent advances in neuro-imaging and the impact on neuro-ophthalmology. Curr Opin Ophthalmol. 1994; 5(6):52–62

[287] Davis PC, Newman NJ. Advances in neuroimaging of the visual pathways. Am J Ophthalmol. 1996; 121(6):690–705

[288] Wong GK, Boet R, Poon WS, Yu S, Lam JM. A review of isolated third nerve palsy without subarachnoid hemorrhage using computed tomographic angiography as the first line of investigation. Clin Neurol Neurosurg. 2004; 107(1):27–31

[289] Anderson GB, Steinke DE, Petruk KC, Ashforth R, Findlay JM. Computed tomographic angiography versus digital subtraction angiography for the diagnosis and early treatment of ruptured intracranial aneurysms. Neurosurgery. 1999; 45(6):1315–1320, discussion 1320–1322

[290] Rustemi O, Alaraj A, Shakur SF, et al. Detection of unruptured intracranial aneurysms on noninvasive imaging. Is there still a role for digital subtraction angiography? Surg Neurol Int. 2015; 6:175

[291] Cox TA, Goldberg RA, Rootman J. Tonic pupil and Czarnecki's sign following third nerve palsy. J Clin Neuroophthalmol. 1991; 11(1):55–56, discussion 57

[292] Vaphiades MS, Cure J, Kline L. Management of intracranial aneurysm causing a third cranial nerve palsy: MRA, CTA or DSA? Semin Ophthalmol. 2008; 23(3):143–150

[293] Lee MS, Egan RA, Shults WT, Lessell S. Idiopathic repetitive oculomotor nerve palsies in otherwise normal patients. Ophthalmology. 2005; 112(12): 2225–2226

[294] Custer PL. Lagophthalmos: an unusual manifestation of oculomotor nerve aberrant regeneration. Ophthal Plast Reconstr Surg. 2000; 16(1):50–51

[295] Barr D, Kupersmith M, Turbin R, Yang S, Iezzi R. Synkinesis following diabetic third nerve palsy. Arch Ophthalmol. 2000; 118(1):132–134

[296] Lee SH, Yeow YK, Tan CB, Tjia H. Transient oculomotor nerve synkinesis in non-Hodgkin's lymphoma. J Clin Neuroophthalmol. 1992; 12(3):203–206

[297] Landau K, Lepore FE. Discovering a dys-covering lid. Surv Ophthalmol. 1997; 42(1):87–91

[298] Mehkri IA, Awner S, Olitsky SE, Dias MS, Elmer TR, Jr. Double vision in a child. Surv Ophthalmol. 1999; 44(1):45–51, discussion 51–52

[299] Varma R, Miller NR. Primary oculomotor nerve synkinesis caused by an extracavernous intradural aneurysm. Am J Ophthalmol. 1994; 118(1):83–87

[300] Cohen DA, Bosley TM, Savino PJ, Sergott RC, Schatz NJ. Primary aberrant regeneration of the oculomotor nerve. Occurrence in a patient with abetalipoproteinemia. Arch Neurol. 1985; 42(8):821–823

12 Fourth Nerve Palsies

William J. Hertzing, Alec L. Amram, and Andres S. Parra

Abstract

A fourth nerve palsy results from an injury to the trochlear nerve, and typically causes a binocular vertical diplopia. There is also excyclotorsion of the affected eye that many patients compensate for by tilting their head in the contralateral direction. The trochlear nerve has the longest intracranial course for a cranial nerve, and the presence or absence of additional neurological features may help localize the lesion. This chapter discusses the clinical pathways in localizing and diagnosing fourth nerve palsies, by reviewing the literature in detail.

Keywords: fourth nerve palsy, trochlear nerve, vertical diplopia, head tilt, three-step test

12.1 What Is the Topographic Anatomy of the Fourth Nerve?

The fourth nerve nucleus is located in the midbrain beneath the inferior colliculus. The fourth nerve is the only cranial nerve that exits dorsally from the brainstem. It has the longest intracranial course of any cranial nerve and crosses in the anterior medullary velum. It passes between the superior cerebellar artery and the posterior cerebral artery, runs in the subarachnoid space, travels within the lateral wall of the cavernous sinus, and enters the orbit via the superior orbital fissure to innervate the superior oblique muscle.

12.2 How Does One Diagnose a Fourth Nerve Palsy (FNP)?

The criteria for diagnosis of FNPs includes binocular vertical and/or torsional diplopia or misalignment, ipsilateral hyperdeviation in primary position worsened by contralateral gaze and ipsilateral head tilt (the three-step test), variable ipsilateral excyclotorsion, anomalous compensatory head or face position, and/or weakness of the involved superior oblique muscle on duction testing. The Parks-Bielschowsky test is a three-step test consisting of (1) determining which eye is hypertrophic in the primary position; (2) determining if hypertropia increases in left gaze or right gaze; and (3) determining if hypertropia increases on left head tilt or right head tilt (Bielschowsky head-tilt test). FNP may be categorized as isolated or nonisolated. A "fourth step" involves using the double Maddox rod test to specifically measure cyclodeviation of the eye.

Skew deviation, a vertical strabismus caused by a posterior fossa supranuclear lesion, may mimic FNP and may be difficult to differentiate from a true FNP. Wong described a highly specific, novel clinical test to differentiate the two, the "upright-supine test." They report a sensitivity of 80% and a specificity of 100% for diagnosing skew deviation in their clinical test of 125 patients. As a "fifth step," the three-step test can be repeated with the patient in the supine position to differentiate a skew deviation from a trochlear nerve palsy. A vertical strabismus

that decreases by greater than 50% from the upright to supine position is considered a positive test result for skew deviation. This finding would prompt neuroimaging to investigate the posterior fossa for the cause of vertical diplopia. The authors note that this is a simple and quick test to perform at the bedside to rule out skew deviation even if the patient displays other symptoms of trochlear nerve palsy.[1,2] This testing for vertical diplopia is also described in detail in Chapter 10.

12.3 What Are the Clinical Features of Fourth Nerve Palsies?

Fourth cranial nerve palsies may present with the following[3]:

1. Incomitant hypertropia, as demonstrated with the three-step maneuver. The hypertropia increases on head tilt toward the paralyzed side (positive Bielschowsky test). Usually, the unaffected eye fixates and the hypertropia occurs in the involved eye. Hypotropia may occur in the normal eye if the affected eye is fixating. The hypertropia is usually most prominent in the field of gaze of the involved superior oblique muscle, especially in cases of acute or recent onset. The hypertropia may also be most prominent in the field of gaze of the ipsilateral overacting inferior oblique muscle in subacute or chronic cases. In palsies of longer duration, the hypertropia may be relatively equal in the various gaze positions due to spread of comitance.

2. Underaction of the ipsilateral superior oblique muscle, overaction of the ipsilateral inferior oblique muscle, or overaction of the contralateral superior oblique muscle on duction testing.

3. Impaired motility in the contralateral eye. Pseudo-overaction of the superior oblique muscle in the uninvolved eye may occur with spread of comitance. Secondary contracture of the superior rectus muscle in the involved eye may cause hypertropia involving the entire lower field of gaze. In a patient with a superior oblique muscle paralysis who habitually fixates with the paretic eye and in whom overaction of the ipsilateral inferior oblique muscle has developed, less than the normal amount of innervation will be required when the patient looks up and to the contralateral side. Because the innervation flowing to the opposite superior rectus is linked to that of the overacting ipsilateral inferior oblique (Hering's law), the opposite superior rectus muscle will seem paretic (inhibitional palsy of the contralateral antagonist). In these cases, the head tilt test will correctly determine which of the two eyes is paretic.

4. Excyclotropia due to loss of incyclotorsion of the superior oblique muscle. This torsion may be evident on fundus exam and can be measured using double Maddox rod testing ("fourth step" of the three-step test). The excyclotropia is usually symptomatic in acquired cases but is often asymptomatic in congenital cases. The degree of excyclotropia is correlated to the severity of superior oblique muscle weakness in acute FNP, but not in presumed congenital FNP.[4]

5. Anomalous head tilt, which eliminates the hypertropia but rarely eliminates the cyclotropia.[5] This head tilt is present in approximately 70% of patients and is usually away from the involved side but may be paradoxical (toward the involved side) in about 3%.

It is important to differentiate patients with decompensation of a congenital FNP from those with an acquired FNP. In patients with congenital FNPs:

1. Old photos may show a long-standing head tilt.
2. Patients often have cyclotropia on examination but are asymptomatic, as are some patients with acquired FNPs.
3. Patients have abnormally large vertical fusional amplitudes (> 8 prism diopters) in primary gaze.
4. Patients have facial asymmetry, with hypoplasia ipsilateral to the side of head turn.
5. Degree of excyclotropia does not correlate to the severity of superior oblique muscle weakness.[4]

Bilateral FNPs are suggested by the following:

1. Alternating or reversing hypertropia: right hypertropia in left gaze and left hypertropia in right gaze.
2. A positive Bielschowsky test on tilt to either shoulder ("double Bielschowsky head-tilt test").
3. Large excyclotropia (> 10 degrees).
4. V-pattern esotropia (15 prism diopters or more difference in esotropia between upward and downward gaze). The V pattern is caused by a decrease of the abducting effect of the superior oblique(s) in depression and secondary overaction of the abducting effect of the inferior oblique muscle(s).
5. Underaction of both superior oblique muscles and/or overaction of both inferior oblique muscles on duction testing.
6. Lesser hypertropia in primary position compared to unilateral FNPs.

12.4 What Are the Types of FNP?

Type 1 FNP is nonisolated, meaning that it occurs in the setting of additional neurological deficits. For diagnostic classification based on topographic localization, nonisolated FNP may be grouped into the following four syndromes:

1. Midbrain (nucleus/fascicle syndrome) FNP.
2. Subarachnoid space FNP.
3. Cavernous sinus FNP.
4. Orbital FNP.

Type 1 FNP with findings that localize to the brainstem, subarachnoid space, cavernous sinus, or orbit, should undergo a directed neuroimaging study.[6,7,8,9,10,11,12,13] ▶ Table 12.1 outlines the clinical features of FNP by location of the responsible lesion. Box 12.1 lists the etiologies for FNP based on clinical topographic localization.

Table 12.1 The localization of trochlear nerve lesions

Structure involved	Clinical manifestation
A: Lesions affecting the trochlear nucleus and/or fascicles (superior oblique palsy contralateral to lesions)	
Nucleus/fascicles alone	Isolated trochlear palsy (rare)
Pretectal region	Vertical gaze palsy (dorsal midbrain syndrome)
Superior cerebellar peduncle	Dysmetria on side of lesion
Descending sympathetic fibers	Horner syndrome on side of lesion
Medial longitudinal fasciculus (MLF)	Ipsilateral paresis of adduction with nystagmus of contralateral abducting eye
Brachium of superior colliculus	Contralateral relative afferent pupillary defect (RAPD) without visual impairment
Anterior medullary velum	Bilateral trochlear nerve palsies
B: Lesions affecting the trochlear nerve within the subarachnoid space (superior oblique palsy usually ipsilateral to lesion unless mesencephalon compressed)	
Trochlear nerve alone	Isolated trochlear palsy
Superior cerebellar peduncle	Ipsilateral dysmetria
Cerebral peduncle	Contralateral hemiparesis
C: Lesions affecting the trochlear nerve within the cavernous sinus and/or superior orbital fissure	
Trochlear nerve alone	Isolated trochlear palsy (rare)
Cranial nerves III, VI, sympathetic	Ophthalmoplegia, pupil small, large, or spared, ptosis
Cranial nerve V (ophthalmic division)	Facial/retro-orbital pain; sensory loss (forehead)
Increased venous pressure	Proptosis; chemosis
D: Lesions affecting the trochlear nerve within the orbit	
Trochlear nerve, trochlea, superior oblique muscle or tendon	Superior oblique palsy
Mechanical restriction of superior oblique tendon	Brown superior oblique tendon sheath syndrome
Other ocular motor nerves/extraocular muscles	Ophthalmoplegia, ptosis, restricted ocular movements
Optic nerve	Visual loss; optic disc swelling/atrophy
Mass effect	Proptosis (occasionally enophthalmos), chemosis, eyelid swelling, etc.

Source: Modified from Brazis et al[14] with permission from Lippincott Williams & Wilkins.

Box 12.1 Etiologies for a Fourth Nerve Palsy Based on Clinical Topographic Localization

- Midbrain (nuclear/fascicular).[10,15]
  - Aplasia of the nucleus.
  - Arteriovenous malformation.[11,16]
  - Demyelination.[17]
  - Hemorrhage.[18,19,20,21,22,23]
  - Ischemia/infarction.[19,23,24]
  - Tumor (e.g., glioma).[25,26,27]

- ○ Trauma (including surgical).
- ○ Sarcoidosis.[28]
- ○ Arachnoid cyst of quadrigeminal cistern.[29]
- • Subarachnoid space.
  - ○ Aneurysm (e.g., superior cerebellar artery).[30,31]
  - ○ Hydrocephalus.
  - ○ Infections (e.g., mastoiditis, meningitis).[32,33,34,35,36]
  - ○ Granulomatosis with polyangitis.[37]
  - ○ Sarcoidosis.[38]
  - ○ Superficial siderosis of central nervous system.[39,40]
  - ○ Postlumbar puncture or spinal anesthesia.
  - ○ Pseudotumor cerebri.[41,42,43]
  - ○ Trauma, including surgical.[44,45,46,47,48,49]
  - ○ Neoplasm.
    - – Carcinomatous meningitis.
    - – Cerebellar hemangioblastoma.
    - – Solitary trochlear nerve hemangioblastoma.[50]
    - – Ependymoma.
    - – Meningioma.
    - – Metastasis.
    - – Neurilemmoma/schwannoma.[51,52,53,54,55]
    - – Pineal tumors.
    - – Trochlear nerve sheath tumors.
  - ○ Miller Fisher syndrome.[56]
  - ○ Churg–Strauss syndrome.[57]
- • Cavernous sinus
  - ○ Neoplasm (e.g., meningioma, pituitary adenoma).[58,59,60]
  - ○ Infectious: Herpes zoster,[34,36,61,62] mucormycosis.[59]
  - ○ Inflammation: Tolosa–Hunt syndrome, granulomatosis with polyangitis.[63]
  - ○ Internal carotid artery aneurysm.[59,64,65,66,67,68]
  - ○ Dural carotid-cavernous sinus fistula.[69]
  - ○ Superior ophthalmic vein thrombosis.[70]
  - ○ Foramen ovale electrode placement.[71]
  - ○ Balloon test occlusion of cervical internal carotid artery (cavernous sinus syndrome).[72]
  - ○ Cavernous malformation of the trochlear nerve.[73]
- • Orbit.
  - ○ Neoplasm.
  - ○ Infection.
  - ○ Infiltration.
  - ○ Waldenström macroglobulinemia.
  - ○ Inflammation (orbital pseudotumor).
  - ○ Progressive systemic sclerosis.
  - ○ Trauma (orbital floor fracture).
  - ○ Disruption of medial orbital periosteum (e.g., surgical dissection).[55]
- • Other (unknown or varied localization).
  - ○ Migraine.[74]
  - ○ Congenital.[75,76]
    - – Trochlear nerve agenesis.[77,78]
    - – Superior oblique hypoplasia.[79]
  - ○ Congenital unmasked by botulinum toxin therapy for cervical torticollis.[80]
  - ○ Cephalic tetanus.[81]
  - ○ Basilar artery dolichoectasia.[82]

Type 2 FNP is traumatic and includes isolated, unilateral, or bilateral FNPs that have a clearly established temporal relationship to previous head trauma and do not progress. Patients must have no other neurologic deficits besides those associated with the traumatic event.

Type 3 FNP is congenital and may show large vertical fusional amplitudes (greater than 8 prism diopters), facial asymmetry or sternocleidomastoid muscle hypertrophy, and/or long-standing anomalous head position variably present in old photographs.

Type 4 FNP is vasculopathic and occurs in patients older than 50 years of age with or without known hypertension or diabetes, or in younger patients with known vasculopathic risk factors.

Type 5 FNP is nonvasculopathic. Patients without vasculopathic risk factors and not classified as any of the above types are classified as nonvasculopathic FNP.

Type 6 FNP is progressive or unresolved. FNPs that worsen after the acute stage (greater than 1 week) as defined by a significant increase in the measured ocular vertical deviation are considered to be progressive, and patients without improvement in the measured ocular vertical deviation after 6 to 8 weeks are considered unresolved.

12.5 Localization

12.5.1 Is the FNP due to a Midbrain Lesion?

A midbrain (i.e., nuclear/fascicular) FNP is defined by the "company it keeps"; other brainstem signs are usually present, including hemisensory loss, hemiparesis, a central Horner syndrome, or other brainstem cranial neuropathies (e.g., third nerve palsy). The differential diagnosis includes midbrain ischemia, hemorrhage, demyelination, and neoplasm. Neuroimaging (preferably magnetic resonance imaging [MRI]) should be directed to the midbrain (class II–III, level B).

12.5.2 Is the FNP the Result of a Subarachnoid Space Lesion?

Lesions of the subarachnoid space are rarely associated with an isolated FNP. Patients with subarachnoid space lesions usually have associated signs and symptoms including headache, stiff neck, and other cranial neuropathies. Neuroimaging (MRI) should be directed to the brainstem and subarachnoid space. Computed tomography (CT) imaging should be considered in cases of acute trauma, to evaluate bone lesions, or in the evaluation of acute vascular processes (e.g., subarachnoid hemorrhage). Lumbar puncture following negative neuroimaging should be considered in these cases (class II–III, level B). Isolated trochlear nerve palsy due to a cisternal trochlear nerve schwannoma has been reported and should be followed with serial MRI scans. In these cases, neurosurgical intervention is not recommended unless patients develop signs of brainstem compression.[83]

12.5.3 Is the FNP Due to a Cavernous Sinus Lesion?

Cavernous sinus lesions are usually associated with other cranial neuropathies (e.g., third, fifth, or sixth nerve paresis) and/or Horner syndrome. Neuroimaging (preferably MRI) should be directed to the cavernous sinus (class II–III, level B).

12.5.4 Is the FNP Caused by an Orbital Lesion?

Orbital lesions usually produce signs such as proptosis, chemosis, and orbital or conjunctival edema. Neuroimaging (preferably MRI) should be directed to the orbit (class II–III, level B).

12.6 Is the FNP Due to Trauma?

At least 23 retrospective studies of traumatic FNP (type 2) have recommended that isolated, traumatic, unilateral, or bilateral FNP do not require additional neuroimaging or further evaluation.[6,8,12,44,46,49] FNP after mild head trauma and out of proportion to the deficit have been observed in association with an underlying asymptomatic basal intracranial tumor in at least three reports.[84,85,86] Neetens and Van Aerde reported three such cases, but two cases had other neuro-ophthalmologic signs as well.[86] Although uncommon, neuroimaging may be warranted in patients with FNP after minimal or trivial head trauma to exclude a mass lesion (class III, level C). It has been proposed that the early use of galantamine in the treatment of posttraumatic oculomotor and trochlear nerve palsy may accelerate the resolution of ophthalmic symptoms.[87]

12.7 Is the FNP Congenital?

Clearly congenital unilateral or bilateral FNP (type 3) are not associated with intracranial lesions in isolation and therefore do not require further diagnostic evaluation such as neuroimaging studies (class III–IV, level C).[3,8,88,89]

12.8 Is the FNP Vasculopathic?

Vasculopathic FNP (type 4) does not require any initial neuroimaging studies, and observation for improvement over the next 6 to 8 weeks is recommended.[8] Type 4 FNP often resolves spontaneously within 4 to 6 months. Rush and Younge reported an overall recovery rate for FNP of 53.5% in 172 nonselected cases and an accelerated recovery rate of 71% in 166 patients with diabetes mellitus, hypertension, or atherosclerosis.[90] Another report by Ksiazek et al described improvement in 90% of 39 patients with microvascular and idiopathic FNP within 6 months.[91] Vasculopathic FNP usually improves within a few months,[3,8,90] and patients with progressive or unresolved FNP, or with new neurologic signs or symptoms, should have neuroimaging (class II–III, level B).[8,30,53,64,85,90] Patients with spontaneously resolving palsies do not require any further neuroimaging (class II–III, level B). It is recommended that elderly patients who present with headache, scalp tenderness, jaw claudication, or vision loss undergo an appropriate evaluation for giant cell arteritis, including an erythrocyte sedimentation rate, C-reactive protein, and a temporal artery biopsy (class III–IV, level B).[8,85,92] There is insufficient evidence to recommend evaluation for giant cell arteritis in every patient with motility suggesting an isolated FNP (class IV, level U).

12.9 What Is the Evaluation of Nonvasculopathic FNP?

Nonvasculopathic FNP (type 5) may be observed for improvement over the next 6 to 8 weeks (class III, level B). Patients with resolution of symptoms and signs do not require further evaluation (class III, level B). Patients with progression or lack of resolution should undergo neuroimaging (preferably MRI). Myasthenia gravis may mimic FNP, and patients with variable or fatigable motility findings and/or ptosis should be evaluated for myasthenia gravis (see Chapter 15) (class III–IV, level B).[8,85]

Testing for vasculopathic risk factors in type 4 or type 5 FNP should be considered, even in the absence of a history of previous diabetes or hypertension. Green et al reported an isolated third nerve palsy as the initial clinical manifestation of diabetes in almost half of 25 patients.[93] Shrader and Schlezinger reported that almost 50% of diabetic sixth nerve palsies were the presenting clinical manifestation of the disease.[94] The results of these studies concerning vasculopathic third and sixth nerve palsies may well be applicable to vasculopathic FNP (class III, level C).

▶ Table 12.2 summarizes the etiologies of FNP in 11 large retrospective series.[3,12,91,95,96,97,98,99,100,101,102] Traumatic FNP occurred in 35%, idiopathic FNP in 34%, vasculopathic FNP in 16%, neoplasm was reported in 3%, aneurysm in 0.5%, and a wide variety of miscellaneous conditions including myasthenia gravis, infections, thyroid disease, and inflammation in 11% of patients.

Younger patients, or those without vasculopathic risk factors (type 5), may require initial neuroimaging, but the data suggest that observation for spontaneous improvement may be sufficient (class III, level C). Isolated, idiopathic FNPs very rarely have been found to have an underlying etiology after prolonged follow-up, and most resolve spontaneously within several weeks to months.[91,103,104] Two retrospective case series with follow-up greater than 6 months described the prognosis of isolated, idiopathic FNP. Coppeto and Lessell reported that 12 of 15 cases had resolved by 4 months after a mean follow-up of 5.5 years.[103] Nemet et al described 13 cases with a follow-up ranging from 4 to 7 years, and all had resolved by 10 weeks.[104] None of the patients in either series developed new neurologic disease over an extensive follow-up period. Although type 5 FNP patients who improve may not require neuroimaging, the clinical certainty of such a recommendation is not sufficiently strong in our opinion to obviate the need for neuroimaging in these nonvasculopathic patients (class III, level U). However, neuroimaging should be considered for patients who do not improvement in 2 months (class III, level C). Some reports have described intracranial aneurysm as an extremely rare cause for isolated FNP,[12,30,31,64,90,101] and cerebral angiography is not recommended unless an aneurysm is suggested by other neuroimaging studies (class III, level B). Agostinis et al and Collins et al reported isolated FNP due to superior cerebellar aneurysms, but both patients described headaches.[30,31] In these cases, neuroimaging studies confirmed the presence of the aneurysm before angiography. There is insufficient data to draw conclusions regarding the utility of MR angiography in FNP (class III–IV, level U).

Although MRI is generally felt to be more sensitive and specific than CT in the evaluation of cranial neuropathies, no conclusive evidence demonstrates an increased yield when performing MRI rather than CT for the specific evaluation of FNP. Richards et al reported an etiologic diagnosis in 69 of 144 (48%) FNP using MRI and in 289 of 684 (42%) cases using CT. These authors felt that "multiplanar CT may be a sufficient noninvasive study, especially when clinical suspicion is high [or] in patients with other neurologic findings."[12] Nevertheless, we believe that MRI is the study of choice for patients with FNP (class II–III, level B).

A number of cases have been reported documenting intracranial lesions in patients with FNP. ▶ Table 12.3 summarizes 87 cases of "isolated" FNP due to an intracranial lesion. Of these 87

patients, only 6 (5.8%) did not have other neurologic signs or symptoms and thus would be considered truly isolated by our criteria. One developed other neurologic signs after a short follow-up period, and in the remaining five patients persistence or progression of symptoms would have eventually resulted in a neuroimaging study. Of the remaining 81 patients, 6 had headache or pain (7%), 31 had other neurologic signs (38%), and the clinical information was insufficient to determine if the FNP was truly isolated in 44 patients (54%). Keane reported intracranial tumor as an etiology in 12 of 95 unilateral cases, but all 12 (100%) had other neuro-ophthalmic signs, and none of the 81 isolated FNP later reported by Keane had an intracranial tumor.[97] This would suggest that the yield for evaluation of an isolated FNP is low (class III, level C).

All patients with progressive FNP (type 6) should undergo neuroimaging (preferably MRI). Lumbar puncture should be considered if neuroimaging is normal or if there are signs or symptoms of meningeal irritation (class III, level C).

An approach to FNP evaluation is outlined in ▶ Fig. 12.1.

Table 12.2 Etiologies for acquired isolated fourth nerve palsy

Author (First)	Cases	Trauma	Tumor	Vascular	Aneurysm	Unknown	Other
Rucker et al[101]	40	12	1	8	1	15	3
Rucker[99]	67	24	3	24	0	9	7
Rucker[100]	84	23	7	13	0	28	13
Mittelman and Folk [98]	64	22	–	–	–	42	–
Ellis and Helveston[95]	104	32	0	–	1	63	8
Wright and Hansotia[102]	23	9	0	8	0	3	3
Harley[96]	18	5	0	0	0	12	1
Richards et al[12]	578	169	28	103	5	186	87
von Noorden et al[3]	141	73	–	–	0	62	6[a]
Ksiazek et al[91]	88	24	2	39	–	23	–
Keane[97]	81	64	0	8	–	–	9
Total	1,288	457	41	203	7	443	137
	100%	35%	3%	16%	0.5%	34%	11%

[a]"Other" in this study included tumor, vascular, and myasthenia gravis.

Table 12.3 "Isolated" Fourth nerve palsy due to intracranial lesion

Author (First)	Cases	Pathology	Other neurologic signs
Suzuki et al[105]	4	Pinealomas	Yes
Rucker et al[101]	2	Frontal lobe glioma	Unknown
		Aneurysm of circle of Willis	Unknown
Rucker[99]	3	Primary brain tumor (1)	Unknown
		Metastatic (2)	Unknown
Wise and Palubinskas[106]	1	Persistent trigeminal artery	Headache
Rucker[100]	7	Midbrain gliomas (2)	Unknown
		Meningioma (1)	Unknown
		Primary brain tumors (3)	Unknown
Khawam et al[107]	1	"Brain tumor"	Unknown
Burger et al[108]	8	Cerebellopontine angle (CPA) tumors (4)	Yes
		Cerebellar tumor (1)	Yes
		Nasopharyngeal cancer (1)	Yes
		Metastatic lung cancer (1)	Yes
		Aneurysm (1)	Yes

Table 12.3 continued

Author (First)	Cases	Pathology	Other neurologic signs
Robert et al[109]	2	Pituitary tumors	Yes
Ellis and Helveston[95]	1	"Intracranial aneurysm"	Unknown
King[110]	1	Schwannoma	No
Scully et al[111]	1	Medulloblastoma	Yes
Younge and Sutula[112]	4	Gliomas (2)	Unknown
		Metastatic breast cancer (1)	Unknown
		Metastatic ovarian cancer (1)	Unknown
Wray[113]	2	Pituitary tumors	Yes
Coppeto and Lessell[103]	3	Ependymoma (1)	Yes
		Medulloblastoma (1)	Yes
		Acoustic neuroma (1)	Yes
Boggan et al[51]	1	Schwannoma	Yes
Rush and Younge[90]	10	Meningiomas (2)	Unknown
		Primary brain tumor (1)	Unknown
		Metastatic tumors (4)	Unknown
		Intracavernous aneurysm (1)	Yes
		Basilar aneurysm (1)	Unknown
		Aneurysm/subarachnoid hemorrhage (1)	Yes
Ho[114]	1	Schwannoma	No
Neetens and Van Aerde[86]	3	Skull base tumors	Yes
Krohel et al[115]	1	Juvenile pilocytic astrocytoma	Yes
Leunda et al[116]	1	Schwannoma	Yes
McKinna[117]	3	Aneurysms	Unknown
Mansour and Reinecke[118]	1	Reported in Krohel et al	Yes
Jacobson et al[84]	1	Vascular malformation	Yes
Slavin[119]	1	Cavernous meningioma	a
Yamamoto et al[120]	1	Schwannoma	Headache
Ksiazek et al[91]	2	"Compressive etiologies"	Unknown
Maurice-Williams and Harvey[121]	1	Intracavernous aneurysm	Headache
Gonyea[16]	1	Brainstem arteriovenous malformation (AVM)	Headache
Arruga et al[64]	1	Intracavernous aneurysm	No
Agostinis et al[30]	1	Superior cerebellar aneurysm	Headache
Collins et al[31]	1	Superior cerebellar aneurysm	Headache
Richards et al[12]	14	Meningioma (7)	Unknown
		Metastatic (1)	Unknown
		Glioma (4)	Unknown
		Acoustic neuroma (1)	Unknown
		Other primary (1)	Unknown
Kim et al[19]	1	Brainstem stroke	Yes
Mon[20]	1	Midbrain hemorrhage	No
Galetta and Balcer[18]	1	Midbrain hemorrhage	No
Petermann and Newman[60]	1	Pituitary tumor	Headache
Feinberg and Newman[52]	6	Trochlear schwannoma	No
Thömke and Ringel[23]	3	Brainstem lacunes (2)	No
		Hemorrhage (1)	No
Mielke et al[27]	1	Metastatic bronchial cancer	No
Tailor et al[122]	1	Intracranial dermoid cyst	No
Elmalem et al[83]	1	Trochlear schwannoma	No
Kawasaki and Purvin[82]	1	Basilar artery dolichoectasia	No
Lanza et al[68]	1	Cavernous carotid aneurysm	No

aPatient developed progression of deviation after 2 years.

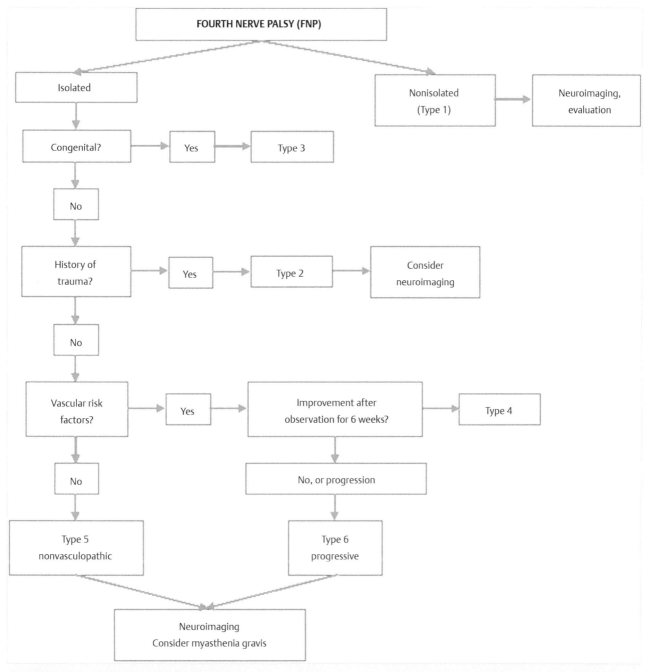

Fig. 12.1 Evaluation of fourth nerve palsy (FNP).

References

[1] Wong AM. Understanding skew deviation and a new clinical test to differentiate it from trochlear nerve palsy. J AAPOS. 2010; 14(1):61–67

[2] Wong AM, Colpa L, Chandrakumar M. Ability of an upright-supine test to differentiate skew deviation from other vertical strabismus causes. Arch Ophthalmol. 2011; 129(12):1570–1575

[3] von Noorden GK, Murray E, Wong SY. Superior oblique paralysis. A review of 270 cases. Arch Ophthalmol. 1986; 104(12):1771–1776

[4] Sheeley M, Arnoldi K. Cyclotropia to differentiate longstanding and acute fourth cranial nerve palsy. Am Orthopt J. 2014; 64:105–111

[5] Kushner BJ. The influence of head tilt on ocular torsion in patients with superior oblique muscle palsy. J AAPOS. 2009; 13(2):132–135

[6] Berlit P. Isolated and combined pareses of cranial nerves III, IV and VI. A retrospective study of 412 patients. J Neurol Sci. 1991; 103(1):10–15

[7] Brazis PW. Palsies of the trochlear nerve: diagnosis and localization–recent concepts. Mayo Clin Proc. 1993; 68(5):501–509

[8] Burde RM, Savino PJ, Trobe JD. Clinical Decisions in Neuro-ophthalmology. 2nd ed. St. Louis: Mosby Year Book; 1992:289–311

[9] Celli P, Ferrante L, Acqui M, Mastronardi L, Fortuna A, Palma L. Neurinoma of the third, fourth, and sixth cranial nerves: a survey and report of a new fourth nerve case. Surg Neurol. 1992; 38(3):216–224

[10] Eliott D, Cunningham ET, Jr, Miller NR. Fourth nerve paresis and ipsilateral relative afferent pupillary defect without visual sensory disturbance. A sign of contralateral dorsal midbrain disease. J Clin Neuroophthalmol. 1991; 11 (3):169–172, discussion 173–174

[11] Kim JS, Kang JK. Contralateral trochlear nerve palsy and facial sensory change due to a probable brainstem vascular malformation. Neuroophthalmology. 1992; 12:59–62

[12] Richards BW, Jones FR, Jr, Younge BR. Causes and prognosis in 4,278 cases of paralysis of the oculomotor, trochlear, and abducens cranial nerves. Am J Ophthalmol. 1992; 113(5):489–496

[13] Vanooteghem P, Dehaene I, Van Zandycke M, Casselman J. Combined trochlear nerve palsy and internuclear ophthalmoplegia. Arch Neurol. 1992; 49(1):108–109

[14] Brazis PW, Masdeu JC, Biller J. Localization in Clinical Neurology. 4th ed. Philadelphia: Lippincott Williams & Wilkins; 2001

[15] Thömke F, Hopf HC. Isolated superior oblique palsies with electrophysiologically documented brainstem lesions. Muscle Nerve. 2000; 23(2):267–270

[16] Gonyea EF. Superior oblique palsy due to a midbrain vascular malformation. Neurology. 1990; 40(3 Pt 1):554–555

[17] Jacobson DM, Moster ML, Eggenberger ER, Galetta SL, Liu GT. Isolated trochlear nerve palsy in patients with multiple sclerosis. Neurology. 1999; 53(4):877–879

[18] Galetta SL, Balcer LJ. Isolated fourth nerve palsy from midbrain hemorrhage: case report. J Neuroophthalmol. 1998; 18(3):204–205

[19] Kim JS, Kang JK, Lee SA, Lee MC. Isolated or predominant ocular motor nerve palsy as a manifestation of brain stem stroke. Stroke. 1993; 24(4):581–586

[20] Mon Y. Midbrain hemorrhage presenting with trochlear nerve palsy–a case report [in Japanese]. Rinsho Shinkeigaku. 1996; 36(1):71–73

[21] Müri RM, Baumgartner RW. Horner's syndrome and contralateral trochlear nerve palsy. Neuroophthalmology. 1995; 15:161

[22] Tachibana H, Mimura O, Shiomi M, Oono T. Bilateral trochlear nerve palsies from a brainstem hematoma. J Clin Neuroophthalmol. 1990; 10(1):35–37

[23] Thömke F, Ringel K. Isolated superior oblique palsies with brainstem lesions. Neurology. 1999; 53(5):1126–1127

[24] Ulrich A, Kaiser HJ. Bilateral trochlear nerve palsy in systemic lupus erythematosus (SLE). Neuroophthalmology. 1998; 20:28

[25] Barr DB, McFadzean RM, Hadley D, Ramsay A, Houston CA, Russell D. Acquired bilateral superior oblique palsy: a localising sign in the dorsal midbrain. Eur J Ophthalmol. 1997; 7(3):271–276

[26] Landolfi JC, Thaler HT, DeAngelis LM. Adult brainstem gliomas. Neurology. 1998; 51(4):1136–1139

[27] Mielke C, Alexander MSM, Anand N. Isolated bilateral trochlear nerve palsy as the first clinical sign of a metastatic bronchial carcinoma. Am J Ophthalmol. 2001; 132:593–594

[28] Leiba H, Siatkowski RM, Culbertson WW, Glaser JS. Neurosarcoidosis presenting as an intracranial mass in childhood. J Neuroophthalmol. 1996; 16(4):269–273

[29] Ohtsuka K, Hashimoto M, Nakamura Y. Bilateral trochlear nerve palsy with arachnoid cyst of the quadrigeminal cistern. Am J Ophthalmol. 1998; 125 (2):268–270

[30] Agostinis C, Caverni L, Moschini L, Rottoli MR, Foresti C. Paralysis of fourth cranial nerve due to superior-cerebellar artery aneurysm. Neurology. 1992; 42(2):457–458

[31] Collins TE, Mehalic TF, White TK, Pezzuti RT. Trochlear nerve palsy as the sole initial sign of an aneurysm of the superior cerebellar artery. Neurosurgery. 1992; 30(2):258–261

[32] Carter N, Miller NR. Fourth nerve palsy caused by Ehrlichia chaffeensis. J Neuroophthalmol. 1997; 17(1):47–50

[33] Ferreira RC, Phan G, Bateman JB. Favorable visual outcome in cryptococcal meningitis. Am J Ophthalmol. 1997; 124(4):558–560

[34] Mansour AM, Bailey BJ. Ocular findings in Ramsay Hunt syndrome. J AAPOS. 1997; 1(3):199–201

[35] Sadun F, De Negri AM, Santopadre P, Pivetti Pezzi P. Bilateral trochlear nerve palsy associated with cryptococcal meningitis in human immunodeficiency virus infection. J Neuroophthalmol. 1999; 19(2):118–119

[36] Keane JR. Delayed trochlear nerve palsy in a case of zoster oticus. Arch Ophthalmol. 1975; 93(5):382–383

[37] Ne, wman NJ, Slamovits TL, Friedland S, Wilson WB. Neuro-ophthalmic manifestations of meningocerebral inflammation from the limited form of Wegener's granulomatosis. Am J Ophthalmol. 1995; 120(5):613–621

[38] Frohman LP, Grigorian R, Bielory L. Neuro-ophthalmic manifestations of sarcoidosis: clinical spectrum, evaluation, and management. J Neuroophthalmol. 2001; 21(2):132–137

[39] Hashimoto M, Hoyt WF. Superficial siderosis and episodic fourth nerve paresis. Report of a case with clinical and magnetic resonance imaging findings. J Neuroophthalmol. 1996; 16(4):277–280

[40] Shinmei Y, Harada T, Ohashi T, Yoshida K, Moriwaka F, Matsuda H. Trochlear nerve palsy associated with superficial siderosis of the central nervous system. Jpn J Ophthalmol. 1997; 41(1):19–22

[41] Lee AG. Fourth nerve palsy in pseudotumor cerebri. Strabismus. 1995; 3(2): 57–59

[42] Patton N, Beatty S, Lloyd IC. Bilateral sixth and fourth cranial nerve palsies in idiopathic intracranial hypertension. J R Soc Med. 2000; 93(2):80–81

[43] Speer C, Pearlman J, Phillips PH, Cooney M, Repka MX. Fourth cranial nerve palsy in pediatric patients with pseudotumor cerebri. Am J Ophthalmol. 1999; 127(2):236–237

[44] Baker RS, Epstein AD. Ocular motor abnormalities from head trauma. Surv Ophthalmol. 1991; 35(4):245–267

[45] Hara N, Kan S, Simizu K. Localization of post-traumatic trochlear nerve palsy associated with hemorrhage at the subarachnoid space by magnetic resonance imaging. Am J Ophthalmol. 2001; 132(3):443–445

[46] Hoya K, Kirino T. Traumatic trochlear nerve palsy following minor occipital impact–four case reports. Neurol Med Chir (Tokyo). 2000; 40(7):358–360

[47] Jacobson DM, Warner JJ, Ruggles KH. Transient trochlear nerve palsy following anterior temporal lobectomy for epilepsy. Neurology. 1995; 45(8): 1465–1468

[48] Lepore FE. Disorders of ocular motility following head trauma. Arch Neurol. 1995; 52(9):924–926

[49] Sabates NR, Gonce MA, Farris BK. Neuro-ophthalmological findings in closed head trauma. J Clin Neuroophthalmol. 1991; 11(4):273–277

[50] Tang Z, Wang C, Shi J. A solitary hemangioblastoma located on the trochlear nerve. J Clin Neurosci. 2014; 21(2):333–335

[51] Boggan JE, Rosenblum ML, Wilson CB. Neurilemmoma of the fourth cranial nerve. Case report. J Neurosurg. 1979; 50(4):519–521

[52] Feinberg AS, Newman NJ. Schwannoma in patients with isolated unilateral trochlear nerve palsy. Am J Ophthalmol. 1999; 127(2):183–188

[53] Gentry LR, Mehta RC, Appen RE, Weinstein JM. MR imaging of primary trochlear nerve neoplasms. AJNR Am J Neuroradiol. 1991; 12(4):707–713

[54] Santoreneos S, Hanieh A, Jorgensen RE. Trochlear nerve schwannomas occurring in patients without neurofibromatosis: case report and review of the literature. Neurosurgery. 1997; 41(1):282–287

[55] Grabe HM, McKean EL, Eggenberger ER, Trobe JD. Persistent diplopia and superior oblique muscle dysfunction following dissection of the orbital periosteum in cranial base surgery. Br J Ophthalmol. 2013; 97(10):1330–1332

[56] Tanaka H, Yuki N, Hirata K. Trochlear nerve enhancement on three-dimensional magnetic resonance imaging in Fisher syndrome. Am J Ophthalmol. 1998; 126(2):322–324

[57] Vitali C, Genovesi-Ebert F, Romani A, Jeracitano G, Nardi M. Ophthalmological and neuro-ophthalmological involvement in Churg-Strauss syndrome: a case report. Graefes Arch Clin Exp Ophthalmol. 1996; 234(6):404–408

[58] Eisenberg MB, Al-Mefty O, DeMonte F, Burson GT. Benign nonmeningeal tumors of the cavernous sinus. Neurosurgery. 1999; 44(5):949–954, discussion 954–955

[59] Keane JR. Cavernous sinus syndrome. Analysis of 151 cases. Arch Neurol. 1996; 53(10):967–971

[60] Petermann SH, Newman NJ. Pituitary macroadenoma manifesting as an isolated fourth nerve palsy. Am J Ophthalmol. 1999; 127(2):235–236

[61] Chang-Godinich A, Lee AG, Brazis PW, Liesegang TJ, Jones DB. Complete ophthalmoplegia after zoster ophthalmicus. J Neuroophthalmol. 1997; 17 (4):262–265

[62] Ryu WY, Kim NY, Kwon YH, Ahn HB. Herpes zoster ophthalmicus with isolated trochlear nerve palsy in an otherwise healthy 13-year-old girl. J AAPOS. 2014; 18(2):193–195

[63] Hermann M, Bobek-Billewicz B, Bullo B, Hermann A, Rutkowski B. Wegener's granulomatosis with unusual cavernous sinus and sella turcica extension. Eur Radiol. 1999; 9(9):1859–1861

[64] Arruga J, De Rivas P, Espinet HL, Conesa G. Chronic isolated trochlear nerve palsy produced by intracavernous internal carotid artery aneurysm. Report of a case. J Clin Neuroophthalmol. 1991; 11(2):104–108

[65] Fitzsimon JS, Toland J, Philips J, et al. Trends and developments: giant aneurysms in the cavernous sinus. Neuroophthalmology. 1995; 15(2):59–65

[66] Hahn CD, Nicolle DA, Lownie SP, Drake CG. Giant cavernous carotid aneurysms: clinical presentation in fifty-seven cases. J Neuroophthalmol. 2000; 20(4):253–258

[67] Shimo-oku M, Izaki A, Shim-myo A. Fourth nerve palsy as an initial sign of internal carotid-posterior communicating artery aneurysm. Neuro-ophthalmology. 1998; 19:185–190

[68] Lanza G, Vinciguerra L, Puglisi V, et al. Acute isolated trochlear nerve palsy in a patient with cavernous carotid aneurysm and visit-to-visit variability in systolic blood pressure. Int J Stroke. 2015; 10(6):E61

[69] Tsai RK, Chen HY, Wang HZ. Painful fourth cranial nerve palsy caused by posteriorly-draining dural carotid-cavernous sinus fistula. J Formos Med Assoc. 2000; 99(9):730–732

[70] Polito E, Leccisotti A. Painful ophthalmoplegia caused by superior ophthalmic vein thrombosis. Neuro-ophthalmology. 1996; 16(3):189–192

[71] Herrendorf G, Steinhoff BJ, Vadokas V, et al. Transitory fourth cranial nerve palsy due to foramen ovale electrode placement. Acta Neurochir (Wien). 1997; 139(8):789–790

[72] Lopes DK, Mericle RA, Wakhloo AK, Guterman LR, Hopkins LN. Cavernous sinus syndrome during balloon test occlusion of the cervical internal carotid artery. Report of two cases. J Neurosurg. 1998; 89(4):667–670

[73] Manjila S, Moon K, Weiner MA, et al. Cavernous malformation of the trochlear nerve: case report and review of the literature on cranial nerve cavernomas. Neurosurgery. 2011; 69(1):E230–E238, discussion E238

[74] Wong AMF, Sharpe JA. Fourth nerve palsy in migraine. Neuro-ophthalmology. 1996; 16:51–54

[75] Botelho PJ, Giangiacomo JG. Autosomal-dominant inheritance of congenital superior oblique palsy. Ophthalmology. 1996; 103(9):1508–1511

[76] Holmes JM, Mutyala S, Maus TL, Grill R, Hodge DO, Gray DT. Pediatric third, fourth, and sixth nerve palsies: a population-based study. Am J Ophthalmol. 1999; 127(4):388–392

[77] Lee S, Kim SH, Yang HK, et al. Imaging demonstration of trochlear nerve agenesis in superior oblique palsy emerging during the later life. Clin Neurol Neurosurg. 2015; 139:269–271

[78] Yang HK, Kim JH, Hwang JM. Congenital superior oblique palsy and trochlear nerve absence: a clinical and radiological study. Ophthalmology. 2012; 119 (1):170–177

[79] Kim JH, Hwang JM. Absence of the trochlear nerve in patients with superior oblique hypoplasia. Ophthalmology. 2010; 117(11):2208–13.e1, 2

[80] Varrato J, Galetta S. Fourth nerve palsy unmasked by botulinum toxin therapy for cervical torticollis. Neurology. 2000; 55(6):896

[81] Orwitz JI, Galetta SL, Teener JW. Bilateral trochlear nerve palsy and downbeat nystagmus in a patient with cephalic tetanus. Neurology. 1997; 49(3):894–895

[82] Kawasaki A, Purvin V. Isolated IVth (trochlear) nerve palsy due to basilar artery dolichoectasia. Klin Monatsbl Augenheilkd. 2006; 223(5):459–461

[83] Elmalem VI, Younge BR, Biousse V, et al. Clinical course and prognosis of trochlear nerve schwannomas. Ophthalmology. 2009; 116(10):2011–2016

[84] Jacobson DM, Warner JJ, Choucair AK, Ptacek LJ. Trochlear nerve palsy following minor head trauma. A sign of structural disorder. J Clin Neuroophthalmol. 1988; 8(4):263–268

[85] Miller NR. Walsh and Hoyt's Clinical Neuro-ophthalmology. 4th ed. Baltimore: Williams & Wilkins; 1989:686

[86] Neetens A, Van Aerde F. Extra-ocular muscle palsy from minor head trauma. Initial sign of intracranial tumour. Bull Soc Belge Ophtal. 1981; 193:161–167

[87] Tokarz-Sawińska E, Lachowicz E, Gosławski W. The use of galantamine in the treatment of post-traumatic oculomotor and trochlear nerve palsy. Klin Oczna. 2013; 115(4):275–279

[88] Robb RM. Idiopathic superior oblique palsies in children. J Pediatr Ophthalmol Strabismus. 1990; 27(2):66–69

[89] von Noorden GK, Helveston EM. Strabismus: A Decision Making Approach. St. Louis: Mosby; 1994:162–169

[90] Rush JA, Younge BR. Paralysis of cranial nerves III, IV, and VI. Cause and prognosis in 1,000 cases. Arch Ophthalmol. 1981; 99(1):76–79

[91] Ksiazek S, Behar R, Savino PJ, et al. Isolated acquired fourth nerve palsies. Neurology. 1988; 38 Suppl 1:246

[92] Reich KA, Giansiracusa DF, Strongwater SL. Neurologic manifestations of giant cell arteritis. Am J Med. 1990; 89(1):67–72

[93] Green WR, Hackett ER, Schlezinger NS. Neuro-ophthalmic evaluation of oculomotor nerve paralysis. Arch Ophthalmol. 1964; 72:154–167

[94] Shrader EC, Schlezinger NS. Neuro-ophthalmologic evaluation of abducens nerve paralysis. Arch Ophthalmol. 1960; 63:84–91

[95] Ellis FD, Helveston EM. Superior oblique palsy: diagnosis and classification. Int Ophthalmol Clin. 1976; 16(3):127–135

[96] Harley RD. Paralytic strabismus in children. Etiologic incidence and management of the third, fourth, and sixth nerve palsies. Ophthalmology. 1980; 87(1):24–43

[97] Keane JR. Fourth nerve palsy: historical review and study of 215 inpatients. Neurology. 1993; 43(12):2439–2443

[98] Mittelman D, Folk ER. The evaluation and treatment of superior oblique muscle palsy. Trans Sect Ophthalmol Am Acad Ophthalmol Otolaryngol. 1976; 81(5):893–898

[99] Rucker CW. Paralysis of the third, fourth and sixth cranial nerves. Am J Ophthalmol. 1958; 46(6):787–794

[100] Rucker CW. The causes of paralysis of the third, fourth and sixth cranial nerves. Am J Ophthalmol. 1966; 61(5 Pt 2):1293–1298

[101] Rucker CW, Dyer JA, Smith DC, Taub RG. The causes of acquired paralysis of the ocular muscles. Am J Ophthalmol. 1956; 41(6):950–955

[102] Wright H, Hansotia P. Isolated fourth cranial nerve palsies: etiology and prognosis. Wis Med J. 1977; 76(2):26–28

[103] Coppeto JM, Lessell S. Cryptogenic unilateral paralysis of the superior oblique muscle. Arch Ophthalmol. 1978; 96(2):275–277

[104] Nemet P, Godel V, Baruch E, Lazar M. Benign palsy of superior oblique muscle. J Pediatr Ophthalmol Strabismus. 1980; 17(5):320–322

[105] Suzuki J, Wada T, Kowada M. Clinical observations on tumors of the pineal region. J Neurosurg. 1962; 19:441–445

[106] Wise BL, Palubinskas AJ. Persistent trigeminal artery (carotid-basilar anastomosis). J Neurosurg. 1964; 21:199–206

[107] Khawam E, Scott AB, Jampolsky A. Acquired superior oblique palsy. Diagnosis and management. Arch Ophthalmol. 1967; 77(6):761–768

[108] Burger LJ, Kalvin NH, Smith JL. Acquired lesions of the fourth cranial nerve. Brain. 1970; 93(3):567–574

[109] Robert CM, Jr, Feigenbaum JA, Stern EW. Ocular palsy occurring with pituitary tumors. J Neurosurg. 1973; 38(1):17–19

[110] King JS. Trochlear nerve sheath tumor; case report. J Neurosurg. 1976; 44 (2):245–247

[111] Scully RE, Galdabini JJ, McNeely BU. Case records of the Massachusetts General Hospital. Weekly clinicopathological exercises. Case 36–1976. N Engl J Med. 1976; 295(10):553–561

[112] Younge BR, Sutula F. Analysis of trochlear nerve palsies. Diagnosis, etiology, and treatment. Mayo Clin Proc. 1977; 52(1):11–18

[113] Wray SH. Neuro-ophthalmologic manifestations of pituitary and parasellar lesions. Clin Neurosurg. 1977; 24:86–117

[114] Ho KL. Schwannoma of the trochlear nerve. Case report. J Neurosurg. 1981; 55(1):132–135

[115] Krohel GB, Mansour AM, Petersen WL, Evenchik B. Isolated trochlear nerve palsy secondary to a juvenile pilocytic astrocytoma. J Clin Neuroophthalmol. 1982; 2(2):119–123

[116] Leunda G, Vaquero J, Cabezudo J, Garcia-Uria J, Bravo G. Schwannoma of the oculomotor nerves. Report of four cases. J Neurosurg. 1982; 57(4):563–565

[117] McKinna AJ. Eye signs in 611 cases of posterior fossa aneurysms: their diagnostic and prognostic value. Can J Ophthalmol. 1983; 18(1):3–6

[118] Mansour AM, Reinecke RD. Central trochlear palsy. Surv Ophthalmol. 1986; 30(5):279–297

[119] Slavin ML. Isolated trochlear nerve palsy secondary to cavernous sinus meningioma. Am J Ophthalmol. 1987; 104(4):433–434

[120] Yamamoto M, Jimbo M, Ide M, Kubo O. Trochlear neurinoma. Surg Neurol. 1987; 28(4):287–290

[121] Maurice-Williams RS, Harvey PK. Isolated palsy of the fourth cranial nerve caused by an intracavernous aneurysm. J Neurol Neurosurg Psychiatry. 1989; 52(5):679

[122] Tailor R, Mollan SP, Burdon MA. Intracranial dermoid cyst presenting as an isolated fourth nerve palsy. J Neurol. 2009; 256(5):820–821

13 Sixth Nerve Palsies

Stacy V. Smith, Andrew G. Lee, and Paul W. Brazis

Abstract

A sixth nerve palsy results from an injury to the abducens nerve, and typically causes a binocular horizontal diplopia, an abduction deficit, and an incomitant esotropia. While ischemia is the most common cause of an isolated, acute sixth nerve palsy in adults, many other etiologies can produce an abducens lesion (e.g., trauma, increased intracranial pressure, compressive lesions). This chapter discusses the clinical pathways in localizing and diagnosing sixth nerve palsies, by reviewing the literature in detail.

Keywords: sixth nerve palsy, abducens nerve, ischemic cranial neuropathy, horizontal diplopia, vasculopathy

13.1 Acknowledgment

The authors gratefully acknowledge the input of Joseph Hough, MD in reviewing this chapter.

13.2 What Is the Epidemiology of Sixth Nerve Palsy?

The incidence of sixth nerve palsy (SNP) is 11.3 in 100,000.[1] In an interesting population-based study, Patel et al found equal incidence of SNP among males and females, with peak incidence within the seventh decade of life.[2,3] While SNP of undetermined origin accounted for 26% of all the cases, hypertension alone accounted for 16%. The combined existence of hypertension and diabetes was the underlying cause of another 12% of the cases. Trauma was implicated in another 12%. Only 2% of the cases, presenting with SNP as the only physical sign, had an underlying neoplasia.[1,2,3]

13.3 What Is the Anatomy of the Sixth Nerve?

The paired abducens nuclei are located in the dorsal lower portion of the pons, separated from the floor of the fourth ventricle by the genu of the facial nerve (facial colliculus). The nucleus contains motor neurons for the lateral rectus muscle and interneurons traveling via the medial longitudinal fasciculus (MLF) to the contralateral medial rectus subnucleus of the third nerve. The sixth nerve nucleus thus contains all the neurons responsible for horizontal conjugate gaze. The nerve fascicle leaves the nucleus and travels within the substance of the pontine tegmentum, adjacent to the medial lemniscus and the corticospinal tract. The sixth nerve leaves the brainstem in the horizontal sulcus between the pons and medulla (lateral to the corticospinal bundles). It enters the subarachnoid space, ascends along the base of the pons in the prepontine cistern, courses nearly vertically along the clivus, and travels over the petrous apex of the temporal bone where it is tethered at the petroclinoid

(Grüber's) ligament in Dorello's canal beneath. It enters the substance of the cavernous sinus lateral to the internal carotid artery and medial to the ophthalmic division of the trigeminal nerve (V1) to enter the orbit via the superior orbital fissure. In their course from the pericarotid plexus to the ophthalmic branch of the trigeminal nerve, the pupil's sympathetic fibers join the abducens nerve for a few millimeters.

13.4 What Are the Types of Sixth Nerve Palsy?

Seven types of SNP can be identified:
- Type 1—Isolated: Possible causes of isolated SNP include ipsilateral abduction deficit, Duane's syndrome, spasm of near reflex, unilateral orbital disease, myasthenia gravis, systemic diseases (e.g., systemic lupus), or infection diseases (e.g., viral encephalitis).
- Type 2—Traumatic: SNPs that have a clearly established temporal relationship to significant previous head trauma and do not progress are considered traumatic in origin; patients with SNP following minor head trauma are excluded.
- Type 3—Congenital SNP.
- Type 4—Vasculopathic SNPs: This form occurs in patients older than age 55 or those with known vasculopathic risk factors (e.g., hypertension or diabetes).
- Type 5—Nonvasculopathic: Patients without vasculopathic risk factors.
- Type 6—Progressive: Progressive SNPs are SNPs that worsen after the acute stage (more than 2 weeks) as defined by a significant increase in the measured ocular deviation or who develop new neurologic findings. Also, patients without resolution in the measured horizontal deviation after 12 to 16 weeks are considered progressive.
- Type 7—Benign recurrent SNP: It mainly affects children. It accounts for almost 13% of all SNPs in children.[4,5] The following clinical factors "favor" benign recurrent SNP: Children under 14 months of age, female gender, postvaccination, and initial left eye involvement. Imaging and other evaluation (e.g., myasthenia gravis) might still be necessary in these patients as this is a diagnosis of exclusion.[4,5]

13.5 Where Does a Lesion Causing a Sixth Nerve Palsy Localize?

Box 13.1 gives an overview of the CNS lesions commonly involved in SNP and their possible clinical presentation. Due to the many possible locations of lesions that can all result in the same neurological finding of an SNP, the SNP is considered a "nonlocalizing" finding on clinical exam. However, additional neurologic findings (e.g., additional cranial nerve palsies) may help identify the most likely lesion location.

- Nuclear lesions.
  - Abducens nucleus.
    - Horizontal gaze palsy (sixth nerve and MLF input).
    - Möbius syndrome (gaze palsy with facial diplegia).
    - Duane retraction syndrome (gaze palsy with globe retraction and narrowing of palpebral fissure with adduction).
  - Dorsolateral pons.
    - Ipsilateral gaze palsy, facial paresis, dysmetria; occasionally with contralateral hemiparesis (Foville syndrome).
- Lesions of the abducens fascicle.
  - Abducens fascicle.
    - Isolated CN VI palsy.
  - Anterior paramedial pons.
    - Ipsilateral CN VI palsy, ipsilateral CN VII palsy, contralateral hemiparesis (Millard–Gubler).
  - Prepontine cistern.
    - May have contralateral hemiparesis.
- Lesion of abducens nerve (subarachnoid, petrous).
  - Petrous apex (Dorello's canal).
    - CN VI palsy, deafness, facial (especially retro-orbital) pain (Gradenigo).
  - Cavernous sinus.
    - Isolated CN VI palsy; CN VI palsy plus Horner syndrome; also may affect CN III, IV, VI.
  - Superior orbital fissure syndrome.
    - CN VI palsy with variable affection of CN III, IV, VI; proptosis.
  - Orbit.
    - CN VI palsy; visual loss; variable proptosis, chemosis, lid swelling.

Source: Modified from Brazis et al[6] with permission from Lippincott Williams & Wilkins.

Nuclear (horizontal gaze).
- Congenital.[7]
  - Möbius syndrome.[7,8]
  - Isolated.[9]
- Demyelinating.
- Infarction or ischemia.
- Neoplasm (pontine and cerebellar).
- Glioma.
- Metastasis.
- Histiocytosis X.
- Trauma.
- Wernicke–Korsakoff syndrome.

Fascicular.
- Demyelination.[10,11]
- Infarction.[10,12,13]
- Neoplasm.[10,14,15]
- Trauma.
- Hematoma.[10]
- Migraine.[16,17]
- Cluster headache.[18]
- Anti-Hu antibody-mediated paraneoplastic brainstem encephalitis.[19]

Subarachnoid.
- Aneurysm or vascular abnormality.[12]
  - Persistent primitive trigeminal artery.[20]
  - Posterior inferior cerebellar aneurysm.
  - Vertebral artery, including elongated vessel.[21,22]
- Carcinomatous or leukemic meningitis.[23]
- Chiari malformation or basilar impression.[12,24,25]
- Following procedures.
  - Cervical traction.[26]
  - Lumbar puncture (LP) or myelography.[27,28,29,30,31,32]
  - Microvascular decompression for trigeminal neuralgia.[33]
  - Postvaccination.[34]
  - Radiculography.[35,36]
  - Shunting for hydrocephalus (ventriculoperitoneal, lumboperitoneal).
  - Spinal or epidural anesthesia and pain management.[37,38,39]
  - Intrathecal glucocorticoid injection.[40]
- Inflammatory.
  - Retropharyngeal space inflammation.[41]
  - Necrotizing vasculitis.
  - Sarcoidosis.[42,43]
  - Systemic lupus erythematosus.
  - Granulomatosis with polyangiitis (GPA) and formerly Wegener granulomatosis.[44]
  - Miller Fisher syndrome.[45]
  - Idiopathic hypertrophic cranial pachymeningitis.[46,47]
- Infectious.
  - Lyme disease.[48,49]
  - Syphilis.[50,51]
  - Tuberculosis.
  - Cryptococcal meningitis.

13.5.1 Is the Nonisolated Sixth Nerve Palsy Due to a Pontine (Lower Pons) Lesion?

Sixth nerve nuclear lesions cause a horizontal gaze palsy, rather than an isolated abduction deficit. An ipsilateral facial palsy may occur because of the close proximity of the facial and abducens nerve in the pons. Nuclear lesions are usually associated with other brainstem signs (e.g., hemiparesis, hemisensory loss, a central Horner syndrome). Likewise, lesions of the sixth nerve fascicle involve adjacent structures (e.g., cranial nerves V, VII, and VIII; cerebellar ataxia; a central Horner syndrome; or contralateral hemiplegia). Patients with a presumed nuclear or fascicular SNP should undergo neuroimaging (usually magnetic resonance imaging [MRI]) directed to the pons. The etiologies of nuclear or fascicular lesions in the pons are listed in Box 13.2.

- ○ Cysticercosis.[52]
- ○ HIV-CMV encephalitis.
- ○ Epstein-Barr virus meningitis.[53]
- ○ West Nile Virus meningoencephalitis.[54]
- ○ Pseudomonas osteomyelitis of the clivus.[55]
- • Neoplasm.[56]
  - ○ Abducens nerve tumor.[57,58,59]
  - ○ Cerebellopontine angle tumor.
  - ○ Clivus tumor (e.g., chordoma, chondrosarcoma, plasmacytoma).[14,60,61,62,63,64]
  - ○ Leukemia.[65]
  - ○ Metastatic.[66]
  - ○ Skull base tumor.[52,67]
  - ○ Nasopharyngeal carcinoma.[52]
  - ○ Trigeminal nerve tumor.
  - ○ Capillary hemangioma of Meckel's cave.[68]
  - ○ Diffuse leptomeningeal gliomatosis.[69,70,71,72]
  - ○ Diffuse leptomeningeal neurocytoma.[73]
  - ○ Diffuse leptomeningeal dissemination of mixed glioneuronal neoplasm.[74]
- • Nonlocalizing sign of increased intracranial pressure.[75]
  - ○ Pseudotumor cerebri.[76,77]
  - ○ Venous sinus thrombosis.[78]
  - ○ Meningeal irritation of any type.
  - ○ Intracranial mass.
  - ○ Syndrome of headache, neurologic deficits, and cerebrospinal fluid lymphocytosis (HaNDL).[79]
- • Spontaneous cerebrospinal fluid leak with intracranial hypotension.[80,81,82,83,84,85,86,87]
- • Trauma (excluding surgical).[88,89,90]
- • Epidural hematoma of clivus.[91]

Petrous apex.
- • Neoplasm (e.g., nasopharyngeal carcinoma, trigeminal neurinoma[92]).
- • Paget disease.[93]
- • Infection.
  - ○ Complicated otitis media.[94]
  - ○ Mastoiditis (Gradenigo syndrome).[95]
- • Thrombosis of inferior petrosal or transverse/sigmoid sinus.[96]
- • Trauma.[97,98]
  - ○ Balloon compression and thermal injury during Gasserian ganglion ablation for trigeminal neuralgia.[99,100,101,102,103]
  - ○ Basilar skull fracture.
- • Inflammatory.

Cavernous sinus.[104]
- • Cavernous sinus thrombosis.[105]
- • Cavernous sinus fistula.[12,106,107,108]
- • Superior ophthalmic vein thrombosis.[109]
- • Neoplasm.[110]
  - ○ Nasopharyngeal carcinoma.[104]
  - ○ Pituitary adenoma.
  - ○ Plasmacytoma.[111]
  - ○ Lymphoma.[104,112,113]
  - ○ Hodgkin disease.[114]
  - ○ Hemangioma.[68,115]
  - ○ Hemangioendothelioma.[116]
  - ○ Meningioma.[117]
  - ○ Rhabdomyosarcoma.[118]
  - ○ Sixth nerve tumors.
  - ○ Trigeminal neurinoma.[92]
  - ○ Malignant trigeminal nerve sheath tumor.[119]
  - ○ Sphenoid sinus tumors.
  - ○ Skull base tumors.
  - ○ Squamous cell cancer of pterygopalatine fossa.
- • Subarachnoid diverticulum.
- • Sphenoid sinus mucocele.[120]
- • Arachnoid cyst of Meckel's cave.[121]
- • Ischemia.
- • Inflammatory or infectious.
  - ○ Herpes zoster.[122,123,124]
  - ○ Herpes simplex 1.
  - ○ Actinomycoses.[125]
  - ○ Actinobacillus actinomycetemcomitans.[126]
  - ○ Tolosa–Hunt syndrome.
  - ○ Idiopathic hypertrophic cranial pachymeningitis.[47,127]

Internal carotid artery diseases.
- • Aneurysm.[104,128,129,130]
- • Dissection.[131,132]
- • Dolichoectasia.[133,134,135]
- • Balloon test occlusion.[136]
  - ○ Toxicity/medication-associated.
    - – Cisplatin infusion.[137,138]

Orbital lesions.
- • Neoplastic (orbital schwannoma).
- • Inflammation (orbital inflammatory pseudotumor).
- • Infectious.
- • Traumatic.[139]

Localization uncertain.
- • Infectious mononucleosis.
- • *Mycoplasma pneumoniae* infection.[140]
- • Lyme disease.[141]
- • *Campylobacter jejuni* enteritis.[142]
- • Creutzfeldt–Jakob disease.[143]
- • Progressive multifocal leukoencephalopathy (PML) in AIDS.[144]
- • Lymphoma.[145]
- • Bing-Neel syndrome with Waldenstrom macroglobulinemia.[146]
- • Wernicke encephalopathy.
- • Guillain–Barré syndrome.[147]
- • Miller Fisher syndrome.[148,149,150,151,152]
- • Associated with anti-GQ1b immunoglobulin G (IgG) antibody.[153]
- • Chronic inflammatory demyelinating polyradiculoneuropathy (CIDP).[154,155]
- • Unintentional subdural catheter.[156]
- • Pregnancy.[157]
- • Toxicity/medication-associated.
  - ○ Vincristine.[158]
  - ○ Acitretin.[159,160,161]
  - ○ Methotrexate.[162]
  - ○ Capecitabine.[163]

- Antivascular endothelial growth factor agents.[164,165,166]
- Interferon[167] and pegylated interferon (one case with pegylated interferon and ribavirin concomitant therapy).[168,169]
- Cyclosporine and ganciclovir therapy for bone marrow transplantation.[170]
- 3,4-Methyl-enedioxymetamphetamine (MDMA, or "ecstasy") abuse.[171]
- Dental anesthesia (e.g., lidocaine injection).[172,173,174,175,176]

13.5.2 Is the Sixth Nerve Palsy Due to a Subarachnoid Space Lesion?

Lesions of the subarachnoid space may result in unilateral or bilateral SNP. This SNP is a nonlocalizing finding because any cause of increased intracranial pressure may result in an SNP (Box 13.2). Patients with a subarachnoid space lesion should undergo neuroimaging directed to this location followed by an LP as needed (class III–IV, level B).

13.5.3 Is the Sixth Nerve Palsy the Result of a Lesion of the Petrous Apex?

Lesions of the petrous apex causing SNP are associated with other neurologic findings, including involvement of other cranial nerves (e.g., fifth, seventh, and eighth) or facial pain. Neuroimaging should be directed toward the petrous apex (MRI or computed tomography [CT] for bone involvement) (class III–IV, level B).

13.5.4 Is Sixth Nerve Palsy Due to a Cavernous Sinus Lesion?

With lesions of the cavernous sinus, SNPs usually occur in association with other cranial neuropathies (e.g., third, fourth, or fifth nerves) or a Horner syndrome. Neuroimaging (usually MRI) should be directed to the cavernous sinus (class III–IV, level B). Box 13.2 lists the etiologies of a cavernous sinus lesion causing an SNP. In their series of 126 patients, Fernández et al found that 58 patients with cavernous sinus lesions presented with SNP.[9] Tumors, vasculopathies, and Tolosa–Hunt syndrome (in that descending order) were the top three causes for SNP in cavernous sinus lesions.[9]

13.5.5 Is the Sixth Nerve Palsy Due to an Orbital Lesion?

Lesions of the orbit causing SNP are usually associated with other orbital signs such as proptosis or chemosis. Neuroimaging (preferably MRI with gadolinium and fat suppression) should be directed to the orbit (class III–IV, level B) in orbital lesions but CT scan can show bony anatomy and sinus disease better than MRI and may be a superior initial or adjunctive imaging study. In addition, some orbital lesions have intracranial involvement or origin and imaging of the entire course of the sixth nerve is generally recommended for SNP.

13.6 What Are the Recommendations for the Evaluation of Sixth Nerve Palsy?

1. Nonisolated SNP (type 1) should undergo neuroimaging and further evaluation (class III–IV, level B). Special attention should be directed to areas suggested topographically by the associated neurologic signs or symptoms (see above).[64,66,67,177,178,179]

2. Traumatic SNP (type 2) should undergo the appropriate acute neuroimaging (CT scanning possibly followed by MRI) as indicated by the trauma-associated neurologic signs and symptoms (class IV, level C). In acute traumatic SNP, failure to recover by 6 months after onset was associated independently with the inability to abduct past midline at presentation and bilaterality.[180] Dhaliwal et al found that SNP results from a milder severity of closed head injury than for injuries causing third and fourth nerves.[181] They also found that SNP recovered faster and needed less intervention than the third and fourth nerve palsies related to closed head injuries. In the same vein, a retrospective study by Sharma et al associated a higher frequency of SNP following head parietal region trauma (Class III evidence).[182]

3. Congenital SNPs (type 3) are rare, and there are insufficient data from our review of the literature to make a strong recommendation for the management of congenital isolated SNPs (class IV, level U). Nevertheless, if the SNP can be clearly demonstrated to be congenital in origin, additional neuroimaging is not generally required (class IV, level U). Transient SNPs may occur following birth trauma in newborns. Galbraith reported the incidence of SNP in a group of 6,886 neonates as being 0.4%.[177] All of these SNPs (type 3) resolved within 6 weeks, and we recommend that imaging may be deferred in these patients. The incidence of SNP increased with "complexity of instrumentation," with 0% prevalence for cesarean section, 0.1% prevalence for spontaneous vaginal delivery, 2.4% prevalence for forceps delivery, and 3.2% for vacuum extraction. Leung reported three cases of right SNP after vaginal delivery that all resolved after 4 to 12 weeks.[183] Observation for improvement is a reasonable approach in these cases (class IV, level C).

4. Many authors believe that neurologically isolated, presumed vasculopathic SNPs (type 4) may be observed (without neuroimaging) for improvement for 4 to 12 weeks (class III, level C),[67,184] as most patients experience a complete recovery.[185,186] However, this recommendation remains controversial due to a lack of sufficient prospective studies.[184,187,188,189,190] The clinical history and examination will help determine which patients may be safely observed for a short period, such as those patients with multiple vasculopathic risk factors found to have a truly isolated SNP on clinical exam.[187,188,189,191,192] If the SNP does not resolve, worsens, or the patient develops new symptoms or signs during the observation period, then further evaluation including neuroimaging (e.g., MRI) should be performed.[184,187] Although several compressive lesions have been reported in isolated SNP, many of these lesions are benign and delaying imaging for an observation period probably did not change treatment or final outcome (e.g., meningioma, schwannoma, chondroma).[67,188,193]

In contrast, several retrospective studies support the alternate recommendation that all SNP, including isolated and presumed vasculopathic SNP, should undergo neuroimaging. The diagnostic yield for a nonvasculopathic etiology may be up to 14%.[184,191,192,194] In addition, patients with vasculopathic risk factors may merit imaging to rule out other significant etiologies such as brainstem ischemic stroke.

Rush and Younge reported a recovery rate of 49.6% in 419 nonselected SNP cases, and a higher rate of 71% in 419 patients with diabetes mellitus, hypertension, or atherosclerosis.[195] Some authors have recommended observing vasculopathic isolated SNP beyond a 3-month interval of recovery if the esotropia and the abduction deficit were decreasing.[194,196] Elderly patients who present with an isolated SNP and headache, scalp tenderness, jaw claudication, or visual loss should undergo an appropriate evaluation for giant cell arteritis (class IV, level C). We recommend checking the erythrocyte sedimentation rate and, when clinically indicated, doing a temporal artery biopsy.[197] Patients with progression or lack of improvement (type 6) should undergo neuroimaging (class IV, level C).

It should be noted that early progression of paresis over the course of 1 week in vasculopathic SNP is not uncommon.[198] In one study, only 2 of 35 patients with ischemic SNP had initial complete abduction deficits.[19,8] Of 33 patients with initial incomplete deficits, 18 (55%) showed progression over a 1-week period. We do not consider progression over the first week after onset to be a sign of nonvasculopathic SNP (class IV, level C).

5. We recommend that nonvasculopathic SNP (type 5) should undergo neuroimaging (class III–IV, level C).[41,43,50,56,59,66,96,108,177,179,195,199] Younger patients, or those without vasculopathic risk factors (type 5), could also undergo a more extensive evaluation including a fasting blood glucose, complete blood cell count, and a blood pressure check for underlying vasculopathy (class IV, level C). Other testing, including neuroimaging (MRI) and if necessary LP, is recommended (class IV, level C). Type 5 SNPs have a significant (27%) chance of harboring an underlying malignant neoplasm.[200] Evaluation for myasthenia gravis as well as sarcoidosis and other connective tissue diseases should also be considered in these patients (class IV, level C).[201,202]

6. Testing for vasculopathic risk factors in type 4 or type 5 SNP should be performed, even in the absence of a previous history of diabetes or hypertension.[196,203,204] Ocular motor cranial neuropathies may be the presenting sign or only sign of underlying vasculopathy in these patients (class IV, level C).

7. Patients with progressive or unresolved SNP (type 6) and patients with new neurologic signs or symptoms should undergo neuroimaging.[196,200,203,205] Patients with progressive or unresolved SNP should probably undergo neuroimaging (class IV, level C). Galetta and Smith described 13 patients with chronic SNP, that is, an SNP lasting 6 months or longer. Of these, four were idiopathic, four due to tumor, two were traumatic, one was postspinal anesthesia, one was temporal

arteritis, and one was intracavernous aneurysm.[206] Savino et al reviewed 38 patients with chronic SNP.[203] Fourteen (37%) were discovered to have an intracranial lesion. These authors specifically recommended neuroradiologic investigation at onset in any patient with a history of carcinoma.

Moster et al commented on the lack of truly isolated SNP reported in the literature.[205] Most reports do not distinguish unilateral from bilateral SNP, or isolated SNP from those associated with other neurologic or cranial nerve defects.[200] Our review of the literature on SNP revealed 31 case reports and case series describing 237 patients with presumed isolated SNP. Of these 237 patients, 31 were traumatic, none were congenital, 60 were vasculopathic, 47 were idiopathic, and the remainder had a number of miscellaneous etiologies (7 post-LP, 19 multiple sclerosis, 2 postimmunizations, 5 "infectious," 5 aneurysms, 1 sarcoidosis, 6 "presumed inflammation," 1 orbital amyloidosis, and 1 diverticulum of the cavernous sinus). Fifty-two cases were the result of tumors (including chordomas, chondrosarcomas, meningiomas, cylindroma, lymphomatous meningitis, schwannomas, nasopharyngeal carcinoma, metastases, trigeminal neurilemmoma, pontine glioma, pituitary adenomas, and miscellaneous tumors). The remaining SNPs in the literature review were associated with other neurologic signs or symptoms, such as headache, tinnitus, disc edema, or nystagmus, or there were insufficient clinical data in the report to determine if the SNP was truly isolated.[27,35,41,43,46,48,50,59,65,66,67,97,177,178,179,183,195,196,199,200,203,204,205,207,208,209,210,211,212,213,214]

SNPs that occur after LP, postmyelographic LP, and spinal anesthesia have been reported in the literature.[213] Thorsen reported 229 cases of SNP after spinal anesthesia and LP.[215] Most of these SNPs occurred at the 10th day following LP, were unilateral, associated with headache, and occurred in young patients.[213,215] These patients may be followed for resolution without imaging (class IV, level C).

Aneurysm is a rare cause of acquired SNP. Rucker reported 924 cases of SNP, and only 31 (3.4%) were due to aneurysm.[216] Rush and Younge described 419 cases of SNP, and only 15 (3.6%) were due to aneurysm.[213] Other authors did not find any cases of aneurysm presenting with an isolated SNP in their series on cerebral aneurysms with ocular involvement,[179] and others have reported similar findings. We do not typically recommend evaluation for aneurysm in isolated SNP (class IV, level C), but aneurysm can cause SNP in patients with signs of subarachnoid hemorrhage, papilledema, or other cranial neuropathies. Unruptured internal carotid artery aneurysms in the cavernous sinus typically have multiple ocular motor cranial neuropathies or other cavernous sinus symptoms and signs. They rarely present as isolated SNP and we do not recommend routine angiography (e.g., CT angiography [CTA], MR angiography [MRA], or digital subtraction angiography [DSA]) studies for evaluating patients with isolated SNP (in contrast to third cranial nerve palsies).[217]

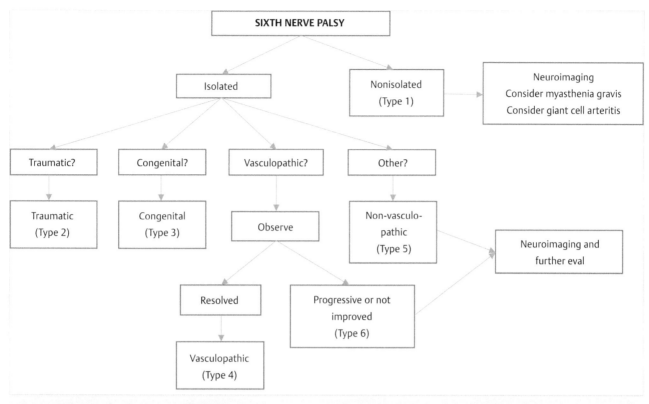

Fig. 13.1 Evaluation of sixth nerve palsy (SNP).

A suggested approach to the evaluation of SNP is presented in ▶ Fig. 13.1.

References

[1] Goodwin D. Differential diagnosis and management of acquired sixth cranial nerve palsy. Optometry. 2006; 77(11):534–539

[2] Patel SV, Holmes JM, Hodge DO, Burke JP. Diabetes and hypertension in isolated sixth nerve palsy: a population-based study. Ophthalmology. 2005; 112(5):760–763

[3] Patel SV, Mutyala S, Leske DA, Hodge DO, Holmes JM. Incidence, associations, and evaluation of sixth nerve palsy using a population-based method. Ophthalmology. 2004; 111(2):369–375

[4] Mahoney NR, Liu GT. Benign recurrent sixth (abducens) nerve palsies in children. Arch Dis Child. 2009; 94(5):394–396

[5] Yousuf SJ, Khan AO. Presenting features suggestive for later recurrence of idiopathic sixth nerve paresis in children. J AAPOS. 2007; 11(5):452–455

[6] Brazis PW, Masdeu JC, Biller J. Localization in Clinical Neurology. 4th ed. Philadelphia: Lippincott Williams & Wilkins; 2001

[7] Carr MM, Ross DA, Zuker RM. Cranial nerve defects in congenital facial palsy. [review]. J Otolaryngol. 1997; 26(2):80–87

[8] Pedraza S, Gámez J, Rovira A, et al. MRI findings in Möbius syndrome: correlation with clinical features. Neurology. 2000; 55(7):1058–1060

[9] Fernández S, Godino O, Martínez-Yélamos S, et al. Cavernous sinus syndrome: a series of 126 patients. Medicine (Baltimore). 2007; 86(5):278–281

[10] Thömke F. Isolated abducens palsies due to pontine lesions. Neuro-ophthalmology. 1998; 20:91–100

[11] Thömke F, Lensch E, Ringel K, Hopf HC. Isolated cranial nerve palsies in multiple sclerosis. J Neurol Neurosurg Psychiatry. 1997; 63(5):682–685

[12] King AJ, Stacey E, Stephenson G, Trimble RB. Spontaneous recovery rates for unilateral sixth nerve palsies. Eye (Lond). 1995; 9(Pt 4):476–478

[13] Lopez JM, Pego Reigosa R, Alonso Losada G, Lopez Facal S, Marin Sanchez M, Martinez Muñiz A. Bilateral infarction of the rostral pontine tegmentum as a cause of isolated bilateral supranuclear sixth nerve palsy related to hypertension. J Neurol Neurosurg Psychiatry. 1996; 60(2):238–239

[14] Balcer LJ, Galetta SL, Cornblath WT, Liu GT. Neuro-ophthalmologic manifestations of Maffucci's syndrome and Ollier's disease. J Neuroophthalmol. 1999; 19(1):62–66

[15] Landolfi JC, Thaler HT, DeAngelis LM. Adult brainstem gliomas. Neurology. 1998; 51(4):1136–1139

[16] Lee TG, Choi W-S, Chung K-C. Ophthalmoplegic migraine with reversible enhancement of intraparenchymal abducens nerve on MRI. Headache. 2002; 42(2):140–141

[17] Margari L, Legrottaglie AR, Craig F, Petruzzelli MG, Procoli U, Dicuonzo F. Ophthalmoplegic migraine: migraine or oculomotor neuropathy? Cephalalgia. 2012; 32(16):1208–1215

[18] Grosberg BM, Vollbracht S, Robbins MS, Lipton RB. Cephalgia. 2011; 31:122–125

[19] Hammam T, McFadzean RM, Ironside JW. Anti-Hu paraneoplastic syndrome presenting as bilateral sixth cranial nerve palsies. J Neuroophthalmol. 2005; 25(2):101–104

[20] Kalidindi RS, Balen F, Hassan A, Al-Din A. Persistent trigeminal artery presenting as intermittent isolated sixth nerve palsy. Clin Radiol. 2005; 60(4):515–519

[21] Narai H, Manabe Y, Deguchi K, Iwatsuki K, Sakai K, Abe K. Isolated abducens nerve palsy caused by vascular compression. Neurology. 2000; 55(3):453–454

[22] Ohtsuka K, Sone A, Igarashi Y, Akiba H, Sakata M. Vascular compressive abducens nerve palsy disclosed by magnetic resonance imaging. Am J Ophthalmol. 1996; 122(3):416–419

[23] Wolfe GI, Galetta SL, Mollman JE. Spontaneous remission of papilledema and sixth nerve palsy in acute lymphoblastic leukemia. J Neuroophthalmol. 1994; 14(2):91–94

[24] Chavis PS, Mullaney PB, Bohlega S. Fluctuating oculomotor signs in Arnold-Chiari malformation. Diagnostic pitfalls. Neuroophthalmology. 1998; 19:215–221

[25] Hirose Y, Sagoh M, Mayanagi K, Murakami H. Abducens nerve palsy caused by basilar impression associated with atlanto-occipital assimilation. Neurol Med Chir (Tokyo). 1998; 38(6):363–366

[26] Pinches E, Thompson D, Noordeen H, Liasis A, Nischal KK. Fourth and sixth cranial nerve injury after halo traction in children: a report of two cases. J AAPOS. 2004; 8(6):580–585

[27] Bell JA, Dowd TC, McIlwaine GG, Brittain GP. Postmyelographic abducent nerve palsy in association with the contrast agent iopamidol. J Clin Neuroophthalmol. 1990; 10(2):115–117

[28] Thömke F, Mika-Grüttner A, Visbeck A, Brühl K. The risk of abducens palsy after diagnostic lumbar puncture. Neurology. 2000; 54(3):768–769

[29] Cain RB, Patel NP, Hoxworth JM, Lal D. Abducens palsy after lumbar drain placement: a rare complication in endoscopic skull base surgery. Laryngoscope. 2013; 123(11):2633–2638

[30] Niedermüller U, Trinka E, Bauer G. Abducens palsy after lumbar puncture. Clin Neurol Neurosurg. 2002; 104(1):61–63

[31] Béchard P, Perron G, Larochelle D, Lacroix M, Labourdette A, Dolbec P. Case report: epidural blood patch in the treatment of abducens palsy after a dural puncture. Can J Anaesth. 2007; 54(2):146–150

[32] Hofer JE, Scavone BM. Cranial nerve VI palsy after dural-arachnoid puncture. Anesth Analg. 2015; 120(3):644–646

[33] Choudhari KA. Isolated abducent nerve palsy after microvascular decompression for trigeminal neuralgia: case report. Neurosurgery. 2005; 57(6):E1317–, discussion E1317

[34] Manzotti F, Menozzi C, Porta MR, Orsoni JG. Partial third nerve palsy after Measles Mumps Rubella vaccination. Ital J Pediatr. 2010; 36:59

[35] Dinakaran S, Desai SP, Corney CE. Case report: sixth nerve palsy following radiculography. Br J Radiol. 1995; 68(808):424

[36] Lloyd MN. Sixth nerve palsy following radiculography. Br J Radiol. 1995; 68 (813):1039–1040 [letter; comment]

[37] De Veuster I, Smet H, Vercauteren M, Tassignon MJ. The time course of a sixth nerve paresis following epidural anesthesia. Bull Soc Belge Ophtalmol. 1994; 252:45–47

[38] Corbonnois G, O'Neill T, Brabis-Henner A, Schmitt E, Hubert I, Bouaziz H. Unrecognized dural puncture during epidural analgesia in obstetrics later confirmed by brain imaging. Ann Fr Anesth Reanim. 2010; 29(7–8):584–588

[39] Sudhakar P, Trobe JD, Wesolowski J. Dural puncture-induced intracranial hypotension causing diplopia. J Neuroophthalmol. 2013; 33(2):106–112

[40] Dumont D, Hariz H, Meynieu P, Salama J, Dreyfus P, Boissier MC. Abducens palsy after an intrathecal glucocorticoid injection. Evidence for a role of intracranial hypotension. Rev Rhum Engl Ed. 1998; 65(5):352–354– (English edition)

[41] Fanous MM, Margo CE, Hamed LM. Chronic idiopathic inflammation of the retropharyngeal space presenting with sequential abducens palsies. J Clin Neuroophthalmol. 1992; 12(3):154–157

[42] Frohman LP, Grigorian R, Bielory L. Neuro-ophthalmic manifestations of sarcoidosis: clinical spectrum, evaluation, and management. J Neuroophthalmol. 2001; 21(2):132–137

[43] Sachs R, Kashii S, Burde RM. Sixth nerve palsy as the initial manifestation of sarcoidosis. Am J Ophthalmol. 1990; 110(4):438–440

[44] Newman NJ, Slamovits TL, Friedland S, Wilson WB. Neuro-ophthalmic manifestations of meningocerebral inflammation from the limited form of Wegener's granulomatosis. Am J Ophthalmol. 1995; 120(5):613–621

[45] Nagaoka U, Kato T, Kurita K, et al. Cranial nerve enhancement on three-dimensional MRI in Miller Fisher syndrome. Neurology. 1996; 47(6):1601–1602

[46] Hamilton SR, Smith CH, Lessell S. Idiopathic hypertrophic cranial pachymeningitis. J Clin Neuroophthalmol. 1993; 13(2):127–134

[47] Miwa H, Koshimura I, Mizuno Y. Recurrent cranial neuropathy as a clinical presentation of idiopathic inflammation of the dura mater: a possible relationship to Tolosa-Hunt syndrome and cranial pachymeningitis. J Neurol Sci. 1998; 154(1):101–105

[48] Lesser RL, Kornmehl EW, Pachner AR, et al. Neuro-ophthalmologic manifestations of Lyme disease. Ophthalmology. 1990; 97(6):699–706

[49] Mastrianni JA, Galetta SL, Raps EC, Liu GT, Volpe NJ. Isolated fascicular abducens nerve palsy and Lyme disease. J Neuroophthalmol. 1994; 14(1):2–5

[50] Slavin ML, Haimovic I, Patel M. Sixth nerve palsy and pontocerebellar mass due to luetic meningoencephalitis. Arch Ophthalmol. 1992; 110(3):322

[51] Stepper F, Schroth G, Sturzenegger M. Neurosyphilis mimicking Miller-Fisher syndrome: a case report and MRI findings. Neurology. 1998; 51(1):269–271

[52] Keane JR. Combined VIth and XIIth cranial nerve palsies: a clival syndrome. Neurology. 2000; 54(7):1540–1541

[53] Gavin C, Langan Y, Hutchinson M. Cranial and peripheral neuropathy due to Epstein-Barr virus infection. Postgrad Med J. 1997; 73(861):419–420

[54] Ross JJ, Worthington MG. Bilateral sixth nerve palsy in West Nile meningoencephalitis. J Neuroophthalmol. 2004; 24(1):97–98

[55] Kulkarni S, Lee A, Lee JH. Sixth and tenth nerve palsy secondary to pseudomonas infection of the skull base. Am J Ophthalmol. 2005; 139(5):918–920

[56] Hashimoto M, Ohtsuka K. Compressive lesions of the abducens nerve in the subarachnoid space disclosed by thin-slice magnetic resonance imaging. Ophthalmologica. 1998; 212(3):188–189

[57] Ichimi K, Yoshida J, Inao S, Wakabayashi T. Abducens nerve neurinoma–case report. Neurol Med Chir (Tokyo). 1997; 37(2):197–200

[58] Okada Y, Shima T, Nishida M, Okita S. Large sixth nerve neuroma involving the prepontine region: case report. Neurosurgery. 1997; 40(3):608–610

[59] Tung H, Chen T, Weiss MH. Sixth nerve schwannomas. Report of two cases. J Neurosurg. 1991; 75(4):638–641

[60] Forsyth PA, Cascino TL, Shaw EG, et al. Intracranial chordomas: a clinicopathological and prognostic study of 51 cases. J Neurosurg. 1993; 78(5):741–747

[61] Harada T, Ohashi T, Ohki K, et al. Clival chordoma presenting as acute esotropia due to bilateral abducens palsy. Ophthalmologica. 1997; 211(2):109–111

[62] Mekari-Sabbagh ON, DaCunha RP. Crossed eyes in a six-year-old girl. Surv Ophthalmol. 2001; 45(4):331–334

[63] Movsas TZ, Balcer LJ, Eggenberger ER, Hess JL, Galetta SL. Sixth nerve palsy as a presenting sign of intracranial plasmacytoma and multiple myeloma. J Neuroophthalmol. 2000; 20(4):242–245

[64] Volpe NJ, Liebsch NJ, Munzenrider JE, Lessell S. Neuro-ophthalmologic findings in chordoma and chondrosarcoma of the skull base. Am J Ophthalmol. 1993b; 115(1):97–104

[65] Averbuch-Heller L, Gillis S, Ben-Hur T. Transient sixth-nerve palsy as the first presentation of acute leukaemia. J Neurol Neurosurg Psychiatry. 1994; 57(4):506

[66] O'Boyle JE, Gardner TA, Oliva A, Enzenauer RW. Sixth nerve palsy as the initial presenting sign of metastatic prostate cancer. A case report and review of the literature. J Clin Neuroophthalmol. 1992; 12(3):149–153

[67] Volpe NJ, Lessell S. Remitting sixth nerve palsy in skull base tumors. Arch Ophthalmol. 1993a; 111(10):1391–1395

[68] Brazis PW, Wharen RE, Czervionke LF, Witte RJ, Jones AD. Hemangioma of the mandibular branch of the trigeminal nerve in the Meckel cave presenting with facial pain and sixth nerve palsy. J Neuroophthalmol. 2000; 20(1):14–16

[69] Kosker M, Sener D, Kilic O, et al. Primary diffuse leptomeningeal gliomatosis mimicking tuberculous meningitis. J Child Neurol. 2014; 29(12):NP171–NP175

[70] Noval S, Ortiz-Pérez S, Sánchez-Dalmau BF, Ruiz-Ares G, Arpa J, Adán A. Neuro-ophthalmological features of primary diffuse leptomeningeal gliomatosis. J Neuroophthalmol. 2011; 31(4):299–305

[71] Somja J, Boly M, Sadzot B, Moonen G, Deprez M. Primary diffuse leptomeningeal gliomatosis: an autopsy case and review of the literature. Acta Neurol Belg. 2010; 110(4):325–333

[72] Ishige S, Iwadate Y, Ishikura H, Saeki N. Primary diffuse leptomeningeal gliomatosis followed with serial magnetic resonance images. Neuropathology. 2007; 27(3):290–294

[73] Arias M, Alberte-Woodward M, Arias S, Dapena D, Prieto A, Suárez-Peñaranda JM. Primary malignant meningeal melanomatosis: a clinical, radiological and pathologic case study. Acta Neurol Belg. 2011; 111(3):228–231

[74] Psarros TG, Swift D, Mulne AF, Burns DK. Neurocytoma-like neoplasm of the thoracic spine in a 15-month-old child presenting with diffuse leptomeningeal dissemination and communicating hydrocephalus. Case report. J Neurosurg. 2005; 103(2) Suppl:184–190

[75] Aroichane M, Repka MX. Outcome of sixth nerve palsy or paresis in young children. J Pediatr Ophthalmol Strabismus. 1995; 32(3):152–156

[76] Krishna R, Kosmorsky GS, Wright KW. Pseudotumor cerebri sine papilledema with unilateral sixth nerve palsy. J Neuroophthalmol. 1998; 18(1):53–55

[77] Patton N, Beatty S, Lloyd IC. Bilateral sixth and fourth cranial nerve palsies in idiopathic intracranial hypertension. J R Soc Med. 2000; 93(2):80–81

[78] Biousse V, Ameri A, Bousser M-G. Isolated intracranial hypertension as the only sign of cerebral venous thrombosis. Neurology. 1999; 53(7):1537–1542

[79] Morrison DG, Phuah HK, Reddy AT, Dure LS, Kline LB. Ophthalmologic involvement in the syndrome of headache, neurologic deficits, and cerebrospinal fluid lymphocytosis. Ophthalmology. 2003; 110(1):115–118

[80] Apte RS, Bartek W, Mello A, Haq A. Spontaneous intracranial hypotension. Am J Ophthalmol. 1999; 127(4):482–485

[81] Case Records of the Massachusetts General Hospital. Case records of the Massachusetts General Hospital. Weekly clinicopathological exercises. Case 2-1998. A 50-year-old woman with increasing headache and a left abducent-nerve palsy. N Engl J Med. 1998; 338(3):180–188

[82] Ferrante E, Savino A, Brioschi A, Marazzi R, Donato MF, Riva M. Transient oculomotor cranial nerves palsy in spontaneous intracranial hypotension. J Neurosurg Sci. 1998; 42(3):177–179, discussion 180

[83] Horton JC, Fishman RA. Neurovisual findings in the syndrome of spontaneous intracranial hypotension from dural cerebrospinal fluid leak. Ophthalmology. 1994; 101(2):244–251

[84] Mokri B, Piepgras DG, Miller GM. Syndrome of orthostatic headaches and diffuse pachymeningeal gadolinium enhancement. Mayo Clin Proc. 1997; 72 (5):400–413

[85] O'Carroll CP, Brant-Zawadzki M. The syndrome of spontaneous intracranial hypotension. Cephalalgia. 1999; 19(2):80–87

[86] Schievink WI, Meyer FB, Atkinson JLD, Mokri B. Spontaneous spinal cerebrospinal fluid leaks and intracranial hypotension. J Neurosurg. 1996; 84(4):598–605

[87] Khemka S, Mearza AA. Isolated sixth nerve palsy secondary to spontaneous intracranial hypotension. Eur J Neurol. 2006; 13(11):1264–1265

[88] Hollis GJ. Sixth cranial nerve palsy following closed head injury in a child. J Accid Emerg Med. 1997; 14(3):172–175

[89] Holmes JM, Droste PJ, Beck RW. The natural history of acute traumatic sixth nerve palsy or paresis. J AAPOS. 1998; 2(5):265–268

[90] Lepore FE. Disorders of ocular motility following head trauma. Arch Neurol. 1995; 52(9):924–926

[91] Mizushima H, Kobayashi N, Sawabe Y, et al. Epidural hematoma of the clivus. Case report. J Neurosurg. 1998; 88(3):590–593

[92] Qasho R, Vangelista T, Rocchi G, Ferrante L, Delfini R. Abducens nerve paresis as first symptom of trigeminal neurinoma. Report of two cases and review of the literature. J Neurosurg Sci. 1999; 43(3):223–228

[93] Pane A. Paget disease manifesting with compressive sixth-nerve palsy that resolved with intravenous zoledronic acid therapy. Arch Ophthalmol. 2007; 125(10):1440–1441

[94] Homer JJ, Johnson IJ, Jones NS. Middle ear infection and sixth nerve palsy. J Laryngol Otol. 1996; 110(9):872–874

[95] Davé AV, Diaz-Marchan PJ, Lee AG. Clinical and magnetic resonance imaging features of Gradenigo syndrome. Am J Ophthalmol. 1997; 124(4):568–570

[96] Kuehnen J, Schwartz A, Neff W, Hennerici M. Cranial nerve syndrome in thrombosis of the transverse/sigmoid sinuses. Brain. 1998; 121(Pt 2): 381–388

[97] Antoniades K, Karakasis D, Taskos N. Abducent nerve palsy following transverse fracture of the middle cranial fossa. J Craniomaxillofac Surg. 1993; 21(4):172–175

[98] Mutyala S, Holmes JM, Hodge DO, Younge BR. Spontaneous recovery rate in traumatic sixth-nerve palsy. Am J Ophthalmol. 1996; 122(6):898–899

[99] Harrigan MR, Chandler WF. Abducens nerve palsy after radiofrequency rhizolysis for trigeminal neuralgia: case report. Neurosurgery. 1998; 43(3): 623–625

[100] Stomal-Słowińska M, Słowiński J, Lee TK, et al. Correlation of clinical findings and results of percutaneous balloon compression for patients with trigeminal neuralgia. Clin Neurol Neurosurg. 2011; 113(1):14–21

[101] Kefalopoulou Z, Markaki E, Constantoyannis C. Avoiding abducens nerve palsy during the percutaneous balloon compression procedure. Stereotact Funct Neurosurg. 2009; 87(2):101–104

[102] Brown JA, Preul MC. Percutaneous trigeminal ganglion compression for trigeminal neuralgia. Experience in 22 patients and review of the literature. J Neurosurg. 1989; 70(6):900–904

[103] Chatterjee N, Chatterjee S, Roy C. Abducens nerve palsy after percutaneous radiofrequency ablation of Gasserian ganglion. J Neurosurg Anesthesiol. 2014; 26(1):89–90

[104] Keane JR. Cavernous sinus syndrome. Analysis of 151 cases. Arch Neurol. 1996; 53(10):967–971

[105] Kriss TC, Kriss VM, Warf BC. Cavernous sinus thrombophlebitis: case report. Neurosurgery. 1996; 39(2):385–389

[106] Eggenberger E, Lee AG, Forget TR, Jr, Rosenwasser R. A bruital headache and double vision. Surv Ophthalmol. 2000; 45(2):147–153

[107] Lee KY, Kim SM, Kim DI. Isolated bilateral abducens nerve palsy due to carotid cavernous dural arteriovenous fistula. Yonsei Med J. 1998; 39(3):283–286

[108] Uehara T, Tabuchi M, Kawaguchi T, Mori E. Spontaneous dural carotid cavernous sinus fistula presenting isolated ophthalmoplegia: evaluation with MR angiography. Neurology. 1998; 50(3):814–816

[109] Polito E, Leccisotti A. Painful ophthalmoplegia caused by superior ophthalmic vein thrombosis. Neuro-ophthalmology. 1996; 16(3):189–192

[110] Eisenberg MB, Al-Mefty O, DeMonte F, Burson GT. Benign nonmeningeal tumors of the cavernous sinus. Neurosurgery. 1999; 44(5):949–954, discussion 954–955

[111] Bachmeyer C, Levy V, Carteret M, et al. Sphenoid sinus localization of multiple myeloma revealing evolution from benign gammopathy. Head Neck. 1997; 19(4):347–350

[112] Liu GT, Kay MD, Byrne GE, Glaser JS, Schatz N. Ophthalmoparesis due to Burkitt's lymphoma following cardiac transplantation. Neurology. 1993; 43 (10):2147–2149

[113] Roman-Goldstein SM, Jones A, Delashaw JB, McMenomey S, Neuwelt EA. Atypical central nervous system lymphoma at the cranial base: report of four cases. Neurosurgery. 1998; 43(3):613–615, discussion 615–616

[114] Kasner SE, Galetta SL, Vaughn DJ. Cavernous sinus syndrome in Hodgkin's disease. J Neuroophthalmol. 1996; 16(3):204–207

[115] Lee AG, Miller NR, Brazis PW, Benson ML. Cavernous sinus hemangioma. Clinical and neuroimaging features. J Neuroophthalmol. 1995; 15(4):225–229

[116] Phookan G, Davis AT, Holmes B. Hemangioendothelioma of the cavernous sinus: case report. Neurosurgery. 1998; 42(5):1153–1155, discussion 1155–1156

[117] Kawase T, Shiobara R, Ohira T, Toya S. Developmental patterns and characteristic symptoms of petroclival meningiomas. Neurol Med Chir (Tokyo). 1996; 36(1):1–6

[118] Arita K, Sugiyama K, Tominaga A, Yamasaki F. Intrasellar rhabdomyosarcoma: case report. Neurosurgery. 2001; 48(3):677–680

[119] Rodríguez JA, Hedges TR, III, Heilman CB, Strominger MB, Laver NM. Painful sixth cranial nerve palsy caused by a malignant trigeminal nerve sheath tumor. J Neuroophthalmol. 2007; 27(1):29–31

[120] Muneer A, Jones NS. Unilateral abducens nerve palsy: a presenting sign of sphenoid sinus mucocoeles. J Laryngol Otol. 1997; 111(7):644–646

[121] Jacob M, Gujar S, Trobe J, Gandhi D. Spontaneous resolution of a Meckel's cave arachnoid cyst causing sixth cranial nerve palsy. J Neuroophthalmol. 2008; 28(3):186–191

[122] Chang-Godinich A, Lee AG, Brazis PW, Liesegang TJ, Jones DB. Complete ophthalmoplegia after zoster ophthalmicus. J Neuroophthalmol. 1997; 17 (4):262–265

[123] Mansour AM, Bailey BJ. Ocular findings in Ramsay Hunt syndrome. J Neuroophthalmol. 1997; 17(3):199–201

[124] Smith EF, Santamarina L, Wolintz AH. Herpes zoster ophthalmicus as a cause of Horner syndrome. J Clin Neuroophthalmol. 1993; 13(4):250–253

[125] Holland NR, Deibert E. CNS actinomycosis presenting with bilateral cavernous sinus syndrome. J Neurol Neurosurg Psychiatry. 1998; 64(1):4

[126] Tobias S, Lee JH, Tomford JW. Rare Actinobacillus infection of the cavernous sinus causing painful ophthalmoplegia: case report. Neurosurgery. 2002; 51 (3):807–809, discussion 809–810

[127] van Toorn R, Esser M, Smit D, Andronikou S. Idiopathic hypertrophic cranial pachymeningitis causing progressive polyneuropathies in a child. Eur J Paediatr Neurol. 2008; 12(2):144–147

[128] Fitzsimon JS, Toland J, Philips J, et al. Trends and developments: giant aneurysms in the cavernous sinus. Neuro-ophthalmology. 1995; 15:59–65

[129] Hahn CD, Nicolle DA, Lownie SP, Drake CG. Giant cavernous carotid aneurysms: clinical presentation in fifty-seven cases. J Neuroophthalmol. 2000; 20(4):253–258

[130] Silva MN, Saeki N, Hirai S, Yamaura A. Unusual cranial nerve palsy caused by cavernous sinus aneurysms. Clinical and anatomical considerations reviewed. Surg Neurol. 1999; 52(2):143–148, discussion 148–149

[131] Kerty E. The ophthalmology of internal carotid artery dissection. Acta Ophthalmol Scand. 1999; 77(4):418–421

[132] Lemesle M, Beuriat P, Becker F, Martin D, Giroud M, Dumas R. Head pain associated with sixth-nerve palsy: spontaneous dissection of the internal carotid artery. Cephalalgia. 1998; 18(2):112–114

[133] Blumenthal EZ, Gomori JM, Dotan S. Recurrent abducens nerve palsy caused by dolichoectasia of the cavernous internal carotid artery. Am J Ophthalmol. 1997; 124(2):255–257

[134] Neugebauer A, Kirsch A, Fricke J, Rüssmann W. New onset of crossed eyes in an adult. Surv Ophthalmol. 2001; 45(4):335–344

[135] Foroozan R. Spontaneous resolution of sixth nerve palsy with ipsilateral cavernous carotid dolichoectasia. Br J Ophthalmol. 2004; 88(4):586–587

[136] Lopes DK, Mericle RA, Wakhloo AK, Guterman LR, Hopkins LN. Cavernous sinus syndrome during balloon test occlusion of the cervical internal carotid artery. Report of two cases. J Neurosurg. 1998; 89(4):667–670

[137] Alderson LM, Noonan PT, Choi IS, Henson JW. Regional subacute cranial neuropathies following internal carotid cisplatin infusion. Neurology. 1996; 47(4):1088–1090

[138] Wu HM, Lee AG, Lehane DE, Chi TL, Lewis RA. Ocular and orbital complications of intraarterial cisplatin. A case report. J Neuroophthalmol. 1997; 17(3):195–198

[139] Lazow SK, Izzo SR, Feinberg ME, Berger JR. Bilateral abducens nerve palsy secondary to maxillofacial trauma: report of case with proposed mechanism of injury. J Oral Maxillofac Surg. 1995; 53(10):1197–1199

[140] Wang CH, Chou ML, Huang CH. Benign isolated abducens nerve palsy in Mycoplasma pneumoniae infection. Pediatr Neurol. 1998; 18(1):71–72

[141] Mikkilä HO, Seppälä IJT, Viljanen MK, Peltomaa MP, Karma A. The expanding clinical spectrum of ocular Lyme borreliosis. Ophthalmology. 2000; 107(3): 581–587

[142] Roberts BN, Mills PV, Hawksworth NJ. Bilateral ptosis, tonic pupils and abducens palsies following Campylobacter jejuni enteritis. Eye (Lond). 1995; 9(Pt 5):657–658

[143] Ifergane G, Merkin S, Valdman I, et al. Ocular manifestations of Jakob-Creutzfeldt disease (CJD). Neuroophthalmology. 1998; 20:21

[144] Ormerod LD, Rhodes RH, Gross SA, Crane LR, Houchin KW. Ophthalmologic manifestations of acquired immune deficiency syndrome-associated progressive multifocal leukoencephalopathy. Ophthalmology. 1996; 103(6): 899–906

[145] Shaw JA, Strachan FM, Sawers HA, Bevan JS. Non-Hodgkin lymphoma with panhypopituitarism, hyperprolactinaemia and sixth nerve palsy. J R Soc Med. 1997; 90(5):274–275

[146] Bhatti MT, Yuan C, Winter W, McSwain AS, Okun MS. Bilateral sixth nerve paresis in the Bing-Neel syndrome. Neurology. 2005; 64(3):576–577

[147] Ropper AH. Four new variants of Guillain-Barré syndrome. Ann Neurol. 1993; 34:306

[148] al-Din SN, Anderson M, Eeg-Olofsson O, Trontelj JV. Neuro-ophthalmic manifestations of the syndrome of ophthalmoplegia, ataxia and areflexia: a review. Acta Neurol Scand. 1994; 89(3):157–163

[149] Chiba A, Kusunoki S, Obata H, Machinami R, Kanazawa I. Serum anti-GQ1b IgG antibody is associated with ophthalmoplegia in Miller Fisher syndrome and Guillain-Barré syndrome: clinical and immunohistochemical studies. Neurology. 1993; 43(10):1911–1917

[150] Chiba A, Kusunoki S, Shimizu T, Kanazawa I. Serum IgG antibody to ganglioside GQ1b is a possible marker of Miller Fisher syndrome. Ann Neurol. 1992; 31(6):677–679

[151] Igarashi Y, Takeda M, Maekawa H, Ohguro H, Ohyachi H, Ogasawara K. Fisher's syndrome without total ophthalmoplegia. Ophthalmologica. 1992; 205(3):163–167

[152] Suzuki T, Chiba A, Kusunoki S, Chikuda M, Fujita T, Misu K. Anti-GQ1b ganglioside antibody and ophthalmoplegia of undetermined cause. Br J Ophthalmol. 1998; 82(8):916–918

[153] Sato K, Yoshikawa H. Bilateral abducens nerve paresis associated with anti-GQ1b IgG antibody. Am J Ophthalmol. 2001; 131(6):816–818

[154] Ropper AH, Wijdisks EFM, Truax BT. Guillain-Barre Syndrome. Philadelphia: FA Davis; 1991

[155] Wokke JH, van den Berg LH, van Schaik JP. Sixth nerve palsy from a CNS lesion in chronic inflammatory demyelinating polyneuropathy. J Neurol Neurosurg Psychiatry. 1996; 60(6):695–696

[156] Haughton AJ, Chalkiadis GA. Unintentional paediatric subdural catheter with oculomotor and abducens nerve palsies. Paediatr Anaesth. 1999; 9(6):543–548

[157] Fung TY, Chung TK. Abducens nerve palsy complicating pregnancy: a case report. Eur J Obstet Gynecol Reprod Biol. 1999; 83(2):223–224

[158] Lash SC, Williams CP, Marsh CS, Crithchley C, Hodgkins PR, Mackie EJ. Acute sixth-nerve palsy after vincristine therapy. J AAPOS. 2004; 8(1):67–68

[159] Arnault JP, Petitpain N, Granel-Brocard F, Cuny JF, Barbaud A, Schmutz JL. Acitretin and sixth nerve palsy. J Eur Acad Dermatol Venereol. 2007; 21(9): 1258–1259

[160] Chroni E, Tsambaos D. Isolated sixth nerve palsy during acitretin treatment: a retinoid side effect or a mere coincidence? J Eur Acad Dermatol Venereol. 2008; 22(8):1024–1025, author reply 1025

[161] Parkins GJ, Brennan KM, Wylie G. Sixth cranial nerve palsy due to acitretin. Clin Exp Dermatol. 2016; 41(2):213–214

[162] Greenblatt D, Sheth N, Teixeira F, Acland K. Isolated sixth nerve palsy following low dose oral methotrexate. Dermatol Online J. 2007; 13(4):19

[163] Dasgupta S, Adilieje C, Bhattacharya A, Smith B, Sheikh Mu. Capecitabine and sixth cranial nerve palsy. J Cancer Res Ther. 2010; 6(1):80–81

[164] Cakmak HB, Toklu Y, Yorgun MA, Simşek S. Isolated sixth nerve palsy after intravitreal bevacizumab injection. Strabismus. 2010; 18(1):18–20

[165] Micieli JA, Santiago P, Brent MH. Third nerve palsy following intravitreal anti-VEGF therapy for bilateral neovascular age-related macular degeneration. Acta Ophthalmol. 2011; 89(1):e99–e100

[166] Park HJ, Guy J. Sixth nerve palsy post intravitreal bevacizumab for AMD: a new possibly causal relationship and complication? Binocul Vis Strabismus Q. 2007; 22(4):209

[167] Fukumoto Y, Shigemitsu T, Kajii N, Omura R, Harada T, Okita K. Abducent nerve paralysis during interferon alpha-2a therapy in a case of chronic active hepatitis C. Intern Med. 1994; 33(10):637–640

[168] Oishi A, Miyamoto K, Kashii S, Yoshimura N. Abducens palsy and Sjogren's syndrome induced by pegylated interferon therapy. Br J Ophthalmol. 2007; 91(6):843–844

[169] Mellon G, Stitou H, Aoun O, et al. Lateral rectus muscle paralysis induced by ribavirin and pegylated interferon-α2a in a patient with HIV/HCV co-infection. J Infect Chemother. 2012; 18(6):937–938

[170] Openshaw H, Slatkin NE, Smith E. Eye movement disorders in bone marrow transplant patients on cyclosporin and ganciclovir. Bone Marrow Transplant. 1997; 19(5):503–505

[171] Schroeder B, Brieden S. Bilateral sixth nerve palsy associated with MDMA ("ecstasy") abuse. Am J Ophthalmol. 2000; 129(3):408–409

[172] Scott JK, Moxham BJ, Downie IP. Upper lip blanching and diplopia associated with local anaesthesia of the inferior alveolar nerve. Br Dent J. 2007; 202(1): 32–33

[173] Kocer B, Ergan S, Nazliel B. Isolated abducens nerve palsy following mandibular block articaine anesthesia, a first manifestation of multiple sclerosis: a case report. Quintessence Int. 2009; 40(3):251–256

[174] Balaji SM. Transient diplopia in dental outpatient clinic: an uncommon iatrogenic event. Indian J Dent Res. 2010; 21(1):132–134

[175] Sarma CM, Babu BV, Manjulamma M. Sixth nerve palsy following dental anaesthesia. Indian J Ophthalmol. 1989; 37(1):27

[176] Walker M, Drangsholt M, Czartoski TJ, Longstreth WT, Jr. Dental diplopia with transient abducens palsy. Neurology. 2004; 63(12):2449–2450

[177] Galbraith RS. Incidence of neonatal sixth nerve palsy in relation to mode of delivery. Am J Obstet Gynecol. 1994; 170(4):1158–1159

[178] Nemzek W, Postma G, Poirier V, Hecht S. MR features of pachymeningitis presenting with sixth-nerve palsy secondary to sphenoid sinusitis. AJNR Am J Neuroradiol. 1995; 16(4) Suppl:960–963

[179] Steel TR, Bentivoglio PB, Garrick R. Vascular neurofibromatosis affecting the internal carotid artery: a case report. Br J Neurosurg. 1994; 8(2): 233–237

[180] Holmes JM, Beck RW, Kip KE, Droste PJ, Leske DA, Pediatric Eye Disease Investigator Group. Predictors of nonrecovery in acute traumatic sixth nerve palsy and paresis. Ophthalmology. 2001; 108(8):1457–1460

[181] Dhaliwal A, West AL, Trobe JD, Musch DC. Third, fourth, and sixth cranial nerve palsies following closed head injury. J Neuroophthalmol. 2006; 26(1): 4–10

[182] Sharma B, Gupta R, Anand R, Ingle R. Ocular manifestations of head injury and incidence of post-traumatic ocular motor nerve involvement in cases of head injury: a clinical review. Int Ophthalmol. 2014; 34(4):893–900

[183] Leung AKC. Transient sixth cranial nerve palsy in newborn infants. Br J Clin Pract. 1987; 41(4):717–718

[184] Volpe NJ, Lee AG. Do patients with neurologically isolated ocular motor cranial nerve palsies require prompt neuroimaging? J Neuroophthalmol. 2014; 34(3):301–305

[185] Tiffin PA, MacEwen CJ, Craig EA, Clayton G. Acquired palsy of the oculomotor, trochlear and abducens nerves. Eye (Lond). 1996; 10(Pt 3): 377–384

[186] Sanders SK, Kawasaki A, Purvin VA. Long-term prognosis in patients with vasculopathic sixth nerve palsy. Am J Ophthalmol. 2002; 134(1):81–84

[187] Miller RW, Lee AG, Schiffman JS, et al. A practice pathway for the initial diagnostic evaluation of isolated sixth cranial nerve palsies. Med Decis Making. 1999; 19(1):42–48

[188] Murchison AP, Gilbert ME, Savino PJ. Neuroimaging and acute ocular motor mononeuropathies: a prospective study. Arch Ophthalmol. 2011; 129(3): 301–305

[189] Mehta S, Loevner LA, Mikityansky I, et al. The diagnostic and economic yield of neuroimaging in neuro-ophthalmology. J Neuroophthalmol. 2012; 32(2): 139–144

[190] Tamhankar MA, Biousse V, Ying GS, et al. Isolated third, fourth, and sixth cranial nerve palsies from presumed microvascular versus other causes: a prospective study. Ophthalmology. 2013; 120(11):2264–2269

[191] Chou KL, Galetta SL, Liu GT, et al. Acute ocular motor mononeuropathies: prospective study of the roles of neuroimaging and clinical assessment. J Neurol Sci. 2004; 219(1–2):35–39

[192] Bendszus M, Beck A, Koltzenburg M, et al. MRI in isolated sixth nerve palsies. Neuroradiology. 2001; 43(9):742–745

[193] Frassanito P, Massimi L, Rigante M, et al. Recurrent and self-remitting sixth cranial nerve palsy: pathophysiological insight from skull base chondrosarcoma. J Neurosurg Pediatr. 2013; 12(6):633–636

[194] Akagi T, Miyamoto K, Kashii S, Yoshimura N. Cause and prognosis of neurologically isolated third, fourth, or sixth cranial nerve dysfunction in cases of oculomotor palsy. Jpn J Ophthalmol. 2008; 52(1):32–35

[195] Rush JA, Younge BR. Paralysis of cranial nerves III, IV, and VI. Cause and prognosis in 1,000 cases. Arch Ophthalmol. 1981; 99(1):76–79

[196] Burde RM, Savino PJ, Trobe JD. Clinical Decisions in Neuro-ophthalmology. 2nd ed. St. Louis: Mosby Year Book; 1992:289–311

[197] Reich KA, Giansiracusa DF, Strongwater SL. Neurologic manifestations of giant cell arteritis. Am J Med. 1990; 89(1):67–72

[198] Jacobson DM. Progressive ophthalmoplegia with acute ischemic abducens nerve palsies. Am J Ophthalmol. 1996; 122(2):278–279

[199] Straussberg R, Cohen AH, Amir J, Varsano I. Benign abducens palsy associated with EBV infection. J Pediatr Ophthalmol Strabismus. 1993; 30(1):60

[200] Savino PJ. Diplopia and sixth nerve palsies. Semin Neurol. 1986; 6(2): 142–146

[201] Doss M, Araneta R, III, Fiel-Gan M, Edelheit B. Cranial nerve VI palsy as an initial presentation of necrotizing sarcoid granulomatosis in a 14-year-old female: case report and literature review. Semin Arthritis Rheum. 2015; 44 (4):456–460

[202] Shioya A, Takuma H, Shiigai M, Ishii A, Tamaoka A. Sixth nerve palsy associated with obstruction in Dorello's canal, accompanied by nodular type muscular sarcoidosis. J Neurol Sci. 2014; 343(1–2):203–205

[203] Savino PJ, Hilliker JK, Casell GH, Schatz NJ. Chronic sixth nerve palsies. Are they really harbingers of serious intracranial disease? Arch Ophthalmol. 1982; 100(9):1442–1444

[204] Watanabe K, Hagura R, Akanuma Y, et al. Characteristics of cranial nerve palsies in diabetic patients. Diabetes Res Clin Pract. 1990; 10(1):19–27

[205] Moster ML, Savino PJ, Sergott RC, Bosley TM, Schatz NJ. Isolated sixth-nerve palsies in younger adults. Arch Ophthalmol. 1984; 102(9):1328–1330

[206] Galetta SL, Smith JL. Chronic isolated sixth nerve palsies. Arch Neurol. 1989; 46(1):79–82

[207] Barry-Kinsella C, Milner M, McCarthy N, Walshe J. Sixth nerve palsy: an unusual manifestation of preeclampsia. Obstet Gynecol. 1994; 83(5 Pt 2): 849–851

[208] Depper MH, Truwit CL, Dreisbach JN, Kelly WM. Isolated abducens nerve palsy: MR imaging findings. AJR Am J Roentgenol. 1993; 160(4):837–841

[209] Fujioka T, Segawa F, Ogawa K, Kurihara T, Kinoshita M. Ischemic and hemorrhagic brain stem lesions mimicking diabetic ophthalmoplegia. Clin Neurol Neurosurg. 1995; 97(2):167–171

[210] Lee J. Modern management of sixth nerve palsy. Aust N Z J Ophthalmol. 1992; 20(1):41–46

[211] Lee J, Harris S, Cohen J, Cooper K, MacEwen C, Jones S. Results of a prospective randomized trial of botulinum toxin therapy in acute unilateral sixth nerve palsy. J Pediatr Ophthalmol Strabismus. 1994; 31 (5):283–286

[212] Lewis AI, Tomsick TA, Tew JM, Jr. Management of 100 consecutive direct carotid-cavernous fistulas: results of treatment with detachable balloons. Neurosurgery. 1995; 36(2):239–244, discussion 244–245

[213] Simcock PR, Kelleher S, Dunne JA. Neuro-ophthalmic findings in botulism type B. Eye (Lond). 1994; 8(Pt 6):646–648

[214] Yang MC, Bateman JB, Yee RD, Apt L. Electrooculography and discriminant analysis in Duane's syndrome and sixth-cranial-nerve palsy. Graefes Arch Clin Exp Ophthalmol. 1991; 229(1):52–56

[215] Thorsen G. Neurological complications after spinal anesthesia. Acta Chir Scand. 1947; 5 Suppl 121:l–272

[216] Rucker CW. The causes of paralysis of the third, fourth and sixth cranial nerves. Am J Ophthalmol. 1966; 61(5 Pt 2):1293–1298

[217] Tso MK, Macdonald RL. Neuro-ophthalmic assessment in unruptured intracranial aneurysms. World Neurosurg. 2015; 84(1):12–14

14 Supranuclear Disorders of Gaze

Alison K. Yoder

Abstract

Supranuclear structures coordinate the ocular motor movements of the eyes. As suggested by the name, supranuclear disorders of gaze are due to lesions higher in the neurological pathways than the cranial nerve nuclei that control the extraocular movements. This chapter discusses the clinical pathways in localizing and diagnosing horizontal and vertical gaze palsies, as well as internuclear ophthalmoplegia and similar syndromes. Reported etiologies from the literature are reviewed in detail.

Keywords: supranuclear gaze palsy, horizontal gaze palsy, vertical gaze palsy, internuclear ophthalmoplegia, one-and-a-half syndrome

14.1 What Is the Anatomy of Horizontal Conjugate Gaze?

Supranuclear structures coordinate the action of muscle groups and control two types of eye movements: conjugate movements (both eyes move in the same direction) and vergence movements (both eyes move in opposite directions). The vergence movements can either turn in (converge) or turn out (diverge).[1] All of the supranuclear components act through a "final common pathway" for horizontal conjugate gaze. This final common pathway starts in the abducens nucleus (composed of two types of intermingled neurons: motor neurons and internuclear neurons). The axons of the internuclear neurons cross to the contralateral side in the lower pons, ascend in the medial longitudinal fasciculus (MLF), and synapse in the portion of the oculomotor nucleus that innervates the medial rectus muscle. The final common pathway is modulated by several inputs: the vestibular, optokinetic, smooth pursuit, and saccadic systems. As an example, an excitatory horizontal vestibulo-ocular impulse originating in the horizontal canal is relayed from the ipsilateral medial vestibular nucleus to the contralateral abducens nucleus, resulting in conjugate horizontal deviation of the eyes to the contralateral side.[2,3,4]

14.2 Where Are Lesions Causing Horizontal Gaze Palsies Located?

A lesion located anywhere along the supranuclear, nuclear, and infranuclear pathways that control horizontal eye movements may cause a horizontal gaze palsy. Depending on the location of the lesion, horizontal pursuit or saccades, or both, may be impaired. Lesions causing defects in horizontal smooth pursuit are summarized in ▶ Table 14.1. Lesions causing defects in horizontal saccadic eye movements are summarized ▶ Table 14.2. Congenital and familial forms of bilateral horizontal gaze palsy can affect both pursuit and saccadic movements.[5,6,7,8,9] The gaze palsy may occur in isolation[10] or as part of a syndrome of horizontal gaze palsy with progressive scoliosis (HGPPS), an autosomal recessive disorder due to mutations in the ROBO3 gene on

chromosome 11.[11,12] Some patients may have an associated Moebius syndrome, limited abduction of one or both eyes, and nonprogressive facial weakness. Magnetic resonance imaging (MRI) may reveal absence or hypoplasia of the abducens nuclei and atrophy of the pons and/or medulla.[5,10,11,12]

There are reports of bilateral, symmetrical pontine infarcts involving both abducens nuclei, which resulted in the patient's complete inability to make any conjugate horizontal eye movements, smooth pursuit, or saccadic.[42] Bilateral horizontal gaze palsy has also been reported with recurrent ovarian teratoma, and resolved completely following removal of the neoplasm. In this case, a T2 MRI image showed a hyperintense signal in the midline dorsal pons.[43]

14.3 What Studies Are Indicated in a Patient with a Horizontal Gaze Palsy?

In general, unilateral restriction of voluntary horizontal conjugate gaze to one side is usually due to contralateral frontal or ipsilateral pontine damage. At the bedside, pontine lesions can usually be differentiated from supranuclear lesions by associated neurologic findings and by the oculocephalic (doll's-eye) maneuver or caloric stimulation. These latter procedures will overcome gaze deviations induced by supranuclear lesions but will not overcome gaze deviations caused by pontine lesions. Structural lesions, such as infarction, hemorrhage, vascular

Table 14.1 Localization of lesions impairing horizontal pursuit eye movements

Localization	Deficit
Frontal lobe	Impaired ipsilateral horizontal smooth pursuit[13]
Posterior parietal cortex or temporo-occipito-parietal region	Decrease the amplitude and velocity of smooth pursuit toward lesion[14,15,16]
Occipitotemporal areas posteriorly, through the internal sagittal stratum, the posterior and anterior limbs of the internal capsule with adjacent striatum, to the dorsomedial frontal cortex anteriorly	Ipsilesional pursuit deficits[15]
Posterior thalamic lesion	Deficit in smooth pursuit toward lesion[17]
Unilateral midbrain or pontine lesion	Ipsilateral pursuit defects[2,18,19,20,21,22,23,24]
Unilateral cerebellar damage	Transient impairment of pursuit in direction of involved side
Bilateral cerebellar damage	Permanent impairment of smooth pursuit eye movements[25]
Posterior vermal lesion	May impair pursuit[26]
Middle cerebellar peduncle lesions or floccular lesions	Ipsilateral pursuit defect[21,24,27]

Table 14.2 Localization of lesions causing impaired horizontal conjugate saccadic eye movements

Localization	Deficit
Frontal lobe lesions	• Transient neglect contralaterally • Defect in generating voluntary saccades • Transient horizontal gaze deviation ipsilaterally acutely • Gaze palsy overcome with the oculocephalic maneuver or caloric stimulation • Late disorders of saccades (contralateral more than ipsilateral) due to frontal eye field (FEF) lesions[28,29] • Prolonged eye deviation after stroke implies large stroke or preexisting damage to the contralateral frontal region[30] • Impaired ability to make a remembered sequence of saccades to visible targets (supplementary eye field lesions) • Impaired performance of antisaccade tasks (dorsolateral prefrontal lesions) • Epileptogenic lesions in the frontal eye fields • Ipsiversive head and eye movements during a seizure may also occur • Transient deviation of the eyes and head to the contralateral side[31] • Initial forced turning (versive) head and eye movements usually correspond to a contralateral epileptiform focus, but these initial contraversive movements may be followed by late ipsiversive or contraversive nonforced movements during the secondary generalization[32]
Unilateral parietal lesions	• Ipsilateral horizontal gaze preference with acute lesions contralateral inattention with right-sided lesions • Unilateral or bilateral increased saccade latencies • Hypometria for contralateral saccades • Saccadic slowing
Bilateral parietal lesions	Acquired ocular motor apraxia[6,7,33,34]
Lesions in the corona radiata adjacent to the genu of the internal capsule	Contralateral selective saccadic palsy[35]
Lesion (e.g., hemorrhage) deep in a cerebral hemisphere, particularly the thalamus	• Eye deviation to the side of the hemiparesis ("wrong-way eyes")[28] • Paresis of contralateral saccades • Supranuclear contralateral gaze palsies associated with ipsilateral oculomotor palsies
Pontine lesions affecting the abducens nucleus and/or the paramedian pontine reticular formation (PPRF)	• Ipsilateral conjugate gaze palsy[36] • Ipsilateral horizontal gaze palsy with ipsilateral esotropia[37] • Acutely, eyes deviated contralaterally • Doll's-eye maneuver or cold caloric stimulation usually does not overcome gaze palsy • Saccades toward side of lesion are present in contralateral hemifield but are slow with abducens nuclear lesions; ipsilaterally directed saccades from opposite field are small and slow or absent with PPRF lesions[38] • Horizontal gaze-evoked nystagmus on looking contralaterally

Table 14.2 continued

Localization	Deficit
	• Bilateral horizontal gaze palsies with bilateral lesions[9,39,40] • Selective saccadic palsy (bilateral lesions of pons) • Voluntary saccades in both horizontal and vertical planes slow • Smooth pursuit, the vestibulo-ocular reflex, the ability to hold steady eccentric gaze, and vergence eye movements preserved • Paraneoplastic loss of horizontal voluntary eye movements or slow horizontal saccades,[41] associated with persistent muscle spasms of the face, jaw, and pharynx, associated prostate carcinoma
Medial longitudinal fasciculus on one side and the contralateral abducens nerve fascicle	• Pseudo-horizontal gaze palsy

malformations, tumors, demyelination, trauma, or infections, are the usual causes of horizontal gaze palsies (see ▶ Table 14.1, ▶ Table 14.2). As all processes causing horizontal gaze palsies directly or indirectly damage intraparenchymal brain pathways, neuroimaging studies are necessary in all patients. In the acute setting, in patients with altered levels of consciousness, or in patients in whom MRI is contraindicated (e.g., patients with non-MRI compatible pacemakers), computed tomography (CT) is appropriate. Otherwise, MRI is the procedure of choice in evaluating patients with horizontal gaze palsies (class III, level B). In patients with evidence of clinical seizure activity, in patients with intermittent conjugate gaze deviation, or in obtunded or comatose patients with horizontal gaze palsies and evidence for possible contralateral cortical lesions, an electroencephalogram is indicted to evaluate the possibility a seizure disorder (e.g., status epilepticus) (class III, level C). The evaluation of patients with horizontal gaze palsies is outlined in ▶ Fig. 14.1.

14.4 What Is the Anatomy of the Abducens Nucleus and Medial Longitudinal Fasciculus?

The abducens nucleus has two types of intermingled neurons: motor neurons and internuclear neurons. The axons of the internuclear neurons cross to the contralateral side in the lower pons and ascend in the MLF to synapse in the portion of the oculomotor nucleus that innervates the medial rectus muscle.[38] In pontine lesions affecting the abducens nucleus and/or the paramedian pontine reticular formation (PPRF), a conjugate horizontal gaze palsy to the ipsilateral side occurs. Lesions of the MLF result in internuclear ophthalmoplegia (INO), whereas lesions of the MLF plus the ipsilateral abducens nucleus and/or PPRF result in the one-and-a-half syndrome. The clinical characteristics of these latter two syndromes and their evaluation are reviewed below.

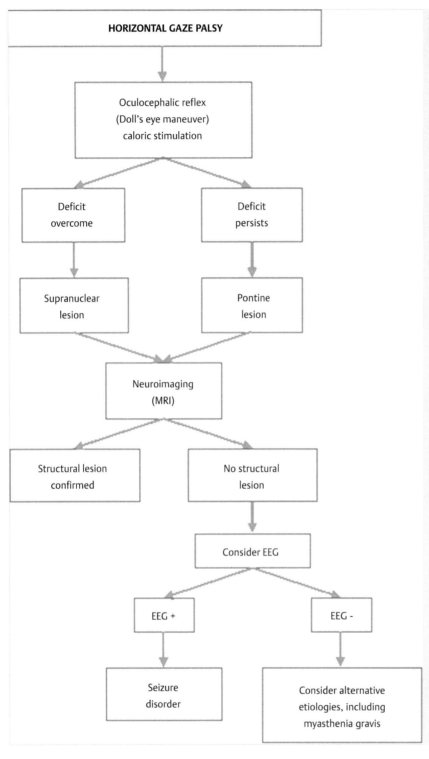

Fig. 14.1 Evaluation of horizontal gaze palsy.

14.5 What Are the Clinical Features of INO?

Clinically, an INO is characterized by adduction weakness on the side of the MLF lesion and monocular horizontal nystagmus of the opposite abducting eye. Convergence is usually preserved unless the responsible lesion is high in the midbrain. Often patients with INO have no visual symptoms, but some complain of diplopia (due to skew deviation or limitation of adduction) or oscillopsia. INO is most evident during horizontal saccadic eye movements, and the "adduction lag" is best detected during optokinetic testing using a tape or drum. For example, with a right INO when the drum is rotated to the right the amplitude and velocity of the adducting quick phase of the right eye is smaller and slower than that of the abducting saccades in the left eye. The pathogenesis of the nystagmus in the abducting eye is unclear but is likely a normal adaptive process that helps overcome the adducting weakness of the fellow eye.[44,45] Other clinical findings noted with unilateral and bilateral INO are outlined in Box 14.1.

Box 14.1 Clinical findings noted with internuclear ophthalmoplegia (INO)

- Unilateral INO.
  - Ipsilateral adduction weakness, especially slow or fractionated adducting saccades ("adduction lag"), and monocular nystagmus in contralateral abducting eye.
  - May have esophoria acutely, suggesting increased vergence tone.
  - Convergence usually spared.
  - Skew deviation with the higher eye on the side of the lesion.
  - Vertical gaze-evoked nystagmus and impaired vestibular and pursuit vertical eye movements (i.e., dissociated vertical nystagmus).[38]
  - Ipsilateral downbeat nystagmus and contralateral incyclorotatory (torsional) nystagmus.[46]
  - Transient (disappearing within 3 days) torsional nystagmus, which is clockwise (examiner's view) in cases of left INO and counterclockwise in right INO.[47]
  - Normal vertical saccades.
  - Rare exotropia (wall-eyed monocular internuclear ophthalmoplegia [WEMINO] syndrome).[48]
  - Rare exotropia in contralateral eye due to overexcitation of contralateral PPRF when fixating with paretic eye.[49]
- Bilateral INO.
  - Bilateral adduction paresis or lag with the eyes generally aligned in primary gaze.
  - Exotropia, with both eyes deviated laterally (wall-eyed bilateral internuclear ophthalmoplegia [WEBINO] syndrome).[50,51,52]
  - Vertical gaze-evoked nystagmus (on looking up or down) and impaired vestibular and pursuit vertical eye movements.[38]
  - Impaired vertical gaze holding.

Vitamin E deficiency syndrome (abetalipoproteinemia) may cause an eye movement disorder that superficially resembles the wall-eyed bilateral internuclear ophthalmoplegia (WEBINO) syndrome.[53] In both of these syndromes, patients demonstrate exotropia with associated adduction limitation and dissociated horizontal nystagmus on lateral gaze. In vitamin E deficiency, however, saccades are slower in the abducting eye than in the adducting eye, and the dissociated nystagmus is of greater amplitude in the adducting eye. This motility impairment is especially noted with abetalipoproteinemia, with other findings including ataxia, weakness, posterior column dysfunction, and pigmentary retinopathy.

What used to be called Lutz posterior INO is now known as INO of abduction.[54,55] In this rare syndrome, abduction is restricted on volition but can be fully effected by reflex maneuvers, such as cold caloric stimulation. Unilateral or bilateral INO of abduction, occasionally associated with adduction nystagmus of the contralateral eye, has been described with ipsilateral rostral pontine or mesencephalic lesions.[55]

14.6 What Is the Cause of the INO?

INO is due to pathologic processes affecting the medial pontine or midbrain parenchyma. Often there are associated brainstem symptoms and signs, although occasionally unilateral or bilateral INO may occur in isolation. The nature of the responsible pathologic process is suggested by the temporal mode of onset of the INO, the general clinical circumstances, and associated signs on neurologic and neuro-ophthalmologic examination. Potential etiologies for INO are listed in Box 14.2.

Box 14.2 Etiologies of internuclear ophthalmoplegia

- Multiple sclerosis.[39,51,56,57,58]
- Brainstem infarction.[36,44,46,52,58,59,60,61,62]
  - Giant cell arteritis.[63,64,65,66,67]
  - Systemic lupus erythematosus (SLE).
  - Neuro-Behçet disease.[68]
  - Sickle cell trait.[69]
  - Polyarteritis nodosa.[70]
  - Eales disease.[71]
  - Pyoderma gangrenosum.[72]
  - Sneddon syndrome.[73]
  - Complication of angiography.
  - Complication of cardiac catheterization.[74]
  - D-penicillamine-induced cerebral vasculitis.[75]
  - Acute myeloid leukemia.[76]
- Brainstem hemorrhage, including hemorrhage due to "crack" cocaine use.[77]
- Brainstem and fourth ventricular tumors.[78]
- Infections.
  - Cryptococcal meningitis.[50,79]
  - Tuberculosis (granuloma or infectious vasculitis).
  - Viral and bacterial meningoencephalitis.[80]
  - Syphilis.
  - Poliomyelitis.[81]
  - AIDS.[82,83]
  - Creutzfeldt–Jakob disease.[84]
  - Neurocysticercosis.[85]
- Head trauma.[86,87,88,89,90]
- Cervical injury by hyperextension or manipulation.
- Cancer-related.
  - Carcinomatous meningitis.
  - Remote effect of cancer.
  - Brainstem demyelination due to chemotherapy/radiation therapy.
  - Nutritional and metabolic disorders.
  - Wernicke encephalopathy.[91]
  - Pernicious anemia.
  - Hepatic encephalopathy.
  - Maple syrup urine disease.
  - Abetalipoproteinemia.
  - Fabry disease.
  - Hexosaminidase A deficiency.[92]
- Degenerative diseases.
  - Progressive supranuclear palsy (PSP).[93,94,95,96]
  - Familial spinocerebellar degeneration.[97]

- Arnold–Chiari malformation and associated hydrocephalus or syringobulbia.[98,99,100]
- Drug intoxications.
  - Narcotics.
  - Phenothiazines.
  - Tricyclic antidepressants.
  - Propranolol.
  - Barbiturates.
  - Lithium.
  - Antiobesity treatments.[101]
  - Toluene.[102]
- Miscellaneous causes.
  - Hydrocephalus.
  - Pseudotumor cerebri.[103]
  - Mesencephalic midline clefts.[104]
  - Subdural hematoma.
  - Subdural hygroma with an arachnoid cyst in the middle cranial fossa.[105]
  - After external ventricular drainage of a benign aqueductal cyst.[106]
  - Supratentorial arteriovenous malformations.
  - Partial seizures.[107]
- Pseudo-INO.
  - Myasthenia gravis (may be associated with downshoot of adducting eye).[108]
  - Fisher syndrome.[109,110,111]
  - Guillain–Barré syndrome.
  - Myotonic muscular dystrophy.[112,113]
  - Surgical paresis of the medial rectus muscle.

Although bilateral INO is more common with multiple sclerosis than with vascular insults, bilateral INO may occur with stroke as well as many other pathologic processes, and thus the presence of a unilateral or bilateral INO cannot be used as a differential feature for etiologic diagnosis (class III–IV, level C). For example, in a series of 100 patients with multiple sclerosis, 34 had INO, which was bilateral in 14 and unilateral in 20.[114] In another study of 51 patients with INO, 28 had multiple sclerosis and 23 had a lacunar infarction; INO was bilateral in 23 patients and unilateral in 28.[58] Most patients with nutritional, metabolic, degenerative, and drug-induced intoxication have bilateral INOs. Bilateral MLF involvement with the pathologic process subsequently extending laterally to the region of the two abducens fascicles has been described as explaining complete bilateral horizontal gaze paralysis in two patients with multiple sclerosis.[39] The pattern of extraocular muscle weakness with myasthenia gravis (including penicillamine-induced myasthenia) can mimic INO (pseudo-INO).[108] Myasthenic pseudo-INO is not uncommon and may be associated with downshoot in the adducting eye.[108] Other etiologies of pseudo-INO are listed in Box 14.2.

14.7 What Studies Should Be Ordered in a Patient with INO?

In general, the investigation of a patient with INO depends on the clinical circumstances. For example, in a patient with known multiple sclerosis, the appearance of INO as part of an exacerbation of the disease may not require neuroimaging (class IV, level C), whereas INO in isolation or with associated unexplained brainstem signs and symptoms usually requires neuroimaging (class III–IV, level C). If there is variability of the adduction deficit, associated fluctuating ptosis, or other variable ocular motor signs suggestive of myasthenia gravis, a myasthenic pseudo-INO should be considered (class III–IV, level C). If the evaluation for myasthenia (i.e., acetylcholine receptor antibody testing, electromyography) is normal or if the clinical situation does not suggest myasthenia and there are no signs of an associated degenerative process (e.g., progressive supranulear palsy) on clinical examination, neuroimaging is usually warranted (class III–IV, level C).

MRI is superior to CT scan in evaluating patients with INO.[56,58,59,87,90,115] For example, in a study of 11 patients with INO (nine with multiple sclerosis and two with infarct), CT in all nine tested failed to show a responsible lesion, whereas appropriate MRI abnormalities were documented in 10 of 11 patients.[115] In another study, CT did not detect abnormalities of the MLF in two patients with INO who had abnormal brainstem T2-weighted hyperintense signals on MRI.[116] In a study of chronic INO in 58 multiple sclerosis patients, proton density imaging (PDI) revealed a hyperintensity in the MLF in all patients, whereas T2-weighted imaging and fluid-attenuated inversion recovery (FLAIR) imaging showed these lesions in 88% and 48% of patients, respectively.[56] Thus, PDI sequences may be more sensitive for an MLF lesion in patients with multiple sclerosis and INO. Diffusion tensor imaging (DTI) sequences can also detect injury to white matter tracts, including the MLF region, in multiple sclerosis patients.[117] CT imaging in a patient with INO is reserved only for acute situations (e.g., brainstem hemorrhage) or for patients in whom MRI is contraindicated (e.g., non-MRI compatible pacemakers, etc.). MRI may give useful diagnostic data by also giving information about supratentorial processes likely to be involved in the etiology of the INO, such as multiple sclerosis, multiple cerebral infarcts, etc. If an infarct is detected as the cause of INO in a patient older than 50 years, giant cell arteritis should be considered as an etiology, especially if other stroke risk factors are not evident (class III, level C). Thus, a sedimentation rate and C-reactive protein are warranted, and if these are elevated or the patient has other systemic symptoms of giant cell arteritis (e.g., jaw claudication, headache, polymyalgia rheumatica symptoms, etc.), a temporal artery biopsy should be obtained. There is insufficient evidence to recommend an evaluation for giant cell arteritis in every INO in the elderly (class III–IV, level U).

If MRI in nontraumatic cases is normal, then rarer etiologies for the INO should be considered (class III–IV, level C). If the INO is bilateral, drug intoxication should be suspected. Because pernicious anemia has rarely been reported to cause INO, a B_{12} level should be considered (class IV, level C). Syphilis may rarely cause INO, so serology for syphilis should be considered (class III–IV, level U). If MRI reveals meningeal enhancement or if meningeal signs or symptoms are present, spinal fluid examination is warranted to search for infectious or carcinomatous meningitis (class III–IV, level C). The suggested evaluation of a patient with INO is outlined in ▶ Fig. 14.2.

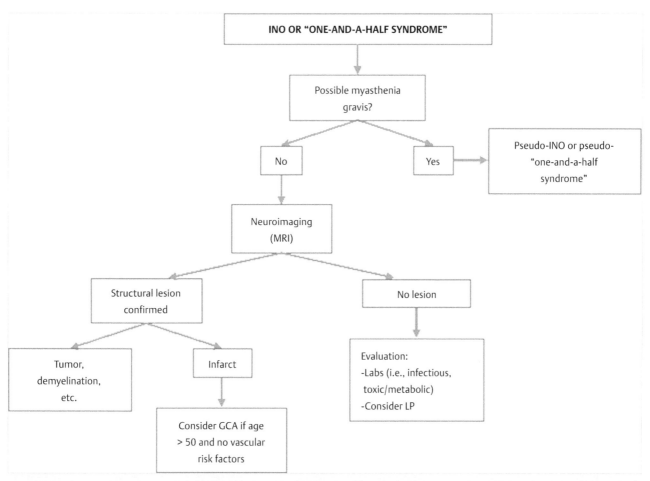

Fig. 14.2 Evaluation of internuclear ophthalmoplegia (INO) and the one-and-a-half syndrome.

14.8 What Is the One-and-a-Half Syndrome?

In the one-and-a-half syndrome, there is a conjugate gaze palsy to one side ("one") and impaired adduction on looking to the other side ("and-a-half").[118,119,120] As a result, the only horizontal movement remaining is abduction of one eye, which may exhibit nystagmus in abduction. The responsible lesion involves the PPRF or abducens nucleus and the adjacent MLF on the side of the complete gaze palsy. Patients with the one-and-a-half syndrome often have exotropia of the eye opposite the side of the lesion (paralytic pontine exotropia). Rarely, a primary position esotropia occurs, most likely due to the involvement of the abducens nerve fascicle superimposed upon lesions of the PPRF and MLF.[120]

The one-and-a-half syndrome may be associated with ocular bobbing and, more often, facial nerve palsy (the "eight-and-a-half syndrome").[121] Patients with the one-and-a-half syndrome and facial nerve palsies may develop oculopalatal myoclonus months to years after the onset of the ocular motility problem.[122]

The one-and-a-half syndrome may also be associated with supranuclear facial weakness on the same side as the gaze palsy and an INO. The lesion is in the paramedian aspect of the dorsal pontine tegmentum, providing evidence for the existence of corticofugal fibers that extend to the facial nucleus in the dorsal paramedian pontine tegmentum.[123]

Another type of one-and-a-half syndrome may result from two separate lesions involving both MLFs and the fascicles of the abducens nerve on the side of the unilateral horizontal "gaze" palsy. In this case, however, if the "gaze" palsy is incomplete, the eyes would move dysconjugately in the direction of the gaze palsy.[124] A true gaze palsy due to unilateral PPRF damage causes concomitant paresis of both eyes. Another form of one-and-a-half syndrome consists of a horizontal conjugate gaze palsy to ipsilateral side (e.g., the left side). This is associated with abduction paralysis of the eye contralateral to the lesion and to the gaze palsy (e.g., the right eye) and adduction nystagmus in the ipsilateral eye (e.g., in left eye).[119] This form of the one-and-a-half syndrome may be seen with rostral brainstem infarction. A fourth type of (pseudo) one-and-a-half syndrome has been described in a patient with mucormycosis of the cavernous sinus.[125] The patient had an ipsilateral sixth nerve palsy due to cavernous sinus involvement and a contralateral horizontal gaze palsy due to simultaneous carotid artery occlusion with infarction of the frontal lobe. Contrary to the pontine one-and-a-half syndrome, in which abduction in one eye is the preserved horizontal movement, this patient had only preserved adduction in one eye (contralateral to the sixth nerve palsy). Myasthenia gravis or the Miller Fisher syndrome may also produce findings that mimic a one-and-a-half syndrome ("pseudo-one-and-a-half syndrome").

14.9 What Etiologies Should Be Considered as a Cause of the One-and-a-Half Syndrome and What Evaluation Is Indicated?

Brainstem infarction is the most common cause of the one-and-a-half syndrome in the elderly, whereas multiple sclerosis is the most common cause of the one-and-a-half syndrome in young adults. In fact, the one-and-a-half syndrome may be the presenting sign of multiple sclerosis.[126] Rarer causes of one-and-a-half syndrome include immune complex deposition in SLE,[127] brainstem encephalitis with parenchymal lesions in Vogt–Koyanagi–Harada disease,[128] and neurocysticercosis.[85] Infarction can also cause a one-and-a-half syndrome in patients with SLE[129] or acute myeloid leukemia (AML).[76] Additional etiologies of one-and-a-half syndrome are discussed in Box 14.3.

Most patients with a one-and-a-half syndrome have other signs and symptoms of brainstem involvement. A patient with findings suggestive of a one-and-a-half syndrome with variable ocular motor paresis or ptosis should be evaluated for myasthenia gravis (class III, level C). All others should have MRI with attention to posterior fossa structures to investigate structural etiologies.[126,130,131] The evaluation of patients with the one-and-a-half syndrome is outlined in ▶ Fig. 14.2 (class III–IV, level B).

Box 14.3 Differential diagnosis of the etiology of a one-and-a-half syndrome

- Brainstem infarction.[36,76,119,120,122,123,129,131,132]
- Brainstem hemorrhage.
- Multiple sclerosis.
- Tumors (primary or metastatic) of the brainstem, fourth ventricle, or cerebellum.[133]
- Postoperatively after the removal of tumors of the posterior fossa.[133]
- Basilar artery aneurysms or brainstem arteriovenous malformations.[120]
- Trauma.
- Mucormycosis of the cavernous sinus.
- Pseudo-one-and-a-half syndrome (myasthenia gravis, Miller Fisher syndrome[134]).
- Brainstem encephalitis (Vogt–Koyanagi–Harada disease).[128]
- Neurocysticercosis.[85]
- Systemic lupus erythematosus.[127,129]
- Brainstem tuberculoma.[135]

14.10 What Is the Anatomy of Vertical Gaze?

The ocular motor neurons concerned with vertical gaze and torsional eye movements lie in the oculomotor and trochlear nuclei. These nuclei receive afferents from the vestibular, smooth pursuit, optokinetic, and saccadic systems.[4,38]

14.11 Where Are the Lesions Responsible for Vertical Gaze Palsies Localized?

The localization of lesions causing vertical gaze palsies is outlined in ▶ Table 14.3. The constellation of neuro-ophthalmologic findings seen with pretectal lesions has been variously designated as Parinaud syndrome, the Sylvian aqueduct syndrome, the pretectal syndrome, the dorsal midbrain syndrome, and the Koerber–Salus–Elschnig syndrome. The ophthalmic findings of Parinaud syndrome are discussed in Box 14.4.

Table 14.3 The localization of lesions causing vertical gaze palsies

Lesion	Deficit
Unilateral right hemispheric lesions[136]	• Upgaze palsy, associated with bilateral ptosis • May reflect the special contribution that the nondominant hemisphere makes to attention
Thalamic lesions may be associated with vertical gaze palsies	• Likely due to concomitant midbrain involvement • Occasionally due to medial thalamic lesions without midbrain involvement[137,138,139]
Unilateral lesions of the rostral interstitial nucleus of the medial longitudinal fasciculus (riMLF)[38,140]	• Slowing of downward saccades or downgaze palsy • Defect of torsional saccades (e.g., lesion of right riMLF impairs extorsion of right eye and intorsion of left eye)[141] • Torsional nystagmus beating contralesionally • Pseudo-abducens palsy in opposite eye[142]
Bilateral lesions of the riMLF[38,143,144]	• Downgaze saccadic palsy • Paralysis of upward and downward saccades
Lesions of the interstitial nucleus of Cajal (INC)[38]	• Impaired vertical gaze holding • Impaired vertical saccades, especially upward • Vertical gaze palsy, especially downward gaze, with bilateral lesions[145] • Ocular tilt reaction with unilateral lesions • Upbeat nystagmus and neck retroflexion with bilateral lesions
Posterior commissure lesions[38,143,144,146]	• Dorsal midbrain syndrome • Paresis of upward gaze • Paresis of downward gaze • Paresis of upward and downward gaze
Unilateral mesencephalic lesions (probably damage afferent and efferent connections to posterior commissure)[144,147]	• Bilateral upgaze palsy[144] • Palsy of upward and downward saccades[144] • Palsy of upward and downward gaze

- Vertical gaze abnormalities, especially upgaze limitation, with or without associated limitation of downgaze.
  - Downward vestibulo-ocular movements may be spared.
  - Bell's phenomenon may be spared.
- Downward gaze preference or a tonic downward deviation of the eyes ("setting sun sign").
- Primary position downbeat nystagmus.
- Impaired convergence and divergence; the patient thus may be exotropic or esotropic with A or V patterns.
- Excessive convergence tone may result in slow or restricted abduction ("midbrain pseudo-sixth palsy") during horizontal refixations.
- Convergence-retraction nystagmus, with quick adducting-retraction jerks predominantly on upgaze.
- Pretectal pseudobobbing (nonrhythmic, rapid combined downward and adducting movements, often preceded by a blink, with movement followed by slow return to midline).
- Skew deviation often with the higher eye on the side of the lesion.
- Alternating adduction hypertropia or alternating adduction hypotropia.
- Fixation instability with square wave jerks.
- Eyelid abnormalities.
  - Bilateral upper eyelid retraction, baring the sclera above the cornea (Collier "tucked lid" sign).
  - Bilateral ptosis (lesion of ventral caudal nucleus of third nerve).
- Pupillary abnormalities (large with light-near dissociation).

14.12 What Etiologies Cause Vertical Gaze Impairment?

Impaired upward gaze often occurs as a "physiologic" finding in the elderly. However, when it presents with accompanying signs of neurodegeneration, the most common etiology is progressive supranuclear palsy (PSP), a degenerative brain disease whose hallmarks consist of supranuclear ophthalmoplegia, pseudobulbar palsy, and dystonia. Generally, patients are unable to direct their gaze downward.[148] There are two well-recognized subtypes of PSP, Richardson syndrome, where the main presentation is falls, instability, vertical gaze palsy, and dementia, and PSP-parkinsonism, where patients present with symptoms similar to that of Parkinson disease, with accompanied vertical gaze palsy.[149] Other etiologies causing impaired vertical gaze are outlined in Box 14.5. Characteristics of PSP are described in Box 14.6

- Primary and secondary tumors of the pineal, thalamus, midbrain, aqueduct of Sylvius, or third ventricle.[146,150,151,152]
- Midbrain or thalamic infarction or hemorrhage.[137,138,139,140, 142,143,144,146,153,154,155,156,157,158,159,160,161,162]

- Hydrocephalus, especially when dilatation of the third ventricle and aqueduct or enlargement of the suprapineal recess cause pressure on and deformity of the posterior commissure.[146,163,164,165,166]
- Infectious or inflammatory etiologies.
  - Encephalitis.[143,146]
  - Syphilis.
  - Toxoplasmosis.[146]
  - Neurocyticercosis.[167]
  - Disseminated histoplasmosis.[168]
  - Tuberculosis.[146]
  - Whipple disease.[169,170,171]
  - Creutzfeldt–Jakob disease.[172,173,174,175,176,177]
  - Sarcoidosis.[178]
  - Postencephalitic parkinsonism.[179]
  - Paraneoplastic encephalomyelitis (e.g., seminoma with positive anti-Ta antibody and encephalomyelitis with anti-Hu antibodies[180,181,182,183]; testicular germ cell tumor and atypical medullary breast carcinoma with anti-Ma2 antibody[184,185]; tonsillar carcinoma[186]).
  - Stiff person syndrome (anti-glutamic acid decarboxylase [GAD] antibodies).[187]
  - Miller Fisher syndrome.[109,110]
  - Progressive encephalomyelitis with rigidity and myoclonus (PERM syndrome) (anti-glycine antibodies).[188]
  - Rheumatoid arthritis causing rheumatoid meningitis.[189]
- Multiple sclerosis.[190]
- Degenerative diseases.
  - Progressive supranuclear palsy[148,149,177,191,192] (and with comorbid chronic traumatic encephalopathy[193]).
  - Motor neuron disease[194,195,196,197,198] (and with cerebral amyloid angiopathy[199]).
  - Parkinson disease[177,200] (including early-onset disease with ATP13A2 mutation related[201]).
  - Parkinsonism (progressive autosomal dominant disease with pallido-ponto-nigral degeneration,[202,203] c9orf72 expansion related,[204] Guamanian neurodegenerative disease/lytico-bodig[205]).
  - Frontotemporal dementia[198,206,207] (including TDP-43 inclusions[208,209]).
  - Multiple system atrophy.[177,200]
  - Alzheimer disease.[200]
  - Corticobasal ganglionic degeneration.[177,210,211]
  - Huntington disease.[177]
  - Diffuse Lewy body disease.[212,213,214,215]
  - Olivopontocerebellar degeneration.[216]
  - Spastic paraplegia type 7.[217]
  - Hereditary spastic ataxia.[218]
  - Spinocerebellar ataxia (type 1,[219] type 7, type 34).
  - Autosomal recessive cerebellar ataxia syndrome with upward gaze palsy, neuropathy, and seizures.
  - Joubert syndrome.[220]
  - Perry syndrome.[221,222]
  - Kufor–Rakeb disease.[223]
  - Childhood onset neurodegeneration due to SQSTM1/p62 absence.[224]
  - Autosomal recessive spastic ataxia of Charlevoix-Saguenay (ARSACS).[225]
- Idiopathic striopallidodentate calcifications syndrome.[226]

- Pantothenate kinase-associated neurodegeneration.[227]
  - Dentatorubral-pallidoluysian atrophy.[228]
- Arteriovenous malformations and posterior fossa aneurysms.[146]
- Metabolic diseases.
  - Bassen–Kornzweig syndrome.[146]
  - Niemann-Pick C disease and variants, including sea-blue histiocytosis syndrome, juvenile dystonic lipidoses, and the DAF (downgaze paralysis, ataxia/athetosis, and foam cells) syndrome.[229,230]
  - Tay–Sachs disease.
  - Gaucher disease.[229]
  - Maple syrup urine disease.
  - Hyperglycinuria.[231]
  - Hexosaminidase A deficiency.
  - Wilson disease.[232]
  - Kernicterus.[146]
  - Wernicke encephalopathy.[146]
  - Vitamin B_{12} deficiency.
  - Leigh disease.[229]
  - Fatty acid amide hydrolase 2 deficiency.[233]
- Trauma, including neurosurgical procedures from catheter compression and deep brain stimulation placement.[146,234,235,236]
- Drugs.
  - Barbiturates.
  - Neuroleptics.
  - Carbamazepine.
  - Organophosphates (Diazinon).[237]
  - Sodium valproate.[238]
  - Drugs most often affect vertical gaze by causing oculogyric crisis, an episodic, spasmodic, conjugate ocular deviation that usually occurs in an upward and lateral direction.
- Miscellaneous causes.
  - Subdural hematoma.
  - Superficial central nervous system (CNS) siderosis with hydrocephalus.[239]
  - Pseudotumor cerebri.[103]
  - Subdural fluid collection over the cerebellar hemisphere.[240]
  - Tentorial herniation.[146]
  - Congenital defects.[146,241]
  - Cerebral palsy.[229]
  - Wolfram syndrome (hereditary diabetes mellitus with brainstem and optic atrophy, diabetes insipidus, and deafness).[242]
  - Benign transient form in childhood (benign paroxysmal tonic upgaze of neonates and children); may be associated with developmental delay, intellectual disability, or language delay.[243,244,245]
  - Migraine.
  - Porencephalic cyst.[246]
  - Mesencephalic clefts.[104]
  - Neurofibromatosis type 2.[247]
  - Moebius syndrome.[134]
  - Xeroderma pigmentosum.[248]

Box 14.6 Common ophthalmic signs and symptoms of progressive supranuclear palsy:[148]

- Vertical supranuclear gaze palsy; downgaze affected before upgaze.
- Abnormal vertical saccades, slowing of horizontal saccades.
- Impaired smooth pursuit movements.
- Abnormal fixation.
- Lid retraction, eyelid mobility impaired.

14.13 What Studies Are Indicated for the Evaluation of a Patient with Impaired Vertical Gaze?

Occasionally, peripheral eye movement abnormalities, such as myasthenia gravis, Lambert–Eaton myasthenic syndrome, thyroid eye disease, or the Miller Fisher variant of Guillain–Barré syndrome may simulate upgaze palsy or even convergence nystagmus.[146] Retractory nystagmus, for example, may be mimicked by bilateral thyroid eye disease with bilateral involvement of both medial recti and inferior recti; saccadic upgaze attempts may cause convergence and retraction due to limitation of eye movements.[249] Most of these peripheral processes are associated with other peripheral neurologic findings suggesting the appropriate localization. If vertical gaze paresis fluctuates and there are no other signs of neurologic or systemic disease, evaluation for myasthenia gravis should be considered (class III–IV, level C).

The evaluation of patients with vertical gaze impairments due to supranuclear etiologies depends on the clinical situation, especially if signs or symptoms of neurologic or systemic disease are present. For example, the presence of isolated impaired upward gaze in an elderly individual is a common "physiologic" finding and requires no further evaluation. Vertical gaze disorders in the setting of other clinical manifestations of metabolic diseases of childhood or adolescence require appropriate biochemical investigation of the metabolic derangement. Also, if a vertical gaze impairment occurs as part of degenerative process (e.g., progressive supranuclear palsy), further neuroimaging may not be required (class III, level C). If there is no evidence of a generalized metabolic or degenerative process on clinical examination to explain the findings, then further evaluation is typically warranted.

Vertical gaze impairment, either in isolation or with other neurologic findings localized to the meso-diencephalon, generally requires cranial MRI with contrast (class IV, level C). PSP patients typically have prominent midbrain atrophy. If MRI is performed on a patient with PSP with vertical gaze palsy, the axial views may show the "morning glory sign." This is a specific atrophic pattern of the midbrain where there is a concavity of the lateral margin of the tegmentum.[250] Sagittal views may show the "hummingbird sign" or "penguin sign" due to flattening of the superior aspect of the midbrain. Though not normally performed, an fluorodeoxyglucose-positron emission tomography (FDG-PET) study of patients with PSP and vertical gaze palsy was done. In this study, metabolic changes in bilateral anterior cingulate gyri and the right lingual gyrus were associated with a downward gaze palsy.[251] If a pretectal syndrome develops in a patient with shunted hydrocephalus and neuroimaging reveals no ventricular dilatation, shunt dysfunction should still be suspected, and neurosurgical consultation should be obtained to consider shunt revision or third ventriculostomy (class III–IV, level C).[164] If MRI is normal and there are signs suggestive of infection, especially signs of meningeal irritation, or if MRI reveals diffuse meningeal enhancement by contrast agent, then a lumbar puncture should be considered (class IV, level C). Finally, if MRI is normal and no other etiologies are evident, a B_{12} level should be obtained and thiamine supplementation considered (class III–IV, level C). Evaluation for Whipple disease (e.g., biopsy of intestine for histology and polymerase chain reaction [PCR] or cerebrospinal fluid PCR for *Tropheryma whippelii*),[252,253] syphilis, or a paraneoplastic process (e.g., seminoma with anti-Ta or anti-Ma2 antibodies)[180,186,254] should be considered (class III–IV, level C). A proposed evaluation of the patient with vertical gaze impairment is outlined in ▶ Fig. 14.3.

14.14 What Are the Characteristics of Supranuclear Monocular Elevation Paresis, the Vertical One-and-a-Half Syndrome, and Skew Deviation?

Monocular elevation paresis may occur on a peripheral basis (e.g., due to primary inferior rectus restriction, primary superior rectus palsy, myasthenia gravis, or a fascicular third nerve lesion) or with pretectal supranuclear lesions. "Double elevator palsy" implies impairment in both elevators, the superior rectus and the inferior oblique. Supranuclear monocular elevation paresis may be congenital[255,256] or acquired. Acquired lesions contralateral or ipsilateral to the paretic eye interrupt efferents from the rostral interstitial nucleus of the MLF to the superior rectus and inferior oblique subnuclei (often Bell's phenomenon is intact).[144,257] An asymmetric upgaze palsy may present clinically as monocular elevation paresis in the more severely affected eye.[257]

A vertical one-and-a-half syndrome, with vertical upgaze palsy and monocular paresis of downgaze on the side of the lesion or contralateral to the lesion, has been described with thalamo-mesencephalic infarction, best explained by selective damage to supranuclear pathways or partial nuclear involvement.[144,155] A neurocysticercosis lesion in the right midbrain extending into the thalamo-mesencephalic junction resulted in vertical one-and-a-half syndrome with associated contralateral horizontal gaze paresis.[167] Another vertical one-and-a-half syndrome due to bilateral mesodiencephalic infarcts has been described. There is impairment of all downward rapid eye movements (including the vestibulo-ocular reflex) and downward smooth pursuit (nondissociated downgaze paralysis)

associated with monocular paralysis of elevation.[258] Monocular elevation paresis of the right eye with contralateral paresis of downward gaze ("crossed vertical gaze paresis") has been described with an infarct involving the left mesodiencephalic junction and medial thalamus.[259] Finally, coexisting vertical and horizontal one-and-a-half syndrome have been described. One patient had an infarct involving the right medial thalamus, left dorsal upper midbrain, and left cerebellum, where the right eye could abduct and had monocular horizontal nystagmus, but the left eye could gaze down only.[260] Another patient had a long, vertical infarct of the brainstem including the bilateral pons and dorsomedial midbrain with bilateral INO, alternating exotropia, bilateral upward, right downward, and conjugate gaze palsies.[52] A patient with dual infarcts, one in the left thalamo-mesencephalic junction and the other in the left infrategmental paramedian area of the rostral midbrain, developed vertical one-and-a-half syndrome with concurrent contralateral pseudo-abducens palsy.[261]

A patient with locked-in syndrome due to pontine infarction had dysconjugate vertical and torsional ocular movements.[262] When the patient was asked to look to the right, the right eye moved upward with intorsion and the left eye moved downward with extorsion. When the patient was asked to look to the left, the reversal cycle, with the left eye moving upward with intorsion and the right eye moving downward with extorsion, was observed. Horizontal gaze was limited to minimal movement. It was thought that this intermittent dysconjugate abnormality was mediated by the interstitial nucleus of Cajal (INC).

The term skew deviation is reserved for vertical misalignment resulting from supranuclear derangements. This skew deviation may be constant or transient. For example, epileptic skew deviation has been described.[263] It occurs whenever peripheral or central lesions cause an imbalance of graviceptive brainstem pathways and can accompany lesions at different areas of the brainstem (mesencephalon to medulla) or cerebellum.[264,265,266,267,268,269] In a study of patients with unilateral brainstem infarcts presenting with skew deviation and ocular torsion, all skew deviations were ipsiversive (ipsilateral eye was undermost) with caudal pontomedullary lesions, and contraversive (contralateral eye was lowermost) with rostral pontomesencephalic lesions.[264] Otolith inputs to the INC from the contralateral vestibular (especially lateral vestibular) nuclei and motor outputs from the INC to cervical and ocular motoneurons are likely involved. In some patients, skew deviation may be associated with ocular torsion and head tilt (the ocular tilt reaction [OTR]).[264,266,267,270] In the OTR, the head tilt, conjugate eye torsion, and hypotropia are all to the same side, suggesting that this reaction is a motor compensation of a lesion-induced apparent eye-head tilt; the contralateral head tilt represents a compensatory response to the perceived tilt of the subjective visual vertical.

A left OTR could be due to a lesion of the left labyrinth, left vestibular nerve, left vestibular nucleus (e.g., Wallenberg syndrome), or right mesodiencephalon, suggesting the existence of a crossed graviceptive pathway (possibly the MLF) between the vestibular nucleus and the contralateral INC.[267,271,272] OTRs have been reported in multiple conditions including vestibular nerve injury (e.g., unilateral vestibular neurectomy and labyrinthectomy), herpes zoster of the vestibular nerve, auditory trauma, Wallenberg syndrome, lateral medullary compression,

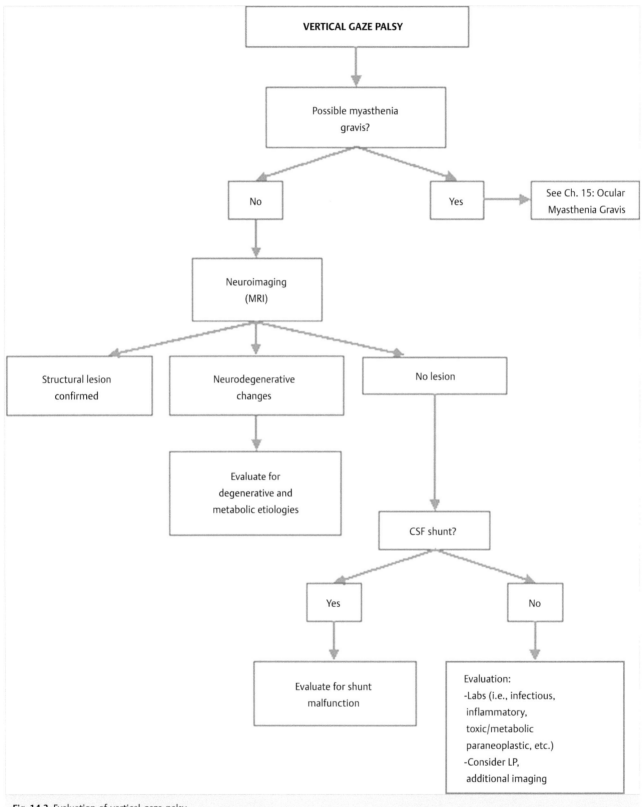

Fig. 14.3 Evaluation of vertical gaze palsy.

pontomedullary ischemia, and mesodiencephalic lesions.[153,220,264,
265,266,267,270,271,272,273,274,275,276,277,278] The absence of brainstem
signs in peripheral OTR helps to exclude a central cause for the
vertical diplopia. OTR has been described secondary to paraneoplastic encephalitis in a patient with seminoma and anti-Ta
antibodies.[180]

A contraversive OTR may rarely be due to unilateral cerebellar
lesions (the OTR may be under inhibitory control by the posterior cerebellum, possibly the nodulus).[279] Rarely, increased intracranial pressure (e.g., from benign intracranial hypertension or
pseudotumor cerebri), Miller Fisher syndrome,[280] or hepatic
coma may cause skew deviation. Finally, a patient with a dorsal
midbrain syndrome with an ipsilateral skew deviation has been
described due to a right paramedian thalamic infarct that perhaps impaired the tonic input of the thalamus on the INC.[153]

A tonic OTR may simulate superior oblique (SO) palsy.[281] Five
patients with OTR had a three-step test suggesting SO palsy
(bilateral in one patient). No patient, however, had the expected
excyclotorsion of the hypertropic eye. Two patients had conjugate ocular torsion (intorsion of the hypertropic eye and extorsion of the hypotropic eye) and two patients had only intorsion
of the hypotropic eye. All had neurologic deficits consistent
with more widespread brainstem disease. The authors concluded that vertical ocular deviations that three-step to a SO
palsy are not always caused by fourth nerve weakness. When a
patient with an apparent fourth nerve palsy has ocular torsion
inconsistent with a SO palsy, OTR should be suspected, especially if posterior fossa or vestibular dysfunction coexist.
Because results of the Bielschowsky head-tilt test may be positive in patients with the OTR, the feature distinguishing OTR
from SO palsy is the direction of torsion. The authors advocate a
fourth step—evaluation of ocular torsion using a double Maddox rod—in addition to the standard three steps.

References

[1] Cassidy L, Taylor D, Harris C. Abnormal supranuclear eye movements in the child: a practical guide to examination and interpretation. Surv Ophthalmol. 2000; 44(6):479–506

[2] Johnston JL, Sharpe JA, Morrow MJ. Paresis of contralateral smooth pursuit and normal vestibular smooth eye movements after unilateral brainstem lesions. Ann Neurol. 1992; 31(5):495–502

[3] Pierrot-Deseilligny C, Rivaud S, Gaymard B, Müri R, Vermersch AI. Cortical control of saccades. Ann Neurol. 1995; 37(5):557–567

[4] Tusa RJ, Ungerleider LG. Fiber pathways of cortical areas mediating smooth pursuit eye movements in monkeys. Ann Neurol. 1988; 23(2):174–183

[5] Aribal ME, Karaman ZC, Özkan SB, Söylev MF. Bilateral congenital horizontal gaze palsy: MR findings. Neuro-ophthalmology. 1998; 19:69–74

[6] Harris CM, Shawkat F, Russell-Eggitt I, Wilson J, Taylor D. Intermittent horizontal saccade failure ('ocular motor apraxia') in children. Br J Ophthalmol. 1996; 80(2):151–158

[7] Shawkat FS, Harris CM, Taylor DSI, Kriss A. The role of ERG/VEP and eye movement recordings in children with ocular motor apraxia. Eye (Lond). 1996; 10(Pt 1):53–60

[8] Stavrou P, Willshaw HE. Familial congenital horizontal gaze palsy. J Pediatr Ophthalmol Strabismus. 1999; 36(1):47–49

[9] Rucker JC, Webb BD, Frempong T, Gaspar H, Naidich TP, Jabs EW. Characterization of ocular motor deficits in congenital facial weakness: Moebius and related syndromes. Brain. 2014; 137(Pt 4):1068–1079

[10] Vrushali D, Muralidhar R, Vijayalakshmi P, Srinivasan KG. Isolated horizontal gaze palsy with congenital pontine hypoplasia. J Neuroophthalmol. 2013; 33(3):312–313

[11] Volk AE, Carter O, Fricke J, et al. Horizontal gaze palsy with progressive scoliosis: three novel ROBO3 mutations and descriptions of the phenotypes of four patients. Mol Vis. 2011; 17:1978–1986

[12] Jen JC, Chan WM, Bosley TM, et al. Mutations in a human ROBO gene disrupt hindbrain axon pathway crossing and morphogenesis. Science. 2004; 304 (5676):1509–1513

[13] Morrow MJ, Sharpe JA. Deficits of smooth-pursuit eye movement after unilateral frontal lobe lesions. Ann Neurol. 1995; 37(4):443–451

[14] Barton JJS, Sharpe JA, Raymond JE. Directional defects in pursuit and motion perception in humans with unilateral cerebral lesions. Brain. 1996; 119(Pt 5):1535–1550

[15] Lekwuwa GU, Barnes GR. Cerebral control of eye movements. I. The relationship between cerebral lesion sites and smooth pursuit deficits. Brain. 1996; 119(Pt 2):473–490

[16] Morrow MJ, Sharpe JA. Retinotopic and directional deficits of smooth pursuit initiation after posterior cerebral hemispheric lesions. Neurology. 1993; 43(3, Pt 1):595–603

[17] Brigell M, Babikian V, Goodwin JA. Hypometric saccades and low-gain pursuit resulting from a thalamic hemorrhage. Ann Neurol. 1984; 15(4):374–378

[18] Furman JMR, Hurtt MR, Hirsch WL. Asymmetrical ocular pursuit with posterior fossa tumors. Ann Neurol. 1991; 30(2):208–211

[19] Gaymard B, Pierrot-Deseilligny C, Rivaud S, Velut S. Smooth pursuit eye movement deficits after pontine nuclei lesions in humans. J Neurol Neurosurg Psychiatry. 1993; 56(7):799–807

[20] Johkura K, Matsumoto S, Komiyama A, Hasegawa O, Kuroiwa Y. Unilateral saccadic pursuit in patients with sensory stroke: sign of a pontine tegmentum lesion. Stroke. 1998; 29(11):2377–2380

[21] Kato I, Watanabe J, Nakamura T, Harada K, Hasegawa T, Kanayama R. Mapping of brainstem lesions by the combined use of tests of visually-induced eye movements. Brain. 1990; 113(Pt 4):921–935

[22] Malessa S, Gaymard B, Rivaud S, et al. Role of pontine nuclei damage in smooth pursuit impairment of progressive supranuclear palsy: a clinical-pathologic study. Neurology. 1994; 44(4):716–721

[23] Thier P, Bachor A, Faiss J, Dichgans J, Koenig E. Selective impairment of smooth-pursuit eye movements due to an ischemic lesion of the basal pons. Ann Neurol. 1991; 29(4):443–448

[24] Waespe W. Deficits of smooth-pursuit eye movements in two patients with a lesion in the (para-)floccular or dorsolateral pontine region. Neuro-ophthalmology. 1992; 12(2):91–96

[25] Waterston JA, Barnes GR, Grealy MA. A quantitative study of eye and head movements during smooth pursuit in patients with cerebellar disease. Brain. 1992; 115(Pt 5):1343–1358

[26] Pierrot-Deseilligny C, Amarenco P, Roullet E, Marteau R. Vermal infarct with pursuit eye movement disorders. J Neurol Neurosurg Psychiatry. 1990; 53(6):519–521

[27] Yee RD, Farlow MR, Suzuki DA, Betelak KF, Ghetti B. Abnormal eye movements in Gerstmann-Sträussler-Scheinker disease. Arch Ophthalmol. 1992; 110(1):68–74

[28] Tijssen CC. Contralateral conjugate eye deviation in acute supratentorial lesions. Stroke. 1994; 25(7):1516–1519

[29] Tijssen CC, van Gisbergen JAM. Conjugate eye deviation after hemispheric stroke. A contralateral saccadic palsy? Neuro-ophthalmology. 1993; 13(2):107–118

[30] Steiner I, Melamed E. Conjugate eye deviation after acute hemispheric stroke: delayed recovery after previous contralateral frontal lobe damage. Ann Neurol. 1984; 16(4):509–511

[31] Godoy J, Lüders H, Dinner DS, Morris HH, Wyllie E. Versive eye movements elicited by cortical stimulation of the human brain. Neurology. 1990; 40(2):296–299

[32] Kernan JC, Devinsky O, Luciano DJ, Vazquez B, Perrine K. Lateralizing significance of head and eye deviation in secondary generalized tonic-clonic seizures. Neurology. 1993; 43(7):1308–1310

[33] Dehaene I, Lammens M. Acquired ocular motor apraxia. A clinicopathologic study. Neuro-ophthalmology. 1991; 11:117–122

[34] Prasad P, Nair S. Congenital ocular motor apraxia: sporadic and familial. Support for natural resolution. J Neuroophthalmol. 1994; 14(2):102–104

[35] Fukutake T, Hirayama K, Sakakibara R. Contralateral selective saccadic palsy after a small haematoma in the corona radiata adjacent to the genu of the internal capsule. J Neurol Neurosurg Psychiatry. 1993; 56 (2):221

[36] Kataoka S, Hori A, Shirakawa T, Hirose G. Paramedian pontine infarction. Neurological/topographical correlation. Stroke. 1997; 28(4):809–815

[37] Coats DK, Avilla CW, Lee AG, Paysse EA. Etiology and surgical management of horizontal pontine gaze palsy with ipsilateral esotropia. J AAPOS. 1998; 2(5):293–297

[38] Leigh RJ, Zee DS. The Neurology of Eye Movements. 3rd ed. New York: Oxford University Press; 1999

[39] Milea D, Napolitano M, Dechy H, Le Hoang P, Delattre JY, Pierrot-Deseilligny C. Complete bilateral horizontal gaze paralysis disclosing multiple sclerosis. J Neurol Neurosurg Psychiatry. 2001; 70(2):252–255

[40] Shimura M, Kiyosawa M, Tominaga T, Tamai M. Bilateral horizontal gaze palsy with pontine cavernous hemangioma: a case report. Ophthalmologica. 1997; 211(5):320–322

[41] Baloh RW, DeRossett SE, Cloughesy TF, et al. Novel brainstem syndrome associated with prostate carcinoma. Neurology. 1993; 43(12):2591–2596

[42] Kunchok A, Todd MJ, Halmagyi GM. Selective total conjugate horizontal gaze paralysis due to bilateral abducens nucleus lesions. J Neurol. 2016; 263(12): 2538–2539

[43] Muni RH, Wennberg R, Mikulis DJ, Wong AM. Bilateral horizontal gaze palsy in presumed paraneoplastic brainstem encephalitis associated with a benign ovarian teratoma. J Neuroophthalmol. 2004; 24(2):114–118

[44] Getenet JC, Ventre J, Vighetto A, Tadary B. Saccades in internuclear ophthalmoplegia: are abduction disorders related to interocular disconjugacy? J Neurol Sci. 1993; 114(2):160–164

[45] Thömke F. Some observations on abduction nystagmus in internuclear ophthalmoplegia. Neuro-ophthalmology. 1996; 16(1):27–38

[46] Marshall RS, Sacco RL, Kreuger R, Odel JG, Mohr JP. Dissociated vertical nystagmus and internuclear ophthalmoplegia from a midbrain infarction. Arch Neurol. 1991; 48(12):1304–1305

[47] Fantin A. Torsional nystagmus in unilateral internuclear ophthalmoplegia. Presented at the annual meeting of the North American Neuro-Ophthalmology Society, Tuscon, Arizona, 1995

[48] Johnston JL, Sharpe JA. The WEMINO syndrome—wall-eyed monocular internuclear ophthalmoplegia: an oculographic and neuropathologic characterization. Neurology. 1994; 44 Suppl 2:A311

[49] Komiyama A, Takamatsu K, Johkura K, et al. Internuclear ophthalmoplegia and contralateral exotropia Nonparalytic pontine exotropia and WEBINO syndrome. Neuro-ophthalmology. 1998; 19 1:33–44

[50] Fay PM, Strominger MB. Wall-eyed bilateral internuclear ophthalmoplegia in central nervous system cryptococcosis. J Neuroophthalmol. 1999; 19(2): 131–135

[51] Flitcroft DI, Saidlear CA, Stack JP, Eustace P. A proposed neuroanatomical and neurophysiological basis for WEBDMO. Neuroophthalmology. 1996; 16:280

[52] Nakajima N, Ueda M, Katayama Y. Brainstem infarction with wall-eyed bilateral internuclear ophthalmoplegia syndrome and vertical one-and-a-half syndrome. J Stroke Cerebrovasc Dis. 2014; 23(4):e291–e293

[53] Yee RD, Cogan DG, Zee DS. Ophthalmoplegia and dissociated nystagmus in adetalipoproteinemia. Arch Ophthalmol. 1976; 94(4):571–575

[54] Oliveri RL, Bono F, Quattrone A. Pontine lesion of the abducens fasciculus producing so-called posterior internuclear ophthalmoplegia. Eur Neurol. 1997; 37(1):67–69

[55] Thömke F, Hopf HC, Krämer G. Internuclear ophthalmoplegia of abduction: clinical and electrophysiological data on the existence of an abduction paresis of prenuclear origin. J Neurol Neurosurg Psychiatry. 1992; 55(2): 105–111

[56] Frohman EM, Zhang H, Kramer PD, et al. MRI characteristics of the MLF in MS patients with chronic internuclear ophthalmoparesis. Neurology. 2001; 57(5):762–768

[57] Gass A, Hennerici MG. Neurological picture. Bilateral internuclear ophthalmoplegia in multiple sclerosis. J Neurol Neurosurg Psychiatry. 1997; 63(5):564

[58] Hopf HC, Thömke F, Gutmann L. Midbrain vs. pontine medial longitudinal fasciculus lesions: the utilization of masseter and blink reflexes. Muscle Nerve. 1991; 14(4):326–330

[59] Alexander JA, Castillo M, Hoffman JC, Jr. Magnetic resonance findings in a patient with internuclear ophthalmoplegia. Neuroradiological-clinical correlation. J Clin Neuroophthalmol. 1991; 11(1):58–61

[60] Nagasaka S, Fukushima T, Utsumomiya H, et al. Internuclear ophthalmoplegia caused by a lesion in the isthmus of the midbrain. Neuroophthalmology. 1999; 21:113–116

[61] Okuda B, Tachibana H, Sugita M, Maeda Y. Bilateral internuclear ophthalmoplegia, ataxia, and tremor from a midbrain infarction. Stroke. 1993; 24(3):481–482

[62] Sierra-Hidalgo F, Moreno-Ramos T, Villarejo A, et al. A variant of WEBINO syndrome after top of the basilar artery stroke. Clin Neurosurg. 2010; 112(9):801–804

[63] Ahmad I, Zaman M. Bilateral internuclear ophthalmoplegia: an initial presenting sign of giant cell arteritis. J Am Geriatr Soc. 1999; 47(6):734–736

[64] Askari A, Jolobe OM, Shepherd DI. Internuclear ophthalmoplegia and Horner's syndrome due to presumed giant cell arteritis. J R Soc Med. 1993; 86(6):362

[65] Hughes TA, Wiles CM, Hourihan M. Cervical radiculopathy and bilateral internuclear ophthalmoplegia caused by temporal arteritis. J Neurol Neurosurg Psychiatry. 1994; 57(6):764–765

[66] Johnston JL, Thomson GT, Sharpe JA, Inman RD. Internuclear ophthalmoplegia in giant cell arteritis. J Neurol Neurosurg Psychiatry. 1992; 55(1):84–85

[67] Trend P, Graham E. Internuclear ophthalmoplegia in giant-cell arteritis. J Neurol Neurosurg Psychiatry. 1990; 53(6):532–533

[68] Masai H, Kashii S, Kimura H, Fukuyama H. Neuro-Behçet disease presenting with internuclear ophthalmoplegia. Am J Ophthalmol. 1996; 122(6): 897–898

[69] Leavitt JA, Butrus SI. Internuclear ophthalmoplegia in sickle cell trait. J Neuroophthalmol. 1994; 14(1):49–51

[70] Kirkali P, Topaloglu R, Kansu T, Bakkaloglu A. Third nerve palsy and internuclear ophthalmoplegia in periarteritis nodosa. J Pediatr Ophthalmol Strabismus. 1991; 28(1):45–46

[71] Atabay C, Erdem E, Kansu T, Eldem B. Eales disease with internuclear ophthalmoplegia. Ann Ophthalmol. 1992; 24(7):267–269

[72] Lana MA, Moreira PR, Neves LB. Wall-eyed bilateral internuclear ophthalmoplegia (Webino syndrome) and myelopathy in pyoderma gangrenosum. Arq Neuropsiquatr. 1990; 48(4):497–501

[73] Rehany U, Kassif Y, Rumelt S. Sneddon's syndrome: neuro-ophthalmologic manifestations in a possible autosomal recessive pattern. Neurology. 1998; 51(4):1185–1187

[74] Mihaescu M, Brillman J, Rothfus W. Midbrain ptosis caused by periaqueductal infarct following cardiac catheterization: early detection with diffusion-weighted imaging. J Neuroimaging. 2000; 10(3):187–189

[75] Pless M, Sandson T. Chronic internuclear ophthalmoplegia. A manifestation of D-penicillamine cerebral vasculitis. J Neuroophthalmol. 1997; 17(1): 44–46

[76] Hsu WH, Chu SJ, Tsai WC, Tsao YT. Acute myeloid leukemia presenting as one-and-a-half syndrome. Am J Emerg Med. 2008; 26(4):513.e1–513.e2

[77] Díaz-Calderón E, Del Brutto OH, Aguirre R, Alarcón TA. Bilateral internuclear ophthalmoplegia after smoking "crack" cocaine. J Clin Neuroophthalmol. 1991; 11(4):297–299

[78] Arnold AC. Internuclear ophthalmoplegia from intracranial tumor. J Clin Neuroophthalmol. 1990; 10(4):278–286

[79] Sung JY, Cheng PN, Lai KN. Internuclear ophthalmoplegia in cryptococcal meningitis. J Trop Med Hyg. 1991; 94(2):116–117

[80] Luis Guerrero-Peral A, Mohamed Buskri A, Angel Ponce Villares M, Bueno V. Internuclear ophthalmoplegia as a presentation of meningeal infection by the varicella zoster virus [in Spanish]. Med Clin (Barc). 2001; 116(1):36

[81] Wasserstrom R, Mamourian AC, McGary CT, Miller G. Bulbar poliomyelitis: MR findings with pathologic correlation. AJNR Am J Neuroradiol. 1992; 13(1):371–373

[82] Cacciatori M, Dhillon B. Bilateral internuclear ophthalmoplegia in AIDS. Neuro-ophthalmology. 1997; 17:219–222

[83] Sherman MD, Allinson RW, Obbens EA, Darragh JM, Simons KB. Internuclear ophthalmoplegia in acquired immunodeficiency syndrome. Ann Ophthalmol. 1989; 21(8):294–295

[84] Billette de Villemeur T, Deslys J-P, Pradel A, et al. Creutzfeldt-Jakob disease from contaminated growth hormone extracts in France. Neurology. 1996; 47(3):690–695

[85] Ranjith MP, Divya R, Sahni A. Isolated one and a half syndrome: an atypical presentation of neurocysticercosis. Indian J Med Sci. 2009; 63(3):119–120

[86] Chan JW. Isolated unilateral post-traumatic internuclear ophthalmoplegia. J Neuroophthalmol. 2001; 21(3):212–213

[87] Haller KA, Miller-Meeks M, Kardon R. Early magnetic resonance imaging in acute traumatic internuclear ophthalmoplegia. Ophthalmology. 1990; 97(9): 1162–1165

[88] Hsu H-C, Chen HJ, Lu K, Liang C-L. Reversible bilateral internuclear ophthalmoplegia following head injury. Acta Ophthalmol Scand. 2001; 79(1):57–59

[89] Mueller C, Koch S, Toifl K. Transient bilateral internuclear ophthalmoplegia after minor head-trauma. Dev Med Child Neurol. 1993; 35(2):163–166

[90] Strauss S, Ganslandt O, Huk WJ, Jonas JB. Isolated unilateral internuclear ophthalmoplegia following head injury: findings in magnetic resonance imaging. Neuro-ophthalmology. 1995; 15:15–19

[91] De La Paz MA, Chung SM, McCrary JA, III. Bilateral internuclear ophthalmoplegia in a patient with Wernicke's encephalopathy. J Clin Neuroophthalmol. 1992; 12(2):116–120

[92] Barnes D, Misra VP, Young EP, Thomas PK, Harding AE. An adult onset hexosaminidase A deficiency syndrome with sensory neuropathy and internuclear ophthalmoplegia. J Neurol Neurosurg Psychiatry. 1991; 54(12): 1112–1113

[93] Friedman DI, Jankovic J, McCrary JA, III. Neuro-ophthalmic findings in progressive supranuclear palsy. J Clin Neuroophthalmol. 1992; 12(2): 104–109

[94] Matsumoto H, Ohminami S, Goto J, Tsuji S. Progressive supranuclear palsy with wall-eyed bilateral internuclear ophthalmoplegia syndrome. Arch Neurol. 2008; 65(6):827–829

[95] Ushio M, Iwasaki S, Chihara Y, Murofushi T. Wall-eyed bilateral internuclear ophthalmoplegia in a patient with progressive supranuclear palsy. J Neuroophthalmol. 2008; 28(2):93–96

[96] Flint AC, Williams O. Bilateral internuclear ophthalmoplegia in progressive supranuclear palsy with an overriding oculocephalic maneuver. Mov Disord. 2005; 20(8):1069–1071

[97] Senanayake N. A syndrome of early onset spinocerebellar ataxia with optic atrophy, internuclear ophthalmoplegia, dementia, and startle myoclonus in a Sri Lankan family. J Neurol. 1992; 239(5):293–294

[98] Arnold AC, Baloh RW, Yee RD, Hepler RS. Internuclear ophthalmoplegia in the Chiari type II malformation. Neurology. 1990; 40(12):1850–1854

[99] Chavis PS, Mullaney PB, Bohlega S. Fluctuating oculomotor signs in Arnold-Chiari malformation. Diagnostic pitfalls. Neuro-ophthalmology. 1998; 19(4): 215–221

[100] Lewis AR, Kline LB, Sharpe JA. Acquired esotropia due to Arnold-Chiari I malformation. J Neuroophthalmol. 1996; 16(1):49–54

[101] Lledo Carreres M, Lajo Garrido JL, Gonzalez Rico M, Navarro Polo JN, Escobar Cava P, Aznar Saliente T. Toxic internuclear ophthalmoplegia related to antiobesity treatment. Ann Pharmacother. 1992; 26(11):1457–1458

[102] Hunnewell J, Miller NR. Bilateral internuclear ophthalmoplegia related to chronic toluene abuse. J Neuroophthalmol. 1998; 18(4):277–280

[103] Friedman DI, Forman S, Levi L, Lavin PJ, Donahue S. Unusual ocular motility disturbances with increased intracranial pressure. Neurology. 1998; 50(6): 1893–1896

[104] Lagreze W-D, Warner JEA, Zamani AA, Gouras GK, Koralnik IJ, Bienfang DC. Mesencephalic clefts with associated eye movement disorders. Arch Ophthalmol. 1996; 114(4):429–432

[105] Minamori Y, Yamamoto M, Tanaka A, et al. Medial longitudinal fasciculus syndrome associated with a subdural hygroma and an arachnoid cyst in the middle cranial fossa. Intern Med. 1992; 31(11):1286–1290

[106] Shin M, Nishihara T, Iai S, Eguchi T. Benign aqueductal cyst causing bilateral internuclear ophthalmoplegia after external ventricular drainage. Case report. J Neurosurg. 2000; 92(3):490–492

[107] Rosenberg ML, Jabbari B. Miosis and internal ophthalmoplegia as a manifestation of partial seizures. Neurology. 1991; 41(5):737–739

[108] Ito K, Mizutani J, Murofushi T, Mizuno M. Bilateral pseudo-internuclear ophthalmoplegia in myasthenia gravis. ORL J Otorhinolaryngol Relat Spec. 1997; 59(2):122–126

[109] al-Din SN, Anderson M, Eeg-Olofsson O, Trontelj JV. Neuro-ophthalmic manifestations of the syndrome of ophthalmoplegia, ataxia and areflexia: a review. Acta Neurol Scand. 1994; 89(3):157–163

[110] Mori M, Kuwabara S, Fukutake T, Yuki N, Hattori T. Clinical features and prognosis of Miller Fisher syndrome. Neurology. 2001; 56(8):1104–1106

[111] Diaz Ortuño A, Maeztu C, Muñoz JA, Reigadas R, Rodriguez T, Valdés M. Miller Fisher syndrome associated with Q fever. J Neurol Neurosurg Psychiatry. 1990; 53(7):615–616

[112] Azuara-Blanco A, Katz LJ, Arkfeld DF, Walsh TJ. Myotonic dystrophy mimicking bilateral internuclear ophthalmoplegia. Neuroophthalmology. 1997; 17:11–14

[113] Verhagen WIM, Huygen PLM. Myotonic dystrophy mimicking INO. Neuroophthalmology. 1998; 20:101–102

[114] Müri RM, Meienberg O. The clinical spectrum of internuclear ophthalmoplegia in multiple sclerosis. Arch Neurol. 1985; 42(9):851–855

[115] Atlas SW, Grossman RI, Savino PJ, et al. Internuclear ophthalmoplegia: MR-anatomic correlation. AJNR Am J Neuroradiol. 1987; 8(2):243–247

[116] Awerbuch G, Brown M, Levin JR. Magnetic resonance imaging correlates of internuclear ophthalmoplegia. Int J Neurosci. 1990; 52(1–2):39–43

[117] Sakaie K, Takahashi M, Remington G, et al. Correlating function and imaging measures of the medial longitudinal fasciculus. PLoS One. 2016; 11(1): e0147863

[118] Bronstein AM, Rudge P, Gresty MA, Du Boulay G, Morris J. Abnormalities of horizontal gaze. Clinical, oculographic and magnetic resonance imaging findings. II. Gaze palsy and internuclear ophthalmoplegia. J Neurol Neurosurg Psychiatry. 1990; 53(3):200–207

[119] Çelebisoy N, Akyürekli Ö. One-and-a-half syndrome, type II: a case with rostral brain stem infarction. Neuroophthalmology. 1996; 16:373–377

[120] Wall M, Wray SH. The one-and-a-half syndrome–a unilateral disorder of the pontine tegmentum: a study of 20 cases and review of the literature. Neurology. 1983; 33(8):971–980

[121] Eggenberger E. Eight-and-a-half syndrome: one-and-a-half syndrome plus cranial nerve VII palsy. J Neuroophthalmol. 1998; 18(2):114–116

[122] Wolin MJ, Trent RG, Lavin PJM, Cornblath WT. Oculopalatal myoclonus after the one-and-a-half syndrome with facial nerve palsy. Ophthalmology. 1996; 103(1):177–180

[123] Anderson CA, Sandberg E, Filley CM, Harris SL, Tyler KL. One and one-half syndrome with supranuclear facial weakness: magnetic resonance imaging localization. Arch Neurol. 1999; 56(12):1509–1511

[124] Pierrot-Deseilligny C, Chain F, Serdaru M, Gray F, Lhermitte F. The 'one-and-a-half' syndrome. Electro-oculographic analyses of five cases with deductions about the Physiological mechanisms of lateral gaze. Brain. 1981; 104(Pt 4):665–699

[125] Carter JE, Rauch RA. One-and-a-half syndrome, type II. Arch Neurol. 1994; 51(1):87–89

[126] Martyn CN, Kean D. The one-and-a-half syndrome. Clinical correlation with a pontine lesion demonstrated by nuclear magnetic resonance imaging in a case of multiple sclerosis. Br J Ophthalmol. 1988; 72(7):515–517

[127] Sasannejad P, Olfati N, Sabi MS, Juibary AG. The one-and-a-half syndrome as the presenting sign of systemic lupus erythematosus. Neurol India. 2014; 62(3):307–308

[128] Hashimoto T, Takizawa H, Yukimura K, Ohta K. Vogt-Koyanagi-Harada disease associated with brainstem encephalitis. J Clin Neurosci. 2009; 16(4): 593–595

[129] Keane JR. Eye movement abnormalities in systemic lupus erythematosus. Arch Neurol. 1995; 52(12):1145–1149

[130] Hirose G, Furui K, Yoshioka A, Sakai K. Unilateral conjugate gaze palsy due to a lesion of the abducens nucleus. Clinical and neuroradiological correlations. J Clin Neuroophthalmol. 1993; 13(1):54–58

[131] Ohta K, Gotoh F, Fukuuchi Y, Tanahashi N, Shinohara T. Midpontine tegmentum infarction with "one-and-a-half syndrome" demonstrated by magnetic resonance imaging. Keio J Med. 1994; 43(3):164–166

[132] Yiğit A, Bingöl A, Mutluer N, Taşçilar N. The one-and-a-half syndrome in systemic lupus erythematosus. J Neuroophthalmol. 1996; 16(4):274–276

[133] Newton HB, Miner ME. "One-and-a-half" syndrome after a resection of a midline cerebellar astrocytoma: case report and discussion of the literature. Neurosurgery. 1991; 29(5):768–772

[134] Bandini F, Faga D, Simonetti S. Ocular myasthenia mimicking a one-and-a-half syndrome. J Neuroophthalmol. 2001; 21(3):210–211

[135] Menon V, Gogoi M, Saxena R, Singh S, Kumar A. Isolated "one and a half syndrome" with brainstem tuberculoma. Indian J Pediatr. 2004; 71(5): 469–471

[136] Averbuch-Heller L, Stahl JS, Remler BF, Leigh RJ. Bilateral ptosis and upgaze palsy with right hemispheric lesions. Ann Neurol. 1996; 40(3):465–468

[137] Clark JM, Albers GW. Vertical gaze palsies from medial thalamic infarctions without midbrain involvement. Stroke. 1995; 26(8):1467–1470

[138] Deleu D. Selective vertical saccadic palsy from unilateral medial thalamic infarction: clinical, neurophysiologic and MRI correlates. Acta Neurol Scand. 1997; 96(5):332–336

[139] Onder F, Can I, Coşar CB, Kural G. Correlation of clinical and neuroradiological findings in down-gaze palsy. Graefes Arch Clin Exp Ophthalmol. 2000; 238(4):369–371

[140] Bogousslavsky J, Miklossy J, Regli F, Janzer R. Vertical gaze palsy and selective unilateral infarction of the rostral interstitial nucleus of the medial longitudinal fasciculus (riMLF). J Neurol Neurosurg Psychiatry. 1990; 53(1): 67–71

[141] Riordan-Eva P, Faldon M, Büttner-Ennever JA, Gass A, Bronstein AM, Gresty MA. Abnormalities of torsional fast phase eye movements in unilateral rostral midbrain disease. Neurology. 1996; 47(1):201–207

[142] Pullicino P, Lincoff N, Truax BT. Abnormal vergence with upper brainstem infarcts: pseudoabducens palsy. Neurology. 2000; 55(3):352–358

[143] Green JP, Newman NJ, Winterkorn JS. Paralysis of downgaze in two patients with clinical-radiologic correlation. Arch Ophthalmol. 1993; 111(2): 219–222

[144] Hommel M, Bogousslavsky J. The spectrum of vertical gaze palsy following unilateral brainstem stroke. Neurology. 1991; 41(8):1229–1234

[145] Ohashi T, Nakano T, Harada T, Yoshida K, Fukushima K, Matsuda H. Downward gaze palsy caused by bilateral lesions of the rostral mesencephalon. Ophthalmologica. 1998; 212(3):212–214

[146] Keane JR. The pretectal syndrome: 206 patients. Neurology. 1990; 40(4): 684–690

[147] Albera R, Magnano M, Lacilla M, et al. Vascular dorsal midbrain syndrome. Neuroophthalmology. 1993; 13:207–213

[148] Armstrong RA. Visual signs and symptoms of progressive supranuclear palsy. Clin Exp Optom. 2011; 94(2):150–160

[149] Williams DR, de Silva R, Paviour DC, et al. Characteristics of two distinct clinical phenotypes in pathologically proven progressive supranuclear palsy: Richardson's syndrome and PSP-parkinsonism. Brain. 2005; 128(Pt 6): 1247–1258

[150] Chang SM, Lillis-Hearne PK, Larson DA, Wara WM, Bollen AW, Prados MD. Pineoblastoma in adults. Neurosurgery. 1995; 37(3):383–390, discussion 390–391

[151] Maranhão-Filho P, Campos JC, Lima MA. Bilateral ptosis and supranuclear downgaze paralysis. Arq Neuropsiquiatr. 2007; 65 4A:1007–1009

[152] Skarbez K, Fanciullo L. Metastatic melanoma from unknown primary presenting as dorsal midbrain syndrome. Optom Vis Sci. 2012; 89(12): e112–e117

[153] Anderson DF, Morris RJ. Parinaud's syndrome and ipsilateral tonic ocular skew deviation from unilateral right paramedian thalamic infarct. Neuro-ophthalmology. 1998; 19(1):13–15

[154] Lee AG, Brown DG, Diaz PJ. Dorsal midbrain syndrome due to mesencephalic hemorrhage. Case report with serial imaging. J Neuroophthalmol. 1996; 16(4):281–285

[155] Tatemichi TK, Steinke W, Duncan C, et al. Paramedian thalamopeduncular infarction: clinical syndromes and magnetic resonance imaging. Ann Neurol. 1992; 32(2):162–171

[156] Tijssen CC, De Letter MACJ, Op de Coul AAW. Convergence-retraction nystagmus. Neuro-ophthalmology. 1996; 16:215–218

[157] Serino J, Martins J, Páris L, Duarte A, Ribeiro I. Parinaud's syndrome due to an unilateral vascular ischemic lesion. Int Ophthalmol. 2015; 35(2):275–279

[158] Caruso P, Manganotti P, Moretti R. Complex neurological symptoms in bilateral thalamic stroke due to Percheron artery occlusion. Vasc Health Risk Manag. 2016; 13:11–14

[159] Sánchez Fernández I, Fernández Carbonell C, Vázquez Ortiz M, González Álvarez V. Vertical ophthalmoplegia due to a unilateral periaqueductal gray matter infarct in an adolescent. J Child Neurol. 2010; 25(12):1552–1554

[160] Alemdar M, Kamaci S, Budak F. Unilateral midbrain infarction causing upward and downward gaze palsy. J Neuroophthalmol. 2006; 26(3): 173–176

[161] Kim HT, Shields S, Bhatia KP, Quinn N. Progressive supranuclear palsy-like phenotype associated with bilateral hypoxic-ischemic striopallidal lesions. Mov Disord. 2005; 20(6):755–757

[162] Jadhav AP, Zenonos G, Pless M, Jovin TG, Wechsler L. A variant of the anterior opercular syndrome with supranuclear gaze palsy. JAMA Neurol. 2013; 70 (6):800–801

[163] Bleasel AF, Ell JJ, Johnston I. Pretectal syndrome and ventricular shunt dysfunction. Neuroophthalmology. 1992; 12:193–196

[164] Cinalli G, Sainte-Rose C, Simon I, Lot G, Sgouros S. Sylvian aqueduct syndrome and global rostral midbrain dysfunction associated with shunt malfunction. J Neurosurg. 1999; 90(2):227–236

[165] Katz DM, Trobe JD, Muraszko KM, Dauser RC. Shunt failure without ventriculomegaly proclaimed by ophthalmic findings. J Neurosurg. 1994; 81(5):721–725

[166] Suzuki H, Matsubara T, Kanamaru K, Kojima T. Chronic hydrocephalus presenting with bilateral ptosis after minor head injury: case report. Neurosurgery. 2000; 47(4):977–979, discussion 979–980

[167] Mesraoua B, Deleu D, D'souza A, Imam YZ, Melikyan G. Neurocysticercosis presenting as a vertical one-and-a-half syndrome with associated contralesional horizontal gaze paresis. J Neurol Sci. 2012; 323(1–2):250–253

[168] Perry JD, Girkin CA, Miller NR, Mann RB. Disseminated histoplasmosis causing reversible gaze palsy and optic neuropathy. J Neuroophthalmol. 1999; 19(2):140–143

[169] Averbuch-Heller L, Paulson GW, Daroff RB, Leigh RJ. Whipple's disease mimicking progressive supranuclear palsy: the diagnostic value of eye movement recording. J Neurol Neurosurg Psychiatry. 1999; 66(4):532–535

[170] Magherini A, Pentore R, Grandi M, Leone ME, Nichelli PF. Progressive supranuclear gaze palsy without parkinsonism: a case of neuro-Whipple. Parkinsonism Relat Disord. 2007; 13(7):449–452

[171] Panegyres PK, Edis R, Beaman M, Fallon M. Primary Whipple's disease of the brain: characterization of the clinical syndrome and molecular diagnosis. QJM. 2006; 99(9):609–623

[172] Grant MP, Cohen M, Petersen RB, et al. Abnormal eye movements in Creutzfeldt-Jakob disease. Ann Neurol. 1993; 34(2):192–197

[173] Ifergane G, Merkin S, Valdman I, et al. Ocular manifestations of Jakob-Creutzfeldt disease (CJD). Neuroophthalmology. 1998; 20:21

[174] Petrovic IN, Martin-Bastida A, Massey L, et al. MM2 subtype of sporadic Creutzfeldt-Jakob disease may underlie the clinical presentation of progressive supranuclear palsy. J Neurol. 2013; 260(4):1031–1036

[175] Prasad S, Ko MW, Lee EB, Gonatas NK, Stern MB, Galetta S. Supranuclear vertical gaze abnormalities in sporadic Creutzfeldt-Jakob disease. J Neurol Sci. 2007; 253(1–2):69–72

[176] Huber FM, Bour F, Sazdovitch V, et al. Creutzfeldt-Jakob disease with slow progression. A mimickry of progressive supranuclear palsy. Bull Soc Sci Med Grand Duche Luxemb. 2007; 2(2):125–130

[177] Martin WRW, Hartlein J, Racette BA, Cairns N, Perlmutter JS. Pathologic correlates of supranuclear gaze palsy with parkinsonism. Parkinsonism Relat Disord. 2017; 38:68–71

[178] Frohman LP, Grigorian R, Bielory L. Neuro-ophthalmic manifestations of sarcoidosis: clinical spectrum, evaluation, and management. J Neuroophthalmol. 2001; 21(2):132–137

[179] Wenning GK, Jellinger K, Litvan I. Supranuclear gaze palsy and eyelid apraxia in postencephalitic parkinsonism. J Neural Transm (Vienna). 1997; 104(8–9):845–865

[180] Bennett JL, Galetta SL, Frohman LP, et al. Neuro-ophthalmologic manifestations of a paraneoplastic syndrome and testicular carcinoma. Neurology. 1999; 52(4):864–867

[181] Crino PB, Galetta SL, Sater RA, et al. Clinicopathologic study of paraneo-plastic brainstem encephalitis and ophthalmoparesis. J Neuroophthalmol. 1996; 16(1):44–48

[182] Schiff ND, Moore DF, Winterkorn JM. Predominant downgaze ophthalmo-paresis in anti-Hu encephalomyelitis. J Neuroophthalmol. 1996; 16(4): 302–303

[183] Wingerchuk DM, Noseworthy JH, Kimmel DW. Paraneoplastic encephalo-myelitis and seminoma: importance of testicular ultrasonography. Neurology. 1998; 51(5):1504–1507

[184] Waragai M, Chiba A, Uchibori A, Fukushima T, Anno M, Tanaka K. Anti-Ma2 associated paraneoplastic neurological syndrome presenting as encephalitis and progressive muscular atrophy. J Neurol Neurosurg Psychiatry. 2006; 77(1):111–113

[185] Sahashi K, Sakai K, Mano K, Hirose G. Anti-Ma2 antibody related paraneoplastic limbic/brain stem encephalitis associated with breast cancer expressing Ma1, Ma2, and Ma3 mRNAs. J Neurol Neurosurg Psychiatry. 2003; 74(9):1332–1335

[186] Adams C, McKeon A, Silber MH, Kumar R. Narcolepsy, REM sleep behavior disorder, and supranuclear gaze palsy associated with Ma1 and Ma2 antibodies and tonsillar carcinoma. Arch Neurol. 2011; 68(4):521–524

[187] Warren JD, Scott G, Blumbergs PC, Thompson PD. Pathological evidence of encephalomyelitis in the stiff man syndrome with anti-GAD antibodies. J Clin Neurosci. 2002; 9(3):328–329

[188] Peeters E, Vanacker P, Woodhall M, Vincent A, Schrooten M, Vandenberghe W. Supranuclear gaze palsy in glycine receptor antibody-positive progressive encephalomyelitis with rigidity and myoclonus. Mov Disord. 2012; 27(14):1830–1832

[189] Aguilar-Amat MJ, Abenza-Abildúa MJ, Vivancos F, et al. Rheumatoid meningitis mimicking progressive supranuclear palsy. Neurologist. 2011; 17(3):136–140

[190] Quint DJ, Cornblath WT, Trobe JD. Multiple sclerosis presenting as Parinaud syndrome. AJNR Am J Neuroradiol. 1993; 14(5):1200–1202

[191] Bhidayasiri R, Riley DE, Somers JT, Lerner AJ, Büttner-Ennever JA, Leigh RJ. Pathophysiology of slow vertical saccades in progressive supranuclear palsy. Neurology. 2001; 57(11):2070–2077

[192] Collins SJ, Ahlskog JE, Parisi JE, Maraganore DM. Progressive supranuclear palsy: neuropathologically based diagnostic clinical criteria. J Neurol Neurosurg Psychiatry. 1995; 58(2):167–173

[193] Ling H, Kara E, Revesz T, et al. Concomitant progressive supranuclear palsy and chronic traumatic encephalopathy in a boxer. Acta Neuropathol Commun. 2014; 2:24

[194] Averbuch-Heller L, Helmchen C, Horn AKE, Leigh RJ, Büttner-Ennerver JA. Slow vertical saccades in motor neuron disease: correlation of structure and function. Ann Neurol. 1998; 44(4):641–648

[195] Okuda B, Yamamoto T, Yamasaki M, Maya K, Imai T. Motor neuron disease with slow eye movements and vertical gaze palsy. Acta Neurol Scand. 1992; 85(1):71–76

[196] Morris HR, Bronstein AM, Shaw CE, Lees AJ, Love S. Clinical grand round: a rapidly progressive pyramidal and extrapyramidal syndrome with a supranuclear gaze palsy. Mov Disord. 2005; 20(7):826–831

[197] Ushio M, Iwasaki S, Sugasawa K, Murofushi T. Atypical motor neuron disease with supranuclear vertical gaze palsy and slow saccades. Auris Nasus Larynx. 2009; 36(1):85–87

[198] Paviour DC, Lees AJ, Josephs KA, et al. Frontotemporal lobar degeneration with ubiquitin-only-immunoreactive neuronal changes: broadening the clinical picture to include progressive supranuclear palsy. Brain. 2004; 127 (Pt 11):2441–2451

[199] Weeks RA, Scaravilli F, Lees AJ, Carroll C, Husain M, Rudge P. Cerebral amyloid angiopathy and motor neurone disease presenting with a progressive supranuclear palsy-like syndrome. Mov Disord. 2003; 18(3): 331–336

[200] Murphy MA, Friedman JH, Tetrud JW, Factor SA. Neurodegenerative disorders mimicking progressive supranuclear palsy: a report of three cases. J Clin Neurosci. 2005; 12(8):941–945

[201] Malakouti-Nejad M, Shahidi GA, Rohani M, et al. Identification of p.Gln858* in ATP13A2 in two EOPD patients and presentation of their clinical features. Neurosci Lett. 2014; 577:106–111

[202] Wszolek ZK, Pfeiffer RF, Bhatt MH, et al. Rapidly progressive autosomal dominant parkinsonism and dementia with pallido-ponto-nigral degeneration. Ann Neurol. 1992; 32(3):312–320

[203] Tsuboi Y, Uitti RJ, Delisle MB, et al. Clinical features and disease haplotypes of individuals with the N279K tau gene mutation: a comparison of the pallidopontonigral degeneration kindred and a French family. Arch Neurol. 2002; 59(6):943–950

[204] Wilke C, Pomper JK, Biskup S, Puskás C, Berg D, Synofzik M. Atypical parkinsonism in C9orf72 expansions: a case report and systematic review of 45 cases from the literature. J Neurol. 2016; 263(3):558–574

[205] Oyanagi K, Chen KM, Craig UK, Yamazaki M, Perl DP. Parkinsonism, dementia and vertical gaze palsy in a Guamanian with atypical neuroglial degeneration. Acta Neuropathol. 2000; 99(1):73–80

[206] Moon SY, Lee BH, Seo SW, Kang SJ, Na DL. Slow vertical saccades in the frontotemporal dementia with motor neuron disease. J Neurol. 2008; 255 (9):1337–1343

[207] Soliveri P, Rossi G, Monza D, et al. A case of dementia parkinsonism resembling progressive supranuclear palsy due to mutation in the tau protein gene. Arch Neurol. 2003; 60(10):1454–1456

[208] Rusina R, Kovacs GG, Fiala J, et al. FTLD-TDP with motor neuron disease, visuospatial impairment and a progressive supranuclear palsy-like syndrome: broadening the clinical phenotype of TDP-43 proteinopathies. A report of three cases. BMC Neurol. 2011; 11:50

[209] Kovacs GG, Murrell JR, Horvath S, et al. TARDBP variation associated with frontotemporal dementia, supranuclear gaze palsy, and chorea. Mov Disord. 2009; 24(12):1843–1847

[210] Riley DE, Lang AE, Lewis A, et al. Cortical-basal ganglionic degeneration. Neurology. 1990; 40(8):1203–1212

[211] Rinne JO, Lee MS, Thompson PD, Marsden CD. Corticobasal degeneration. A clinical study of 36 cases. Brain. 1994; 117(Pt 5):1183–1196

[212] Brett FM, Henson C, Staunton H. Familial diffuse Lewy body disease, eye movement abnormalities, and distribution of pathology. Arch Neurol. 2002; 59(3):464–467

[213] Fearnley JM, Revesz T, Brooks DJ, Frackowiak RS, Lees AJ. Diffuse Lewy body disease presenting with a supranuclear gaze palsy. J Neurol Neurosurg Psychiatry. 1991; 54(2):159–161

[214] Lewis AJ, Gawel MJ. Diffuse Lewy body disease with dementia and oculomotor dysfunction. Mov Disord. 1990; 5(2):143–147

[215] Clerici F, Ratti PL, Pomati S, et al. Dementia with Lewy bodies with supra-nuclear gaze palsy: a matter of diagnosis. Neurol Sci. 2005; 26(5):358–361

[216] Wessel K, Moschner C, Wandinger KP, Kömpf D, Heide W. Oculomotor testing in the differential diagnosis of degenerative ataxic disorders. Arch Neurol. 1998; 55(7):949–956

[217] van Gassen KL, van der Heijden CD, de Bot ST, et al. Genotype-phenotype correlations in spastic paraplegia type 7: a study in a large Dutch cohort. Brain. 2012; 135(Pt 10):2994–3004

[218] Grewal KK, Stefanelli MG, Meijer IA, Hand CK, Rouleau GA, Ives EJ. A founder effect in three large Newfoundland families with a novel clinically variable spastic ataxia and supranuclear gaze palsy. Am J Med Genet A. 2004; 131(3): 249–254

[219] Klostermann W, Zühlke C, Heide W, Kömpf D, Wessel K. Slow saccades and other eye movement disorders in spinocerebellar atrophy type 1. J Neurol. 1997; 244(2):105–111

[220] Arbusow V, Dieterich M, Strupp M, et al. Herpes zoster neuritis involving superior and inferior parts of the vestibular nerve causes ocular tilt reaction. Neuroophthalmology. 1998; 19(1):17–22

[221] Chung EJ, Hwang JH, Lee MJ, et al. Expansion of the clinicopathological and mutational spectrum of Perry syndrome. Parkinsonism Relat Disord. 2014; 20(4):388–393

[222] Newsway V, Fish M, Rohrer JD, et al. Perry syndrome due to the DCTN1 G71 R mutation: a distinctive levodopa responsive disorder with behavioral syndrome, vertical gaze palsy, and respiratory failure. Mov Disord. 2010; 25 (6):767–770

[223] Williams DR, Hadeed A, al-Din AS, Wreikat AL, Lees AJ. Kufor Rakeb disease: autosomal recessive, levodopa-responsive parkinsonism with pyramidal degeneration, supranuclear gaze palsy, and dementia. Mov Disord. 2005; 20 (10):1264–1271

[224] Haack TB, Ignatius E, Calvo-Garrido J, et al. Absence of the autophagy adaptor SQSTM1/p62 causes childhood-onset neurodegeneration with ataxia, dystonia, and gaze palsy. Am J Hum Genet. 2016; 99(3):735–743

[225] Stevens JC, Murphy SM, Davagnanam I, et al. The ARSACS phenotype can include supranuclear gaze palsy and skin lipofuscin deposits. J Neurol Neurosurg Psychiatry. 2013; 84(1):114–116

[226] Saver JL, Liu GT, Charness ME. Idiopathic striopallidodentate calcification with prominent supranuclear abnormality of eye movement. J Neuroophthalmol. 1994; 14(1):29–33

[227] Bozi M, Matarin M, Theocharis I, Potagas C, Stefanis L. A patient with pantothenate kinase-associated neurodegeneration and supranuclear gaze palsy. Clin Neurol Neurosurg. 2009; 111(8):688–690

[228] Espay AJ, Bergeron C, Chen R, Lang AE. Rapidly progressive sporadic dentatorubral pallidoluysian atrophy with intracytoplasmic inclusions and no CAG repeat expansion. Mov Disord. 2006; 21(12):2251–2254

[229] Garbutt S, Harris CM. Abnormal vertical optokinetic nystagmus in infants and children. Br J Ophthalmol. 2000; 84(5):451–455

[230] Lossos A, Schlesinger I, Okon E, et al. Adult-onset Niemann-Pick type C disease. Clinical, biochemical, and genetic study. Arch Neurol. 1997; 54(12):1536–1541

[231] Nightingale S, Barton ME. Intermittent vertical supranuclear ophthal-moplegia and ataxia. Mov Disord. 1991; 6(1):76–78

[232] Lee MS, Kim YD, Lyoo CH. Oculogyric crisis as an initial manifestation of Wilson's disease. Neurology. 1999; 52(8):1714–1715

[233] Sirrs S, van Karnebeek CD, Peng X, et al. Defects in fatty acid amide hydrolase 2 in a male with neurologic and psychiatric symptoms. Orphanet J Rare Dis. 2015; 10:38–48

[234] Shults WT, Hamby S, Corbett JJ, Kardon R, Winterkorn JS, Odel JG. Neuro-ophthalmic complications of intracranial catheters. Neurosurgery. 1993; 33(1):135–138

[235] Fleury V, Spielberger S, Wolf E, et al. Vertical supranuclear gaze palsy induced by deep brain stimulation: report of two cases. Parkinsonism Relat Disord. 2014; 20(11):1295–1297

[236] Ackermans L, Temel Y, Bauer NJ, Visser-Vandewalle V, Dutch-Flemish Tourette Surgery Study Group. Vertical gaze palsy after thalamic stimulation for Tourette syndrome: case report. Neurosurgery. 2007; 61(5):E1100–, discussion E1100

[237] Liang T-W, Balcer LJ, Solomon D, Messé SR, Galetta SL. Supranuclear gaze palsy and opsoclonus after Diazinon poisoning. J Neurol Neurosurg Psychiatry. 2003; 74(5):677–679

[238] Gosala Raja Kukkuta S, Srinivas M, Raghunandan N, Thomas M, Prabhu A, Laly M. Reversible vertical gaze palsy in sodium valproate toxicity. J Neuroophthalmol. 2013; 33(2):202–203

[239] Janss AJ, Galetta SL, Freese A, et al. Superficial siderosis of the central nervous system: magnetic resonance imaging and pathological correlation. Case report. J Neurosurg. 1993; 79(5):756–760

[240] Rismondo V, Borchert M. Position-dependent Parinaud's syndrome. Am J Ophthalmol. 1992; 114(1):107–108

[241] Magli A, De Marco R, Di Maio S, Nunziata L, Villani S, Calace PL. A case of Parinaud's syndrome in a boy with delayed puberty. Ophthalmologica. 1991; 202(3):132–137

[242] Scolding NJ, Kellar-Wood HF, Shaw C, Shneerson JM, Antoun N. Wolfram syndrome: hereditary diabetes mellitus with brainstem and optic atrophy. Ann Neurol. 1996; 39(3):352–360

[243] Campistol J, Prats JM, Garaizar C. Benign paroxysmal tonic upgaze of childhood with ataxia. A neuro-ophthalmological syndrome of familial origin? Dev Med Child Neurol. 1993; 35(5):436–439

[244] Gieron MA, Korthals JK. Benign paroxysmal tonic upward gaze. Pediatr Neurol. 1993; 9(2):159

[245] Hayman M, Harvey AS, Hopkins IJ, Kornberg AJ, Coleman LT, Shield LK. Paroxysmal tonic upgaze: a reappraisal of outcome. Ann Neurol. 1998; 43(4):514–520

[246] Chaudhuri Z, Saxena R. Vertical gaze palsy in a case with growing skull fracture and porencephalic cyst. Eye (Lond). 2005; 19(2):232–234

[247] Feucht M, Griffiths B, Niemüller I, Haase W, Richard G, Mautner VF. Neurofibromatosis 2 leads to higher incidence of strabismological and neuro-ophthalmological disorders. Acta Ophthalmol. 2008; 86(8):882–886

[248] Ganos C, Biskup S, Kleinmichel S, et al. Progressive ataxia associated with scarring skin lesions and vertical gaze palsy. Mov Disord. 2013; 28(4):443–445

[249] Burde RM, Savino PJ, Trobe JD. Clinical Decisions in Neuro-Ophthalmology. 2nd ed. St. Louis: Mosby; 1985:204–205

[250] Adachi M, Kawanami T, Ohshima H, Sugai Y, Hosoya T. Morning glory sign: a particular MR finding in progressive supranuclear palsy. Magn Reson Med Sci. 2004; 3(3):125–132

[251] Amtage F, Maurer C, Hellwig S, et al. Functional correlates of vertical gaze palsy and other ocular motor deficits in PSP: an FDG-PET study. Parkinsonism Relat Disord. 2014; 20(8):898–906

[252] Lynch T, Odel J, Fredericks DN, et al. Polymerase chain reaction-based detection of Tropheryma whippelii in central nervous system Whipple's disease. Ann Neurol. 1997; 42(1):120–124

[253] von Herbay A, Ditton H-J, Schuhmacher F, Maiwald M. Whipple's disease: staging and monitoring by cytology and polymerase chain reaction analysis of cerebrospinal fluid. Gastroenterology. 1997; 113(2):434–441

[254] Voltz R, Gultekin SH, Rosenfeld MR, et al. A serologic marker of paraneoplastic limbic and brain-stem encephalitis in patients with testicular cancer. N Engl J Med. 1999; 340(23):1788–1795

[255] Bell JA, Fielder AR, Viney S. Congenital double elevator palsy in identical twins. J Clin Neuroophthalmol. 1990; 10(1):32–34

[256] Ziffer AJ, Rosenbaum AL, Demer JL, Yee RD. Congenital double elevator palsy: vertical saccadic velocity utilizing the scleral search coil technique. J Pediatr Ophthalmol Strabismus. 1992; 29(3):142–149

[257] Thömke F, Hopf HC. Acquired monocular elevation paresis. An asymmetric upgaze palsy. Brain. 1992; 115(Pt 6):1901–1910

[258] Deleu D, Ebinger G. Vertical one-and-a-half syndrome. Clinical, oculographic and radiologic findings. Neuroophthalmology. 1991; 11:99–101

[259] Wiest G, Baumgartner C, Schnider P, Trattnig S, Deecke L, Mueller C. Monocular elevation paresis and contralateral downgaze paresis from unilateral mesodiencephalic infarction. J Neurol Neurosurg Psychiatry. 1996; 60(5):579–581

[260] Terao S, Osano Y, Fukuoka T, Miura N, Mitsuma T, Sobue G. Coexisting vertical and horizontal one and a half syndromes. J Neurol Neurosurg Psychiatry. 2000; 69(3):401–402

[261] Deleu D, Imam YZB, Mesraoua B, Salem KY. Vertical one-and-a-half syndrome with contralesional pseudo-abducens palsy in a patient with thalamomesencephalic stroke. J Neurol Sci. 2012; 312(1–2):180–183

[262] Park S-H, Na DL, kim M. Disconjugate vertical ocular movement in a patient with locked-in syndrome. Br J Ophthalmol. 2001; 85(4):497–498

[263] Galimberti CA, Versino M, Sartori I, Manni R, Martelli A, Tartara A. Epileptic skew deviation. Neurology. 1998; 50(5):1469–1472

[264] Brandt T, Dieterich M. Skew deviation with ocular torsion: a vestibular brainstem sign of topographic diagnostic value. Ann Neurol. 1993; 33(5):528–534

[265] Brandt T, Dieterich M. Vestibular syndromes in the roll plane: topographic diagnosis from brainstem to cortex. Ann Neurol. 1994; 36(3):337–347

[266] Brandt T, Dieterich M. Central vestibular syndromes in the roll, pitch, and yaw planes: topographic diagnosis of brainstem disorders. Neuroophthalmology. 1996; 15:291–303

[267] Halmagyi GM, Brandt T, Dieterich M, Curthoys IS, Stark RJ, Hoyt WF. Tonic contraversive ocular tilt reaction due to unilateral meso-diencephalic lesion. Neurology. 1990; 40(10):1503–1509

[268] Hamed LM, Maria BL, Briscoe ST, Shamis D. Intact binocular function and absent ocular torsion in children with alternating skew on lateral gaze. J Pediatr Ophthalmol Strabismus. 1996; 33(3):164–166

[269] Suzuki T, Nishio M, Chikuda M, Takayanagi K. Skew deviation as a complication of cardiac catheterization. Am J Ophthalmol. 2001; 132(2):282–283

[270] Brandt T, Dieterich M. Two types of ocular tilt reaction: the "ascending" pontomedullary VOR-OTR and the "descending" mesencephalic integrator-OTR. Neuro-ophthalmology. 1998; 19(2):83–92

[271] Brazis PW. Ocular motor abnormalities in Wallenberg's lateral medullary syndrome. Mayo Clin Proc. 1992; 67(4):365–368

[272] Keane JR. Ocular tilt reaction following lateral pontomedullary infarction. Neurology. 1992; 42(1):259–260

[273] Averbuch-Heller L, Rottach KG, Zivotofsky AZ, et al. Torsional eye movements in patients with skew deviation and spasmodic torticollis: responses to static and dynamic head roll. Neurology. 1997; 48(2):506–514

[274] Dieterich M, Brandt T. Ocular torsion and tilt of subjective visual vertical are sensitive brainstem signs. Ann Neurol. 1993; 33(3):292–299

[275] Ohashi T, Fukushima K, Chin S, et al. Ocular tilt reaction with vertical eye movement palsy caused by localized unilateral midbrain lesion. J Neuroophthalmol. 1998; 18(1):40–42

[276] Riordan-Eva P, Harcourt JP, Faldon M, Brookes GB, Gresty MA. Skew deviation following vestibular nerve surgery. Ann Neurol. 1997; 41(1):94–99

[277] Safran AB, Vibert D, Issoua D, Häusler R. Skew deviation after vestibular neuritis. Am J Ophthalmol. 1994; 118(2):238–245

[278] Vibert D, Häusler R, Safran AB, Koerner F. Diplopia from skew deviation in unilateral peripheral vestibular lesions. Acta Otolaryngol. 1996; 116(2):170–176

[279] Mossman S, Halmagyi GM. Partial ocular tilt reaction due to unilateral cerebellar lesion. Neurology. 1997; 49(2):491–493

[280] Esaki H, Shinji O. Skew deviation in Fisher's syndrome. Neuro-ophthalmol Jpn. 1992; 9:66

[281] Donahue SP, Lavin PJ, Hamed LM. Tonic ocular tilt reaction simulating a superior oblique palsy: diagnostic confusion with the 3-step test. Arch Ophthalmol. 1999; 117(3):347–352

15 Ocular Myasthenia Gravis

John D. Eatman and Stacy V. Smith

Abstract

Myasthenia gravis in adults is an acquired autoimmunity to the motor endplate, and the ocular form of the disease results in fatigable weakness of the levator palpebrae superioris (producing ptosis), the extraocular muscles, and the orbicularis oculi. In systemic disease, the weakness can involve all voluntary muscles in the body. This chapter discusses the clinical pathways in evaluating and treating ocular myasthenia gravis, by reviewing the literature in detail.

Keywords: ocular myasthenia gravis, fatigable weakness, ptosis, diplopia, neuromuscular disease

15.1 What Are the Clinical Findings in Myasthenia Gravis?

Myasthenia gravis (MG) is a chronic disorder of neuromuscular transmission characterized clinically by varying degrees of weakness and fatigue of voluntary muscles. MG is caused by an acquired autoimmunity to the motor endplate and is associated with antibodies that block or cause increased degradation of acetylcholine receptors (AChRs). There is abnormal weakness in some or all voluntary muscles. The most commonly affected muscles are the levator palpebrae superioris, the extraocular muscles, the orbicularis oculi, triceps, quadriceps, and the tongue. Other voluntary muscles innervated by cranial nerves (facial, masticatory, pharyngeal, and laryngeal muscles) and cervical, pectoral girdle, and hip flexor muscles are also frequently affected. The weakness increases with repeated or sustained exertion and over the course of the day, but is improved by rest; it also may be worsened by elevation of body temperature and is often improved by cold.[1,2]

15.2 What Are the Clinical Features of Ocular Myasthenia Gravis and Generalized Myasthenia Gravis?

The levator palpebrae superioris and extraocular muscles are involved initially in approximately 50 to 70% of cases, and these muscles are eventually affected in about 90% of patients. Ocular myasthenia (OM) is a form of MG confined to the extraocular, levator palpebrae superioris, and/or orbicularis oculi muscles. Various studies put the conversion rate from OM to generalized MG from 50 to 64%, but a more recent retrospective multicenter analysis by Nagia et al showed an overall conversion rate of 20.9%.[3,4,5] Of the patients with purely ocular symptoms and signs at onset that go on to develop generalized MG, most, but not all, develop generalized symptoms within 2 to 3 years of onset of the disorder. Bever et al performed a retrospective study and found that 226 (84%) of 269 myasthenics displayed

ocular findings at onset of disease and 142 (53%) demonstrated only ocular involvement.[3] Follow-up (average 14 years, range 1–39 years) of 108 patients with MG who had only ocular symptoms and signs at onset showed that 43 (40%) remained ocular and 53 (49%) became generalized. Of the 53 patients who became generalized, 44 (83%) did so within 2 years of onset of the disease. Age of onset in their patients was of prognostic significance. Patients older than 50 years of age at onset had a greater risk of generalized MG and severe complications, whereas patients who were younger at onset had a more benign outcome. In another study of 1,487 myasthenic patients, 53% presented with ocular MG and 202 (4%) continued to demonstrate purely ocular involvement for up to 45 years of follow-up (mean, 17 years).[4] Of those patients with strictly ocular signs and symptoms during the first month after onset (40% of the 1487 patients), 66% subsequently developed clinically generalized disease; of these, 78% became generalized within 1 year after onset of symptoms and 94% within 3 years. Nagia et al did a retrospective chart review on 158 patients who presented with OM which showed that 33 (20.9%) converted to generalized MG. Of those that converted, 23 (69.3%) converted within the first 2 years.[5]

Ptosis in MG may occur as an isolated sign or in association with extraocular muscle involvement. Evoli et al studied 48 patients with OM and noted that 10% had ptosis only, 90% had ptosis and extraocular muscle involvement, and 25% had weakness of the orbicularis oculi.[6] Ptosis may be unilateral or bilateral and, when bilateral, is usually asymmetric. The ptosis may be absent when the patient awakens and appear later in the day, becoming more pronounced as the day progresses. Prolonged upward gaze may increase the ptosis. Enhanced or seesaw ptosis may be demonstrated (i.e., a worsening of ptosis on one side when the opposite eyelid is elevated and held in a fixed position). Enhancement of ptosis is not specific for MG and may rarely be seen with the Lambert–Eaton myasthenic syndrome, senile ptosis, ocular myopathy, Miller Fisher syndrome, and even third nerve palsy.[7,8,9] During refixation (a vertical saccade) from down to the primary position, the upper eyelid may either slowly begin to droop or twitch several times before settling in a stable position (Cogan lid-twitch sign). This sign is characteristic, but not diagnostic, of MG.[10,11] For example, Kao et al described two patients with fatigable ptosis due to intracranial mass lesions (hematoma and metastasis) likely causing compression of the central caudal nucleus of the dorsal midbrain.[12] MG may also be associated with three types of eyelid retraction[13]: (1) contralateral eyelid retraction due to bilateral excessive innervation (Hering's law) to raise the ptotic lid; (2) brief eyelid retraction lasting only seconds following a saccade from downgaze to primary position (Cogan lid twitch sign); and (3) transient eyelid retraction lasting seconds or minutes after staring straight ahead or looking upward for several seconds.

Involvement of extraocular muscles with MG usually occurs in association with ptosis, though not always. MG should be considered in any case of ocular motor weakness without pupil involvement because MG may mimic any pattern of neurogenic paresis. Any extraocular muscle may be selectively impaired, especially the medial rectus, and weakness characteristically increases with sustained effort.[2,13,14] Myasthenia can mimic painless, pupil-sparing third nerve palsies, superior division third nerve palsies, and fourth or sixth nerve palsies.[2,13,15] Myasthenia may mimic an internuclear ophthalmoplegia (pseudo-INO),[16] the one-and-a-half syndrome,[17] horizontal or vertical gaze palsy,[13] divergence paresis,[18] double elevator palsy, and complete external ophthalmoplegia. MG may also be associated with abnormalities of saccadic eye movements[13] including (1) hypermetric saccades; (2) hypometric saccades that begin with normal velocity but ultimately show a decrease in velocity (intersaccadic fatigue) and undershoot the target; (3) small, jerky, quivering eye movements; and (4) gaze-evoked nystagmus. Patients with MG often have weakness of the orbicularis oculi muscles. In some cases, a "peek sign" may occur. In an attempt to sustain forceful eye closure, the orbicularis oculi may fatigue, resulting in the patient "peeking" through the partially opened palpebral fissure. Lower eyelid ectropion may occur in myasthenic patients, and become especially noticeable as the day progresses.[13] Finally, although abnormalities of pupillary function and accommodation have been described in MG, this dysfunction is not clinically significant.[2,13]

There is a higher percentage of OM in the prepubertal onset juvenile MG cases (between 26 and 50%) compared to pubertal and postpubertal onset juvenile MG.[19,20] In a study of 25 children with MG, more than half had had ocular symptoms.[21] Generalization occurred in 5 of the 14 patients; ocular progression to systemic involvement developed on average in 7.8 months (range 1–23 months). Long-term permanent damage to the extraocular muscles as a result of juvenile MG is rare.[21] A 2-year surveillance study in Canada identified 52 cases of acquired myasthenia in children, of which 34 generalized MG and 18 OM. Ptosis was the most common presenting symptom in both groups. Children in the generalized group were predominantly Caucasian (59%), while those in the ocular group were predominantly Asian (44%). A greater ratio of females to males was seen overall, and more pronounced in the ocular group as well as in the puberty/postpuberty group. Treatment history indicated a high response rate of OM to both steroid (100%) and pyridostigmine (94%) therapy.[20]

15.3 What Studies Are Suggested to Diagnose Ocular Myasthenia Gravis?

The diagnosis of OM is based on the clinical history and exam (fatigue, rest, or sleep test), serologic testing (e.g., antibody testing), electrophysiology (e.g., electromyography [EMG], single fiber EGM [SFEMG]), and pharmacologic testing (e.g., rapid-onset, short-acting acetylcholinesterase inhibitor trial). EMG investigations include study of the decremental response, conventional needle EMG, and single-fiber recordings. In some instances, in vitro microelectrode studies of neuromuscular transmission and ultrastructural studies of the neuromuscular junction may be required to establish the diagnosis.[1] In general, microelectrode and ultrastructural studies are reserved for patients with generalized MG and are not discussed here.

The diagnosis of OM should be considered in any patient with ptosis and/or ocular motor weakness without pupillary involvement. Weakness and fatigue confined to the extraocular muscles or lids combined with orbicularis oculi paresis is especially suggestive of OM. Significant clinical involvement of the pupil, eye pain or headaches, proptosis, visual loss, or involvement of trigeminal sensation are not seen in MG.

15.4 What Studies Are Used in the Pharmacologic Testing for Ocular MG?

A positive edrophonium hydrochloride (traditionally known as the "Tensilon test") or neostigmine methylsulfate test is usually, but not always, indicative of OM. The improvement of extraocular muscle function should be quantified with prisms, a Hess screen, or the Lancaster red-green test.[22] Ptosis tends to respond better to anticholinesterases than does ophthalmoparesis.[13] Evoli et al studied 43 OM patients with both ptosis and diplopia and found that edrophonium relieved only the ptosis in 15 (35%) patients.[6] False-positive responses to anticholinesterases have been described with brainstem and parasellar tumors, aneurysms, metastasis to the orbital apex, multiples sclerosis, Lambert–Eaton myasthenic syndrome, poliomyelitis, Guillain–Barré syndrome, motor neuron disease, botulism, orbital myositis, congenital ptosis, snake bites, diabetic sixth nerve palsy, and dermatomyositis.[2,11,13,23,24] In most of these reports, the correct diagnosis was evident by associated neurologic signs and symptoms. Moorthy et al, however, described eight cases originally diagnosed as having MG in whom an intracranial lesion instead of, or in addition to, MG was later identified.[25] Four of these patients probably had both MG and an intracranial lesion, but the other four had only intracranial lesions with clinical "pseudomyasthenic" features, including fatigable weakness, Cogan lid twitch sign, and positive pharmacologic tests. Three had pupil-sparing third nerve palsies and one had a third nerve palsy associated with a sixth nerve palsy. These authors suggested that patients with clinical features consistent with MG restricted to the ocular or cranial muscles should be carefully evaluated for intracranial lesions using computed tomography (CT) or magnetic resonance imaging (MRI). Miller suggests that it is advisable to rule out an intracranial lesion by CT or MR imaging in all patients with isolated, unilateral, pupil-sparing ophthalmoparesis even when the diagnosis of MG seems assured by antibody testing, response to acetylcholinesterase inhibitors, or other studies (class IV, level C).[13]

A negative edrophonium or neostigmine test does not rule out MG.[2,6,13] For example, Spector and Daroff noted negative responses to edrophonium in 2 of 11 (18%) OM and in 6 of 21 (29%) of patients with both OM and generalized MG.[26] Paradoxical responses to edrophonium may also occur in OM patients, including paresis of previously nonparetic muscles and increased eye misalignment due to further weakening of paretic muscles.

While edrophonium testing is considered a safe diagnostic tool, it must be used with caution in patients with heart disease, or patients on atrioventricular (AV) nodal blocking drugs. The test can also be uncomfortable for the patient causing nausea and vomiting. Pharmacologic testing is best utilized for the patient where other testing (such as clinical examination, ice pack test, antibody testing, repetitive stimulation on single fiber

EMG) is negative or equivocal and the results of the test will impact the management plan.[27] The ice and rest tests have largely supplanted the use of edrophonium testing in our clinic for the diagnosis of ocular MG.

15.5 What Nonpharmacologic Testing Is Helpful in the Diagnosis of Myasthenia Gravis?

The "sleep test" may also be incorporated to demonstrate objective improvement in MG symptoms after rest.[28] The patient is kept in a quiet, darkened room and instructed to close the eyes and rest for 30 minutes. The ptosis and ocular motility are quantified before and after the rest period. This study may be positive in some patients that fail pharmacologic testing, but may also be negative in edrophonium-responsive patients.[2]

Another noninvasive test is the ice-pack test, which may be useful in the diagnosis of OM in the patient with ptosis.[29,30,31] Ice in a surgical glove is placed over one lightly closed eye for 2 minutes or to the limit of patient tolerance. In cases of bilateral ptosis, the opposite (uncooled) eye serves as control. The palpebral fissures are measured before and after the ice is applied. Sethi et al noted improvement of ptosis in 8 of 10 MG patients,[31] and Golnik et al found the test to be positive in 16 of 20 (80%) of patients with MG and none of 20 patients with ptosis not due to MG.[29] In four patients with MG and complete ptosis, however, the ice-pack test was negative, and thus the sensitivity of the test in patients with complete ptosis decreases considerably. It is thought that the decreased temperature may inhibit acetylcholinesterase function.[29] Improvement of eyelid elevation after the ice test is in part caused by rest, but the ice significantly improved ptosis more than rest alone in one study.[30] In another study, however, myasthenic ptosis was markedly improved in four patients regardless of local cooling or warming, with the common denominator of these tests being rest rather than temperature per se.[32]

Electrophysiologic testing might establish the diagnosis of MG. EMG findings include fluctuations in the amplitude and duration of motor unit potentials recorded during voluntary activity, decremental responses of evoked compound muscle action potentials to repetitive supramaximal motor nerve stimulation, and single-fiber EGM (SFEMG) abnormalities (e.g., impulse blocking and increased "jitter").[1,13,28,33] Repetitive nerve stimulation (RNS) studies should include proximal and facial nerves to increase diagnostic yield.[34,35] While RNS studies are more widely available than SFEMG and the decrement is specific (up to 100%), the sensitivity remains low (18–36%).[34,36,37] Due to this low sensitivity, some authors recommend against RNS in OM with a preference for the SFEMG.[38]

If RNS studies are negative in a patient with suspected MG, SFEMG studies might be useful due to increased sensitivity. SFEMG is positive in 75% of myasthenic patients in remission, 80 to 88% of those with ocular signs and symptoms only, 91 to 100% of patients with generalized symptoms, and 88 to 94% of patients with myasthenia overall.[2,39,40] For example, in one study SFEMG in limb muscles was abnormal in 17 of 20 patients with OM.[39] SFEMG is quite sensitive for detecting abnormalities of the neuromuscular junction but is not specific for MG. In another study of OM, SFEMG showed the highest sensitivity

(100%), whereas AChR antibodies studies showed the highest specificity (100%) for diagnosis.[41] SFEMG of the frontalis muscle may be a sensitive technique for the diagnosis of OM.[42] SFEMG is a highly specialized test that is not available in all care settings, and thus the EMG/RNS is more commonly performed in many facilities.

15.6 What Is the Diagnostic Utility of Antiacetylcholine Receptor Antibodies in the Diagnosis of Myasthenia Gravis?

AChR antibody titers are quite useful in the diagnosis of MG. A retrospective observational cohort study of 223 OM patients by Peeler et al found that 158 (70.9) patients had positive AChR antibody testing. Previous studies showed the percentage of AChR antibody positivity in OM to be 40 to 70%.[43] Testing for AChR binding, blocking, and modulating antibodies increases the assay yield in patients with generalized MG and OM. In OM, the antibody titer tends to be low, and the serum antibody titer correlates poorly with the severity of MG when a group of patients is studied.[1] If AChR antibodies are negative, consider testing for additional neuromuscular antibodies such as muscle-specific kinase (MuSK) antibodies.

15.7 Summary of Testing for Ocular Myasthenia Gravis

No test is specific for OM, and its diagnosis should not be based exclusively on any single test. Kelly et al advised that all patients with suspected MG should have serum assays of AChR antibodies, repetitive stimulation studies, and, if indicated, SFEMG and pharmacologic testing.[44] These procedures confirm the diagnosis in at least 95% of patients. Muscle biopsy with receptor assay, in addition to these studies, should diagnose close to 100% of patients, including those with OM,[13] although the invasive nature of this procedure makes it uncommon in clinical practice. Oh et al studied 20 patients diagnosed with OM and found SFEMG positive in 80%, AChR antibodies present in 70%, and RNS studies positive in 35 to 45%.[45] These authors advised initial AChR antibody assay and RNS studies, and follow-up SFEMG if the first two studies are normal. Evoli et al studied 48 patients with OM and found edrophonium tests positive in 47, RNS of the limb muscles positive in 50% (24 of 48), and elevated AChR antibody titers in 45% (20 of 44).[6] In another study of 19 edrophonium-responsive OM patients, Tsujihata et al found that 6 of 16 (38%) were seronegative for AChR antibodies. Eight of 13 (62%) had normal SFEMG of arm muscles, and 15 of 17 (88%) had normal RNS study of the facial nerve to the orbicularis oculi muscles.[46]

15.8 Should CT Imaging of the Chest for Thymoma Be Performed in MG?

Because there is an increased risk of thymoma in patients with MG, all patients with the diagnosis of MG should undergo CT or

MRI of the mediastinum. Thymoma occurs in 5 to 20% of myasthenic patients overall. Conversely, 15 to 20% of thymoma patients have clinical MG, with an additional 25% positive for AChR antibodies but asymptomatic.[47] The risk of thymoma in patients with OM is probably lower: 4% in patients with OM compared to 12% in those with generalized MG in one series.[48] Thymoma is more common in older patients and in patients with high AChR antibody titers.[49] In a large series of patients with MG, striated muscle antibodies were present in 84% of patients with thymoma.[50] In those without thymoma, striational antibodies were found in 5 or 47%, respectively, of patients in whom the onset of MG was before or after the age of 40.

15.9 What Is the Association of Thyroid Disease and MG?

Thyroid disease may be associated with MG. A systematic review of the literature found that 13% of MG patients reported another coexisting autoimmune disease, with autoimmune thyroid disease (Graves disease and Hashimoto disease) the most common comorbid disorder. A second autoimmune disease occurred more often in female and seropositive MG patients.[51] A prevalence study in Norway found other autoimmune diseases in 11 of 48 patients (23%), with 10.4% having autoimmune thyroiditis.[52] A retrospective review of patients in a MG clinic in Taiwan suggests that MG patients with autoimmune disease are predominantly female, have a younger onset of MG symptoms, a milder MG course (including OM), a higher incidence of thymic hyperplasia, and lower levels of seropositive AChR antibodies. Similar to a prior study, it found an association between thyroid eye disease and OM.[53,54] However, the clinical signs and symptoms of OM and thyroid eye disease can overlap and may confound the interpretation of this data. In OM patients, thyroid-stimulating hormone (TSH) levels might detect subclinical or asymptomatic associated thyroid disease (class IV, level C). An approach to the diagnosis and evaluation of patients with possible OM is outlined in ▸ Fig. 15.1.

15.10 What Is the Suggested Management of OM?

Patients with pure OM must be warned of the possibility of generalization of the disease process and should specifically be instructed to inform their physician immediately if symptoms such as dysphagia, respiratory involvement, or extremity weakness develop. Good diet (e.g., potassium), adequate rest, and avoidance of precipitants (e.g., heat, medications that worsen MG) are reasonable.

For patients with OM, if the diplopia or ptosis is mild, then observation or patching one eye may be sufficient. Ptosis may be eliminated in some patients by temporarily taping the lid up or having a crutch attachment placed on a spectacle frame for one or both eyes, although this often causes irritation of the eyes from exposure.[13,55] Ptosis surgery may be performed in some patients, particularly those who are refractory to medical therapy or in whom ptosis is a predominant finding.[13] However, they must be cautioned that ptosis can reoccur postoperatively

as the underlying disease process is still present. In some patients, prisms can alleviate diplopia, particularly when there is a relatively comitant deviation.

For more severe ocular motor weakness, anticholinesterase agents, such as pyridostigmine bromide, are warranted, although these agents often do not succeed in correcting the diplopia. Diplopia is often more refractory to treatment than ptosis. If moderate or large doses of anticholinesterase drugs fail or cannot be tolerated and symptoms are troublesome, then corticosteroids, often at relatively low alternate-day doses, are usually effective in correcting the diplopia (class III, level B–C).[6,55,56,57,58] Some authors, however, suggest that corticosteroids be used for OM only if patients demand their use, or if there is severe bilateral ptosis or severe ophthalmoplegia that precludes useful vision.[59] However, others suggest that steroids could modify the course of the disease in OM and prevent generalization.[58] A randomized controlled trial by Benatar et al attempting to determine the efficacy of prednisone for the treatment of OM (the EPITOME trial) was closed early due to slow enrollment.[60] Despite only enrolling 11 subjects, the study showed a clinical and statistical benefit of prednisone compared to placebo, administered as a slowly escalating dose.[60] Some authors have suggested azathioprine or mycophenolate for MG that is inadequately controlled on low-dose steroids or for those patients with intolerable steroid side effects (class IV, level C).[2,55,58] Cyclophosphamide, cyclosporine, intravenous immunoglobulin, and plasmapheresis have also been used but are not usually recommended for OM because their benefit–risk ratios have not been adequately studied (class IV, level U).

15.11 What about Thymectomy for OM?

The presence of a thymoma in any patient with MG is an indication for thymectomy (class III, level B).[1] Wolfe et al completed a randomized clinical trial on thymectomy for generalized MG in 126 patients without thymoma.[61] Patients who underwent thymectomy in addition to alternate-day prednisone therapy had lower time-weighted average Quantitative Myasthenia Gravis scores at 3 years. The patients also required lower average prednisone doses, a lower rate of immunosuppression use, and fewer hospitalizations for MG exacerbations. This study excluded patients with purely ocular symptoms.[61] Patients with OM should be evaluated with mediastinal CT or MRI. Although thymectomy can be effective in OM without thymoma and may prevent generalization of the disease, most clinicians are reluctant to recommend this procedure for purely ocular symptoms.[62] Transsternal thymectomy was studied in 22 cases of purely OM. Remission was defined as complete freedom from symptoms without medications for more than 3 months. The remission rates increased with time from 11.8% at 3 years to 23.1% at 5 years and 33.3% at 10 years.[63] Those patients undergoing thymectomy within 12 months of symptom onset showed a significantly earlier and better chance of remission compared to patients undergoing thymectomy longer than 12 months after symptom onset. The authors concluded that thymectomy for OM in the earlier stages of the disease is the preferred treatment, just as for generalized MG. Another study reviewed 61 patients with OM who underwent thymectomy

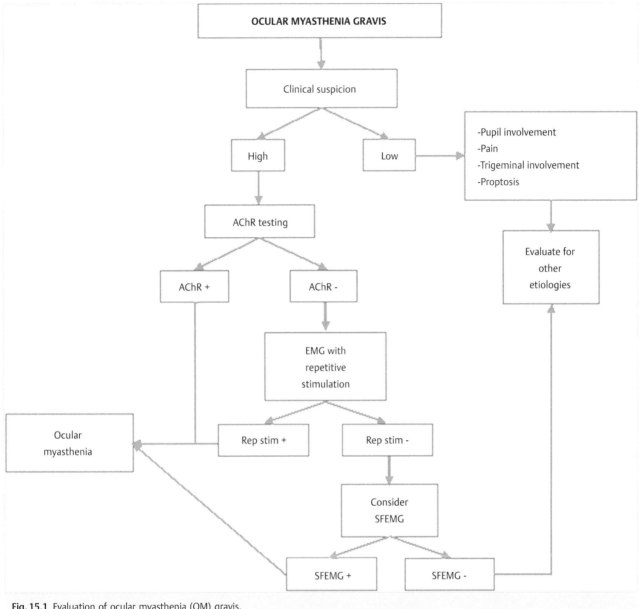

Fig. 15.1 Evaluation of ocular myasthenia (OM) gravis.

and who were followed for a mean of 9 years.[64] Thymoma was present in 12 patients. Overall, 71% were cured (51%) or improved (20%) by thymectomy, with 16 patients (26%) unchanged, 1 worsening, and 1 dying in the postoperative period. Improvement or cure was noted in 67% of the thymoma group. The authors concluded that thymectomy is safe and effective for OM.

We do not generally recommend thymectomy (without thymoma) for OM (class IV, level C). From 20 to 50% of patients with OM go into remission without thymectomy, and no controlled studies have compared this to a surgical group. The argument for thymectomy will remain unconvincing unless a prospective trial comparing thymectomy to medical management is performed.[65]

15.12 What Is the Prognosis of OM? Does the Use of Corticosteroids Alter the Prognosis?

About 10 to 20% of patients with OM undergo spontaneous remission that may be temporary or permanent. Although corticosteroid treatment produces a higher incidence of remission and improvement, there is no evidence that anticholinesterase agents affect the course of the disease.[57] Kupersmith et al reported a retrospective review of 32 patients with OM who were treated with corticosteroids and followed for a minimum of 2 years.[57] Diplopia was initially present in the primary position in 29 patients and in downgaze position in 26. Ptosis was present in 24 patients (unilateral in 13 and bilateral in 11). Patients were treated with one or more courses of daily prednisone (the highest initial dose, 40–80 mg) gradually withdrawn over 4 to 6 weeks. Subsequently, in six patients, 2.5 to 20 mg of prednisone was given on alternate days for more than 6 months. No patients had major steroid complications. Two years after diagnosis, diplopia was found in primary position in 11 patients and in downward gaze in 11 patients (9 had diplopia in primary gaze), and 66% of patients had normal ocular function. Ptosis was found in seven patients. Generalized MG had developed in three patients (9.4%) at 2 years. Of the 16 patients who had follow-up for 3 years and the 13 for 4 or longer, ocular motility was normal in 56% at 3 years and 62% at 4 years, with 2 additional patients developing generalized MG at 4 years. The authors concluded that moderate-dose daily prednisone for 4 to 6 weeks, followed by low-dose, alternate-day therapy as needed, can control the diplopia of OM, and that the frequency of deterioration to generalized MG at 2 years may be reduced.

Sommer et al retrospectively analyzed 78 patients with OM with a mean disease duration of 8.3 years.[66] In 54 patients (69%), symptoms and signs remained confined to the extraocular muscles during the observation period, whereas the remaining 24 patients (31%) developed symptoms of generalized myasthenia (50% of them within 2 years and 75% within 4 years after onset). There was a slightly reduced risk of generalization for patients with mild symptoms, normal repetitive stimulation studies, and low or absent AChR antibodies. Patients receiving immunosuppressive treatment (corticosteroids and/or azathioprine) rarely developed generalized MG (6 of 50 [12%]). Those without such treatment, usually due to uncertain diagnosis and late referral, converted into generalized MG significantly more often (18 of 28 [64%]). The authors concluded that short-term corticosteroids and long-term azathioprine seemed adequate for achieving remission in most patients. The proportion of patients developing generalized MG was smaller in this population compared to previously published groups and early immunosuppressive treatment was thought to be at least partially responsible for this finding. Thymectomy (performed in 12 patients with an abnormal chest CT) also correlated with a good outcome, but had no apparent advantage over medical treatment alone.[66] Until a prospective clinical trial of corticosteroids or other immunosuppressive is performed in patients with OM, the value of these agents in the prevention of the development of generalized MG remains undefined (class III–IV, level C). Finally, stable disabling diplopia may occasionally respond favorably to strabismus surgery.[67] Due to the neuromuscular blockade action of botulinum toxin, it should never be used for symptom management in a patient with confirmed or suspected MG, regardless of the disease stability.

References

[1] Engel AG. Disturbances of neuromuscular transmission. Acquired auto-immune myasthenia gravis. In: Engel AG, Franzini-Armstrong C, eds. Myology. Basic and Clinical. 2nd ed. New York: McGraw-Hill; 1994:1769–1797

[2] Weinberg DA, Lesser RL, Vollmer TL. Ocular myasthenia: a protean disorder. Surv Ophthalmol. 1994; 39(3):169–210

[3] Bever CT, Jr, Aquino AV, Penn AS, Lovelace RE, Rowland LP. Prognosis of ocular myasthenia. Ann Neurol. 1983; 14(5):516–519

[4] Oosterhuis HJ. The ocular signs and symptoms of myasthenia gravis. Doc Ophthalmol. 1982; 52(3–4):363–378

[5] Nagia L, Lemos J, Abusamra K, Cornblath WT, Eggenberger ER. Prognosis of ocular myasthenia gravis: retrospective multicenter analysis. Ophthalmology. 2015; 122(7):1517–1521

[6] Evoli A, Tonali P, Bartoccioni E, Lo Monaco M. Ocular myasthenia: diagnostic and therapeutic problems. Acta Neurol Scand. 1988; 77(1):31–35

[7] Averbuch-Heller L, Poonyathalang A, von Maydell RD, Remler BF. Hering's law for eyelids: still valid. Neurology. 1995; 45(9):1781–1783

[8] Brazis PW. Enhanced ptosis in Lambert-Eaton myasthenic syndrome. J Neuroophthalmol. 1997; 17(3):202–203

[9] Ishikawa H, Wakakura M, Ishikawa S. Enhanced ptosis in Fisher's syndrome after Epstein-Barr virus infection. J Clin Neuroophthalmol. 1990; 10(3):197–200

[10] Phillips PH, Newman NJ. Here today … gone tomorrow. Surv Ophthalmol. 1997; 41(4):354–356

[11] Ragge NK, Hoyt WF. Midbrain myasthenia: fatigable ptosis, 'lid twitch' sign, and ophthalmoparesis from a dorsal midbrain glioma. Neurology. 1992; 42(4):917–919

[12] Kao Y-F, Lan M-Y, Chou M-S, Chen W-H. Intracranial fatigable ptosis. J Neuroophthalmol. 1999; 19(4):257–259

[13] Miller NR. Walsh and Hoyt's Clinical Neuro-ophthalmology. 4th ed. Baltimore: Williams & Wilkins; 1985:841–891

[14] Odel J. Ocular myasthenia. Presented at the North American Neuro-Ophthalmology Society meeting, Rancho Bernardo, California, February 1992

[15] Dehaene I, van Zandijcke M. Isolated paralysis of the superior division of the ocular motor nerve mimicked by myasthenia gravis. Neuro-ophthalmology. 1995; 15(5):257–258

[16] Ito K, Mizutani J, Murofushi T, Mizuno M. Bilateral pseudo-internuclear ophthalmoplegia in myasthenia gravis. ORL J Otorhinolaryngol Relat Spec. 1997; 59(2):122–126

[17] Bandini F, Faga D, Simonetti S. Ocular myasthenia mimicking a one-and-a-half syndrome. J Neuroophthalmol. 2001; 21(3):210–211

[18] Lepore FE. Divergence paresis: a nonlocalizing cause of diplopia. J Neuroophthalmol. 1999; 19(4):242–245

[19] Ionita CM, Acsadi G. Management of juvenile myasthenia gravis. Pediatr Neurol. 2013; 48(2):95–104

[20] VanderPluym J, Vajsar J, Jacob FD, Mah JK, Grenier D, Kolski H. Clinical characteristics of pediatric myasthenia: a surveillance study. Pediatrics. 2013; 132(4):e939–e944

[21] Mullaney P, Vajsar J, Smith R, Buncic JR. The natural history and ophthalmic involvement in childhood myasthenia gravis at the hospital for sick children. Ophthalmology. 2000; 107(3):504–510

[22] Coll GE, Demer JL. The edrophonium-Hess screen test in the diagnosis of ocular myasthenia gravis. Am J Ophthalmol. 1992; 114(4):489–493

[23] Shams PN, Waldman A, Plant GT. B Cell lymphoma of the brain stem masquerading as myasthenia. J Neurol Neurosurg Psychiatry. 2002; 72(2):271–273

[24] Straube A, Witt TN. Oculo-bulbar myasthenic symptoms as the sole sign of tumour involving or compressing the brain stem. J Neurol. 1990; 237(6):369–371

[25] Moorthy G, Behrens MM, Drachman DB, et al. Ocular pseudomyasthenia or ocular myasthenia 'plus': a warning to clinicians. Neurology. 1989; 39(9):1150–1154

[26] Spector RH, Daroff RB. Edrophonium infrared optokinetic nystagmography in the diagnosis of myasthenia gravis. Ann N Y Acad Sci. 1976; 274:642–651

[27] Okun MS, Charriez CM, Bhatti MT, Watson RT, Swift T. Tensilon and the diagnosis of myasthenia gravis: are we using the Tensilon test too much? Neurologist. 2001; 7(5):295–299

[28] Odel JG, Winterkorn JM, Behrens MM. The sleep test for myasthenia gravis. A safe alternative to Tensilon. J Clin Neuroophthalmol. 1991; 11(4):288–292

[29] Golnik KC, Pena R, Lee AG, Eggenberger ER. An ice test for the diagnosis of myasthenia gravis. Ophthalmology. 1999; 106(7):1282–1286

[30] Kubis KC, Danesh-Meyer HV, Savino PJ, Sergott RC. The ice test versus the rest test in myasthenia gravis. Ophthalmology. 2000; 107(11):1995–1998

[31] Sethi KD, Rivner MH, Swift TR. Ice pack test for myasthenia gravis. Neurology. 1987; 37(8):1383–1385

[32] Movaghar M, Slavin ML. Effect of local heat versus ice on blepharoptosis resulting from ocular myasthenia. Ophthalmology. 2000; 107(12):2209–2214

[33] Hermann RC Jr. Repetitive stimulation studies. In: Daube JR, ed. Clinical Neurophysiology. Philadelphia, FA Davis; 1996:237–247

[34] Chiou-Tan FY, Gilchrist JM. Repetitive nerve stimulation and single-fiber electromyography in the evaluation of patients with suspected myasthenia gravis or Lambert-Eaton myasthenic syndrome: review of recent literature. Muscle Nerve. 2015; 52(3):455–462

[35] Witoonpanich R, Barakul S, Dejthevaporn C. Relative fatigability of muscles in response to repetitive nerve stimulation in myasthenia gravis. J Med Assoc Thai. 2006; 89(12):2047–2049

[36] Benatar M. A systematic review of diagnostic studies in myasthenia gravis. Neuromuscul Disord. 2006; 16(7):459–467

[37] Zinman LH, O'Connor PW, Dadson KE, Leung RC, Ngo M, Bril V. Sensitivity of repetitive facial-nerve stimulation in patients with myasthenia gravis. Muscle Nerve. 2006; 33(5):694–696

[38] Costa J, Evangelista T, Conceição I, de Carvalho M. Repetitive nerve stimulation in myasthenia gravis–relative sensitivity of different muscles. Clin Neurophysiol. 2004; 115(12):2776–2782

[39] Emeryk B, Rowińska-Marcińska K, Nowak-Michalska T. Pseudoselectivity of the neuromuscular block in ocular myasthenia: a SFEMG study. Electromyogr Clin Neurophysiol. 1990; 30(1):53–59

[40] Sanders DB, Howard JF. Single fiber EMG in myasthenia gravis. Muscle Nerve. 1986; 9:809–819

[41] Padua L, Stalberg E, LoMonaco M, Evoli A, Batocchi A, Tonali P. SFEMG in ocular myasthenia gravis diagnosis. Clin Neurophysiol. 2000; 111(7):1203–1207

[42] Valls-Canals J, Montero J, Pradas J. Stimulated single fiber EMG of the frontalis muscle in the diagnosis of ocular myasthenia. Muscle Nerve. 2000; 23(5):779–783

[43] Peeler CE, De Lott LB, Nagia L, Lemos J, Eggenberger ER, Cornblath WT. Clinical utility of acetylcholine receptor antibody testing in ocular myasthenia gravis. JAMA Neurol. 2015; 72(10):1170–1174

[44] Kelly JJ, Jr, Daube JR, Lennon VA, Howard FM, Jr, Younge BR. The laboratory diagnosis of mild myasthenia gravis. Ann Neurol. 1982; 12(3):238–242

[45] Oh SJ, Kim DE, Kuruoglu R, Bradley RJ, Dwyer D. Diagnostic sensitivity of the laboratory tests in myasthenia gravis. Muscle Nerve. 1992; 15(6):720–724

[46] Tsujihata M, Yoshimura T, Satoh A, et al. Diagnostic significance of IgG, C3, and C9 at the limb muscle motor end-plate in minimal myasthenia gravis. Neurology. 1989; 39(10):1359–1363

[47] Fujii Y. Thymus, thymoma and myasthenia gravis. Surg Today. 2013; 43(5):461–466

[48] Papatestas AE, Alpert LI, Osserman KE, Osserman RS, Kark AE. Studies in myasthenia gravis: effects of thymectomy. Results on 185 patients with nonthymomatous and thymomatous myasthenia gravis, 1941–1969. Am J Med. 1971; 50(4):465–474

[49] Oger JJF. Thymus histology and acetylcholine receptor antibodies in generalized myasthenia gravis. Ann N Y Acad Sci. 1993; 681:110–112

[50] Limburg PC, The TH, Hummel-Tappel E, Oosterhuis HJ. Anti-acetylcholine receptor antibodies in myasthenia gravis. Part 1. Relation to clinical parameters in 250 patients. J Neurol Sci. 1983; 58(3):357–370

[51] Mao ZF, Yang LX, Mo XA, et al. Frequency of autoimmune diseases in myasthenia gravis: a systematic review. Int J Neurosci. 2011; 121(3):121–129

[52] Thorlacius S, Aarli JA, Riise T, Matre R, Johnsen HJ. Associated disorders in myasthenia gravis: autoimmune diseases and their relation to thymectomy. Acta Neurol Scand. 1989; 80(4):290–295

[53] Chen YL, Yeh JH, Chiu HC. Clinical features of myasthenia gravis patients with autoimmune thyroid disease in Taiwan. Acta Neurol Scand. 2013; 127(3):170–174

[54] Marinó M, Ricciardi R, Pinchera A, et al. Mild clinical expression of myasthenia gravis associated with autoimmune thyroid diseases. J Clin Endocrinol Metab. 1997; 82(2):438–443

[55] Haines SR, Thurtell MJ. Treatment of ocular myasthenia gravis. Curr Treat Options Neurol. 2012; 14(1):103–112

[56] Agius MA. Treatment of ocular myasthenia with corticosteroids: yes. Arch Neurol. 2000; 57(5):750–751

[57] Kupersmith MJ, Moster M, Bhuiyan S, Warren F, Weinberg H. Beneficial effects of corticosteroids on ocular myasthenia gravis. Arch Neurol. 1996; 53(8):802–804

[58] Kerty E, Elsais A, Argov Z, Evoli A, Gilhus NE. EFNS/ENS Guidelines for the treatment of ocular myasthenia. Eur J Neurol. 2014; 21(5):687–693

[59] Kaminski HJ, Daroff RB. Treatment of ocular myasthenia: steroids only when compelled. Arch Neurol. 2000; 57(5):752–753

[60] Benatar M, Mcdermott MP, Sanders DB, et al. Muscle Study Group (MSG). Efficacy of prednisone for the treatment of ocular myasthenia (EPITOME): a randomized, controlled trial. Muscle Nerve. 2016; 53(3):363–369

[61] Wolfe GI, Kaminski HJ, Aban IB, et al. MGTX Study Group. Randomized trial of thymectomy in myasthenia gravis. N Engl J Med. 2016; 375(6):511–522

[62] Lanska DJ. Indications for thymectomy in myasthenia gravis. Neurology. 1990; 40(12):1828–1829

[63] Nakamura H, Taniguchi Y, Suzuki Y, et al. Delayed remission after thymectomy for myasthenia gravis of the purely ocular type. J Thorac Cardiovasc Surg. 1996; 112(2):371–375

[64] Roberts PF, Venuta F, Rendina E, et al. Thymectomy in the treatment of ocular myasthenia gravis. J Thorac Cardiovasc Surg. 2001; 122(3):562–568

[65] Cea G, Benatar M, Verdugo RJ, Salinas RA. Thymectomy for non-thymomatous myasthenia gravis. Cochrane Database Syst Rev. 2013; 2013(10):CD008111

[66] Sommer N, Sigg B, Melms A, et al. Ocular myasthenia gravis: response to long-term immunosuppressive treatment. J Neurol Neurosurg Psychiatry. 1997; 62(2):156–162

[67] Bentley CR, Dawson E, Lee JP. Active management in patients with ocular manifestations of myasthenia gravis. Eye (Lond). 2001; 15(Pt 1):18–22

16 Thyroid Eye Disease: Graves Ophthalmopathy

Grecia Rico

Abstract

Thyroid eye disease (Graves ophthalmopathy) is a syndrome of ocular symptoms and signs associated with autoimmune thyroid disease. In some cases, the orbital tissue enlargement and proptosis can cause a vision-threatening optic neuropathy. This chapter discusses the clinical pathways in evaluating and treating thyroid eye disease, by reviewing the literature in detail.

Keywords: thyroid eye disease, Graves ophthalmopathy, proptosis, extraocular muscle enlargement, lid retraction

16.1 What Are the Typical Clinical Features of Thyroid Eye Disease (TED)?

Thyroid eye disease (TED), also known as Graves ophthalmopathy, is characterized clinically by symptoms of dry or red eyes, eye pain, proptosis, lid edema, blurred vision, diplopia, photopsias, and lid retraction (the most common clinical feature of TED).[1,2,3,4] The signs of TED include lid edema, lid retraction, stare, lid lag in downgaze, increased intraocular pressure, exposure keratopathy, conjunctival injection and chemosis, exophthalmos, ophthalmoplegia, and visual loss (e.g., compressive optic neuropathy).[5,6,7,8,9,10] Radiographically, there can be soft tissue edema, enlargement of extraocular muscles with tendon sparing,[11] increased orbital fat volume,[12] and orbital apex compression of the optic nerve from apical crowding.[13,14,15,16,17,18] Alternatively, visual loss in TED can be due to stretching of the optic nerve due to proptosis rather than compression optic neuropathy (CON).[13] It is more common in women, and the peak incidence is the mid-to-late 40 s for both women and men.[19,20]

Patients without the typical features of TED should undergo further evaluation for other etiologies of their signs: proptosis (e.g., orbital tumor or pseudotumor), strabismus (e.g., myasthenia gravis), and lid retraction (see Chapter 19). Although we do not typically perform neuroimaging in typical cases of TED without compressive optic neuropathy, we do recommend neuroimaging and/or orbital imaging for patients with atypical features for TED (class IV, level C).

16.2 What Are the Imaging Findings in Thyroid Eye Disease?

Orbital imaging, such as orbital computed tomography (CT) and magnetic resonance imaging (MRI) scans, often demonstrate proptosis, extraocular muscle (EOM) enlargement sparing the tendons,[21,22,23] increased orbital fat volume,[24,25,26] and sometimes engorgement of the superior ophthalmic vein. MRI may be superior to CT scan in differentiating EOM edema (with elevated T2 relaxation times) from fibrosis but CT is faster and cheaper.[16,21,27] Serial short tau inversion recovery (STIR) sequence MRI correlates with the clinical activity score (CAS).[28] MRI, however, is usually more costly than CT imaging. CT is also useful for evaluating the paranasal sinuses and bony orbit anatomy and for measuring the orbit angles and orbit wall length,[29] especially if surgery is being considered. No contrast is typically needed for a CT orbit for thyroid ophthalmopathy, which is an important consideration as iodinated contrast is contraindicated in hyperthyroid patients due to risk of thyrotoxicosis. Ultrasonography of the orbit can also demonstrate EOM enlargement consistent with TED. It is a noninvasive, accessible, inexpensive study useful in measuring the EOMs and evaluation of disease activity by the presence of inflammation and edema. Unfortunately, high-quality ultrasound of the orbit is not as universally available as CT or MR scans.[30]

Apical compression of the optic nerve in CON may be seen on CT or MRI. Coronal as well as axial images are useful in the radiographic diagnosis of CON in TED.[31] We recommend orbital imaging in patients with clinical evidence of an optic neuropathy and in cases where the diagnosis is uncertain or atypical features are present (class IV, level C).

Newer technologies such as 1H-magnetic resonance spectroscopy of the retrobulbar tissues have been used to estimate the concentration of chondroitin sulfate proteoglycan in retrobulbar tissue. Because the concentration of glycosaminoglycans is increased in patients with TED, this clinical tool may thus assist in the evaluation of patients with thyroid orbitopathy.[32] Octreotide scintigraphy may also be a useful test for determining activity of disease by demonstrating orbital uptake in TED.[33,34,35]

16.3 What Is the Relationship between Thyroid Eye Disease and Systemic Thyroid Status?

Although TED is often associated with systemic Graves hyperthyroidism, TED may occur in primary hypothyroidism, Hashimoto thyroiditis, and sometimes in euthyroid individuals.[36,37,38,39] It is believed that low TSH levels, a positive thyroid-stimulating hormone antibody titer, and a previous history of Graves disease are associated to relapse and levels are directly proportional to signs and symptoms.[40,41,42,43]

16.4 What Is the Treatment for Thyroid Eye Disease ?

Treatment of the underlying systemic thyroid abnormalities is the logical first step in the management of TED.[44] The evidence, however, is controversial regarding the effect of the degree of thyroid abnormality or the speed, type (medical or surgical), or completeness of systemic therapy[45] on the incidence or severity of TED (class III–IV, level C). Nevertheless, we recommend that systemic thyroid control be achieved and this may improve the signs and symptoms of TED (class III–IV, level B).[46,47] Prummel et al studied 90 patients with TED and hyperthyroidism in whom the severity of TED and thyroid function were assessed. Patients were assigned to four groups with increasingly severe TED. More dysthyroid patients were in the groups with severe TED than in the other groups.[46] Other uncontrolled studies, however, failed to show regression of TED after careful treatment of hyperthyroidism (class III–IV, level C).

The relation between therapy for hyperthyroidism and the course of TED was studied by Bartalena et al[48] Patients with Graves hyperthyroidism and slight or no TED (443 patients) were randomly assigned to receive radioactive iodine (RAI), RAI followed by a 3-month course of prednisone, or methimazole for 18 months. The patients were evaluated at intervals of 1 to 2 months for 12 months. Among the 150 patients treated with RAI, TED developed or worsened in 23 (15%) at 2 to 6 months after treatment. The change was transient in 15 patients, but it persisted in 8 (5%), who subsequently required treatment for TED. None of the 55 other patients in this group who had TED at baseline had improvement. Among the 145 patients treated with RAI and prednisone, 50 (67%) of the 75 with TED at baseline had improvement and no patient had progression. The effects of RAI on thyroid function were similar in these two groups. Among the 148 patients treated with methimazole, 3 (2%) who had TED at baseline improved, 4 (3%) had worsening of eye disease, and the remaining 141 had no change. The authors concluded that RAI therapy for Graves hyperthyroidism is followed by the appearance or worsening of TED more than is therapy with methimazole. Worsening of TED after RAI therapy is often transient and might be prevented by the administration of low-dose prednisone.[49,50] The authors concluded there was worsening of TED in 15% of the patients treated with RAI, but in none of those treated with RAI and prednisone. Only 3% of those treated with methimazole experienced any worsening of TED.[51]

Bartalena et al studied 26 patients treated with RAI alone and 26 treated with RAI and systemic prednisone for 4 months.[52] The initial dose of prednisone was 0.4 to 0.5 mg/kg of body weight for 1 month, with a gradual taper over 3 months. Before RAI, 15 patients had no evidence for TED and none of these developed TED after RAI. Of the patients treated with RAI alone with initial TED, 56% worsened and 44% were unchanged in soft tissue abnormalities and EOM function. Conversely, there was an improvement in TED in 52% and no change in 48% of RAI patients treated with steroids. These authors and others[44,52,53] have recommended systemic corticosteroid treatment to prevent exacerbation of TED in patients undergoing RAI who have some degree of ocular involvement before treatment, but there is some disagreement with this recommendation.[54] We recommend a short course of oral prednisone during RAI therapy for TED (class III–IV, level C).

Some authors believe that patients may experience worsening of TED after any systemic thyroid treatments (e.g., thyroid surgery, RAI, and neck radiotherapy (RT) for nonthyroidal neoplasms). The presumed mechanism for worsening TED is leakage of thyroid antigens and an increase in circulating thyroid autoantibodies. In contrast to RAI, Marcocci et al did not find any effect on TED of near-total thyroidectomy in patients with nonsevere or absent TED.[55]

Several studies have shown that smoking is associated with worsening TED, and we recommend discontinuing tobacco to all of our patients with TED (class III, level B).[56,57,58,59,60,61,62,63,64,65,66,67] Smoking causes oxidative stress which can induce connective tissue growth factor (CNGF) expression in orbital fibroblasts thus worsening the TED signs and symptoms.[68] The studies conducted by Tsai et al propose antioxidative medications as a treatment for TED.[69,70] Insulin-dependent diabetes mellitus is also a risk factor for TED, and optic neuropathy occurs much more frequently (33.3%) in patients with TED and diabetes (and seems to have a worse prognosis) than in a total group of patients with TED (3.9%).[71]

The natural history of the TED is variable, and although most TED appears within a few months of the diagnosis of hyperthyroidism, it may develop many months to years before or after the onset of the systemic diagnosis of thyroid abnormality. Some patients never show clinical or laboratory evidence for systemic thyroid abnormalities (euthyroid TED). In many patients, TED is a self-limited disease that may not require any therapy and the disease often stabilizes within 1 to 3 years. Therefore, treatment is usually directed at short-term control of the inflammatory component of the disease (usually within the first 6 to 36 months), acute intervention for vision-threatening proptosis or CON, and long-term reconstructive management of lid retraction, strabismus, and proptosis.

Medical and other conservative therapy should generally precede consideration of surgical intervention. Shorr and Seiff described a logical stepwise approach to the surgical rehabilitation of TED.[72] These authors proposed the following four stages for TED: (1) orbital decompression, (2) strabismus surgery, (3) lid margin repositioning surgery, and (4) blepharoplasty. The rationale for this sequential approach to TED is that orbital decompression often results in worsening, new, or changed EOM dysfunction as well as changes in lid position. Therefore, orbital decompression should precede strabismus and lid surgery in patients who require all three surgeries (class III–IV, level C).

Patients with CON due to TED should probably undergo treatment to preserve or improve vision (class III–IV, level B). Trobe et al summarized the natural course of untreated CON in three series of 32 eyes with TED. In this report, 21% of these eyes were left with a visual acuity of 20/100 or less, including a final vision of counting fingers to no light perception in five eyes.[17]

16.5 What Therapies Are Suggested for Local Ocular and Orbital Inflammatory Signs?

Patients with lid or ocular irritation, mild inflammation, or exposure keratopathy may benefit from conservative treatments, such as topical artificial tears and/or lubricating ointments, tinted or wrap-around glasses, elevation of the head of the bed, or taping the eyelids shut during sleep.[13] Although some authors have advocated the use of topical, peribulbar, or retrobulbar steroids, we do not usually employ these routes of steroid therapy for periorbital swelling (class IV, level C). The evidence to support the use of steroids in this manner is anecdotal at best, and these treatments may be associated with complications, such as secondary increased intraocular pressure (class III–IV, level U). Treatment with selenium (Se) is also recommended by some authors and a few studies have suggested that Se improves mild orbital inflammatory signs and symptoms.[73,74,75] Se is a cofactor for antioxidant enzymes, it reduces oxidative tissue damage and it may be associated with the regulation of the inflammatory process in autoimmune thyroiditis.[76,77] Similarly, the use of nonsteroidal anti-inflammatory drugs (NSAIDs) may provide benefit by blocking the response of T-lymphocytes via cyclooxygenase-2 pathway, thus decreasing the differentiation and proliferation of orbital fibroblast to adipocytes.[78,79,80,81,82,83]

16.6 Should Immunosuppressive Therapy Be Considered in TED?

Systemic corticosteroids have been employed for TED but there is only modest evidence outlining the specific indications for their use or the results of treatment, except in patients with CON due to TED.[13] In addition, although medical therapy usually consists of prednisone, other immunosuppressive agents (e.g., azathioprine [Imuran], methotrexate, cyclophosphamide [Cytoxan], or cyclosporine) have also been recommended. Experience with these agents is limited (class IV, level U). Perros et al reported negative results with azathioprine for moderate TED in a matched study of 20 patients.[84] Other studies have reported little effect with azathioprine, methotrexate,[85] or cimexone.[86] Anecdotal success has been reported with plasmapheresis and bromocriptine, but the relative efficacy of these therapies compared with traditional treatment for TED remains to be defined.

Prummel et al reported a single-blind randomized clinical trial comparing the efficacy of prednisone (60 mg/day with a tapering dose) versus cyclosporine (7.5 mg/kg of body weight/day).[87] During the 12-week treatment period, 11 prednisone-treated and 4 cyclosporine-treated patients responded to therapy (61 vs. 22%; p = 0.018) as defined by decrease in EOM enlargement and proptosis, improved vision, and subjective eye scores. There were no differences at baseline between the patients who responded later and those who did not, but the prednisone was less well tolerated than the cyclosporine, and combination therapy was better tolerated than prednisone alone. These authors concluded that single-drug therapy with prednisone was more effective than cyclosporine in patients with severe TED, but that the combination may be effective in patients who did not respond to either drug alone.[87]

Corticosteroids have been shown to reduce EOM enlargement in CON.[13] Many authors recommend relatively high doses of prednisone (1–1.5 mg/kg/day) for the treatment of CON.[13] Kazim et al reviewed 84 cases of acute TED treated with either high-dose systemic steroids or RT and reported that RT (1 of 29 required decompression) was more effective than corticosteroids (6 of 16 patients required decompression) and that RT had fewer complications than steroids.[88] Guy et al reported the use of high-dose pulse intravenous (IV) corticosteroids.[89] Macchia et al compared oral (prednisone 60–80 mg/d) and high-dose IV (two weekly injections of 1 g for 6 weeks) corticosteroid therapy for TED in 25 patients. High-dose IV steroids were better tolerated but all patients showed significant improvement in proptosis, inflammation, and diplopia.[90] Many authors believe that improvement in CON following prednisone therapy is usually evident within the first few weeks of treatment and that

there is no justification for maintaining patients with CON on prolonged corticosteroid regimens.[91]

A recent meta-analysis showed that in moderate-to-severe active phase of TED, IV glucocorticoids (IVGC) were beneficial in 78% of the cases and had less adverse effects oral steroids (52%).[92] This benefit was based on the CAS.[93] Claridge et al investigated combined immunosuppression with primary bilateral orbital RT (20 Gy in 10 fractions). These authors studied RT with azathioprine (up to 3 mg/kg/d) and low-dose prednisolone (maximum dose 40 mg/kg/d).[94] Forty consecutive patients with active TED were recruited. Before treatment, 15 had CON, 35 had significant motility restriction, and 38 had marked soft tissue signs. On average, TED became inactive after 1.2 years of immunosuppression, and treatment was well tolerated. Compared with previously reported treatments, the authors thought that this therapy regimen was more effective than either treatment alone and led to fewer side effects than high-dose steroids. In particular, there was more than a fourfold reduction in the requirement for orbital decompression and strabismus surgery. Monoclonal antibodies such as adalimumab, infliximab, and rituximab have also been proposed as an alternative management of severe inflammatory cases of TED that spares the metabolic and psychiatric alterations of steroids.[95,96,97,98,99] It remains to be seen, however, if these treatments will be superior to corticosteroid therapy in TED.

Baschieri et al performed a prospective nonrandomized study of IV immunoglobulin (IVIG) versus corticosteroids for TED.[100] Twenty-seven patients treated with IVIG were followed for an average of 21 months (12–48 months). Soft tissue involvement improved or disappeared in 32 of 35 patients (91%) treated with IVIG and 25 of 27 (93%) of patients treated with steroids. Diplopia improved or disappeared in 22 of 29 (76%) patients treated with IVIG and 16 of 20 (80%) of patients treated with steroids. A significant reduction of EOM thickness on CT imaging was observed after treatment in both groups. Proptosis improved or disappeared in 20 of 31 (65%) of patients treated with IVIG and in 15 of 24 (63%) of patients treated with steroids. The authors suggest that IVIG is safe and effective in reducing the eye changes in patients with TED. Prophet et al used immunoadsorption therapy (20 sessions of Plasmaselect/Therasorp Anti-IgG) in two patients with refractory TED.[101]

Balazs et al performed a pilot study of pentoxifylline on moderately severe TED in 10 patients.[102] At 12 weeks, 80% of patients had improvement of soft tissue involvement, but not of proptosis or EOM involvement. This agent may have a future role in the treatment of TED.

Krassas and Heufelder reviewed the immunosuppressive treatment available for TED, and concluded that cyclosporin A, azathioprine, cyclophosphamide, and cimexone had modest results but with unfavorable risk–benefit ratios.[103] Somatostatin analogs, octreotide, and lanreotide are emerging therapies but remain costly and as yet unproven alternatives.[103] Uysal et al reported a positive response to octreotide in seven of nine patients with TED.[104]

We usually recommend immunosuppression therapy only for TED in the active phase. Typically, the patient is advanced to immunosuppression only if they are unresponsive to less-aggressive therapies such as nonsteroidal anti-inflammatory medications and supplements, if they cannot take these medications, or if the symptoms are too severe at presentation.

Usually, a short course (2- to 4-week trial) of oral corticosteroids (prednisone 1 mg/kg per day) would be a reasonable first-line therapy (class IV, level C). We generally do not recommend long-term corticosteroid therapy in TED because of the systemic side effects. Concomitant corticosteroid treatment, however, may be useful as an adjunct to RT (see below). The evidence for using other immunosuppressive agents in TED is not sufficient to support a definitive recommendation on the indications, drug, dosage, or duration of therapy (class IV, level U).

16.7 What Is the Role of Radiotherapy in TED?

Low-dose orbital RT has been reported with good results for the treatment of acute inflammation (soft tissue signs) and/or CON due to TED. The typical cumulative RT dose of 2,000 cGy is well tolerated and generally considered to be safe (class III, level B). RT may also be useful in reducing the dosage or eliminating the need for corticosteroid or other immunosuppressive treatments.[88,105,106] ► Table 16.1 summarizes selected cases of orbital RT in the treatment of TED.

Tsujino et al reported 121 patients with TED treated with orbital RT (20 Gy in 10 fractions). The clinical response was excellent in 14%, good in 54%, fair in 25%, no response in 6%, and worse in 1%.[115] Kahaly et al reported improvement using three RT dosing protocols: group A (1 Gy weekly for 20 weeks), group B (10 fractions of 1 Gy), and group C (2 Gy daily over 2 weeks). Improvement was noted in 12 patients in group A (67%), 13 in group B (59%), and 12 in group C (55%). They concluded that the response rates were similar in low and high RT dose treatment but that the 1 Gy per week protocol was most effective and better tolerated.[120]

The combination of systemic steroids with orbital RT may be more effective than orbital RT alone.[121] Marcocci et al compared the efficacy and tolerance of IV or oral glucocorticoids and orbital RT in a prospective, single-blind, randomized study of 82 patients with severe TED.[122] There was a significant reduction in proptosis, diplopia, and CON in both groups. These authors concluded that high-dose (15 mg/kg for four cycles, then 7.5 mg/kg for four cycles, each cycle consisted of two infusions on alternate days at 2-week intervals) IV steroids and oral steroids (prednisone 100 mg/d, withdrawal after 5 months) associated with orbital RT were effective in severe TED. IV steroids, however, were more effective, had fewer side effects, and were better tolerated than oral steroids.[122] Mou et al found that retrobulbar steroid injection and orbital RT had fewer side effects than oral glucocorticoids, but there was no improvement in outcome.[92]

Most authors do not believe that RT is indicated for patients with mild TED or for long-standing, fibrotic, noninflammatory TED (class IV, level C). Previous head or orbit RT is probably a contraindication to further RT for TED. No significant morbidity has been reported in patients with appropriate RT dosing for TED, although there is a theoretical risk of RT-induced cataracts or neoplasms, radiation optic neuropathy, or radiation retinopathy (class III–IV, level C). Several cases of radiation retinopathy have been described in patients with inappropriate RT dosing but this is rare.[123] We recommend that only centers with considerable experience with RT perform this treatment for TED.[25]

Gorman et al performed a prospective, randomized, double-blind, placebo-controlled study of orbital RT for TED.[117] The patients had symptomatic TED without optic neuropathy. Forty-two of 53 eligible consecutive patients were treated (20 Gy of external beam therapy to one orbit with sham therapy to other side, followed in 6 months with reversal of the

Table 16.1 Treatment of TED with orbital RT: Summary of selected studies

Author	No. of patients	Response rate (%)	Comments
Donaldson et al[107]	80	67%	>1 -y follow-up
Ravin et al[108]	9 with optic neuropathy	All 9 improved vision	Little effect on soft tissue abnormalities
Brennan et al[109]	14	13/14 (93%) reduced soft tissue inflammation	Myopathy showed the least improvement
Hurbli et al[110]	62	34/46 (74%) improved motility and 10/14 (71%) CON improved	Patients with duration <6 mo responded better
Wiersinga et al[111]	39	25 (64%) improved	
Sandler et al[112]	35	71% improved	
Lloyd et al[113]	36	33/36 (92%) improved	
Kazim et al[88]	29	28/29 (97%) improved	1 required decompression
Mourits et al[114]	30	60% improved	Placebo controlled
		Placebo (31%) improved	Improved diplopia
Rush et al[106]	10 CON	8/10 (80%) improved	Improved vision
Tsujino et al[115]	121	Limited proptosis response	Excellent (14%), good (54%), fair (25%)
Van Ruyven et al[116]	111	No change in proptosis	Improved motility; improved soft tissue signs
Gorman et al[117]	42	No beneficial response	Randomized trial
Prummel et al[118]	48	13 (46%) improved	Randomized trial
Petersen et al[105]	311	94% no progression of disease	
Prummel et al[119]	44	23 (52%) improvement after 1 y	Randomized controlled

Abbreviations: CON, compression optic neuropathy; RT, radiotherapy; TED, thyroid eye disease.

therapies). Every 3 months for 1 year, the authors measured the volume of the EOM and of fat, proptosis, range of EOM motion, area of diplopia fields, and lid fissure width. No clinical statistically significant difference between the treated and untreated orbit was observed in any of the outcome measures at 6 months. At 12 months, muscle volume and proptosis improved slightly more in the orbit that was treated first. The authors concluded that in this group of patients they were unable to demonstrate any beneficial therapeutic effects.[117] The usefulness of this study has been criticized, however, because of its broad patient inclusion criteria that lacked rigor in controlling the issues of timing of therapy, the clinical variability in presentation of the patients, and multiple treatment methods used for individual patients.[124] We recommend that low-dose orbital RT still be considered a valid treatment option for the treatment of active inflammatory TED (class III–IV, level C). Unfortunately, the assessment of which patients have active TED remains difficult and controversial despite multiple proposed grading schemes.[125,126]

16.8 What Is the Treatment for Lid Retraction in TED?

Lid retraction may be due to superior tarsal muscle (sympathetic) or levator overaction, levator contraction (degeneration of the muscle or aponeurosis), levator adhesions, or pseudoretraction.[127] Occasionally, eyelid retraction spontaneously resolves.[128] Upper eyelid retraction may be treated surgically by a number of approaches,[129,130] including levator marginal myotomies, superior tarsal muscle excision, levator stripping, and levator spacers placed into the upper eyelid to create length. Detailed descriptions of these procedures are beyond the scope of this text. Patients with lesser degrees of proptosis may benefit from eyelid procedures more than orbital procedures. Char recommended that patients with exophthalmometry readings of under 23 or 24 with good motility are probably better treated with eyelid procedures.[25,131] The use of topical α-adrenergic agents, such as guanethidine, has been advocated by some authors, but significant corneal toxicity usually limits the use of these agents. Botulinum toxin injections into the lids may also transiently relieve lid retraction but caution be exercised in patients with TED who might have concomitant autoimmune myasthenia gravis before botulinum toxin is used.[132,133,134,135] We generally recommend lid surgery be considered for patients with inactive and stable disease who do not have evidence for optic neuropathy and who are not going to undergo orbital decompression or strabismus surgery in the near future (class IV, level C).

16.9 What Treatments Should Be Considered for Strabismus Due to TED?

Strabismus in TED may be treated with patching, prism therapy, or strabismus surgery.[136,137,138,139] Patients with difficulty in downgaze and the reading position may benefit from simply occluding the lower segment of their bifocal, raising the bifocal height, or using two pairs of spectacles (one pair of single-vision glasses for reading and one pair for distance). The surgical techniques to correct strabismus will vary depending on the severity and distribution of extraocular involvement.[137,140,141,142,143] A detailed description of these procedures is beyond the scope of this text.[14,15,144,145] Limited anecdotal success has been reported with botulinum toxin injections into EOMs, but we do not generally recommend botulinum toxin treatment for TED (class IV, level C). Surgical treatment for strabismus should be deferred until after the acute inflammatory phase of TED has been treated adequately (class III–IV, level C). Although successful long-term alignment may be achieved with strabismus surgery during the active phase of TED in selected patients with marked disability,[146] we generally advocate stable measurements, good thyroid control, and inactive disease before proceeding with strabismus surgery (class IV, level C).

16.10 What Treatments Are Suggested for Proptosis and/or Compressive Optic Neuropathy Due to TED?

The natural history of CON is poorly documented but presumably variable (class IV). Carter et al reviewed the combined reports of 16 untreated patients (26 eyes). There was spontaneous visual improvement to 20/50 acuity or better in 19 eyes (73%), but 6 eyes (23%) did not improve (range, counting fingers to no light perception).[147] CON may be treated with systemic corticosteroids, orbital RT, or orbital surgical decompression.[17,88,148] Kazim et al retrospectively reviewed 84 cases of acute TED and reported that only 1 of 29 patients with CON treated with RT required surgical decompression versus 6 of 16 treated with corticosteroids.[88] Nevertheless, oral or IV corticosteroids may be the first-line treatment for CON.[89] Guy et al reported the use of pulse IV methylprednisolone (1 g daily for 3 days) in five patients with CON. Oral corticosteroids and orbital RT allowed the treatment response to be maintained in all five patients for several months.[89] Patients with CON who fail or cannot tolerate steroid treatment and/or RT should be considered for orbital decompression.

A wide variety of surgical approaches for orbital decompression have been advocated, and may include one, two, three, or even four wall decompression.[15,17,72,147,149,150,151,152,153,154,155,156,157,158,159,160,161,162,163,164,165,166,167,168,169,170,171,172,173,174,175,176,177,178,179,180,181,182,183,184,185,186,187,188,189,190,191,192,193] It is beyond the scope of our intent for this work to cover all of the surgical decompression literature on TED but we include some information for completeness. Wulc et al also advocated lateral wall advancement as an adjunct to orbital decompression to enhance the decompressive effect and provide a potential space for lateral expansion.[194] Gockeln et al described microsurgical liposuction in TED via a lateral canthotomy.[195] Kazim et al performed orbital fat decompression instead of orbital bone decompression on five patients (eight eyes) with dysthyroid optic neuropathy who had an enlarged orbital fat compartment.[196] These patients did not have EOM enlargement as the solitary cause of the optic neuropathy. The optic neuropathy was reversed in all of the patients, and there was no postoperative diplopia, enophthalmos, globe ptosis, or sensory loss. ▶ Table 16.2 summarizes several studies concerning surgical orbital decompression in the treatment of proptosis and/or CON in TED. Although there is no class I evidence, there is consensus class III evidence that orbital decompression is an effective treatment for CON in TED (class III–IV, level B).

Table 16.2 Orbital decompression (results in selected series)

Author/Year	Number of eyes or patients	Surgical approach	Comment
Algvere et al[149]	22 eyes	Pterional	91% improved
Trobe et al[17]	9 eyes (6 patients)	4 temporal decompression, 3 temporal and orbital floor, 2 transfrontal	66% improved, 3/4 steroid failures, 3/5 primary surgery
Linberg and Anderson[167]	11 eyes	Transorbital	82% improved
Leone and Bajandas[165]	14 eyes	Inferior orbital	100% improved
McCord[173]	11 patients	Antral ethmoidal	55% improved with surgery alone, 45% improved after radiotherapy (RT)
Hurwitz and Birt[190]	27 eyes	Inferomedial approach	81% improved
Lamberg et al[163]	27 bilateral and 3 unilateral	Transantral approach	93% improved
Shorr and Seiff[72]	28 patients	Transantral approach	100% improved
Hallin et al[191]	25 patients (48 eyes)	Transantral approach	77% improved visual acuity
Härting et al[158]	28 patients	Variable techniques	50% improved
Leone et al[166]	2 patients	Medial and lateral wall	100% improved
Warren et al[187]	305 patients	Transantral	95% improved
Kennedy et al[161]	4 patients	Endoscopic transnasal	75% improved
Mourits et al[15]	25 patients underwent surgery for optic nerve compression	13 inferomedial, 5 inferomedial + lateral, 7 coronal	76% improved
Carter et al[147]	30 (52 orbits)	Transantral-ethmoidal	92% improved
Leatherbarrow et al[164]	4 patients	3 wall coronal	50% improved
Olivari[178]	10 patients	Intraorbital fat removal	60% improved
Hurwitz et al[159]	25 patients (46 orbits)	Ethmoidectomy (medial wall)	86% improved
Antoszyk[150]	5 orbits	Transorbital 3 wall	80% improved
Garrity et al[154]	217 patients	Transantral	89% improved visual acuity; 91% improved visual field
Neugebauer et al[176]	21	Endoscopic-endonasal	95% improved vision
West and Stranc[188]	22	4 wall coronal	
Goldberg et al[155]	20	3 wall coronal	
Kalmann et al[160]	125	3 wall coronal	
May et al[171]	17 patients (27 orbits)	Microsurgical endonasal	Proptosis reduction 4.1 mm
Ohtsuka and Nakamura[177]	4 patients	Transmedial-canthal ethmoidal (one-wall)	All improved
Ulualp et al[185]	28 orbits	Transnasal endoscopic	Vision improved 9/15 (60%)
Eloy et al[152]	16 patients, 27 orbits	Endoscopic endonasal	Proptosis reduction 3.17 mm
May et al[172]	19 patients, 29 orbits	Endonasal microsurgery	Proptosis reduction 4.2 mm
Paridaens et al[180]	19 patients (35 orbits), 6 with CON	1, 2, or 3 wall by lateral canthotomy and lower fornix incision	6 CON improved
Tallstedt et al[183]	63 patients	Transantral	Proptosis reduction 3.2 mm, 20/21 (95%) vision improved
Michel et al[175]	78 patients (145 eyes)	Transnasal orbital	4 cases required repeat surgery
Linnet et al[168]	50 eyes	Transcranial 2 wall	87% improved vision
Fatourechi et al[192]	34 patients	Transantral	22 (65%) improved
Soares-Welch et al[193]	215 patients	Transantral orbital	88% satisfied after 20-y follow-up

Abbreviation: CON, compression optic neuropathy.

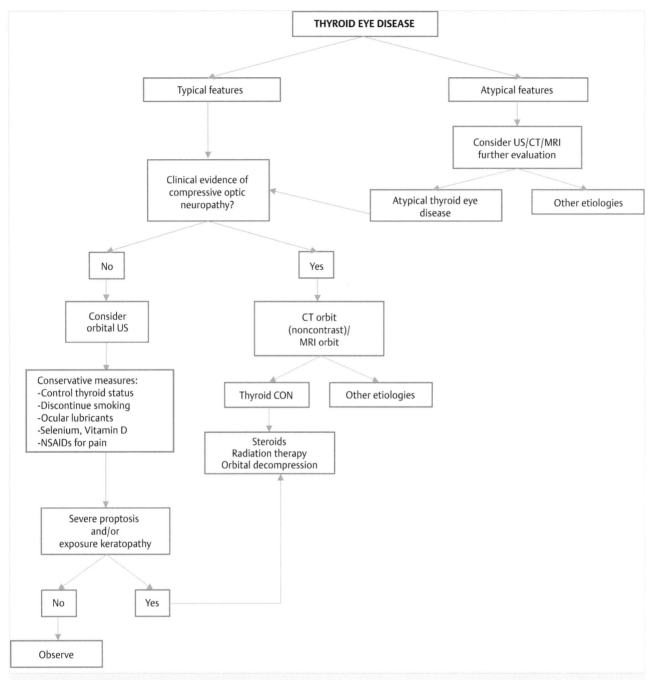

Fig. 16.1 Evaluation and treatment of thyroid eye disease.

16.11 What Is the Treatment for Proptosis without Optic Neuropathy in TED?

McCord in 1985 reported that more than 60% of orbital decompressions were performed for mild to severe exophthalmos to correct corneal exposure or disfigurement, based on a survey of members of the American Society of Ophthalmic Plastic and Reconstructive Surgeons and the Orbital Society. The majority of decompressions were via an antral-ethmoidal decompression

and translid or fornix approach.[197] Kennerdell et al suggested that patients with proptosis of less than 25 to 26 mm, especially if accompanied by lid retraction but without CON, could be treated with lid lengthening procedures alone to disguise the proptosis.[198] Lyons and Rootman reported orbital decompression on 65 orbits (34 patients) for disfiguring exophthalmos and achieved a mean retroplacement of 4 mm (range 21.0–10 mm). Diplopia, however, arose de novo in five (18%) previously asymptomatic patients in this series.[199] Fatourechi et al described 34 patients with TED who underwent transantral orbital decompression primarily for cosmetic reasons.[200] There was a mean reduction in proptosis of 5.2 mm. Persistent diplopia developed in 73% of 15 patients who were asymptomatic preoperatively. Other reports have confirmed that although orbital decompression for primarily cosmetic reasons is successful, ocular motility deficits and diplopia may occur post decompression in a significant number of patients.[147,174,200,201] For example, in a study of 81 patients with TED who underwent orbital decompression, 8 of 41 coronal patients (20%) and 4 of 29 translid patients (14%) experienced aggravation of their motility impairment.[179] Goldberg et al reported that lateral wall decompression produced less new-onset, persistent postoperative strabismus than balanced medial and lateral wall decompression for TED.[202] Seiff et al reported modified orbital decompression with preservation of the anterior periorbita reduced the risk of postoperative diplopia.[203] Bersani and Jian-Seyed-Ahmadi reported surgical placement of a lateral orbital rim implant as an effective method of orbital volume expansion in TED.[204]

In addition to diplopia, orbital decompression may result in loss of vision, globe or eyelid damage, worsening lid retraction, cerebrospinal fluid leakage, infraorbital anesthesia, or sinus complications. Therefore, patients should be counseled appropriately preoperatively regarding these possible complications.

Trokel et al performed orbital fat removal on 81 patients (158 decompressions).[91] These authors reported an average reduction of proptosis of 1.8 mm (range 0–6.0 mm). The greatest reduction in proptosis (3.3 mm) was produced in patients with more than 25 mm of proptosis (Hertel measurements). Trokel et al reserve decompression with bone removal for patients with CON who are unresponsive to medical therapy or patients with persistent deforming exophthalmos following primary orbital fat removal. We recommend orbital decompression for proptosis in patients who have vision-threatening exposure keratopathy or other significant symptoms (e.g., pain, pressure, severe exophthalmos) related to the proptosis (class III–IV, level C).

An approach to the patient with TED is outlined in ▶ Fig. 16.1.

References

[1] Bartley GB. The epidemiologic characteristics and clinical course of ophthalmopathy associated with autoimmune thyroid disease in Olmsted County, Minnesota. Trans Am Ophthalmol Soc. 1994; 92:477–588

[2] Bartley GB. Evolution of classification systems for Graves' ophthalmopathy. Ophthal Plast Reconstr Surg. 1995; 11(4):229–237

[3] Bartley GB. The differential diagnosis and classification of eyelid retraction. Ophthalmology. 1996; 103(1):168–176

[4] Danks JJ, Harrad RA. Flashing lights in thyroid eye disease: a new symptom described and (possibly) explained. Br J Ophthalmol. 1998; 82(11):1309–1311

[5] Bahn RS, Garrity JA, Gorman CA. Clinical review 13: diagnosis and management of Graves' ophthalmopathy. J Clin Endocrinol Metab. 1990; 71(3):559–563

[6] Bahn RS, Heufelder AE. Pathogenesis of Graves' ophthalmopathy. N Engl J Med. 1993; 329(20):1468–1475

[7] Danesh-Meyer HV, Savino PJ, Deramo V, Sergott RC, Smith AF. Intraocular pressure changes after treatment for Graves' orbitopathy. Ophthalmology. 2001; 108(1):145–150

[8] Kalmann R, Mourits MP. Prevalence and management of elevated intraocular pressure in patients with Graves' orbitopathy. Br J Ophthalmol. 1998; 82(7):754–757

[9] Nunery WR. Ophthalmic Graves' disease: a dual theory of pathogenesis. Ophthalmol Clin North Am. 1991; 4:73–87

[10] Srivastava SK, Newman NJ. Pseudo-pseudotumor. Surv Ophthalmol. 2000; 45(2):135–138

[11] Kahaly G. Glycosaminoglycans in Graves' orbitopathy. In: Dutton JJ, Haik BG, eds. Thyroid Eye Disease: Diagnosis and Treatment. New York: Marcel Dekker Inc; 2002:235–242

[12] Hudson HL, Levin L, Feldon SE. Graves exophthalmos unrelated to extraocular muscle enlargement. Superior rectus muscle inflammation may induce venous obstruction. Ophthalmology. 1991; 98(10):1495–1499

[13] Liu D, Feldon SE. Thyroid ophthalmopathy. Ophthalmol Clin North Am. 1992; 5:597–622

[14] Mourits MP, Koorneef L, van Mourik-Noordenbos AM, et al. Extraocular muscle surgery for Graves' ophthalmopathy: does prior treatment influence surgical outcome? Br J Ophthalmol. 1990; 74(8):481–483

[15] Mourits MP, Koornneef L, Wiersinga WM, Prummel MF, Berghout A, van der Gaag R. Orbital decompression for Graves' ophthalmopathy by inferomedial, by inferomedial plus lateral, and by coronal approach. Ophthalmology. 1990; 97(5):636–641

[16] Nagy EV, Toth J, Kaldi I, et al. Graves' ophthalmopathy: eye muscle involvement in patients with diplopia. Eur J Endocrinol. 2000; 142(6):591–597

[17] Trobe JD, Glaser JS, Laflamme P. Dysthyroid optic neuropathy. Clinical profile and rationale for management. Arch Ophthalmol. 1978; 96(7):1199–1209

[18] Wiersinga WM, Bartalena L. Epidemiology and prevention of Graves' ophthalmopathy. Thyroid. 2002; 12(10):855–860

[19] Bartley GB, Fatourechi V, Kadrmas EF, et al. The incidence of Graves' ophthalmopathy in Olmsted County, Minnesota. Am J Ophthalmol. 1995; 120(4):511–517

[20] Kendler DL, Lippa J, Rootman J. The initial clinical characteristics of Graves' orbitopathy vary with age and sex. Arch Ophthalmol. 1993; 111(2):197–201

[21] Just M, Kahaly G, Higer HP, et al. Graves ophthalmopathy: role of MR imaging in radiation therapy. Radiology. 1991; 179(1):187–190

[22] Ozgen A, Alp MN, Ariyürek M, Tütüncü NB, Can I, Günalp I. Quantitative CT of the orbit in Graves' disease. Br J Radiol. 1999; 72(860):757–762

[23] Chatzistefanou KI, Kushner BJ, Gentry LR. Magnetic resonance imaging of the arc of contact of extraocular muscles: implications regarding the incidence of slipped muscles. J AAPOS. 2000; 4(2):84–93

[24] Chang TC, Huang KM, Chang TJ, Lin SL. Correlation of orbital computed tomography and antibodies in patients with hyperthyroid Graves' disease. Clin Endocrinol (Oxf). 1990; 32(5):551–558

[25] Char DH. The ophthalmopathy of Graves' disease. Med Clin North Am. 1991; 75(1):97–119

[26] Firbank MJ, Coulthard A. Evaluation of a technique for estimation of extraocular muscle volume using 2D MRI. Br J Radiol. 2000; 73(876):1282–1289

[27] Müller-Forell W, Pitz S, Mann W, Kahaly GJ. Neuroradiological diagnosis in thyroid-associated orbitopathy. Exp Clin Endocrinol Diabetes. 1999; 107 Suppl 5:S177–S183

[28] Mayer E, Herdman G, Burnett C, Kabala J, Goddard P, Potts MJ. Serial STIR magnetic resonance imaging correlates with clinical score of activity in thyroid disease. Eye (Lond). 2001; 15(Pt 3):313–318

[29] Chan LL, Tan HE, Fook-Chong S, Teo TH, Lim LH, Seah LL. Graves ophthalmopathy: the bony orbit in optic neuropathy, its apical angular capacity, and impact on prediction of risk. AJNR Am J Neuroradiol. 2009; 30(3):597–602

[30] Rabinowitz MP, Carrasco JR. Update on advanced imaging options for thyroid-associated orbitopathy. Saudi J Ophthalmol. 2012; 26(4):385–392

[31] So NM, Lam WW, Cheng G, Metreweli C, Lam D. Assessment of optic nerve compression in Graves' ophthalmopathy. The usefulness of a quick T1-weighted sequence. Acta Radiol. 2000; 41(6):559–561

[32] Ohtsuka K, Hashimoto M. H-magnetic resonance spectroscopy of retrobulbar tissue in Graves ophthalmopathy. Am J Ophthalmol. 1999; 128(6):715–719

[33] Gerding MN, van der Zant FM, van Royen EA, et al. Octreotide-scintigraphy is a disease-activity parameter in Graves' ophthalmopathy. Clin Endocrinol (Oxf). 1999; 50(3):373–379

[34] Krassas GE, Doumas A, Kaltsas T, Halkias A, Pontikides N. Somatostatin receptor scintigraphy before and after treatment with somatostatin analogues in patients with thyroid eye disease. Thyroid. 1999; 9(1):47–52

[35] Krassas GE, Kahaly GJ. The role of octreoscan in thyroid eye disease. Eur J Endocrinol. 1999; 140(5):373–375

[36] Gleeson H, Kelly W, Toft A, et al. Severe thyroid eye disease associated with primary hypothyroidism and thyroid-associated dermopathy. Thyroid. 1999; 9(11):1115–1118

[37] Salvi M, Zhang ZG, Haegert D, et al. Patients with endocrine ophthalmopathy not associated with overt thyroid disease have multiple

thyroid immunological abnormalities. J Clin Endocrinol Metab. 1990; 70(1): 89–94

[38] Weetman AP. Graves' disease. N Engl J Med. 2000; 343(17):1236–1248

[39] Bahn RS. Graves' ophthalmopathy. N Engl J Med. 2010; 362(8):726–738

[40] Liu X, Shi B, Li H. Valuable predictive features of relapse of Graves' disease after antithyroid drug treatment. Ann Endocrinol (Paris). 2015; 76(6): 679–683

[41] Gerding MN, van der Meer JW, Broenink M, Bakker O, Wiersinga WM, Prummel MF. Association of thyrotrophin receptor antibodies with the clinical features of Graves' ophthalmopathy. Clin Endocrinol (Oxf). 2000; 52(3):267–271

[42] Eckstein AK, Plicht M, Lax H, et al. Thyrotropin receptor autoantibodies are independent risk factors for Graves' ophthalmopathy and help to predict severity and outcome of the disease. J Clin Endocrinol Metab. 2006; 91(9): 3464–3470

[43] Wakelkamp IM, Bakker O, Baldeschi L, Wiersinga WM, Prummel MF. TSH-R expression and cytokine profile in orbital tissue of active vs. inactive Graves' ophthalmopathy patients. Clin Endocrinol (Oxf). 2003; 58(3):280–287

[44] Bartalena L, Pinchera A, Marcocci C. Management of Graves' ophthalmopathy: reality and perspectives. Endocr Rev. 2000; 21(2): 168–199

[45] Feldon SE. Graves' ophthalmopathy. Is it really thyroid disease? Arch Intern Med. 1990; 150(5):948–950

[46] Prummel MF, Wiersinga WM, Mourits MP, Koornneef L, Berghout A, van der Gaag R. Effect of abnormal thyroid function on the severity of Graves' ophthalmopathy. Arch Intern Med. 1990; 150(5):1098–1101

[47] Tallstedt L, Lundell G, Tørring O, et al. The Thyroid Study Group. Occurrence of ophthalmopathy after treatment for Graves' hyperthyroidism. N Engl J Med. 1992; 326(26):1733–1738

[48] Bartalena L, Marcocci C, Bogazzi F, et al. Relation between therapy for hyperthyroidism and the course of Graves' ophthalmopathy. N Engl J Med. 1998; 338(2):73–78

[49] Dietlein M, Dederichs B, Weigand A, Schicha H. Radioiodine therapy and thyroid-associated orbitopathy: risk factors and preventive effects of glucocorticoids. Exp Clin Endocrinol Diabetes. 1999; 107 Suppl 5:S190–S194

[50] Marcocci C, Bartalena L, Tanda ML, et al. Graves' ophthalmopathy and 131I therapy. Q J Nucl Med. 1999; 43(4):307–312

[51] Keltner JL. Is Graves ophthalmopathy a preventable disease? Arch Ophthalmol. 1998; 116(8):1106–1107

[52] Bartalena L, Marcocci C, Bogazzi F, Panicucci M, Lepri A, Pinchera A. Use of corticosteroids to prevent progression of Graves' ophthalmopathy after radioiodine therapy for hyperthyroidism. N Engl J Med. 1989; 321(20): 1349–1352

[53] Rasmussen AK, Nygaard B, Feldt-Rasmussen U. (131)I and thyroid-associated ophthalmopathy. Eur J Endocrinol. 2000; 143(2):155–160

[54] Beck RW, DiLoreto DA. Treatment of Graves' ophthalmopathy. N Engl J Med. 1990; 322(15):1088–1089

[55] Marcocci C, Bruno-Bossio G, Manetti L, et al. The course of Graves' ophthalmopathy is not influenced by near total thyroidectomy: a case-control study. Clin Endocrinol (Oxf). 1999; 51(4):503–508

[56] Balazs G, Stenszky V, Farid NR. Association between Graves' ophthalmopathy and smoking. Lancet. 1990; 336(8717):754

[57] Bartalena L, Marcocci C, Tanda ML, et al. Cigarette smoking and treatment outcomes in Graves ophthalmopathy. Ann Intern Med. 1998; 129(8): 632–635

[58] Mann K. Risk of smoking in thyroid-associated orbitopathy. Exp Clin Endocrinol Diabetes. 1999; 107 Suppl 5:S164–S167

[59] Nunery WR, Martin RT, Heinz GW, Gavin TJ. The association of cigarette smoking with clinical subtypes of ophthalmic Graves' disease. Ophthal Plast Reconstr Surg. 1993; 9(2):77–82

[60] Pfeilschifter J, Ziegler R. Smoking and endocrine ophthalmopathy: impact of smoking severity and current vs lifetime cigarette consumption. Clin Endocrinol (Oxf). 1996; 45(4):477–481

[61] Prummel MF, Wiersinga WM. Smoking and risk of Graves' disease. JAMA. 1993; 269(4):479–482

[62] Shine B, Fells P, Edwards OM, Weetman AP. Association between Graves' ophthalmopathy and smoking. Lancet. 1990; 335(8700):1261–1263

[63] Shukla R, Kurinczuk JJ. Graves' ophthalmopathy and smoking. Lancet. 1990; 336(8708):184

[64] Solberg Y, Rosner M, Belkin M. The association between cigarette smoking and ocular diseases. Surv Ophthalmol. 1998; 42(6):535–547

[65] Tallstedt L, Lundell G, Taube A. Graves' ophthalmopathy and tobacco smoking. Acta Endocrinol (Copenh). 1993; 129(2):147–150

[66] Tellez M, Cooper J, Edmonds C. Graves' ophthalmopathy in relation to cigarette smoking and ethnic origin. Clin Endocrinol (Oxf). 1992; 36(3):291–294

[67] Costenbader KH, Karlson EW. Cigarette smoking and autoimmune disease: what can we learn from epidemiology? Lupus. 2006; 15(11):737–745

[68] Cawood TJ, Moriarty P, O'Farrelly C, O'Shea D. Smoking and thyroid-associated ophthalmopathy: A novel explanation of the biological link. J Clin Endocrinol Metab. 2007; 92(1):59–64

[69] Tsai CC, Wu SB, Chang PC, Wei YH. Alteration of connective tissue growth factor (CTGF) expression in orbital fibroblasts from patients with Graves' ophthalmopathy. PLoS One. 2015; 10(11):e0143514

[70] Smith TJ, Tsai CC, Shih MJ, et al. Unique attributes of orbital fibroblasts and global alterations in IGF-1 receptor signaling could explain thyroid-associated ophthalmopathy. Thyroid. 2008; 18(9):983–988

[71] Kalmann R, Mourits MP. Diabetes mellitus: a risk factor in patients with Graves' orbitopathy. Br J Ophthalmol. 1999; 83(4):463–465

[72] Shorr N, Seiff SR. The four stages of surgical rehabilitation of the patient with dysthyroid ophthalmopathy. Ophthalmology. 1986; 93(4):476–483

[73] Drutel A, Archambeaud F, Caron P. Selenium and the thyroid gland: more good news for clinicians. Clin Endocrinol (Oxf). 2013; 78(2):155–164

[74] Marcocci C, Kahaly GJ, Krassas GE, et al. European Group on Graves' Orbitopathy. Selenium and the course of mild Graves' orbitopathy. N Engl J Med. 2011; 364(20):1920–1931

[75] Wertenbruch T, Willenberg HS, Sagert C, et al. Serum selenium levels in patients with remission and relapse of Graves' disease. Med Chem. 2007; 3(3):281–284

[76] Weeks BS, Hanna MS, Cooperstein D. Dietary selenium and selenoprotein function. Med Sci Monit. 2012; 18(8):RA127–RA132

[77] Xue H, Wang W, Li Y, et al. Selenium upregulates CD4(+)CD25(+) regulatory T cells in iodine-induced autoimmune thyroiditis model of NOD.H-2(h4) mice. Endocr J. 2010; 57(7):595–601

[78] Feldon SE, O'loughlin CW, Ray DM, Landskroner-Eiger S, Seweryniak KE, Phipps RP. Activated human T lymphocytes express cyclooxygenase-2 and produce proadipogenic prostaglandins that drive human orbital fibroblast differentiation to adipocytes. Am J Pathol. 2006; 169(4):1183–1193

[79] Kuriyan AE, Phipps RP, O'Loughlin CW, Feldon SE. Improvement of thyroid eye disease following treatment with the cyclooxygenase-2 selective inhibitor celecoxib. Thyroid. 2008; 18(8):911–914

[80] Prabhakar BS, Bahn RS, Smith TJ. Current perspective on the pathogenesis of Graves' disease and ophthalmopathy. Endocr Rev. 2003; 24(6):802–835

[81] Bahn RS. Clinical review 157: pathophysiology of Graves' ophthalmopathy: the cycle of disease. J Clin Endocrinol Metab. 2003; 88(5):1939–1946

[82] Starkey KJ, Janezic A, Jones G, Jordan N, Baker G, Ludgate M. Adipose thyrotrophin receptor expression is elevated in Graves' and thyroid eye diseases ex vivo and indicates adipogenesis in progress in vivo. J Mol Endocrinol. 2003; 30(3):369–380

[83] Konuk EB, Konuk O, Misirlioglu M, Menevse A, Unal M. Expression of cyclooxygenase-2 in orbital fibroadipose connective tissues of Graves' ophthalmopathy patients. Eur J Endocrinol. 2006; 155(5):681–685

[84] Perros P, Weightman DR, Crombie AL, Kendall-Taylor P. Azathioprine in the treatment of thyroid-associated ophthalmopathy. Acta Endocrinol (Copenh). 1990; 122(1):8–12

[85] Smith JR, Rosenbaum JT. A role for methotrexate in the management of non-infectious orbital inflammatory disease. Br J Ophthalmol. 2001; 85(10): 1220–1224

[86] Kahaly G, Lieb W, Müller-Forell W, et al. Ciamexone in endocrine orbitopathy. A randomized double-blind, placebo-controlled study. Acta Endocrinol (Copenh). 1990; 122(1):13–21

[87] Prummel MF, Mourits MP, Berghout A, et al. Prednisone and cyclosporine in the treatment of severe Graves' ophthalmopathy. N Engl J Med. 1989; 321 (20):1353–1359

[88] Kazim M, Trokel S, Moore S. Treatment of acute Graves orbitopathy. Ophthalmology. 1991; 98(9):1443–1448

[89] Guy JR, Fagien S, Donovan JP, Rubin ML. Methylprednisolone pulse therapy in severe dysthyroid optic neuropathy. Ophthalmology. 1989; 96(7):1048–1052, discussion 1052–1053

[90] Macchia PE, Bagattini M, Lupoli G, Vitale M, Vitale G, Fenzi G. High-dose intravenous corticosteroid therapy for Graves' ophthalmopathy. J Endocrinol Invest. 2001; 24(3):152–158

[91] Trokel S, Kazim M, Moore S. Orbital fat removal. Decompression for Graves orbitopathy. Ophthalmology. 1993; 100(5):674–682

[92] Mou P, Jiang LH, Zhang Y, et al. Common immunosuppressive monotherapy for Graves' ophthalmopathy: a meta-analysis. PLoS One. 2015; 10(10): e0139544

[93] Mourits MP, Prummel MF, Wiersinga WM, Koornneef L. Clinical activity score as a guide in the management of patients with Graves' ophthalmopathy. Clin Endocrinol (Oxf). 1997; 47(1):9–14

[94] Claridge KG, Ghabrial R, Davis G, et al. Combined radiotherapy and medical immunosuppression in the management of thyroid eye disease. Eye (Lond). 1997; 11(Pt 5):717–722

[95] Ayabe R, Rootman DB, Hwang CJ, Ben-Artzi A, Goldberg R. Adalimumab as steroid-sparing treatment of inflammatory-stage thyroid eye disease. Ophthal Plast Reconstr Surg. 2014; 30(5):415–419

[96] Durrani OM, Reuser TQ, Murray PI. Infliximab: a novel treatment for sight-threatening thyroid associated ophthalmopathy. Orbit. 2005; 24(2):117–119

[97] Salvi M, Vannucchi G, Campi I, et al. Treatment of Graves' disease and associated ophthalmopathy with the anti-CD20 monoclonal antibody rituximab: an open study. Eur J Endocrinol. 2007; 156(1):33–40

[98] El Fassi D, Banga JP, Gilbert JA, Padoa C, Hegedüs L, Nielsen CH. Treatment of Graves' disease with rituximab specifically reduces the production of thyroid stimulating autoantibodies. Clin Immunol. 2009; 130(3):252–258

[99] Salvi M, Vannucchi G, Campi I, et al. Rituximab treatment in a patient with severe thyroid-associated ophthalmopathy: effects on orbital lymphocytic infiltrates. Clin Immunol. 2009; 131(2):360–365

[100] Baschieri L, Antonelli A, Nardi S, et al. Intravenous immunoglobulin versus corticosteroid in treatment of Graves' ophthalmopathy. Thyroid. 1997; 7(4):579–585

[101] Prophet H, Matic GB, Winkler RE, et al. Two cases of refractory endocrine ophthalmopathy successfully treated with extracorporeal immunoadsorption. Ther Apher. 2001; 5(2):142–146

[102] Balazs C, Kiss E, Vamos A, Molnar I, Farid NR. Beneficial effect of pentoxifylline on thyroid associated ophthalmopathy (TAO)*: a pilot study. J Clin Endocrinol Metab. 1997; 82(6):1999–2002

[103] Krassas GE, Heufelder AE. Immunosuppressive therapy in patients with thyroid eye disease: an overview of current concepts. Eur J Endocrinol. 2001; 144(4):311–318

[104] Uysal AR, Corapçioğlu D, Tonyukuk VC, et al. Effect of octreotide treatment on Graves' ophthalmopathy. Endocr J. 1999; 46(4):573–577

[105] Petersen IA, Kriss JP, McDougall IR, Donaldson SS. Prognostic factors in the radiotherapy of Graves' ophthalmopathy. Int J Radiat Oncol Biol Phys. 1990; 19(2):259–264

[106] Rush S, Winterkorn JM, Zak R. Objective evaluation of improvement in optic neuropathy following radiation therapy for thyroid eye disease. Int J Radiat Oncol Biol Phys. 2000; 47(1):191–194

[107] Donaldson SS, Bagshaw MA, Kriss JP. Supervoltage orbital radiotherapy for Graves' ophthalmopathy. J Clin Endocrinol Metab. 1973; 37(2):276–285

[108] Ravin JG, Sisson JC, Knapp WT. Orbital radiation for the ocular changes of Gravess' disease. Am J Ophthalmol. 1975; 79(2):285–288

[109] Brennan MW, Leone CR, Jr, Janaki L. Radiation therapy for Graves' disease. Am J Ophthalmol. 1983; 96(2):195–199

[110] Hurbli T, Char DH, Harris J, Weaver K, Greenspan F, Sheline G. Radiation therapy for thyroid eye diseases. Am J Ophthalmol. 1985; 99(6):633–637

[111] Wiersinga WM, Smit T, Schuster-Uittenhoeve AL, van der Gaag R, Koornneef L. Therapeutic outcome of prednisone medication and of orbital irradiation in patients with Graves' ophthalmopathy. Ophthalmologica. 1988; 197(2):75–84

[112] Sandler HM, Rubenstein JH, Fowble BL, Sergott RC, Savino PJ, Bosley TM. Results of radiotherapy for thyroid ophthalmopathy. Int J Radiat Oncol Biol Phys. 1989; 17(4):823–827

[113] Lloyd WC, III, Leone CR, Jr. Supervoltage orbital radiotherapy in 36 cases of Graves' disease. Am J Ophthalmol. 1992; 113(4):374–380

[114] Mourits MP, van Kempen-Harteveld ML, García MB, Koppeschaar HP, Tick L, Terwee CB. Radiotherapy for Graves' orbitopathy: randomised placebo-controlled study. Lancet. 2000; 355(9214):1505–1509

[115] Tsujino K, Hirota S, Hagiwara M, et al. Clinical outcomes of orbital irradiation combined with or without systemic high-dose or pulsed corticosteroids for Graves' ophthalmopathy. Int J Radiat Oncol Biol Phys. 2000; 48(3):857–864

[116] Van Ruyven RL, Van Den Bosch WA, Mulder PG, Eijkenboom WM, Paridaens AD. The effect of retrobulbar irradiation on exophthalmos, ductions and soft tissue signs in Graves' ophthalmopathy: a retrospective analysis of 90 cases. Eye (Lond). 2000; 14(Pt 5):761–764

[117] Gorman CA, Garrity JA, Fatourechi V, et al. A prospective, randomized, double-blind, placebo-controlled study of orbital radiotherapy for Graves' ophthalmopathy. Ophthalmology. 2001; 108(9):1523–1534

[118] Prummel MF, Mourits MP, Blank L, Berghout A, Koornneef L, Wiersinga WM. Randomized double-blind trial of prednisone versus radiotherapy in Graves' ophthalmopathy. Lancet. 1993; 342(8877):949–954

[119] Prummel MF, Terwee CB, Gerding MN, et al. A randomized controlled trial of orbital radiotherapy versus sham irradiation in patients with mild Graves' ophthalmopathy. J Clin Endocrinol Metab. 2004; 89(1):15–20

[120] Kahaly GJ, Rösler HP, Pitz S, Hommel G. Low- versus high-dose radiotherapy for Graves' ophthalmopathy: a randomized, single blind trial. J Clin Endocrinol Metab. 2000; 85(1):102–108

[121] Marcocci C, Bartalena L, Bogazzi F, Bruno-Bossio G, Lepri A, Pinchera A. Orbital radiotherapy combined with high dose systemic glucocorticoids for Graves' ophthalmopathy is more effective than radiotherapy alone: results of a prospective randomized study. J Endocrinol Invest. 1991; 14(10):853–860

[122] Marcocci C, Bartalena L, Tanda ML, et al. Comparison of the effectiveness and tolerability of intravenous or oral glucocorticoids associated with orbital radiotherapy in the management of severe Graves' ophthalmopathy: results of a prospective, single-blind, randomized study. J Clin Endocrinol Metab. 2001; 86(8):3562–3567

[123] Kinyoun JL, Kalina RE, Brower SA, Mills RP, Johnson RH. Radiation retinopathy after orbital irradiation for Graves' ophthalmopathy. Arch Ophthalmol. 1984; 102(10):1473–1476

[124] Feldon SE. Radiation therapy for Graves' ophthalmopathy: trick or treat? Ophthalmology. 2001; 108(9):1521–1522

[125] Cockerham KP, Kennerdell JS. Does radiotherapy have a role in the management of thyroid orbitopathy? View 1. Br J Ophthalmol. 2002; 86(1):102–104

[126] Dickinson AJ, Perros P. Controversies in the clinical evaluation of active thyroid-associated orbitopathy: use of a detailed protocol with comparative photographs for objective assessment. Clin Endocrinol (Oxf). 2001; 55(3):283–303

[127] Lemke BN. Management of thyroid eyelid retraction. Focal Point 9. Module. 1991; 6:1–9

[128] von Brauchitsch DK, Egbert J, Kersten RC, Kulwin DR. Spontaneous resolution of upper eyelid retraction in thyroid orbitopathy. J Neuroophthalmol. 1999; 19(2):122–124

[129] Mourits MP, Sasim IV. A single technique to correct various degrees of upper lid retraction in patients with Graves' orbitopathy. Br J Ophthalmol. 1999; 83(1):81–84

[130] Olver JM, Rose GE, Khaw PT, Collin JRO. Correction of lower eyelid retraction in thyroid eye disease: a randomised controlled trial of retractor tenotomy with adjuvant antimetabolite versus scleral graft. Br J Ophthalmol. 1998; 82(2):174–180

[131] Char DH. Advances in thyroid orbitopathy. Neuro-ophthalmology. 1992; 12:25–39

[132] Ceisler EJ, Bilyk JR, Rubin PA, Burks WR, Shore JW. Results of Müllerotomy and levator aponeurosis transposition for the correction of upper eyelid retraction in Graves' disease. Ophthalmology. 1995; 102(3):483–492

[133] Olver JM. Botulinum toxin A treatment of overactive corrugator supercilii in thyroid eye disease. Br J Ophthalmol. 1998; 82(5):528–533

[134] Ozkan SB, Can D, Söylev MF, Arsan AK, Duman S. Chemodenervation in treatment of upper eyelid retraction. Ophthalmologica. 1997; 211(6):387–390

[135] Träisk F, Tallstedt L. Thyroid associated ophthalmopathy: botulinum toxin A in the treatment of upper eyelid retraction–a pilot study. Acta Ophthalmol Scand. 2001; 79(6):585–588

[136] Prendiville P, Chopra M, Gauderman WJ, Feldon SE. The role of restricted motility in determining outcomes for vertical strabismus surgery in Graves' ophthalmology. Ophthalmology. 2000; 107(3):545–549

[137] Al Qahtani ES, Rootman J, Kersey J, Godoy F, Lyons CJ. Clinical pearls and management recommendations for strabismus due to thyroid orbitopathy. Middle East Afr J Ophthalmol. 2015; 22(3):307–311

[138] Buckley EG, Plager DA, Plager DA, et al. Strabismus surgery: basic and advanced strategies. Am Orthopt J. 2005; 55:166–167

[139] Kerr NC. Practical management of strabismus and diplopia in thyroid eye disease. In: Dutton JJ, Haik BG, eds. Thyroid Eye Disease: Diagnosis and Treatment. New York: Marcel Dekker Inc; 2002:389–405

[140] Nardi M. Squint surgery in TED – hints and fints, or why Graves' patients are difficult patients. Orbit. 2009; 28(4):245–250

[141] Pratt-Johnson J, Tillson G. Management of Strabismus and Amblyopia: A Practical Guide. 2nd ed. New York: Thieme; 2001:221

[142] Kerr NC. The role of thyroid eye disease and other factors in the overcorrection of hypotropia following unilateral adjustable suture recession of the inferior rectus (an American Ophthalmological Society thesis). Trans Am Ophthalmol Soc 2011;109:168–200

[143] Black BC. Treatment of incomitant hypertropia and diplopia with recession of the inferior rectus and superior rectus muscles of the same eye. J AAPOS. 2007; 11(3):262–265

[144] Schotthoefer EO, Wallace DK. Strabismus associated with thyroid eye disease. Curr Opin Ophthalmol. 2007; 18(5):361–365

[145] Volpe NJ, Mirza-George N, Binenbaum G. Surgical management of vertical ocular misalignment in thyroid eye disease using an adjustable suture technique. J AAPOS. 2012; 16(6):518–522

[146] Coats DK, Paysse EA, Plager DA, Wallace DK. Early strabismus surgery for thyroid ophthalmopathy. Ophthalmology. 1999; 106(2):324–329

[147] Carter KD, Frueh BR, Hessburg TP, Musch DC. Long-term efficacy of orbital decompression for compressive optic neuropathy of Graves' eye disease. Ophthalmology. 1991; 98(9):1435–1442

[148] Kubis KC, Danesh-Meyer HV, Pribitkin EA, Bilyk JR. Progressive visual loss and ophthalmoplegia. Surv Ophthalmol. 2000; 44(5):433–441

[149] Algvere P, Almqvist S, Backlund EO. Pterional orbital decompression in progressive ophthalmopathy of Graves' disease II. A follow-up study. Acta Ophthalmol (Copenh). 1973; 51(4):475–482

[150] Antoszyk JH, Tucker N, Codère F. Orbital decompression for Graves' disease: exposure through a modified blepharoplasty incision. Ophthalmic Surg. 1992; 23(8):516–521

[151] Coday MP, Dallow RL. Managing Graves' orbitopathy. Int Ophthalmol Clin. 1998; 38(1):103–115

[152] Eloy P, Trussart C, Jouzdani E, Collet S, Rombaux P, Bertrand B. Transnasal endoscopic orbital decompression and Graves' ophtalmopathy. Acta Otorhinolaryngol Belg. 2000; 54(2):165–174

[153] Fatourechi V, Garrity JA, Bartley GB, Bergstralh EJ, Gorman CA. Orbital decompression in Graves' ophthalmopathy associated with pretibial myxedema. J Endocrinol Invest. 1993; 16(6):433–437

[154] Garrity JA, Fatourechi V, Bergstralh EJ, et al. Results of transantral orbital decompression in 428 patients with severe Graves' ophthalmopathy. Am J Ophthalmol. 1993; 116(5):533–547

[155] Goldberg RA, Weinberg DA, Shorr N, Wirta D. Maximal, three-wall, orbital decompression through a coronal approach. Ophthalmic Surg Lasers. 1997; 28(10):832–843

[156] Gormley PD, Bowyer J, Jones NS, Downes RN. The sphenoidal sinus in optic nerve decompression. Eye (Lond). 1997; 11(Pt 5):723–726

[157] Graham SM, Carter KD. Combined endoscopic and subciliary orbital decompression for thyroid-related compressive optic neuropathy. Rhinology. 1997; 35(3):103–107

[158] Härting F, Koornneef L, Peeters HJF, Gillisen JP. Decompression surgery in Graves' orbitopathy–a review of 14 years' experience at the Orbita Centrum, Amsterdam. Dev Ophthalmol. 1989; 20:185–198

[159] Hurwitz JJ, Freeman JL, Eplett CJ, Fliss DM, Avram DR. Ethmoidectomy decompression for the treatment of Graves' optic neuropathy. Can J Ophthalmol. 1992; 27(6):283–287

[160] Kalmann R, Mourits MP, van der Pol JP, Koornneef L. Coronal approach for rehabilitative orbital decompression in Graves' ophthalmopathy. Br J Ophthalmol. 1997; 81(1):41–45

[161] Kennedy DW, Goodstein ML, Miller NR, Zinreich SJ. Endoscopic transnasal orbital decompression. Arch Otolaryngol Head Neck Surg. 1990; 116(3):275–282

[162] Kulwin DR, Cotton RT, Kersten RC. Combined approach to orbital decompression. Otolaryngol Clin North Am. 1990; 23(3):381–390

[163] Lamberg BA, Grahne B, Tommila V, et al. Orbital decompression in endocrine exophthalmos of Graves' disease. Acta Endocrinol (Copenh). 1985; 109(3):335–340

[164] Leatherbarrow B, Lendrum J, Mahaffey PJ, Noble JL, Kwartz J, Davies H. Three wall orbital decompression for Graves' ophthalmopathy via a coronal approach. Eye (Lond). 1991; 5(Pt 4):456–465

[165] Leone CR, Jr, Bajandas FJ. Inferior orbital decompression for dysthyroid optic neuropathy. Ophthalmology. 1981; 88(6):525–532

[166] Leone CR, Jr, Piest KL, Newman RJ. Medial and lateral wall decompression for thyroid ophthalmopathy. Am J Ophthalmol. 1989; 108(2):160–166

[167] Linberg JV, Anderson RL. Transorbital decompression. Indications and results. Arch Ophthalmol. 1981; 99(1):113–119

[168] Linnet J, Hegedüs L, Bjerre P. Results of a neurosurgical two-wall orbital decompression in the treatment of severe thyroid associated ophthalmopathy. Acta Ophthalmol Scand. 2001; 79(1):49–52

[169] Lund VJ, Larkin G, Fells P, Adams G. Orbital decompression for thyroid eye disease: a comparison of external and endoscopic techniques. J Laryngol Otol. 1997; 111(11):1051–1055

[170] Mann W, Kahaly G, Lieb W, Rothoff T, Springborn S. Orbital decompression for endocrine ophthalmopathy: the endonasal approach. Dev Ophthalmol. 1993; 25:142–150

[171] May A, Fries U, Reimold I, Weber A. Microsurgical endonasal decompression in dysthyroid orbitopathy. Acta Otolaryngol. 1999; 119(7):826–831

[172] May A, Fries U, von Ilberg C, Weber A. Indication and technique of transnasal microscopic orbital decompression for endocrine ophthalmopathy. ORL J Otorhinolaryngol Relat Spec. 2000; 62(3):128–133

[173] McCord CD, Jr. Orbital decompression for Graves' disease. Exposure through lateral canthal and inferior fornix incision. Ophthalmology. 1981; 88(6):533–541

[174] McNab AA. Orbital decompression for thyroid orbitopathy. Aust N Z J Ophthalmol. 1997; 25(1):55–61

[175] Michel O, Oberländer N, Neugebauer P, Neugebauer A, Rüssmann W. Follow-up of transnasal orbital decompression in severe Graves' ophthalmopathy. Ophthalmology. 2001; 108(2):400–404

[176] Neugebauer A, Nishino K, Neugebauer P, Konen W, Michel O. Effects of bilateral orbital decompression by an endoscopic endonasal approach in dysthyroid orbitopathy. Br J Ophthalmol. 1996; 80(1):58–62

[177] Ohtsuka K, Nakamura Y. Results of transmedial-canthal ethmoidal decompression for severe dysthyroid optic neuropathy. Jpn J Ophthalmol. 1999; 43(5):426–432

[178] Olivari N. Transpalpebral decompression of endocrine ophthalmopathy (Graves' disease) by removal of intraorbital fat: experience with 147 operations over 5 years. Plast Reconstr Surg. 1991; 87(4):627–641, discussion 642–643

[179] Paridaens D, Hans K, van Buitenen S, Mourits MP. The incidence of diplopia following coronal and translid orbital decompression in Graves' orbitopathy. Eye (Lond). 1998; 12(Pt 5):800–805

[180] Paridaens DA, Verhoeff K, Bouwens D, van Den Bosch WA. Transconjunctival orbital decompression in Graves' ophthalmopathy: lateral wall approach ab interno. Br J Ophthalmol. 2000; 84(7):775–781

[181] Ruttum MS. Effect of prior orbital decompression on outcome of strabismus surgery in patients with thyroid ophthalmopathy. J AAPOS. 2000; 4(2):102–105

[182] Sillers MJ, Cuilty-Siller C, Kuhn FA, Porubsky ES, Morpeth JF. Transconjunctival endoscopic orbital decompression. Otolaryngol Head Neck Surg. 1997; 117(6):S137–S141

[183] Tallstedt L, Papatziamos G, Lundblad L, Anggård A. Results of transantral orbital decompression in patients with thyroid-associated ophthalmopathy. Acta Ophthalmol Scand. 2000; 78(2):206–210

[184] Thaller SR, Kawamoto HK. Surgical correction of exophthalmos secondary to Graves' disease. Plast Reconstr Surg. 1990; 86(3):411–418, discussion 419–421

[185] Ulualp SO, Massaro BM, Toohill RJ. Course of proptosis in patients with Graves' disease after endoscopic orbital decompression. Laryngoscope. 1999; 109(8):1217–1222

[186] van der Wal KG, de Visscher JG, Boukes RJ, Smeding B. Surgical treatment of Graves orbitopathy: a modified balanced technique. Int J Oral Maxillofac Surg. 2001; 30(4):254–258

[187] Warren JD, Spector JG, Burde R. Long-term follow-up and recent observations on 305 cases of orbital decompression for dysthyroid orbitopathy. Laryngoscope. 1989; 99(1):35–40

[188] West M, Stranc M. Long-term results of four-wall orbital decompression for Graves' ophthalmopathy. Br J Plast Surg. 1997; 50(7):507–516

[189] Wilson WB, Manke WF. Orbital decompression in Graves' disease. The predictability of reduction of proptosis. Arch Ophthalmol. 1991; 109(3):343–345

[190] Hurwitz JJ, Birt D. An individualized approach to orbital decompression in Graves' orbitopathy. Arch Ophthalmol. 1985; 103(5):660–665

[191] Hallin ES, Feldon SE, Luttrell J. Graves' ophthalmopathy: III. Effect of transantral orbital decompression on optic neuropathy. Br J Ophthalmol. 1988; 72(9):683–687

[192] Fatourechi V, Garrity JA, Bartley GB, Bergstralh EJ, DeSanto LW, Gorman CA. Graves ophthalmopathy. Results of transantral orbital decompression performed primarily for cosmetic indications. Ophthalmology. 1994; 101(5):938–942

[193] Soares-Welch CV, Fatourechi V, Bartley GB, et al. Optic neuropathy of Graves' disease: results of transantral orbital decompression and long-term follow-up in 215 patients. Am J Ophthalmol. 2003; 136(3):433–441

[194] Wulc AE, Popp JC, Bartlett SP. Lateral wall advancement in orbital decompression. Ophthalmology. 1990; 97(10):1358–1369

[195] Gockeln R, Winter R, Sistani F, Kretschmann U, Hussein S. Minimal invasive decompression of the orbit in Graves' orbitopathy. Strabismus. 2000; 8(4):251–259

[196] Kazim M, Trokel SL, Acaroglu G, Elliott A. Reversal of dysthyroid optic neuropathy following orbital fat decompression. Br J Ophthalmol. 2000; 84(6):600–605

[197] McCord CD, Jr. Current trends in orbital decompression. Ophthalmology. 1985; 92(1):21–33

[198] Kennerdell JS, Maroon JC, Buerger GF. Comprehensive surgical management of proptosis in dysthyroid orbitopathy. Orbit. 1987; 6(3):153–179

[199] Lyons CJ, Rootman J. Orbital decompression for disfiguring exophthalmos in thyroid orbitopathy. Ophthalmology. 1994; 101(2):223–230

[200] Fatourechi V, Garrity JA, Bartley GB, Bergstralh EJ, DeSanto LW, Gorman CA. Graves ophthalmopathy. Results of transantral orbital decompression performed primarily for cosmetic indications. Ophthalmology. 1994; 101(5): 938–942

[201] Roberts CJ, Murphy MF, Adams GG, Lund VJ. Strabismus following endoscopic orbital decompression for thyroid eye disease. Strabismus. 2003; 11(3):163–171

[202] Goldberg RA, Perry JD, Hortaleza V, Tong JT. Strabismus after balanced medial plus lateral wall versus lateral wall only orbital decompression for dysthyroid orbitopathy. Ophthal Plast Reconstr Surg. 2000; 16(4): 271–277

[203] Seiff SR, Tovilla JL, Carter SR, Choo PH. Modified orbital decompression for dysthyroid orbitopathy. Ophthal Plast Reconstr Surg. 2000; 16(1):62–66

[204] Bersani T, Jian-Seyed-Ahmadi A. Orbital volume expansion of dysthyroid ophthalmopathy by surgical placement of lateral rim implants: a case study. Ophthal Plast Reconstr Surg. 1999; 15(6):429–431

17 Nystagmus and Other Ocular Oscillations

Elsa Rodarte

Abstract

Nystagmus is a rhythmic oscillation movement of the eyes, and it is often associated with the clinical symptom of oscillopsia. Nystagmus can occur in a variety of patterns, which can aid in the localization of the central nervous system lesion causing the abnormal eye movements. This chapter discusses the clinical pathways in evaluating and diagnosing abnormal eye movements, including nystagmus, as well as a detailed review of the relevant literature.

Keywords: nystagmus, oscillopsia, opsoclonus, ocular bobbing, periodic alternating gaze

17.1 Anatomical Characterization of Conjugate Eye Movements

17.1.1 What Are the Types of Eye Movements?

Eye movements can be classified as slow or fast. Saccades are rapid, take milliseconds, and bring the fovea rapidly to the target. In contrast, smooth pursuit movements are slow and follow a moving target. Vergences involve disconjugate slow movements. Convergence is coupled with lens accommodation and pupil miosis in order to focus a near target. Vestibulo-ocular and optokinetic movements deal with gaze stabilization during head movement. After the vestibulo-ocular reflex (VOR) induces slow movement, saccades refoveate the target. Retinal images need continuous foveal refixation to be continuously perceived.[1,2] This fixation process starts at age 3 months and matures over childhood.[3]

17.1.2 What is Nystagmus?

Oscillopsia is the sensation of motion in the environment which correlates to the sign of nystagmus. Oscillopsia is the visual perception of the world moving and is result of an inability to fixate on a target, the slow drift of the fovea off of the target, followed by rapid corrective saccades back to the target. Nystagmus is the observed rhythmic to-and-fro (oscillating) movement of the eyes where a drift from fixation occurs and is followed by either a fast refixation saccade (jerk nystagmus) or by slow movement back to fixation (pendular nystagmus).[3] ► Fig. 17.1 illustrates the movement patterns of nystagmus.

17.1.3 What Cortical and Brainstem Pathways Are Involved in Conjugate Eye Movement?

In addition to control of slow movements from the vestibular input on self-position, the following areas activate saccades to refoveate targets, or provide cognitive guidance for these mechanisms.

Cortex

The occipital primary visual area communicates with temporal and parietal areas (constituting the cortical dorsal spatial vision pathway). Motion processing is an important function of the occipital cortex dorsal pathway (areas V1, V2, V6, V5), and area V5 has been hypothesized to influence the perception of oscillopsia.[3,4] The frontal eye field then adds the voluntary attentional and cognitive component to integrate the sensory information with ocular motor planning. Like other motor modulation, it relays information to the basal ganglia and the vestibular nuclei, as well as to the superior colliculi, the thalamomesencephalic vertical gaze center, and the horizontal gaze center in the pontine reticular formation. The substantia nigra and the cerebellum also are indirectly activated by these pathways.[5]

Fasold et al stimulated nystagmus with cold nitrogen and found predominantly right hemisphere activation of the temporoparietal junction, the insula, the parietal lobe, the inferior frontal gyrus, and the ventrolateral occipital lobe.[6] Brandt et al showed how each vestibular stimulus inactivates the contralateral occipital cortex during activation of the parieto-insular cortex.[7]

The cerebellum and brainstem nuclei contain a "velocity storage system" which drives the extended duration of the horizontal VOR after a rotational stimulus. Bronstein et al hypothesized that the vestibular cortex is able to downregulate this mechanism in individuals with congenital blindness, chronic progressive external ophthalmoplegia, and infantile nystagmus. They compared vestibulo-ocular and vestibulo-perceptual pathways by comparing perceived rotation times of subjects manually turning a wheel and measuring nystagmus after the rotational stimulus. The perception of movement of those with abnormal extra ocular movement (EOM) function was reduced compared to controls with intact EOM.[8]

Horizontal Gaze Center

The paramedian pontine reticular formation (PPRF) in the pons sends excitatory projections to the ipsilateral sixth cranial nucleus (the final common pathway for horizontal gaze), which then activates the contralateral third cranial nuclei (via the medial longitudinal fasciculus, MLF) to induce ipsilateral conjugate horizontal gaze.[2]

Vertical Gaze Center

The rostral interstitial nucleus of the MLF in the rostral midbrain is critical for fast downward eye movements[9] and because the innervation is bilateral, lesions must be bilateral to obliterate this response. The upward gaze center is located in the pretectum[10] where the retinal ganglion cells send bilateral projections.[11] Lesions in this area result in Parinaud dorsal midbrain syndrome. In addition, the cerebellar flocculus inhibits the anterior (upward motion) semicircular canal to maintain balance with the posterior (downward motion) semicircular canal.[12]

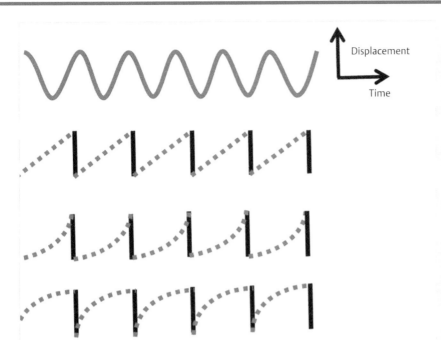

Fig. 17.1 Nystagmus movement patterns. From top to bottom: Pendular nystagmus, linear nystagmus (e.g., peripheral vestibular), accelerating nystagmus (e.g., infantile nystagmus), and decelerating nystagmus (e.g., latent infantile nystagmus and gaze-evoked). The slow phase (dashed gray) and the fast phase (solid black) of biphasic nystagmus are depicted.

Superior Colliculus

The paired superior colliculi contain topographic representations of ocular motor control and visual input, which act together with sensory and motor input from the substantia nigra and the frontal, parietal, and temporal lobes to coordinate saccades to the site of the visual stimulus.[13] Developing these maps requires previous visual experience. Stimulating the anterior areas of the colliculus results in small amplitude nasally directed or ipsiversive saccades, and these progress gradually into large temporal or contraversive saccades in the posterior area of the superior colliculus.[14]

Nucleus Prepositus Hypoglossi

The nucleus prepositus hypoglossi (NPH) contains neurons that are sensitive to specific eye position and velocity, both during saccades and during the VOR.[15] These neurons form connections with the cerebellum to conform the "velocity storage system" where the input of velocity signals is integrated and allows extension of horizontal nystagmus times to optimize responses to low frequency long duration rotational stimuli.

Thalamus

The thalamus, along with the cerebellum and the ocular motor nuclei, receives vestibular input from the perihypoglossal nuclei.

17.1.4 What Is the Vestibulo-ocular Reflex?

The vestibulo-ocular pathway is the best characterized nystagmus-inducing pathway. The vestibular system constantly relays information to the cortex and the cervical spine to integrate position, proprioception, and muscle tone, and to the extraocular muscles to maintain gaze. It is the first structure to react to changes in head position and gravity, and to relay the signal to the nuclei in the rostral medulla. The response to angular acceleration is comprised by the firing sequence of cells in three different rotation axes along the superior, posterior, and horizontal canals and the integration of these, results into "yaw," "pitch," and "roll" axes. Linear acceleration, on the other hand, is detected by hair cells whose kinocilia are polarized in opposing horizontal (utricle) and diverging vertical (saccular) directions within the maculae of the otolith organs (utricle and saccule). Gravity and displacement of the head will move the otoconia on the gelatinous substance and the cilia in the x-, y-, and z-axes.[2]

The kinocilia in the horizontal canals are activated with ipsilateral head turns and the frequency and time at which they fire will determine the characteristics of muscle contraction. A right turn will activate the right horizontal canal, ganglion, and vestibular nucleus. The vestibular nucleus then inhibits the ipsilateral abducens nucleus and excites the contralateral abducens nucleus. The left abducens nucleus will contract the left lateral rectus muscle and orchestrate conjugate gaze by crossing and ascending from the pons to the midbrain via the MLF and activating the contralateral oculomotor nucleus to contract the right medial rectus. The velocity with which they move parallels the velocity at which the head turns. This dynamic process is called the VOR (▶ Fig. 17.2).[2,8]

The VOR is divided into translational and rotational depending on whether structures in the linear or angular planes are activated. Like the horizontal canal, the anterior and posterior canals also relay signals to ocular nuclei for gaze stabilization during forward and backward movements. The anterior

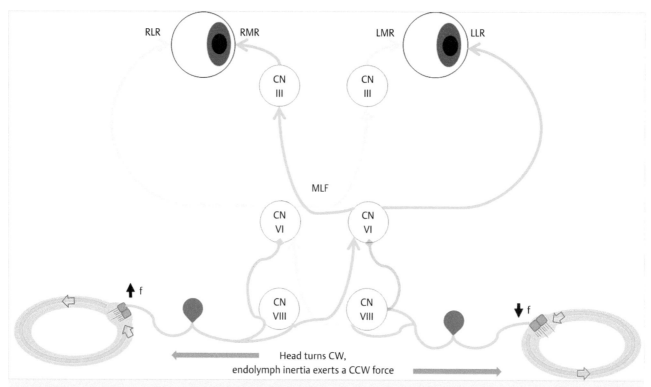

Fig. 17.2 The vestibular-ocular reflex, highlighting the pathways involved in stabilizing gaze following a right head turn. A cross-sectional view of the horizontal semicircular canals is displayed. Brainstem connections are caudal to rostral. Green excitatory projections end with an arrow, black inhibitory projections end with a square, and inactivated projections are shown as gray transparencies. Abbreviations: CCW, counter-clockwise; CN, cranial nerve nucleus; CW, clockwise; f, firing frequency; LLR, left lateral rectus; LMR, left medial rectus; MLF, medial longitudinal fasciculus; RLR, right lateral rectus; RMR, right medial rectus.

Table 17.1 Head thrust or impulse test (HIT)

Canal	Test	Normal response	Contracting muscles	Inhibited muscles
Right horizontal (RH)	Fixate on target while turning the head to the left	• Slow-phase movement toward the right • No correcting saccades	RH: Right LR Left MR	LH: Left MR Right LR
Left anterior right posterior (LARP)	• Align the anterior and posterior canals by tilting the patient's head 30° to the right. • Place one hand on top of the patient's head and one hand below her chin • LA: thrust the head forward • RP: thrust the head backward	• LA: left eye elevation and intorsion + right eye elevation and extorsion • RP: left eye depression and extorsion + right eye depression and intorsion • No overt saccades	LA: Left SR Right IO RP: Left IR Right SO	LP: Right SR Left IO RA: Right IR Left SO
Right anterior left posterior (RALP)	• Align the anterior and posterior canals by tilting the head 30° to the left • Place one hand on top of the patient's head and one hand below her chin • RA: thrust the head forward • LP: thrust the head backward	• RA: right eye elevation and intorsion + left eye elevation and extorsion • LP: right eye depression and extorsion + left eye depression and intorsion • No overt saccades	RA: Right SR Left IO LP: Left SO Right IR	LA: Left SR Right IO RP: Right SO Left IR

Abbreviations: IO, inferior oblique; IR, inferior rectus; LR, lateral rectus; MR, medial rectus; SO, superior oblique; SR, superior rectus

semicircular canal sends excitatory projections to the ipsilateral superior rectus and the contralateral inferior oblique, and it sends inhibitory projections to their opposing cyclovertical yoke muscles: the contralateral inferior rectus and the ipsilat-eral superior oblique. The clinical evaluation of these muscles can be seen in ▶ Table 17.1. The posterior semicircular canals send excitatory and inhibitory projections to the opposing yoke muscles as do the anterior canals.[8,16]

17.1.5 Do the Central Gaze Stability Mechanisms Explain All Forms of Conjugate Abnormal Eye Movements?

No, in addition to eye movement initiation and regulation originating at the central level and vestibular peripheral organs, afferent visual pathologies are associated with nystagmus.[17,18] For example, children with foveal hypoplasia typically present with nystagmus. Likewise, children with severe vision loss from a variety of etiologies (e.g., congenital cataracts, retinopathy, corneal opacities) can also present with nystagmus. Since constant refoveation is necessary for the sustained perception of retinal images,[1] foveal abnormalities may trigger compensatory central mechanisms for refoveation. Any anterior segment or retinal abnormalities may also result in nystagmus. Some examples include ocular albinism type 1,[19] autosomal recessive oculocutaneous albinism,[20] PAX6 gene mutation syndromes,[21] and Forsius–Eriksson syndrome (an X-linked recessive retinal disease).[22]

17.2 Clinical Approach To Nystagmus

What Cues from the History and Physical Examination Are Useful to Define Nystagmus?

It is useful to know whether it is

- Binocular or monocular.
- Symmetrical or asymmetrical.
- Conjugate or disconjugate.
- Horizontal, vertical, or torsional.
- Sine wave (pendular, with both phases having equal amplitude and velocity) or biphasic ("jerk," slow and fast phase). By convention, the fast phase classifies the direction of jerk nystagmus (e.g., "right-beating nystagmus").
- Linear or exponential slow phase.
- Accelerating or decelerating slow phase.
- First degree (present only with eccentric gaze in the direction of the fast phase), second degree (present in primary gaze and increasing with gaze toward the beating direction), or third degree (nystagmus persists on gaze toward the slow component).
- Congenital or acquired.
- Spontaneously appearing or induced.
- Manifest or latent.
- Physiological or pathologic.
- Central or vestibular.
- Sensory or motor.

17.2.1 In Biphasic or "Jerk" Nystagmus, Which Phase Is More Informative?

The slow phase reflects the underlying abnormality causing the nystagmus (even though by convention jerk nystagmus is named for the fast phase). The slow component may have a uniform velocity or may reduce or gain speed as the eyes move in the direction of the slow component. This slow-phase abnormality is usually due to disruption of the mechanisms that normally function to hold gaze steady.[23] Thus, disorders of the

Table 17.2 Localization of suspected lesion by nystagmus type[25,26]

Nystagmus type	Lesion localization
Upbeat nystagmus, increasing in upgaze	Cerebellar vermis
Upbeat nystagmus, increasing in downgaze	Medulla
Downbeat nystagmus	Cervico-medullary junction
Rebound nystagmus	Cerebellum
Periodic alternating nystagmus	Brainstem or cerebellum
Ocular flutter or opsoclonus	Cerebellum, especially dentate nucleus
Ocular bobbing	Pons
Seesaw nystagmus	Anterior third ventricle or parasellar lesion
Convergence-retraction nystagmus	Rostral midbrain, pretectum, posterior commissure, or posterior third ventricle

vestibular system, the gaze-holding mechanisms (e.g., the neural integrator), and visual stabilization and pursuit systems may lead to nystagmus.[24] The fast phase is thought to arise as a rescue mechanism to realign the fovea after the slow phase. It is useful to assess cortical and subcortical structures during the induced caloric vestibular reflex.[2]

17.2.2 How Can Nystagmus Be Classified?

The Classification of Eye Movement Abnormalities and Strabismus (CEMAS) listed below was accorded during a 2001 National Eye Institute workshop (Box 17.1). Certain types of nystagmus may help in localization of a lesion within the nervous system, as shown in ▶ Table 17.2.[25,26] For practical use, ▶ Fig. 17.3 presents a clinical pathway for diagnosing eye oscillations and intrusions.

Box 17.1 Classification of eye movement abnormalities and strabismus (CEMAS): nystagmus

- Physiological nystagmus:
  - Induced vestibular.
  - Optokinetic.
  - Eccentric gaze or endpoint.
- Pathologic nystagmus:
  - Infantile nystagmus syndrome (INS).
  - Fusion maldevelopment nystagmus syndrome (FMNS).
  - Spasmus nutans syndrome (SNS).
  - Vestibular nystagmus:
    - Peripheral vestibular imbalance.
    - Central vestibular imbalance.
    - Central vestibular instability.
  - Gaze-holding deficiency nystagmus:
    - Eccentric gaze nystagmus.
    - Rebound nystagmus.
    - Gaze-instability nystagmus.
  - Vision loss nystagmus:
    - Prechiasmal.

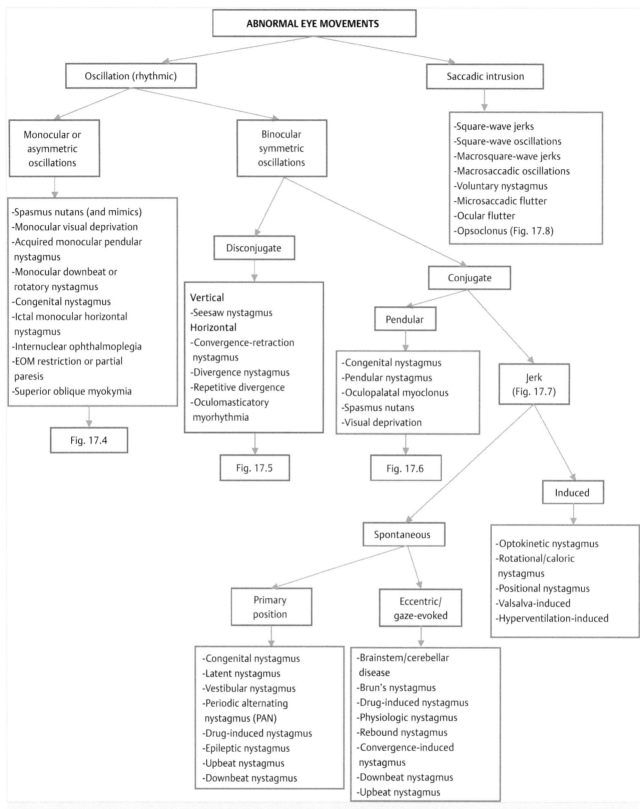

Fig. 17.3 Monocular and binocular eye oscillations and intrusions. Refer to the associated figures and text for evaluation recommendations.

- Chiasmal.
- Postchiasmal.
  ○ Other pendular nystagmus and nystagmus associated with disease of central myelin:
    - Multiple sclerosis, Pelizaeus–Merzbacher, Cockayne peroxisomal disorders, toluene abuse.
    - Pendular nystagmus associated with tremor of the palate.
    - Pendular nystagmus associated with Whipple disease.
  ○ Ocular bobbing (typical and atypical).
  ○ Lid nystagmus.
- Saccadic intrusions and oscillations:
  ○ Square-wave jerks and oscillations.
  ○ Square-wave pulses.
  ○ Saccadic pulses (single and double).
  ○ Induced convergence-retraction.
  ○ Dissociated ocular oscillations.
  ○ Hypermetric saccades.
  ○ Macrosacadic oscillations.
  ○ Ocular flutter.
  ○ Flutter dysmetria.
  ○ Opsoclonus.
  ○ Psychogenic (voluntary) flutter.
  ○ Superior oblique myokymia.
- Generalized disturbances of saccades.
- Generalized disturbance of smooth pursuit.
- Generalized disturbance of vestibular eye movements.
- Generalized disturbance of optokinetic eye movements.

17.2.3 What Are the Three Types of Physiological Nystagmus?

Optokinetic, vestibular, and eccentric gaze-induced are the three physiologic types of nystagmus.

- *Opto* means vision and *kinesis* movement. Slow movements of the visual field induce optokinetic nystagmus. The rotating optokinetic drum is a useful tool to elicit this reflex. Following a moving object involves smooth pursuit and then a saccade brings the eyes back to the beginning of the frame. While optokinetic nystagmus is normal, parietal lesions can cause a pathologic optokinetic nystagmus.[25]
- Self-movement and fast field drifts are the trigger of vestibular nystagmus.[2,8] It can be induced in normal individuals with caloric water testing and rotation in the Barany chair. These slow and fast visual drift triggers have caused some to propose common initiating mechanisms for the optokinetic and the translational VOR, describing an initial "short-latency slow tracking movement evoked by sudden drifting movements of a large field visual stimulus" that does not involve cognitive cues like smooth pursuit does.[27]
- Fine nystagmus for a few seconds on eccentric gaze is normal, but sustained nystagmus on lateral gaze indicates underlying pathology. It can be normal even at 30° of deviation past normal fixation. Features like symmetry on bilateral gaze, the absence of other neurological abnormalities, and abolition by moving the eyes toward primary position, distinguish nonpathologic endpoint nystagmus.[25]

17.2.4 How Does Vestibular System Dysfunction Cause Nystagmus?

Vestibular tone imbalance results in an asymmetric input to the horizontal gaze generator transmitting a false perception of rotation to the brain. Vestibular nystagmus shows linear, constant velocity slow phases reflecting a persistent drive of the eyes toward the damaged vestibular apparatus (labyrinth, nerve, nuclei). Unilateral vestibular lesions display neural compensation with time, but bilateral lesions do not. Because of the bilateral innervation the vestibular nuclei provide to the abducens nuclei, unilateral vestibular lesions do not affect the function of the oculomotor nerves or the MLF permanently. On the other hand, a palsy resulting from abducens, MLF, or oculomotor lesions will affect the structures they innervate and may give the appearance of an apparent monocular nystagmus.

17.2.5 What Role Does the "Leaky Neural Integrator" Hypothesis Play in Gaze-Holding Deficiency Nystagmus?

The neural integrator hypothesis proposes that a common network is responsible for the eye position signal regardless of the type of visional movement.[15] This hypothesis has been tested in perihypoglossal nuclei neurons. These are sensitive (i.e., fire at a reliable rate) when the eye holds a specific position, both during spontaneous intersaccade periods and during VOR slow phases,[15] thus pointing toward a common network for gaze holding.

The initial neural integrator model proposed that the eye velocity command needs to await eye position input for about 20 to 70 ms (leak) plus the time the cerebellum takes to provide feedback. According to the model, the drift velocity was expected to grow linearly with eccentricity. However, observation of human pathology led to a modification of this theory where nonlinearity at eccentric eye positions is accounted for.[28]

Gaze-holding deficiency or gaze-instability nystagmus refers to the oscillation that arises from inaccurate feedback between eye position and eye velocity systems, which tends to bring the eye back to an erroneous centered position when gazing laterally or upward. The occurrence of physiologic endpoint nystagmus shows that gaze-holding is harder at eccentric points.

Cerebellar dysfunction, as seen with alcohol intoxication and cerebellar lesions, magnifies the dysmetria of skeletal movements. In effect, nystagmus at less than 45° is considered a positive test for driving while intoxicated and used by law-enforcement agencies. The observation that alcohol intoxication reduces the eccentric angle at which the nystagmus appears[29] could indicate the importance of the cerebellum for gaze-holding, in a similar way to its function modulating skeletal muscle movements.

An impaired neural integrator ("leaky" integrator) may cause gaze-evoked nystagmus with exponential slow phases. The velocity of the slow phase decreases as the eyes move toward resting primary position and away from the periphery, where the pull of the orbital tissues is greatest.

Muscle weakness (paretic nystagmus) is an additional mechanism contributing to nystagmus. The inability of the gaze-holding mechanisms to keep the eyes eccentric in the orbit is often present with central or peripheral lesions causing weakness of eye movements. For this reason, this type of nystagmus is sometimes referred to as "gaze-paretic" nystagmus.

17.2.6 What Is the Approach to Acute Presentation of Nystagmus and Vertigo?

Acute vertigo and nystagmus could indicate either a peripheral (often benign) or central (potentially life-threatening) vestibulopathy. Normal vestibular tests, including the head-impulse test (HIT), should alert toward etiologies of central origin, such as stroke (refer to ▶ Table 17.1 for additional details on HIT evaluation). Other markers of central origin are skew deviation and multivectorial nystagmus. Skew deviation is more commonly due to central than peripheral causes and it commonly produces diplopia. It is important to distinguish vertical misalignment due to fourth nerve palsy from skew deviation using the Parks–Bielschowsky three-step test.[30] Nystagmus with more than one direction makes central etiologies more likely.[19] This is the basis of the Head Impulse Nystagmus Test of Skew (HINTS) clinical testing sequence, whose sensitivity has been found superior to diffusion weighted magnetic resonance imaging (MRI) sequences.[31] However, neuroimaging with computed tomography (CT) and/or MRI are still indicated if there is suspicion for a central nervous system (CNS) lesion.

17.2.7 What Causes Monocular Eye Oscillations and Asymmetric Binocular Eye Oscillations?

Monocular eye oscillations and asymmetric binocular eye oscillations may be due to spasmus nutans and its mimickers, monocular visual deprivation or loss, monocular pendular nystagmus, internuclear ophthalmoplegia (INO), partial paresis of extraocular muscles, restrictive syndromes of extraocular muscles, or superior oblique myokymia (SOM).

Spasmus nutans is a benign syndrome characterized by a triad of head nodding, nystagmus, and abnormal head posture.[32,33] The onset is typically in the first year of life and remits spontaneously within 1 month to several (up to 8) years. The syndrome is occasionally familial and has been reported in monozygotic twins. The sinusoidal nystagmus is often intermittent, asymmetric, or unilateral, and of high frequency and small amplitude with a "shimmering" quality. The nystagmus is usually horizontal but may have a vertical or torsional component. It may be accentuated by near effort and is usually greater in an abducting eye. Rarely, convergence nystagmus may occur.[34] The irregular head nodding with spasmus nutans has horizontal, vertical, or mixed components. Patients often also demonstrate a head turn or tilt.

In children with spasmus nutans, monocular nystagmus, or asymmetric pendular nystagmus, one must consider tumor of the anterior visual pathway (e.g., optic nerve, chiasm, third ventricle, or thalamus).[35,36,37] These latter patients may also have visual loss, optic atrophy, or other signs of tumor. Other spasmus nutans mimickers include arachnoid cyst, Leigh subacute necrotizing encephalomyelopathy, congenital stationary night blindness,[38,39] retinal dystrophy,[40] and Bardet–Biedl syndrome (characterized by polydactyly, obesity, cognitive delay, and retinal degeneration).[41]

All children with monocular nystagmus or spasmus nutans should undergo a complete ophthalmologic examination. We recommend neuroimaging (preferably MRI) in patients with monocular or predominantly monocular oscillations, spasmus nutans, or a spasmus nutans-like clinical picture (class IV, level C). Although most cases of spasmus nutans are benign, atypical features should prompt further evaluation including older age of onset, associated visual loss, or persistence of symptoms.[36,37] Some authors, however, have stated that the estimated prevalence of tumor in spasmus nutans is less than 1.4%, and have suggested that without other evidence of an intracranial mass lesion, neuroimaging of infants initially diagnosed with spasmus nutans may not be immediately warranted.[35] Electrophysiological testing should be considered for a myopic child suspected of having spasmus nutans to exclude the diagnosis of congenital stationary night blindness[39] or retinal dystrophy (class IV, level C).[40]

Monocular nystagmus may occur in adults or children with acquired monocular visual loss, and consists of small, slow vertical pendular oscillations in primary position of gaze. It may develop years after uniocular visual loss (Heimann–Bielschowsky phenomenon) and may improve if vision is corrected. Monocular, small-amplitude, fast frequency, and predominantly horizontal nystagmus in children may be caused by unilateral anterior visual pathway disease.[42,43]

Acquired monocular pendular nystagmus may also occur with multiple sclerosis, neurosyphilis, and brainstem infarct (thalamus and upper midbrain) and may be vertical, horizontal, or multivectorial. Stahl et al reported that servo-controlled optics could reduce oscillopsia in acquired pendular nystagmus.[44]

Vertical pendular nystagmus, with greater amplitude in the involved eye, has been described in a patient with chronic monocular myositis of the medial and lateral rectus muscles.[45] Monocular downbeat nystagmus may occur with acute infarction of the medial thalamus and upper midbrain and with pontocerebellar degeneration; this abnormality is likely due to dysfunction of the ipsilateral brachium conjunctivum (superior cerebellar peduncle). Contralateral unilateral downbeat nystagmus has been described with a paramedian thalamopeduncular infarction.[46,47] Monocular rotatory nystagmus may occur with brainstem lesions. Infantile nystagmus may rarely be uniocular. One patient has been described who developed ictal monocular horizontal nystagmus during a generalized seizure triggered by photic stimulation.[48] We recommend that neuroimaging for patients with monocular nystagmus (class IV, level C).

Dissociated nystagmus occurs in the abducting eye in INO and in pseudo-INO syndromes. These entities and their evaluation are discussed in Chapter 14. In patients with partial paresis of one of the extraocular muscles, a monocular oscillation may occur in the involved eye or its yoke during an ocular movement into the field of action of the involved muscle.[49] Monocular oscillations may also occur in restrictive syndromes (e.g., thyroid ophthalmopathy) in the field of action in which the tethering is occurring.[49]

SOM is a disorder of unknown etiology characterized symptomatically by oscillopsia, vertical or torsional diplopia, or both. Affected patients show bursts of rotary oscillations of the eye of small amplitude and high-frequency, slow-frequency large-amplitude in torsional movements, or a combination of these paroxysms. Most patients with SOM complain of brief episodes of rapid vertical or torsional movements of the environment or shimmering sensations, usually lasting only a few seconds.

Neuro-ophthalmologic examination of SOM patients often reveals brief episodes of rapid, fine, torsional movements of one eye that are best seen using either the slit-lamp biomicroscope or the direct ophthalmoscope. The abnormal movements can be induced in some patients by movement of the affected eye down and outward, by a head tilt toward the side of the affected eye, by convergence effort, or by movement of the eye downward and back to primary position.

Patients with SOM are usually young adults who are otherwise healthy. Most patients report no precipitating event for the onset of their symptoms. Several cases have followed ipsilateral trochlear nerve palsies, leading some authors to suggest that SOM might be associated with the recovery stage of injury to this nerve.[50] SOM has occurred several months after removal of a cerebellar tumor. In addition, two cases of SOM have occurred in patients with posterior fossa tumors (one an astrocytoma of the rostral cerebellar vermis with midbrain tectal compression and the other a pilocytic astrocytoma expanding within the fourth ventricle and compressing the midbrain tectum).[51,52]

The rare association of SOM with brainstem tectal disease has caused some authors to recommend neuroimaging examination of the course of the trochlear nerve in all patients with this diagnosis[52]; however, the association of SOM with a posterior fossa tumor is extremely uncommon (class IV, level U).[53] In one reported case, SOM may have been due to vascular compression of the trochlear nerve by a branch of the posterior cerebral artery noted on thin-slice MRI.[54] In another study of six patients with SOM, neurovascular contact at the root exit zone of the trochlear nerve was identified in all patients, suggesting that SOM may be a neurovascular compression syndrome.[55] SOM has been described in a patient with a dural arteriovenous fistula,[56] and Neetens and Martin described two cases of SOM, one associated with lead intoxication and the other with adrenoleukodystrophy.[57] Some of these associations may well have been coincidental (class IV). We do not recommend neuroimaging for typical isolated SOM but consider MRI scan in patients with atypical features (class IV, level C).

Rosenberg and Glaser obtained from 1 to 19 years (average 8 years) of follow-up for nine patients with SOM.[58] These authors noted that the natural history of the disorder is one of spontaneous remissions and exacerbations, with untreated patients frequently enjoying months or even years of remission before subsequent relapses. Indeed, seven of their nine patients continued to have some symptoms after prolonged follow-up.

The treatment for a majority of patients with SOM is reassurance, because most are not significantly disabled by their visual symptoms. If the condition disrupts the patient's work and lifestyle, medications such as carbamazepine or propranolol[59] may be considered. In Rosenberg and Glaser's series, 7 of 11 patients were tried on carbamazepine, and 6 noted a prompt decrease or cessation of ocular symptoms.[58] All experienced at least one subsequent relapse days to months after the initial improvement, however, and only three chose to continue the medication. We have tried gabapentin in one patient with SOM without subjective or objective improvement.

Brazis et al investigated the clinical presentations and long-term course of 16 patients with SOM.[53] Follow-up information was obtained for 14 of the 16 patients with time from onset of symptoms to most recent contact 3 to 29 years (mean, 12 years). The SOM gradually improved or resolved, at least temporarily, without treatment in a significant number of patients. Three of the patients had complete spontaneous resolution of symptoms for periods of 6 to 12 months without recurrence. Six of 7 patients treated with carbamazepine reported no significant response. One patient remained on the medication for 3 years with only rare symptoms that worsen when attempts were made to taper the drug. Two of the patients treated with propranolol reported no significant benefit, and a third noted dramatic but transient improvement in symptoms. Four of the patients were cured by superior oblique tenectomy combined with inferior oblique myectomy. All four surgical patients experienced disappearance of oscillopsia, although one patient developed postoperative vertical diplopia that gradually resolved.

Brazis et al concluded that because SOM is a much more chronic disease than formerly realized and because of the poor long-term effects and potential side effects of the medications used for treatment, medical treatment of SOM, at least with currently available medications, may not be the optimum way to manage the disease. These authors reported that surgery is the treatment of choice when symptoms of SOM are intolerable to the patient. Other authors have also reported successful treatment of SOM with surgery.[60,61] For example, Kosmorsky et al performed a Harada–Ito procedure on a woman with SOM.[62] This procedure involves nasally transposing the anterior portion of the superior oblique tendon, which is responsible for the cyclorotation, to create an effective weakening of the anterior portion of the tendon instead of temporal displacement utilized for superior oblique paresis. The SOM was abolished and vertical eye movements, including saccades, were unaffected. Samii et al reported one patient with SOM who responded to microvascular decompression of the fourth nerve at the root exit zone.[63]

The treatment of SOM is usually reassurance and the condition may be self-limiting. When symptoms are intolerable, medical or surgical therapy may be considered. A weakening procedure of the affected superior oblique muscle combined with a weakening procedure of the ipsilateral inferior oblique muscle or the Harada–Ito procedure is an effective treatment for SOM after failure of medical treatment or as an alternative to such treatment, and should be considered in patients with unacceptable visual symptoms. Microvascular decompression of the fourth cranial nerve at the root exit zone may be another approach, but so far there has been little experience with this procedure for SOM.

The evaluation monocular or asymmetric oscillations is outlined in ▶ Fig. 17.4.

17.2.8 What Are the Causes of Disconjugate Bilateral Symmetric Eye Oscillations?

If the ocular oscillations involve both eyes to a relatively equal degree, the next step in evaluation involves determining whether the eye movements are conjugate (both eyes moving in the same direction) or disconjugate (the eyes moving in different directions).[49] When the oscillations are disconjugate,

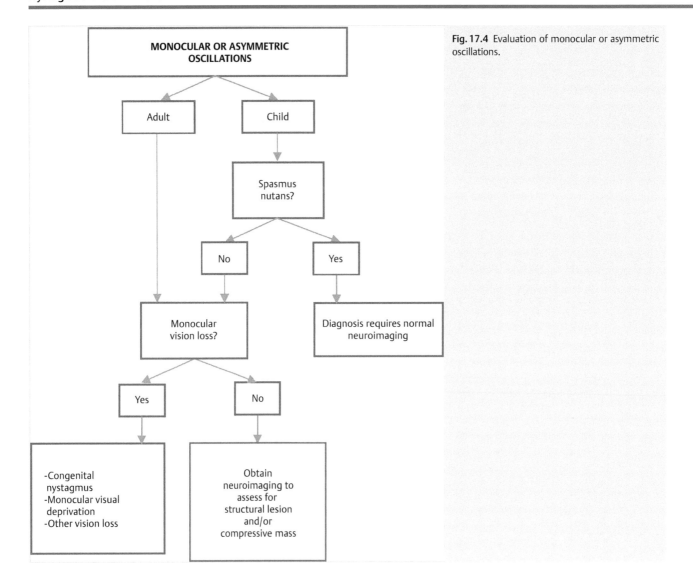

Fig. 17.4 Evaluation of monocular or asymmetric oscillations.

the examiner should determine whether the oscillations are vertical or horizontal. Vertical disconjugate eye oscillations are usually due to seesaw nystagmus. Horizontal disconjugate eye oscillations include convergence-retraction nystagmus (nystagmus retractorius), divergence nystagmus, repetitive divergence, and oculomasticatory myorhythmia.

17.2.9 What Are the Clinical Features and Etiologies of Seesaw Nystagmus?

Seesaw nystagmus is a cyclic movement of the eyes with a conjugate torsional component and a disjunctive vertical component. While one eye rises and intorts, the other falls and extorts; the vertical and torsional movements are then reversed, completing the cycle. This nystagmus is usually pendular and may be due to a large suprasellar lesion compressing or invading the brainstem bilaterally at the mesodiencephalic junction. Pendular seesaw nystagmus may also be congenital.[64]

Seesaw nystagmus may also have an underlying jerk waveform, often due to an intrinsic focal brainstem lesion, either in the lateral medulla (usually on the side opposite the torsional quick phases) or in the mesodiencephalon on the same side as the quick phases.[65,66] Jerk seesaw nystagmus has a slow phase corresponding to one half-cycle of seesaw nystagmus and is thus often called hemi-seesaw nystagmus.

Seesaw nystagmus likely represents oscillations involving central otolithic connections, especially the interstitial nucleus of Cajal, where vertical versions and torsions are computed.[66] Midbrain lesions around this nucleus cause nonpendular, jerk, or hemi-seesaw nystagmus. Seesaw nystagmus may also be in part due to an unstable visuovestibular interaction control system. Lesions in the optic pathways may prevent retinal error signals, essential for vestibulo-ocular reflex adaptation, from reaching the cerebellar flocculus and inferior olivary nucleus, thereby making the system less stable. Reported etiologies responsible for seesaw nystagmus are listed in Box 17.2.

- Parasellar masses.[67]
- Brainstem and thalamic strokes.[65,66]
- Multiple sclerosis.[68]
- Trauma.
- Chiari malformation.
- Hydrocephalus.
- Syringobulbia.
- Paraneoplastic encephalitis (with testicular cancer and anti-Ta antibodies).[69]
- Whole brain irradiation and intrathecal methotrexate.[70]
- Septo-optic dysplasia, retinitis pigmentosa, and cone degeneration.[64]
- VACTERL (vertebral defects, anal atresia, cardiac defects, trachea-esophageal fistula, renal anomalies, and limb abnormalities) association.[71]
- Congenital seesaw nystagmus.[72]

Congenital seesaw nystagmus may lack the torsional component or even present with an opposite pattern, that is, extorsion with eye elevation and intorsion with eye depression. With congenital cases, the binocular torsional eye movements may be in phase with clinically visible head oscillations (i.e., head movements are not compensatory for the torsional eye movements).[72]

Chiari malformation type I may be associated with nystagmus of skew in which one eye beats upward while the other eye beats downward.[73] The evaluation of a patient with seesaw nystagmus includes a complete ophthalmologic and neurologic examination. Patients with parasellar lesions often have bitemporal field defects and "bow-tie" optic atrophy associated with pendular seesaw nystagmus. Jerk seesaw nystagmus usually is associated with other brainstem signs. We recommend neuroimaging (preferably MRI attending to parasellar and posterior fossa regions) for patients with seesaw nystagmus, with particular attention to the third ventricle/parasellar area (class IV, level C). The presence of this nystagmus with a skew deviation requires MRI studies for a Chiari malformation (class IV, level C). The treatment of seesaw nystagmus is directed at the responsible lesion. One patient with intermittent seesaw nystagmus responded to clonazepam, and the nystagmus did not recur after withdrawal of the medication.[74] Also, baclofen, with and without clonazepam, improved both nystagmus and associated oscillopsia in another patient, suggesting a possible γ-aminobutyric acid (GABA)-ergic mechanism influencing the interstitial nucleus of Cajal.

17.2.10 What Are the Causes of Horizontal Disconjugate Eye Oscillations?

Convergence may evoke various forms of nystagmus (i.e., convergence-evoked nystagmus; see below). Convergence-retraction nystagmus is a disorder of ocular motility in which repetitive adducting saccades, which are often accompanied by retraction of the eyes into the orbit, occur spontaneously or on attempted upgaze.[75] Rotating an optokinetic tape or drum

downward may elicit the movements. Convergence-retraction nystagmus is primarily a saccadic disorder as the convergence movements are not normal vergence movements but asynchronous, adducting saccades.

Other authors think that convergence-retraction nystagmus is a disorder of vergence rather than of opposing adducting saccades.[76] Mesencephalic lesions affecting the pretectal region are most likely to cause this type of nystagmus, which is often associated with abnormalities of vertical gaze. The localization and evaluation of these vertical gaze abnormalities and convergence-retraction nystagmus are discussed in Chapter 14. Convergence nystagmus has been described without vertical gaze abnormalities in patients with dorsal midbrain stroke and in patients with Chiari malformation.[77,78] Whipple disease may also cause convergence nystagmus at approximately 1 Hz (pendular vergence oscillations).[79] Convergence nystagmus has been described in a patient with spasmus nutans.[34]

Divergence nystagmus (with divergent quick phases) may occur with hindbrain abnormalities (e.g., Chiari malformation) and is associated with downbeat nystagmus. These patients have slow phases directed upward and inward. Repetitive divergence consists of a slow divergent movement followed by a rapid return to the primary position at regular intervals.[80] This rare disorder has been described with coma from hepatic encephalopathy. A similar disorder, probably related to seizures, was reported in a neonate in association with burst-suppression patterns of the electroencephalogram (EEG).[81]

Oculomasticatory myorhythmia refers to acquired pendular vergence oscillations associated with concurrent contraction of the masticatory muscles.[82,83] If nonfacial skeletal muscles are involved, it is called oculofacial-skeletal myorhythmia. There is a smooth, rhythmic eye convergence, which cycles at a frequency of approximately 1 Hz, followed by divergence back to the primary position. Rhythmic elevation and depression of the mandible is synchronous with the ocular oscillations that persist in sleep and are unaltered by stimuli. The masticatory involvement may occasionally consist of a permanent bruxism leading to severe tooth abrasions.[84] Patients with oculomasticatory myorhythmia may also have paralysis of vertical gaze, progressive somnolence, and intellectual deterioration. This distinct movement disorder has been recognized only in Whipple disease (class III–IV, level B). If this condition is diagnosed, empiric antibiotic treatment should be considered and tissue diagnosis should be attempted. Whipple disease may be diagnosed by endoscopically guided biopsy of multiple jejunal sites.[82,83] Electron microscopy and polymerase chain reaction (PCR)-based testing on intestinal or extraintestinal tissue may also confirm the diagnosis.[83,84] PCR can also be performed on cerebrospinal fluid in CNS Whipple disease.[85,86]

The evaluation of disconjugate bilateral symmetric eye oscillations is outlined in ▶ Fig. 17.5.

17.2.11 What Are the Causes of Binocular Symmetric Conjugate Eye Oscillations?

Binocular symmetric conjugate eye oscillations may be divided into pendular nystagmus, jerk nystagmus, and saccadic intrusions.[49]

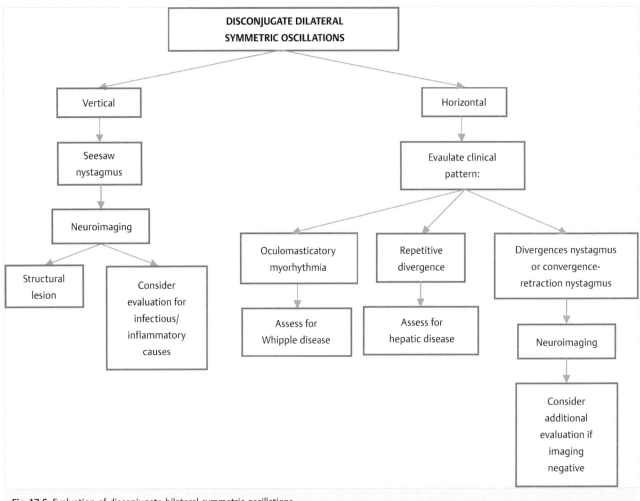

Fig. 17.5 Evaluation of disconjugate bilateral symmetric oscillations.

17.2.12 What Are the Causes of Binocular Symmetric Pendular Conjugate Eye Oscillations?

Binocular symmetric pendular conjugate eye oscillations may be due to infantile nystagmus, pendular nystagmus, oculopalatal tremor, spasmus nutans (discussed above), and visual deprivation nystagmus.

Infantile nystagmus may be noted at birth or in early infancy, or may emerge or enhance in teenage or adult life.[23,87,88] It may be familial, hereditary (X-linked such as FRMD7 mutations in locus Xq26.2 and unknown genes in locus Xp11.4-p11.3, autosomal dominant loci 6p12, 7p11.2, and 13q31–33, or autosomal recessive),[89,90,91,92] or idiopathic. Metabolic derangements and structural anomalies of the brain, including abnormalities of the anterior and posterior visual pathways, may be responsible.[93] Less than 20% of childhood nystagmus cases are acquired and red flags include age older than 4 months, the presence of oscillopsia, asymmetric nystagmus, preserved optokinetic nystagmus, relative afferent pupillary defect, papilledema, and additional neurological symptoms.[3] More importantly, when it is found later in life it must be distinguished from other forms of nystagmus that have a potentially treatable cause.

Infantile nystagmus may be wholly pendular or have both pendular and jerk components. Congenital jerk nystagmus has a slow phase with a velocity that increases exponentially as the eyes move in the direction of the slow phase. Occasionally, infantile nystagmus may be purely vertical or torsional, and although these findings usually implicate an intracranial lesion, these forms of nystagmus may occur in sensory infantile nystagmus.[94] Although irregular, infantile nystagmus is generally conjugate and horizontal, even on upgaze or downgaze (uniplanar), visual fixation accentuates it and active eyelid closure or convergence attenuates it.[87] The nystagmus decreases in an eye position ("null region") that is specific for each patient. Despite the constant eye motion, these patients do not experience oscillopsia. When they are tested with a hand-held optokinetic tape or drum, the quick phase of the elicited nystagmus generally follows the direction of the tape (reversed optokinetic nystagmus).

Symptomatic oscillopsia in patients with infantile nystagmus is unusual but may be precipitated after visual maturation by new or changing-associated visual sensory conditions (e.g., decompensating strabismus or retinal degeneration).[95] Infantile nystagmus has been associated with many disease processes affecting the visual afferent system including ocular and oculocutaneous albinism, achromatopsia, optic nerve hypoplasia, Leber congenital amaurosis, coloboma, aniridia, cone dystrophies, corectopia, congenital stationary night blindness, Chédiak–Higashi syndrome, Joubert syndrome, and peroxisomal disorders. It has also been associated with hypothyroidism. The evaluation of children with infantile nystagmus thus should include a complete ophthalmologic examination, especially attending to symptoms of photophobia and paradoxical pupillary constriction in darkness, and thyroid functions. An electroretinogram (ERG) may be helpful even with a normal afferent exam.[96] For example, 56% of 105 consecutive patients with infantile nystagmus were found to have retinal disease when tested with ERG.[96]

Infantile nystagmus often decreases in an eye position ("null region") that is specific for each patient, and convergence often attenuates the nystagmus. Prisms can be used to take advantage of the dampening effect of convergence and the null region-lens combinations can be adjusted so that an asymmetric arrangement of base-out prisms both converge the eyes and turn them toward the null angle. Leigh et al suggest 7.00-diopter base-out prisms with 1.00-diopter spheres added to compensate for accommodation.[97] Contact lenses may improve vision in patients with infantile nystagmus, possibly due to tactile feedback. Another approach for the treatment of severe nystagmus in general involves employing an optical system to stabilize images on the retina.[97,98] The combination of high "plus" (i.e., converging) spectacle lenses with high "minus" (i.e., diverging) contact lenses is used with the converging system focusing the image at the center of eye rotation (thus, stabilizing the image) and the diverging system moving the image back to focus on the retina. The contact lens moves with the eye so it does not negate the effect of image stabilization produced by the spectacle lens. This imaging system is theoretically beneficial but difficult to maintain in practice, especially as the system disables the VOR and is thus only useful when the patient is stationary.

Infantile nystagmus may also be treated with botulinum toxin injections into the extraocular muscles or surgery. Acuity was restored in four patients, to the extent that they were able to receive daytime drivers licenses, by multiple horizontal recti injections of botulinum toxin.[99] Surgical procedures effectively control infantile nystagmus by attempting to move the attachments of the extraocular muscles so that the null angle corresponds to the new primary position (the null region is shifted and broadened), to decrease nystagmus outside the null region, and to prolong foveation time by changing the waveform and dampening the nystagmus.[100,101,102,103,104] Procedures used include the Anderson–Kestenbaum procedure, which moves the eyes to the null region, divergence procedures, large recessions of the horizontal rectus muscles, and combined procedures.[97,105] Finally, biofeedback has been reported to help some patients with this disorder. Evans et al performed a randomized, double-masked, placebo-controlled trial of various treatments for infantile nystagmus and concluded that these putative therapies should be assumed to be placebos until proven otherwise by randomized trial (class III–IV, level C).[106]

Latent nystagmus (LN), a result of fusion maldevelopment syndromes like strabismus and amblyopia, is common and generally congenital.[107,108,109] It appears or worsens when one eye is covered. Both eyes then develop conjugate jerk nystagmus, with the viewing eye having a slow phase directed toward the nose (i.e., the quick phase of both eyes beat toward the side of the fixating eye). Although present at birth, LN is often not recognized until later in life, when an attempt is made to determine monocular visual acuity during vision screening at school. LN is usually associated with strabismus, especially esotropia; amblyopia may occur and binocular vision with normal stereopsis is rare. In addition to horizontal strabismus, upward deviation of the covered eye (dissociated vertical deviation or alternating sursumduction) and a torsional, occasionally pendular, component to the nystagmus may occur. LN does not indicate progressive structural brain disease.[49] It has been shown that loss of binocular connections within V1 in the first months of life is sufficient to cause LN. In fact, avoiding correction of the unequal cortical input after 2 to 3 months of life leads to LN in 100% of infants.[110]

Manifest LN is an oscillation that occurs in patients with strabismus or acquired visual loss who have a jerk nystagmus in the direction of the fixing eye (i.e., right-beating nystagmus when fixing with the right eye and left-beating nystagmus when fixing with the left eye).[49] Patients with infantile uniocular blindness may have a bilateral horizontal nystagmus that represents a manifest nystagmus of the latent type.[111] These patients often have a family history of strabismus; the monocular blindness (opacity of the media or suppression) acts as an occluder, making manifest what would have been LN. Therapy for LN consists of measures to improve vision, such as patching for amblyopia in children or surgical correction of strabismus.[104]

Voluntary nystagmus (psychogenic flutter) occurs in normal subjects, sometimes as a familial trait, and consists of bursts of high-frequency horizontal oscillations composed of back-to-back saccades.[112,113] The movements may be vertical or torsional as well. This movement will completely disappear if patients are forced to keep their eyes open, because it requires tremendous volitional effort and cannot be sustained for prolonged periods of time.[49] Voluntary nystagmus is often accompanied by a "fixed look" required to produce the symptoms, eyelid flutter, and convergence. Voluntary nystagmus may be associated with spasm of the near reflex[113] and has been described as a component of nonepileptic seizures.[114]

Although pendular nystagmus is often congenital, acquired forms exist. Acquired pendular nystagmus may be wholly horizontal, wholly vertical, or have mixed components (circular, elliptical, or windmill pendular nystagmus). Pendular nystagmus may be symmetric, dissociated, or even monocular and often causes distressing oscillopsia and decreased visual acuity.[115,116,117] Damage to the dentatorubro-olivary pathways (Guillain–Mollaret triangle) is found in some cases of acquired pendular nystagmus, which is most often caused by oculopalatal tremor, multiple sclerosis, stroke, or tumor of the brainstem or other posterior fossa structures.[115,116,117,118,119,120,121,122] In multiple sclerosis, pendular nystagmus may be a sign of cerebellar nuclear involvement or result from optic neuropathy, but the most consistent finding on MRI is a lesion in the dorsal pontine tegmentum, perhaps affecting the central tegmental tract.[116] Though the frequency oscillates between 2 and 4 Hz, similar to nonoculopalatal tremor (OPT) multiple sclerosis-acquired pendular nystagmus, the "dual hypothesis" states that enhancement of gap junctions leads to irregular firing of synchronous olivary neuron patches toward a second learning site: the deep cerebellar nuclei.[123,124] In a study of 27 patients with acquired pendular nystagmus, MRI findings were characterized by multiple areas of abnormal signal with statistically significant ones occurring in areas containing the red nucleus, the central tegmental tract, the medial vestibular nucleus, and the inferior olive.[117] The abundance of abnormal MRI signals, predominantly in the pons but also in the midbrain and the medulla, suggests that large or multiple structural lesions may be required to elicit pendular nystagmus. Acquired convergence-induced pendular nystagmus may occur with multiple sclerosis[118] and we recommend neuroimaging (e.g., cranial MRI) for all unexplained cases of acquired pendular nystagmus (class III–IV, level B). The frequency range in multiple sclerosis-induced APN characteristically oscillates at 3 to 5 Hz.[123]

Other causes of acquired binocular pendular nystagmus include Pelizaeus–Merzbacher disease, mitochondrial cytopathy, Cockayne syndrome, neonatal adrenoleukodystrophy (a peroxisomal disorder), and toluene addiction.[125,126,127] Spontaneous horizontal pendular nystagmus in a patient with a surgically acquired perilymph fistula was found related to the heart rate and may have been caused by pressure transfer of blood pulses to the labyrinth.[128] Congenital, familial, or acquired bilateral paralysis of horizontal gaze may be associated with pendular nystagmus; the familial type may also be associated with progressive scoliosis and facial contractures with myokymia. Pendular nystagmus may also appear with blindness or monocular loss of vision; in the latter case, it may be monocular (see above). Binocular visual loss may cause nystagmus that has both horizontal and vertical components that change direction over seconds or minutes (i.e., a wandering null point).[129] Blind patients may have windmill nystagmus, in which there are repeated oscillations in the vertical plane alternating with repeated oscillations in the horizontal plane.

Horizontal pendular pseudonystagmus has been described in patients with horizontal essential head tremor and bilateral vestibular dysfunction.[130,131] The deficient VOR results in ocular oscillations in space when the head oscillates, and funduscopy reveals a fine pendular motion of the eyes that is reduced by firm support of the head. The oscillopsia improves with treatment of the tremor with propranolol. Yen et al described two renal transplant patients who developed pseudonystagmus and oscillopsia caused by immunosuppressant (tacrolimus)-induced head tremor and gentamicin-induced vestibulopathy.[132] Although the patients were initially thought to have nystagmus, closer observation revealed no true nystagmus but corrective saccades compensating for an absent VOR during the head tremor (pseudonystagmus). Typically, patients with vestibulo-ocular impairment have only head movement-induced oscillopsia, but these patients had constant oscillopsia because the visual tracking system (smooth pursuit) could not compensate for the loss of vestibular function at immunosuppressant-induced head oscillation greater than 1 Hz. Vestibular rehabilitation helped one of these patients.

Palatal myoclonus is a continuous rhythmic involuntary movement of the soft palate that may be accompanied by synchronous movements of other adjacent structures, such as the face, pharynx, larynx, or diaphragm. The association of pendular nystagmus with palatal myoclonus is not infrequent, and the condition is then termed oculopalatal myoclonus or oculopalatal tremor (OPT).[122,133] OPT may be of two types[134]:

1. A lateral form, consisting of jerky, nystagmoid movements with simultaneous oblique and rotatory components associated (and synchronous) with lateralized palatal myoclonus (in this form, the eye on the side of the myoclonus intorts as it rises and extorts as it falls, whereas the opposite eye extorts as it rises and intorts as it falls).
2. A midline form in which vertical to-and-fro pendular eye movements occur synchronous with symmetric bilateral palatal myoclonus.

OPT involves VOR adaption mediated by the cerebellar flocculus, and floccular integrity is preserved in most patients.[134] The lateral form implies unilateral disease, whereas the midline form indicates bilateral disease. Damage to the dentatorubro-olivary pathways (Guillain–Mollaret triangle) is found in cases of OPT, which is most often caused by multiple sclerosis or vascular lesions of the brainstem. MRI often shows enlargement of the inferior olivary nuclei.[122]

There may be an association between the one-and-a-half syndrome (see Chapter 14) and OPT.[135] In five patients with one-and-a-half syndrome and facial nerve palsy, OPT developed in 4 months to 3 years. Involvement of the facial nerve may predict subsequent development of OPT. It may be associated with delayed (tardive) ataxia.[133]

The evaluation of the patient with pendular nystagmus depends on the clinical circumstances and associated neurologic findings. In patients with multiple sclerosis, the diagnosis is usually obvious by a history of remissions and exacerbations of neurologic signs and symptoms associated with abnormalities on neurologic examination, suggesting a disseminated process. Brainstem stroke or tumor is diagnosed by mode of onset of symptoms, associated neurologic signs and symptoms, and MRI. Ophthalmologic exam will reveal blindness as a cause for the nystagmus in some patients. MRI is warranted in all patients with palatal myoclonus (class III–IV, level B).

The neurotransmitters involved in pendular nystagmus are unknown, but cholinergic and GABA-ergic pathways may be involved. Anticholinergic agents have produced variable treatment results.[136,137] In a randomized, double-blind study, trihexyphenidyl improved only one of five patients with pendular elliptical nystagmus. In another double-blind study, intravenous scopolamine reduced nystagmus and improved vision in five patients.[136,138] Isoniazid relieved nystagmus and oscillopsia in two of three patients with pendular elliptical nystagmus due to multiple sclerosis, but others have not found this drug to be helpful.[97,139] Memantine (a glutamate receptor antagonist) caused complete cessation of nystagmus in 11 of 14 patients with acquired pendular nystagmus due to multiple sclerosis.[121] These 11 responders had fixation pendular nystagmus (i.e., nystagmus increased with fixation). A dramatic suppression of pendular nystagmus in a patient with multiple sclerosis was described after smoking cannabis, but not by taking orally administered capsules containing cannabis oil.[120]

Stahl et al have measured the effects of gabapentin on vision and eye movements in acquired pendular nystagmus in two patients with multiple sclerosis and one with brainstem stroke.[140] An oral dose of 600 mg produced improvement of vision due to changes in ocular oscillations in all three patients. The drug was well tolerated and was continued at 900 to 1,500 mg daily in divided doses with long-term benefit. All the patients reported useful visual improvement that enabled them to read, watch television, and recognize faces. In other studies, gabapentin improved acquired pendular nystagmus in 10 of 15 patients[141] and 3 of 8 patients.[142]

Several reports have suggested that injection of botulinum toxin either into selected extraocular muscles or into the retrobulbar space might be effective in the treatment of acquired nystagmus.[99,122,143,144,145,146,147] Leigh et al injected the horizontal rectus muscles of the right eye of two patients with acquired pendular nystagmus.[143] The treatment effectively abolished the horizontal component of the nystagmus in the injected eyes of both patients for 2 months. However, side effects including diplopia, ptosis, and worsening of the oscillopsia in the uninjected eye (attributed to plastic-adaptive changes in response to paresis caused by the botulinum toxin) limited the effectiveness of the treatment. In another study, botulinum toxin injection into the retrobulbar space of three patients with acquired pendular nystagmus abolished or reduced all components of the nystagmus.[147] Again, side effects of the treatment seem to be the limiting factor. Others have reported variable improvement in visual function and oscillopsia with retrobulbar or horizontal recti botulinum injection, with transient ptosis the most common side effect.[145,146] Repka et al injected 25 to 30 units of botulinum toxin into the retrobulbar space of six adults with acquired nystagmus.[144] Each patient had subjective and objective improvement of distance visual acuity following injection with reduction of the amplitude but not the frequency of the nystagmus. Visual improvement lasted no more than 8 weeks but persisted for 6 months in two patients with OPT. The authors concluded that retrobulbar botulinum toxin injection may improve visual function for patients with acquired nystagmus and that improvement seemed to be longer for patients with OPT. Further studies on the safety and efficacy of botulinum toxin injection for acquired nystagmus are warranted (class IV, level U).

Lesions of the Guillain–Mollaret triangle are thought to induce cholinergic denervation supersensitivity of the inferior olive, which results in the oculopalatal tremor. Anticholinergic agents (trihexyphenidyl) have thus been tried effectively in four patients with palatal myoclonus without ocular involvement[138] and in one patient with vertical pendular nystagmus identical to that seen with OPT but without palatal involvement.[148] Valproate and carbamazepine have each been reported to reduce the nystagmus of OPT. Finally, as noted above, the nystagmus in patients with OPT may be especially sensitive to retrobulbar botulinum toxin injection.[144]

The evaluation and treatment of pendular nystagmus is outlined in ▶ Fig. 17.6.

17.2.13 What Are the Causes of Binocular Symmetric Jerk Nystagmus?

Binocular symmetric conjugate jerk nystagmus may be divided into that which is present spontaneously and that which is induced.[49] Spontaneous jerk nystagmus may be further divided into forms present in primary position and forms present predominantly on eccentric gaze.

Spontaneous symmetric conjugate jerk nystagmus that occurs in primary position may be predominantly horizontal, predominantly torsional, or predominantly vertical. Spontaneous symmetric conjugate jerk nystagmus in primary gaze that is predominantly horizontal includes infantile nystagmus (above), LN (above), vestibular nystagmus, periodic alternating nystagmus (PAN), drug-induced nystagmus, and epileptic nystagmus. Spontaneous symmetric conjugate jerk nystagmus in primary gaze that is purely torsional is a form of central vestibular nystagmus. Spontaneous symmetric conjugate jerk nystagmus in primary gaze that is predominantly vertical includes upbeat nystagmus and downbeat nystagmus.

Horizontal nystagmus in the primary position is often the result of peripheral vestibular disease. Vestibular nystagmus has a linear (constant velocity) slow phase. The horizontal component is diminished when the patient lies with the intact ear down and is exacerbated with the affected ear down. Peripheral vestibular lesions induce a tendency for the eyes to drift in a direction parallel to the plane in which the diseased canal lies. Horizontal nystagmus with the slow component toward the lesion (the opposite vestibular nuclei drive the eyes toward the diseased side) results from unilateral horizontal canal or total labyrinthine destruction. In the latter case, there is a torsional slow component causing the upper part of the globe to rotate toward the lesioned side. Although constant for a particular position of gaze, the slow-phase velocity is greater when the eyes are turned in the direction of the quick component (Alexander's law). Nystagmus due to peripheral vestibular disease is most prominent, or only becomes apparent, when fixation is prevented. Both peripheral and central vestibular nystagmus may vary with head position and movement, but peripheral nystagmus changes after a latency period following the postural change and tends to fatigue.

Peripheral vestibular disease is suspected when the nystagmus is associated with subjective vertigo. Central vestibular disease (e.g., brainstem infarction) is suspected when associated neurologic signs and symptoms of brainstem dysfunction are present. We recommend otolaryngologic consultation for peripheral vestibular disease and MRI for central vestibular disorders (class III–IV, level C).

With PAN, the eyes exhibit primary position nystagmus, which, after 60 to 120 seconds, stops for a few seconds and then starts beating in the opposite direction.[149] Horizontal jerk

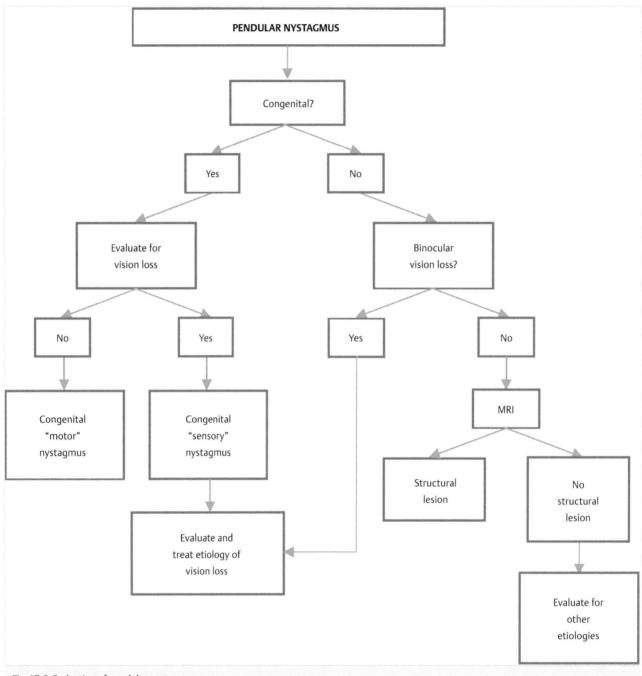

Fig. 17.6 Evaluation of pendular nystagmus.

nystagmus in the primary position not associated with vertigo is usually PAN.[49] This disorder may be associated with periodic alternating oscillopsia, periodic alternating gaze, or periodic alternating skew deviation.[150] PAN may be congenital or acquired. Reported etiologies are listed in Box 17.3. It may be caused by craniocervical junction disease. The nodulus and uvula of the cerebellum maintain inhibitory control over vestibular rotational responses by using gamma aminobutyric acid (GABA).

Following ablation of these structures, the postrotational response is excessively prolonged, so that normal vestibular repair mechanisms act to reverse the direction of the nystagmus, which results in PAN.[137] PAN is thus thought to be produced by dysfunction of the GABA-ergic velocity-storage mechanism and may be controlled in most, but not all, patients by the GABA-B agonist baclofen.[150,151] Patients with congenital PAN may also respond to baclofen or benefit from horizontal recti recessions.[152]

- Congenital (may be associated with albinism and X-linked mutations).[149,152,153,154,155,156]
- Arnold–Chiari malformation and other malformations of the craniocervical junction.[151]
- Cerebellar degenerations.[151,157]
- Ataxia-telangiectasia.
- Cerebellar masses (tumor, abscess, cyst).
- Brainstem infarction.[151]
- Cerebellar infections, including syphilis, HIV,[158] and Creutzfeldt–Jakob disease.[137,159,160]
- Posterior reversible encephalopathy syndrome (PRES) with bilateral cerebellar and temporo-occipital involvement.[161]
- Syndrome of nystagmus and ataxia due to antiganglioside antibodies.[162]
- Late-onset cerebellar ataxia with anti-glutamic acid decarboxylase (GAD) antibodies.[163,164]
- Hepatic encephalopathy.[165]
- Trauma.[137]
- Multiple sclerosis.[137,166]
- Medications (e.g., antiepileptics, lithium).[167]
- Following visual loss (e.g., due to cataract or vitreous hemorrhage).
- Epileptic PAN (after hypoxic encephalopathy).[168]

The evaluation of a patient with PAN includes a complete neurologic and ophthalmologic exam. In many patients, the etiology of the nystagmus is evident by history (e.g., congenital onset, associated albinism, family history of cerebellar degeneration, anticonvulsant use, history of remissions and exacerbations of neurologic signs and symptoms, acute onset of brainstem signs and symptoms, severe visual impairment, etc.). Otherwise, the evaluation should include MRI with attention to the craniocervical junction (class III–IV, level B). If MRI is normal and the patient has a history of the subacute onset of progressive cerebellar signs and symptoms, Creutzfeldt–Jakob disease should be suspected (class IV, level C). Serology for syphilis and hepatic function studies could be considered (class IV, level C).

Drug-induced nystagmus may be horizontal, vertical, rotatory, or (most commonly) mixed.[169] It is most often seen with tranquilizing medications and anticonvulsants. Although drug-induced nystagmus is more often evident with eccentric gaze (see below), it may also be evident in primary gaze.[49,170]

Nystagmus may occur as an epileptic phenomenon. Epileptic nystagmus is usually horizontal, may be seen with epileptiform activity ipsilateral or contralateral to the direction of the slow component of the nystagmus, and often is associated with altered states of consciousness, although consciousness may be preserved during the attacks.[157,171,172,173,174] There are two postulated mechanisms for the eye deviation in epileptic nystagmus. Ipsiversive eye deviation, with eye movement recordings and EEG showing seizure-induced ipsilateral linear slow phases, is postulated to result from stimulation of the smooth pursuit region in the temporo-occipital cortex. If eye velocity is high or the eye reaches a far eccentric portion in the orbit, a normal resetting quick phase eye movement occurs after each slow phase, resulting in nystagmus. Contraversive eye deviations, with eye movement recordings and EEG showing seizure-induced contralateral quick phases, are thought due to stimulation of the saccade-controlling regions of the temporo-occipital or frontal cortex. If gaze-holding is defective (e.g., the neural integration is "leaky"), then velocity-decreasing slow phases bring the eyes back to the midline after each quick phase, resulting in nystagmus.[157,171,172,174]

Epileptic nystagmus is rare and usually seen in patients with a history of epilepsy and in those with the nystagmus associated with altered levels of consciousness.[175] Epileptic PAN has been described after hypoxic encephalopathy.[168] Electroencephalography should be considered in patients with episodic nystagmus and oscillopsia, especially if other findings suggest a seizure disorder as a diagnostic possibility. Episodic vertigo with nystagmus may also be seen in vestibular migraine.[176]

Spontaneous jerk nystagmus that is purely torsional is a rare form of central vestibular nystagmus. Often it is difficult to detect except by observation of the conjunctival vessels or by noting the direction of retinal movements on either side of the fovea. Purely torsional nystagmus may be present in primary gaze or elicited by head positioning or gaze deviation.[177] Purely torsional nystagmus may be seen with brainstem and posterior fossa lesions, such as tumors, syringobulbia, syringomyelia with Arnold–Chiari malformation, lateral medullary syndrome, multiple sclerosis, trauma, vascular anomalies, postencephalitis, and sarcoidosis, and the stiff-person syndrome.[177,178]

Contralesional-beating torsional nystagmus may be due to a midbrain lesion involving the rostral interstitial nucleus of the MLF, whereas lesions of the interstitial nucleus of Cajal in the midbrain cause ipsilesional torsional nystagmus.[179] Torsional nystagmus occurring only during vertical pursuit has been described with cavernous angiomas of the middle cerebellar peduncle.[180] We recommend MRI for unexplained purely torsional nystagmus (class III–IV, level B). Nonrhythmic but continuous torsional eye movements have been reported as a paraneoplastic process.[181]

17.2.14 What Are the Causes of Predominantly Vertical Jerk Nystagmus?

Spontaneous jerk nystagmus in primary gaze that is predominantly vertical includes upbeat nystagmus and downbeat nystagmus.[182] Downbeat nystagmus is usually present in primary position, but is greatest when the patient looks down (Alexander's law) and laterally. On upward gaze, the nystagmus is less pronounced or disappears completely.

Downbeat nystagmus is often associated with horizontal gaze-evoked nystagmus. Convergence may increase, suppress, or convert the nystagmus to upbeat nystagmus. The nystagmus may be disjunctive, more vertical in one eye, and torsional in the other eye. There may be an INO (see Chapter 14). Downbeat nystagmus may occur with cervicomedullary junction disease, midline medullary lesions, posterior midline cerebellar lesions, or diffuse cerebellar disease.[182,183] Most lesions affect the vestibulocerebellum (flocculus, paraflocculus, nodulus, and uvula) and the underlying medulla. Deficient drive by the posterior semicircular canals, whose central projections cross in the floor of the fourth ventricle, or a faulty GABA inhibition of upward motion from the flocculus to the anterior semicircular canal have been postulated as explanations for downbeat nystagmus.

Interruption of downward VOR pathways, which synapse in the medial vestibular nucleus and cross in the medulla (beneath the NPH) to reach the contralateral MLF, would result in upward smooth eye drift and a downward corrective saccade.

Cerebellar, especially floccular and uvulonodular, lesions may cause this nystagmus by disinhibition of the cerebellar effect on the vestibular nuclei. The cerebellar flocculus contains Purkinje cells that send inhibitory projections to the anterior canal but not posterior canal central pathways; therefore, disinhibition would lead to downbeat nystagmus. Damage to the nuclei propositus hypoglossi and the medial vestibular nuclei (the neural integrator) in the medulla has also been suggested as the cause of the nystagmus. A patient with acute multiple sclerosis with a lesion of the caudal medulla (which contains Roller's nucleus and nucleus intercalatus) developed downbeat nystagmus upon horizontal head oscillations (perverted head-shaking nystagmus).[184]

After gaze-evoked nystagmus, downbeat nystagmus was the most frequent fixation nystagmus seen in a neurological dizziness unit and 62% of the cases were secondary to cerebellar degeneration, ischemia, bilateral vestibulopathy, polyneuropathy, or cerebellar ataxia, not necessarily coupled to abnormal MRI/CT findings.[123,185] This is in agreement with recent descriptions of cerebellar ataxia,[186,187] type 1 diabetes mellitus, downbeat nystagmus, stiff person syndrome, and palatal myoclonus.[12,188,189] Paraneoplastic syndromes have also been associated to downbeat nystagmus as the initial presenting symptom.[190,191] Box 17.4 lists additional reported etiologies of downbeat nystagmus.

Box 17.4 Etiologies of downbeat nystagmus

- Craniocervical anomalies, including cerebellar ectopia, Chiari malformation, platybasia, basilar invagination, and Paget disease.[73,192]
- Familial cerebellar degenerations including spinocerebellar ataxia 6.[193,194]
- Stiff person syndrome and cerebellar ataxia with anti-GAD antibodies.[164,195]
- Familial hemophagocytic lymphohistiocytosis.[196]
- Multiple system atrophy.[197]
- Posterior fossa tumors.[198]
- Increased intracranial pressure (e.g., due to supratentorial mass) and hydrocephalus.[198]
- Brainstem or cerebellar hypoperfusion, infarction, anoxia, or hemorrhage.[199,200,201]
- Dolichoectasia of the vertebrobasilar artery.[202,203,204,205]
- Rotational vertebral artery syndrome (RVAS) from hypoplastic right vertebral artery terminating in the posterior inferior cerebellar artery.[206,207,208]
- Intermittent vertebral artery compression by an osteophyte.[209]
- Encephalitis, including herpes simplex encephalitis and human T-cell leukemia virus 1 (HTLV-1) infection.[210]
- Heat stroke.[211]
- Cephalic tetanus.[212]
- Multiple sclerosis and other leukodystrophies.[184]
- Syringomyelia/syringobulbia.[213]
- Trauma.
- Alcohol, including alcohol-induced cerebellar degeneration.

- Wernicke encephalopathy.
- Thiamine deficiency:[214]
  - Alcoholics.
  - Nonalcoholics (vomiting, drastic weight reduction diet, colonic surgery, chronic hemodialysis).[215]
- Paraneoplastic cerebellar degeneration[216,217] (including adenocarcinoma with anti-Ma1 and anti-Ma2 antibodies,[190] small-cell lung cancer (SCLC) with anti-Hu and anti-CV2 antibodies[190] or anti-P/Q-type and N-type VGCC antibodies,[191] and testicular cancer with anti-Ta antibodies[69]).
- Nystagmus and ataxia due to antiganglioside antibodies.[162]
- Anti-AQP-4+ antibodies in neuromyelitis optica (NMO) with vertigo, ataxia, and upper extremity weakness.[218]
- Superficial siderosis of the CNS.[219]
- Congenital.
- MELAS (mitochondrial encephalopathy with lactic acid and stroke-like episodes).[220]
- Vitamin B_{12} deficiency.
- Magnesium deficiency.[221]
- Drugs, including lithium, toluene, intravenous or epidural narcotics, and anticonvulsants (e.g., phenytoin, carbamazepine, felbamate).[222,223,224]
- Transient finding in otherwise normal infants.
- Idiopathic.[199]

The evaluation of downbeat nystagmus depends on the clinical circumstances and associated neurologic findings. We recommend MRI in patients with unexplained downbeat nystagmus (class IV, level C).[203] MRI is normal or shows diffuse cerebellar atrophy in patients with familial cerebellar degenerations. In patients taking anticonvulsants or lithium, drug levels should be measured and adjusted as needed (class IV, level C). If MRI is normal, B_{12} and magnesium levels should be considered (class IV, level C). Thiamine therapy for selected cases should be considered and the possibility of alcohol or toluene abuse investigated (class IV, level C). If there are signs suggestive of CNS infection, a spinal tap may be warranted. In a patient with downbeat nystagmus with the acute or subacute onset of cerebellar signs and symptoms, a paraneoplastic process must be considered, especially due to SCLC, testicular cancer, gynecologic cancers (especially ovarian and breast cancer), and Hodgkin disease. The workup of these patients might include serum anti-Yo (anti-Purkinje cell) antibodies, serum anti-Hu antibodies (antineuronal nuclear antibodies type 1 or ANNA type 1), serum anti-Ta antibodies, chest X-ray and chest CT imaging, gynecologic examination, CT or MRI of the abdomen and pelvis, mammography, and possibly hematologic consultation for bone marrow biopsy (class IV, level C).

Finally, in a significant number of individuals, no etiology for the downbeat nystagmus will be discovered. Young and Huang reported the use of clonazepam (1.0 mg twice daily) in five idiopathic cases of downbeat nystagmus.[225]

Damage to the central projections of the anterior semicircular canals, which tend to deviate the eyes superiorly, has been suggested to explain upbeat nystagmus. Upbeat nystagmus is usually worse in upgaze (Alexander's law) and, unlike downbeat nystagmus, it usually does not increase on lateral gaze. Convergence may increase or decrease the nystagmus, or convert downbeat nystagmus to upbeat nystagmus.[226,227] Damage to the ventral tegmental pathways, which may link the superior vestibular nuclei to the superior rectus and inferior oblique subnuclei of the oculomotor nuclei, may cause the eyes to glide down, resulting in upbeat nystagmus.

Medullary disease may cause upbeat nystagmus as may lesions of the anterior cerebellar vermis, perihypoglossal and inferior olivary nuclei of the medulla, pontine tegmentum, brachium conjunctivum, midbrain, and brainstem diffusely.[182,228,229] Medullary lesions invariably involve the perihypoglossal nucleus and adjacent medial vestibular nucleus, nucleus intercalatus, and ventral tegmentum, which contain projections from vestibular nuclei that receive inputs from the anterior semicircular canals.

Primary position upbeat nystagmus may occur with unilateral medial medullary infarction, likely due to impairment of the vertical position-to-velocity neural integrator in the nucleus intercalatus of Staderini, a structure in the paramedian caudal medulla located caudal to the vestibular nuclei and to the most rostral of the perihypoglossal nuclei (NPH and nucleus of Roller).[230,231] Lesions of this structure may cause primary position upbeat nystagmus increased in downward gaze.[232] Bow-tie nystagmus, in which quick phases are directed obliquely upward with horizontal components alternating to the right and left, is probably a variant of upbeat nystagmus. Box 17.5 lists additional reported etiologies of upbeat nystagmus.

Box 17.5 Etiologies of upbeat nystagmus

- Arnold–Chiari malformation.
- Primary cerebellar degenerations and atrophies.[233,]
- Posterior fossa and central skull base tumors.[234]
- Brainstem or cerebellum infarction or hemorrhage.[200,229,230,235,236]
- Idiopathic intracranial hypertension.[237]
- Osmotic demyelination syndrome.[238]
- Multiple sclerosis.[226,232,235]
- Neuromyelitis optima (NMO).[218]
- Meningitis and brainstem encephalitis.
- Thalamic arteriovenous malformation.
- Wernicke encephalopathy.
- Behçet syndrome.
- Congenital, including cases associated with Leber congenital amaurosis and other congenital anterior visual pathway disorders.[43,129]
- Pelizaeus–Merzbacher disease.[127]
- Antiganglioside antibody syndromes.[162,239]
- Middle ear disease.
- Organophosphate and organoarsenic poisoning.[240]
- Tobacco-induced.
- Anticonvulsant intoxication.
- Cyclosporin A.[241]
- Paraneoplastic syndrome (e.g., testicular cancer with anti-Ta antibodies,[69] pancreatic cancer with anti-Hu antibodies,[227] anti-Ma2 encephalitis with pancreatitis[242]).
- Transient finding in otherwise healthy neonates.[243]

The evaluation of upbeat nystagmus includes a complete neurologic and ophthalmologic examination. MRI is warranted in most cases to investigate the presence of a structural lesion (class III–IV, level B). In children, MRI is indicated to investigate not only posterior fossa lesions but also lesions of the anterior visual pathways. If imaging is normal in children, then ERG should be considered (class IV, level C). Spinal tap is indicated in patients with signs or symptoms suggestive of meningeal irritation or CNS infection. In adults with negative neuroimaging studies, organophosphate or anticonvulsant intoxication should be investigated. Testicular cancer is a consideration in men (anti-Ta antibodies) (class IV, level C).[69]

The treatment of vertical nystagmus is directed at the etiology (e.g., surgical correction of Arnold–Chiari malformation). Clinical evidence suggests involvement of GABA-ergic pathways and cholinergic transmission in vertical VORs.[97] GABA agonists and cholinergic drugs have thus been tried to relieve the visual impairment with vertical nystagmus. Clonazepam, a GABA-A agonist, and baclofen, a GABA-B agonist, have been shown to reduce nystagmus velocity and oscillopsia in some patients with downbeat or upbeat nystagmus.[141,244] Gabapentin may occasionally induce a response[141,142] in acquired nystagmus in multiple sclerosis.

Intravenous physostigmine, an acetylcholinesterase inhibitor, worsened vertical nystagmus in five patients,[244] whereas intravenous scopolamine, an anticholinergic drug, reduced nystagmus and oscillopsia in two patients with downbeat nystagmus.[136] Anticholinergic drugs may thus be considered for patients with upbeat or downbeat nystagmus. Finally, downbeat nystagmus usually is present in primary position but is greatest when the patient looks down (Alexander's law) and subsides in upgaze. Patients may therefore benefit from symmetric base-down prisms that turn the eyes up.

17.2.15 What Are the Causes of Binocular Symmetric Jerk Nystagmus Present in Eccentric Gaze or Induced by Various Maneuvers?

Spontaneous binocular conjugate symmetric jerk nystagmus that is induced by eccentric gaze (gaze-evoked nystagmus) includes nystagmus due to brainstem/cerebellar disease, Bruns nystagmus, drug-induced nystagmus, physiologic nystagmus, rebound nystagmus, and convergence-induced nystagmus. Downbeat nystagmus and upbeat nystagmus may occur only on downward or upward gaze, respectively (see above).

With gaze-evoked nystagmus, the eyes fail to remain in an eccentric position of gaze but drift to midposition. The velocity of the slow component decreases exponentially as the eyes approach midposition. A "leaky" neural integrator or cerebellar (especially vestibulocerebellar) lesion may result in this type of nystagmus, which is more pronounced when the patient looks toward the lesion. Cerebellopontine angle tumors may cause Bruns nystagmus, a combination of ipsilateral large-amplitude, low-frequency nystagmus that is due to impaired gaze holding, and contralateral small-amplitude, high-frequency nystagmus that is due to vestibular impairment.[137] Gaze-evoked nystagmus may be a side effect of medications, including anticonvulsants, sedatives, and alcohol. Gaze-evoked nystagmus has been described with adult-onset Alexander's disease with involvement of the middle cerebellar peduncles and dentate nuclei[245] and is also a feature of familial episodic vertigo and ataxia type 2 that is responsive to acetazolamide.[246,247,248] Physiologic or endpoint nystagmus is a benign low-amplitude jerk nystagmus with the fast component directed toward the field of gaze. It usually ceases when the eyes are brought to a position somewhat less than the extremes of gaze.

Rebound nystagmus is seen in some patients with brainstem and/or cerebellar disease (e.g., olivocerebellar atrophy, brainstem/cerebellar tumor or infarction, Marinesco–Sjögren syndrome, Dandy–Walker cyst, Gerstmann–Straussler–Scheinker disease, adult-onset Alexander disease, etc.).[245,249,250] The original gaze-evoked nystagmus may wane and actually reverse direction so that the slow component is directed centrifugally (centripetal nystagmus). Rebound nystagmus probably reflects an attempt by brainstem or cerebellar mechanisms to correct for the centripetal drift of gaze-evoked nystagmus.[24]

Patients with gaze-evoked nystagmus who are taking anticonvulsant or sedative medications and those with physiologic nystagmus require no further evaluation. Otherwise, patients with gaze-evoked or rebound nystagmus, especially if associated symptoms or signs of brainstem or cerebellar dysfunction or auditory impairment exist, require MRI, with special attention to the cerebellum and cerebello-pontine angle (class IV, level C).[249]

Convergence may change nystagmus by converting downbeat to upbeat, upbeat to downbeat, or pendular to upbeat. Convergence-evoked nystagmus is usually vertical (upbeat is more common than downbeat) and seen most commonly with multiple sclerosis or brainstem infarction.[251] MRI is thus warranted in patients with convergence-induced nystagmus (class IV, level C). Convergence may also increase or decrease the amplitude of nystagmus and may evoke horizontal (congenital or acquired pendular and jerk) or vertical (upbeat or downbeat) nystagmus. Convergence-induced pendular nystagmus has been described as a congenital phenomenon (conjugate) and as an acquired phenomenon (disjunctive) with multiple sclerosis.[118,251] Base-in prisms have been used to alleviate the symptoms of oscillopsia and improve reading acuity in patients with acquired convergence-evoked pendular nystagmus due to multiple sclerosis.[118] The effects of convergence on nystagmus are not to be confused with convergence nystagmus in which a slow abduction of the eyes is followed by quick adduction (see above).

Binocular symmetric conjugate jerk nystagmus that is induced includes optokinetic nystagmus, rotational/caloric vestibular nystagmus, positional nystagmus, Valsalva-induced nystagmus, and hyperventilation-induced nystagmus.[49,137] The first two types of induced nystagmus are physiologic and, although abnormalities of these responses may aid in clinical diagnosis, they are not further discussed here.

Positional vertigo of the benign paroxysmal type, also known as benign paroxysmal positioning vertigo or positional nystagmus, is usually idiopathic and possibly related to degeneration of the macula of the otolith organ or to lesions of the posterior semicircular canal.[252,253,254,255,256,257] It has been proposed that otoconia detached from the otoconial layer (by degeneration or trauma) gravitate and settle on the cupula of the posterior canal causing it to become heavier than the surrounding endolymph and thus sensitive to changes in the direction of gravity (with positional change). After rapid head tilt toward the affected ear or following head extension, when the posterior semicircular

canal is moved in the specific plane of stimulation, an ampullifugal deflection of the cupula occurs, with a rotational vertigo and concomitant nystagmus. Some patients show a strong horizontal nystagmus induced by lateral head positioning suggesting lateral (rather than posterior) semicircular canal irritation (lateral canal or horizontal canal variant of benign paroxysmal positional vertigo).[258,259] Other causes of positional vertigo include trauma, infection, labyrinthine fistula, amiodarone, ischemia, demyelinating disease, Arnold–Chiari malformation, and, rarely, posterior fossa tumors or vascular malformations.[256,260,261]

Besides paroxysmal positional nystagmus, patients often also exhibit static (persistent) positional nystagmus while lying in a lateral position. This static nystagmus is predominantly horizontal with minimal vertical component. Paroxysmal vertigo induced by certain head positions is the most common complaint; the patient is asymptomatic between bouts. The Nylen–Barany or Dix–Hallpike maneuver (briskly tilting the patient's head backward and turning it 45° to one side) allows differentiating a peripheral from a central origin for positional vertigo.

With peripheral lesions, severe rotational vertigo associated with nausea (occasionally vomiting) and nystagmus appear several seconds (2–15 seconds) after the head position is changed. In benign paroxysmal positional (positioning) vertigo, it is unusual for the vertigo to have a duration of more than 1 minute. Cochlear or neurologic symptoms are typically absent. The nystagmus is usually torsional, with the upper pole of the eye beating toward the ground. The vertigo and nystagmus then fatigue and abate within 10 seconds after appearance, and when the patient is rapidly brought back to a sitting position, vertigo recurs and nystagmus develops in the opposite direction (rebound). With repetition of the maneuver, the symptoms and nystagmus become progressively less severe (habituation), and the reproducibility of the abnormalities is inconstant. Mild transient nystagmus in one head position may occasionally be elicited in normal subjects. Patients with benign paroxysmal positional vertigo are often treated successfully with canalith repositioning procedures.[257]

A central lesion should be suspected when (1) the maneuver is positive with the head turned to either side; (2) the nystagmus is direction changing rather than fixed, appearing immediately after the shift in position and remaining for as long as the head is down; (3) the nystagmus is unaccompanied by nausea or a sense of discomfort; if present, vertigo is mild and lasts no longer than 60 seconds; and (4) repetition does not cause blunting of the effects. Typically, there are other associated CNS findings. Patients with the central form of positional nystagmus require MRI to investigate structural posterior fossa lesions (class III–IV, level B). Occasionally, patients with benign paroxysmal positional vertigo will demonstrate findings during the Nylen–Barany maneuver similar to those documented in patients with central lesions.[252]

Nystagmus induced by the Valsalva maneuver may occur with Chiari malformation or perilymph fistulas.[137] Hyperventilation may induce nystagmus in patients with tumors of the eighth cranial nerve (e.g., acoustic neuroma or epidermoid tumors), after vestibular neuritis, or with central demyelinating lesions.[137,262] Hyperventilation-induced nystagmus has the slow phase away from the side of the lesion (an excitatory or recovery nystagmus) and is likely due to the effect of hyperventilation upon serum pH

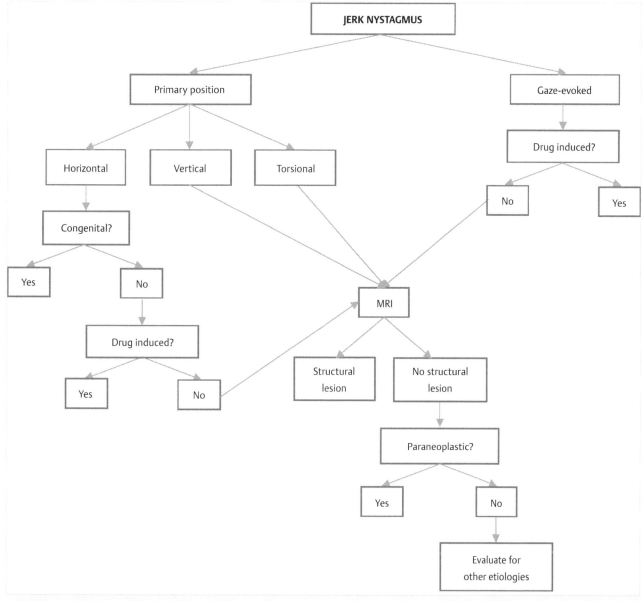

Fig. 17.7 Evaluation of jerk nystagmus.

and calcium concentration, which improves nerve conduction in a marginally functional, demyelinated nerve.[137,262]

The evaluation of patients with jerk nystagmus is outlined in ▶ Fig. 17.7. Medical treatment options for nystagmus are summarized in ▶ Table 17.3.

17.2.16 What Are the Characteristics of Saccadic Intrusions?

Inappropriate saccades, or saccadic intrusions, interfere with macular fixation of an object of interest. The essential difference between nystagmus and saccadic intrusions lies in the initial eye movement that takes the line of sight away from the object of regard.[24] For nystagmus, it is a slow drift or slow phase as opposed to an inappropriate saccadic movement that intrudes on steady fixation. There are several types of saccadic intrusions.

Square-wave jerks take the eyes off the target and are followed after about 200 ms by a corrective saccade.[267] They may appear normally in the young and the elderly, but when larger than 1° or 2° they are pathologic, resulting from disorders including a variety of cerebral or cerebellar lesions, progressive supranuclear palsy, Huntington chorea, Parkinson disease, Wernicke–Korsakoff syndrome, Friedreich ataxia, AIDS dementia complex, Gerstmann–Straussler–Scheinker disease, adult-onset Alexander disease, carbohydrate-deficient glycoprotein syndrome type 1a, schizophrenia, and MELAS.[220,245,250,268,269,270] They may also occur with lithium or tobacco use. An increased frequency of square wave jerks may be noted after unilateral pallidotomy for Parkinson disease.[271] Very frequent square-wave jerks (square wave oscillations) may be mistaken for nystagmus and may occur with cerebellar disease, progressive supranuclear palsy, and cerebral hemispheral disease.[137,268]

Table 17.3 Medical therapy to dampen nystagmus[123,263]

Treatment option	Suggested for nystagmus types
4-aminopyridine, 3,4-diaminopyridine (increase Purkinje cell excitability and inhibition on CN VIII nuclei[264] and their pacemaking[265])	Downbeat nystagmus,[266] upbeat nystagmus
Gabapentin	Gaze-evoked nystagmus, acquired pendular nystagmus, periodic alternating nystagmus (PAN), infantile nystagmus, superior oblique myokymia, oculopalatal tremor
Baclofen (reduced the excitability of premotor vestibular neurons)	Central vestibular nystagmus, acquired pendular nystagmus, periodic alternating nystagmus (PAN), upbeat nystagmus, downbeat nystagmus
Benzodiazepines (e.g., clonazepam, diazepam, lorazepam)	All acute/current nystagmus types
Memantine (decreases the output of Purkinje cells)	Acquired pendular nystagmus (especially multiple sclerosis-related), severe or persistent upbeat nystagmus, infantile nystagmus
Scopolamine	Downbeat nystagmus, disequilibrium symptoms
Carbamazepine	Superior oblique myokymia, oculopalatal tremor
Botulinum toxin injections	Acquired pendular nystagmus, infantile nystagmus, oculopalatal tremor

Macrosquare-wave jerks are similar to square-wave jerks but are of larger amplitude (20–40 degrees). They are occasionally present in the vertical plane and have been noted in multiple sclerosis, cerebellar hemorrhage, olivopontocerebellar atrophy, multiple systems atrophy, and Arnold–Chiari malformation.[137]

Macrosaccadic oscillations are different from square-wave jerks and consist of eye oscillations around the fixation angle with intersaccadic intervals approximately 200 ms.[137] They are usually conjugate, horizontal, and symmetric in both directions of gaze, but may occur in torsional or vertical planes. Macrosaccadic oscillations occur in patients with cerebellar disease, especially affecting the cerebellar midline and underlying nuclei (e.g., cerebellar hemorrhage or spinocerebellar degenerations). Macrosaccadic oscillations after pontine trauma may have been due to dysfunction of pontine omnipause neurons, and thus disinhibition of saccadic burst neurons.[272] Macrosaccadic oscillations may be induced by edrophonium in patients with profound ophthalmoplegia from myasthenia gravis.[273]

Square-wave jerks, square-wave oscillations, macrosquare-wave jerks, and macrosaccadic oscillations usually occur in the context of otherwise evident neurologic diseases. If the nature of the causal degenerative process accounting for these intrusions is not evident on clinical history and neurologic exam, MRI may be needed (class IV, level C). Macrosaccadic oscillations and high-amplitude square-wave jerks may be treated with GABA-A agonists, benzodiazepines, and barbiturates. Square-wave jerks and square-wave oscillations may improve with valproic acid (2,000 mg/day), which may restore GABA-ergic tonic

inhibitory action from the substantia nigra pars reticulata to the superior colliculus.[274]

Occasionally, otherwise normal individuals show intermittent, 15- to 30-Hz frequency, low-amplitude (0.1–0.5 degrees) horizontal oscillations (not detected on visual inspection but seen with the ophthalmoscope) termed *microsaccadic flutter*.[275] Patients with microsaccadic flutter often complain of "shimmering," "jiggling," "wavy," or "laser beams" with paroxysms of visual disturbances lasting seconds to hours. Dizziness or dysequilibrium often accompanies the visual symptoms. Most patients are otherwise normal,[276] although one patient had multiple sclerosis. Clonazepam, propranolol, and verapamil may reduce visual symptoms in some patients.[275]

Ocular flutter is a burst of to-and-fro horizontal saccades without an intersaccadic interval. Opsoclonus (saccadomania) is similar to ocular flutter, except that in opsoclonus there are conjugate, involuntary, large amplitude saccades in all directions. Like ocular flutter, opsoclonus indicates brainstem, especially mesencephalic or pontine, or cerebellar disease.[277] Opsoclonus evident only during eye closure has been described with hereditary cerebellar ataxia.[277] Etiologies for ocular flutter and opsoclonus are listed in Box 17.6.

Box 17.6 Etiologies for ocular flutter and opsoclonus

- Viral encephalitis (e.g., West Nile virus, Coxsackie B3, Epstein-Barr virus, enterovirus, varicella-zoster virus, human immunodeficiency virus/acquired immune deficiency syndrome,[270,278,279] hepatitis A), meningitis (H. influenza, streptococcal), neuroborreliosis (Lyme disease),[280,281,282] and other infections.[283,284,285,286,287,288,289,290]
- GABA-b receptor and NR1 N-methyl-D-aspartate receptor autoantibody encephalitis.[291,292,293]
- Kinsbourne myoclonic encephalopathy or infantile polymyoclonia ("dancing eyes and dancing feet" syndrome).
- Neuroblastoma.[294,295]
- Paraneoplastic effect of other tumors, including SCLC, breast cancer, renal adenocarcinoma, papillary renal cell carcinoma, pancreatic carcinoma, malignant fibrous histiocytoma, and non-Hodgkin lymphoma.[288,296,297,298,299,300,301,302,303,304,305]
- Intracranial tumors or cysts.[299]
- Trauma.
- Hydrocephalus and intracranial hypertension secondary to cerebral venous thrombosis.[306]
- Hereditary cerebellar degeneration.[277]
- Autoimmune disorders (e.g., adult-onset cerebellar ataxia with CSF anti-GAD65 antibodies,[307] opsoclonus with anti-ganglionic acetylcholine receptor antibodies,[308] and opsoclonus with antimitochondrial antibodies[309]).
  - NMO and systemic lupus erythematosus (SLE) with hypothalamic, pontine, cerebellar peduncles, and medullary lesions.[218]
  - Sjögren syndrome.[312]
  - Sarcoidosis.
- Posterior reversible encephalopathy syndrome (PRES) with bilateral dentate nuclei lesions on T2 FLAIR.[310]
- Thalamic, pontine, or cerebellar hemorrhage.
- Vertebrobasilar vascular insufficiency.
- Multiple sclerosis.[311]

- Hyperosmolar stupor and coma.
- Side effects of drugs, including diphenhydramine,[313,314] cyclosporin A,[315,316] lithium, amitriptyline, cocaine, phenytoin and diazepam, phenelzine, and imipramine.[317]
- Toxic exposures, including thallium, toluene, chlordecone, strychnine, dichlorodiphenyltrichloroethane (DDT), and organophosphates.
- Acute polyradiculoneuritis.
- Cherry-red spot myoclonus syndrome.
- Carbohydrate-deficient glycoprotein syndrome type 1a.
- In neonates, as either a transient benign phenomenon or related to brain injury due to anoxia, intracranial hemorrhage, or Leber congenital amaurosis.
- Idiopathic.[297]

In patients with viral encephalitis, meningitis, and other infections, the opsoclonus may occur after a prodromal illness, including gastrointestinal tract symptoms, upper respiratory symptoms, malaise, and fever.[284,285,287] The opsoclonus in these patients is often associated with truncal ataxia and other cerebellar signs, long tract signs, tremulousness, and myoclonus of the trunk and limbs. Spinal fluid studies often show increased protein and a mononuclear pleocytosis. The illness usually resolves in a few weeks or months, although the course may be protracted and recovery incomplete, especially in children (Kinsbourne's myoclonic encephalopathy or dancing eyes and dancing feet or infantile polymyoclonia).

Opsoclonus occurs in 2% of children with neuroblastoma, and conversely 50% of children with opsoclonus/myoclonus have neuroblastoma.[294,295] Opsoclonus appears before the discovery of a neuroblastoma in over 50% of the cases, and neuroblastomas associated with opsoclonus have a tendency to be located within the thorax. Opsoclonus may also develop as a paraneoplastic effect of other tumors, especially SCLC and breast cancer.[296,297,298,299,301,302,303,304,305,318] Approximately 20% of patients with opsoclonus-myoclonus in adults have an underlying tumor.

In patients with SCLC, opsoclonus usually antedates the diagnosis of the neoplasm, whereas in patients with breast cancer, opsoclonus develops before the diagnosis of the tumor in only half the patients. Although opsoclonus in these patients may occur as an isolated sign, it is more often associated with myoclonus, ataxia, and encephalopathy. The cerebrospinal fluid may show an elevated protein and a mild pleocytosis. Patients with breast cancer or SCLC and opsoclonus/myoclonus may have serum anti-Ri antibodies (antineuronal nuclear antibody 2 [ANNA-2]).[303]

Bataller et al analyzed a series of 24 adult patients with idiopathic (10 cases) and paraneoplastic (14 cases) opsoclonus-myoclonus syndrome (OMS) to ascertain possible differences in clinical course and response to immunotherapies between both groups.[297] Associated tumors were SCLC (nine patients), non-SCLC (one patient), breast carcinoma (two patients), gastric adenocarcinoma (one patient), and kidney carcinoma (one patient). Patients with paraneoplastic OMS were older (median age: 66 years versus 40 years of those with idiopathic OMS) and had a higher frequency of encephalopathy (64% versus 10%).

Serum from 10 out of 10 idiopathic and 12 out of 14 paraneoplastic OMS patients showed no specific immunoreactivity on rat or human brainstem or cerebellum, lacked specific antineuronal antibodies (Hu, Yo, Ri, Tr, GAD, amphiphysin, or CV2), and did not contain antibodies to voltage-gated calcium channels. The two paraneoplastic exceptions were a patient with SCLC, whose serum contained both anti-Hu and antiamphiphysin antibodies, and a patient with breast cancer who had serum anti-Ri antibodies.

The clinical course of idiopathic OMS was monophasic except in two elderly women who had relapses of the opsoclonus and mild residual ataxia. Most idiopathic OMS patients made a good recovery, but residual gait ataxia tended to persist in older patients. Immunotherapy (mainly intravenous immunoglobulins or corticosteroids) seemed to accelerate recovery. Paraneoplastic OMS had a more severe clinical course, despite treatment with intravenous immunoglobulins or corticosteroids, and was the cause of death in five patients whose tumors were not treated. By contrast, the eight patients whose tumors were treated showed a complete or partial neurologic recovery. The authors concluded that idiopathic OMS occurs in younger patients, the clinical evolution is more benign, and the effect of immunotherapy appears more effective than in paraneoplastic OMS. In patients aged 50 years and older with OMS who develop encephalopathy, early diagnosis and treatment of a probable underlying tumor, usually SCLC, is indicated to increase the chances of neurologic recovery.

The evaluation of ocular flutter and opsoclonus depends on the age of the patient and the clinical circumstances. In children or adults with prodromal symptoms and signs of systemic or CNS infection, neuroimaging (preferably MRI) followed by spinal tap are warranted (class IV, level C). In children without apparent infection, a search for occult neuroblastoma is indicated, with studies variably including chest X-ray, CT, or MRI of chest and abdomen, skeletal survey, intravenous pyelogram, bone marrow biopsy, and determination of urinary catecholamines (class III–IV, level C). In adults, without signs of infection, an occult malignancy should be sought with workup including gynecologic examination; chest X-ray; CT or MRI of the chest, abdomen, and pelvis; mammogram; possible bone marrow biopsy; and serum anti-Ri antibody (ANNA-2), anti-Hu antibody, and antiamphiphysin antibody studies (class III–IV, level C). MRI of the brain is warranted for most patients (class III–IV, level B). A history of drug or toxic exposures should be sought in all patients. In some circumstances, other blood studies to be considered include serum osmolality, HIV titers, and angiotensin-converting enzyme (ACE) levels for sarcoidosis (class IV, level C).

The treatment of ocular flutter and opsoclonus is initially directed at the underlying etiology (e.g., underlying neoplasm) as some patients improve with tumor removal.[318] Symptomatic reduction of the eye movements has been reported with adrenocorticotropic hormone (ACTH), corticosteroids, clonazepam, baclofen, propranolol, thiamine, reserpine, and valproic acid.[137] High-dose intravenous immunoglobulin has been successful in several cases.[294,319]

The evaluation of opsoclonus is outlined in ▶ Fig. 17.8.

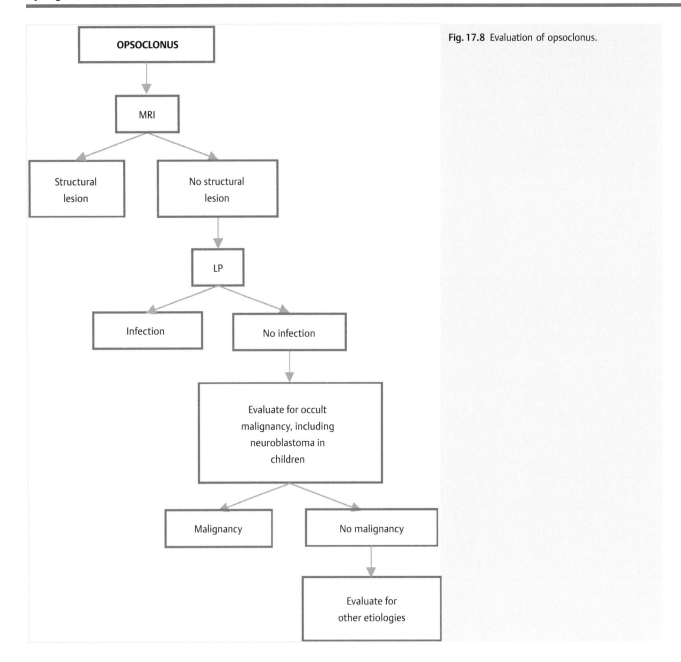

Fig. 17.8 Evaluation of opsoclonus.

17.2.17 What Are the Characteristics of Spontaneous Eye Oscillations in Stuporous and Comatose Patients?

In comatose patients, if the brainstem is intact, the eyelids are closed, and the eyes, slightly divergent, drift slowly from side to side (roving eye movements). The roving eye movements of light coma cannot be voluntarily executed and are therefore incompatible with the diagnosis of feigned unresponsiveness. As coma deepens, roving eye movements disappear.

Other spontaneous eye movements seen in comatose patients include the following (▶ Table 17.4):

1. Short-cycle periodic alternating gaze ("ping-pong gaze"), which consists of roving of the eyes from one extreme of horizontal gaze to the other and back with each oscillating cycle taking 2.5 to 8 seconds.[320] This finding usually indicates bilateral cerebral damage (e.g., bilateral cerebral infarcts) with an intact brainstem, but has also been described with posterior fossa hemorrhage, basal ganglia infarcts, bilateral cerebral peduncle lesions, hydrocephalus, hepatic encephalopathy, diffuse cerebral hypoxia, carbon monoxide intoxication, and overdose of the monoamine oxidase inhibitor trancypromine.[320,321,322] The disorder may occasionally occur in coma with no structural hemispheric lesion. Saccadic (versus smooth waveform) ping-pong gaze may indicate less extensive brain damage.[322]

2. Ping-pong gaze must be differentiated from periodic alternating gaze deviation, which is an alternating horizontal conjugate gaze deviation lasting 1 to 2 minutes in each direction. Periodic alternating gaze deviation usually

Table 17.4 Spontaneous eye movements in comatose patients

Movement	Description	Localization
Periodic alternating gaze (ping-pong gaze)	Cyclic horizontal roving	Bilateral cerebral damage, rarely posterior fossa lesion, hepatic, hypoxic, carbon monoxide, drug intoxication
Repetitive divergence	Slow deviation out, rapid return to primary	Metabolic encephalopathy
Monocular nystagmoid	Vertical, horizontal, or rotatory movements	Middle or low pontine lesion
Status epilepticus	Small-amplitude vertical (occasionally horizontal) movements	Diffuse encephalopathy (hypoxic)
Ocular bobbing	Fast down, slow up	Pontine lesion, extra-axial posterior fossa mass, diffuse encephalopathy
Inverse ocular bobbing (ocular dipping)	Slow down, fast up	Anoxia, post-status epilepticus (diffuse encephalopathy)
Reverse ocular bobbing	Fast up, slow down	Diffuse encephalopathy, rarely pontine
Slow-upward ocular	Slow up, fast down	Diffuse encephalopathy bobbing
Pretectal pseudobobbing	"V-pattern"; down and in	Pretectal (hydrocephalus)
Vertical ocular myoclonus	Pendular, vertical isolated	Pontine

occurs in alert patients with structural lesions involving the cerebellum and brainstem, such as the Arnold–Chiari malformation or medulloblastoma, but has been described in obtunded or comatose patients with hepatic encephalopathy.[165] Creutzfeldt–Jakob disease may be associated with geotropic ocular deviation with skew deviation and absence of saccades.[159] When the head is turned to one side, the eyes very slowly deviate to that side, while the abducting eye moves upward and the adducting eye moves downward. These spontaneous ocular movements are slow with no saccadic component.

3. Repetitive divergence is rarely seen in patients with coma from metabolic encephalopathy (e.g., hepatic encephalopathy).[80] With this disorder, the eyes are midposition or slightly divergent at rest. They then slowly deviate out, become fully deviated for a brief period, and then rapidly return to primary position before repeating the cycle. These motions are synchronous in the two eyes.

4. Nystagmoid jerking of a single eye, in a vertical, horizontal, or rotatory fashion, may occur with mid- to lower pontine damage. Pontine lesions occasionally give rise to disconjugate rotatory and vertical movements of the eyes, in which one eye may rise and intort as the other falls and extorts. This type of movement should not be confused with seesaw nystagmus, which is very seldom seen in comatose patients.

5. Electrographic status epilepticus without appendicular motor manifestations, due to anoxia, may result in brisk, small-amplitude, mainly vertical (occasionally horizontal) eye movements detectable by passive lid elevation.[323]

6. Ocular bobbing refers to intermittent, often conjugate, brisk, bilateral downward movement of the eyes with slow return to midposition. Ocular bobbing has been associated with intrinsic pontine lesions (e.g., hemorrhage, tumor, infarction, central pontine myelinolysis, etc.), extra-axial posterior fossa masses (e.g., aneurysm rupture or cerebellar hemorrhage or infarction), diffuse encephalitis, Creutzfeldt–Jakob disease, and toxic-metabolic encephalopathies (e.g., acute organophosphate poisoning). "Typical" ocular bobbing, which is associated with preserved horizontal eye movements, is thought to be specific but not pathognomonic of acute pontine injury, whereas "atypical"

ocular bobbing, which is associated with absent horizontal eye movements, is thought to be less helpful in predicting the site of abnormality. Monocular bobbing (paretic bobbing), which consists of a quick downward movement of one eye and intorsion or no movement in the other eye, may occur if there is a coexistent unilateral fascicular oculomotor nerve palsy.[324] Disconjugate ocular bobbing, with movements involving sometimes one eye and sometimes the other, may also occur without oculomotor nerve palsy.[325]

7. Inverse ocular bobbing (ocular dipping or fast-upward ocular bobbing) consists of a slow-downward eye movement with fast return to midposition, which may occur in anoxic coma or after prolonged status epilepticus. Ocular dipping has also been described associated with deafness in a patient with pinealoblastoma[326] and with anti-NMDA receptor encephalitis.[327] Inverse/reverse ocular bobbing consists of inverse ocular bobbing in which the eyes do not stop on rapidly returning to primary position but shoot into upgaze and slowly return to midposition.

8. Reverse ocular bobbing (fast-upward ocular bobbing) consists of fast-upward eye movement with a slow return to midposition, which may occur in patients with metabolic encephalopathy, viral encephalitis, or pontine hemorrhage. It has been described with coma due to combined phenothiazine and benzodiazepine poisoning.[328] Occasionally, ocular bobbing, ocular dipping, and reverse bobbing may occur at different times in the same patient.

9. Slow-upward ocular bobbing (converse ocular bobbing or reverse ocular dipping) is characterized by slow-upward eye movements followed by a fast return to midposition. This eye movement disorder has been described with pontine infarction and with metabolic or viral encephalopathy (i.e., diffuse cerebral dysfunction).

10. Pretectal pseudobobbing has been described with acute hydrocephalus[329] and consists of arrhythmic, repetitive downward and inward ("V-pattern") eye movements at a rate ranging from one per 3 seconds to two per second and an amplitude of one-fifth to one-half of the full voluntary range. These movements may be mistaken for ocular bobbing, but their V pattern, their faster rate, and their

pretectal rather than pontine-associated signs distinguish them from true pontine bobbing. Thus, patients with pretectal pseudobobbing may have abnormal pupillary light reactions, intact horizontal eye movements, open and often retracted eyelids, a blink frequently preceding each eye movement, and a mute or stuporous rather than a comatose state. Pretectal pseudobobbing probably represents a variety of convergence nystagmus, and its presence usually indicates the need for prompt surgical attention (e.g., hydrocephalus decompression).[329] Pretectal pseudobobbing has also been described with an expanding posterior fossa cyst.[330] It is possible that some cases of "ocular bobbing" associated with thalamic hemorrhage or tentorial herniation may actually be cases of pretectal pseudobobbing.

11. Vertical ocular myoclonus consists of pendular, vertical isolated movements of the eyes noted in patients either locked-in or comatose after severe pontine strokes.[331] Their frequency is 2 Hz, and other rhythmic body movements at a similar frequency occur after a 6-week to 9-month delay. These movements are generally associated with palatal myoclonus (palatal tremor), with which they share a common mechanism.[331]

References

[1] Coppola D, Purves D. The extraordinarily rapid disappearance of entoptic images. Proc Natl Acad Sci U S A. 1996; 93(15):8001–8004

[2] Purves D, Augustine GJ, Fitzpatrick D, et al. Chapter 14. The Vestibular System. Neuroscience. 4th ed. Sunderland, MA: Sinauer Associates; 2008

[3] Ehrt O. Infantile and acquired nystagmus in childhood. Eur J Paediatr Neurol. 2012; 16(6):567–572

[4] Kim SM, Kim JS, Heo YE, Yang HR, Park KS. Cortical oscillopsia without nystagmus, an isolated symptom of neuromyelitis optica spectrum disorder with anti-aquaporin 4 antibody. Mult Scler. 2012; 18(2):244–247

[5] Krauzlis RJ. The control of voluntary eye movements: new perspectives. Neuroscientist. 2005; 11(2):124–137

[6] Fasold O, von Brevern M, Kuhberg M, et al. Human vestibular cortex as identified with caloric stimulation in functional magnetic resonance imaging. Neuroimage. 2002; 17(3):1384–1393

[7] Brandt T, Glasauer S, Stephan T, et al. Visual-vestibular and visuovisual cortical interaction: new insights from fMRI and pet. Ann N Y Acad Sci. 2002; 956:230–241

[8] Bronstein AM, Patel M, Arshad Q. A brief review of the clinical anatomy of the vestibular-ocular connections-how much do we know? Eye (Lond). 2015; 29(2):163–170

[9] Kömpf D, Pasik T, Pasik P, Bender MB. Downward gaze in monkeys: stimulation and lesion studies. Brain. 1979; 102(3):527–558

[10] Bender MB. Brain control of conjugate horizontal and vertical eye movements: a survey of the structural and functional correlates. Brain. 1980; 103(1):23–69

[11] Gamlin PD. The pretectum: connections and oculomotor-related roles. Prog Brain Res. 2006; 151:379–405

[12] Antonini G, Nemni R, Giubilei F, et al. Autoantibodies to glutamic acid decarboxylase in downbeat nystagmus. J Neurol Neurosurg Psychiatry. 2003; 74(7):998–999

[13] Sparks DL, Mays LE. Signal transformations required for the generation of saccadic eye movements. Annu Rev Neurosci. 1990; 13:309–336

[14] Wang L, Liu M, Segraves MA, Cang J. Visual experience is required for the development of eye movement maps in the mouse superior colliculus. J Neurosci. 2015; 35(35):12281–12286

[15] Godaux E, Cheron G. The hypothesis of the uniqueness of the oculomotor neural integrator: direct experimental evidence in the cat. J Physiol. 1996; 492(Pt 2):517–527

[16] Donahue SP, Lavin PJ, Hamed LM. Tonic ocular tilt reaction simulating a superior oblique palsy: diagnostic confusion with the 3-step test. Arch Ophthalmol. 1999; 117(3):347–352

[17] Harrison JJ, Sumner P, Dunn MJ, Erichsen JT, Freeman TC. Quick phases of infantile nystagmus show the saccadic inhibition effect. Invest Ophthalmol Vis Sci. 2015; 56(3):1594–1600

[18] Perez Y, Gradstein L, Flusser H, et al. Isolated foveal hypoplasia with secondary nystagmus and low vision is associated with a homozygous SLC38A8 mutation. Eur J Hum Genet. 2014; 22(5):703–706

[19] Camand O, Boutboul S, Arbogast L, et al. Mutational analysis of the OA1 gene in ocular albinism. Ophthalmic Genet. 2003; 24(3):167–173

[20] Gargiulo A, Testa F, Rossi S, et al. Molecular and clinical characterization of albinism in a large cohort of Italian patients. Invest Ophthalmol Vis Sci. 2011; 52(3):1281–1289

[21] Dansault A, David G, Schwartz C, et al. Three new PAX6 mutations including one causing an unusual ophthalmic phenotype associated with neurodevelopmental abnormalities. Mol Vis. 2007; 13:511–523

[22] Jalkanen R, Bech-Hansen NT, Tobias R, et al. A novel CACNA1F gene mutation causes Aland Island eye disease. Invest Ophthalmol Vis Sci. 2007; 48(6): 2498–2502

[23] Dell'Osso LF, Weissman BM, Leigh RJ, Abel LA, Sheth NV. Hereditary congenital nystagmus and gaze-holding failure: the role of the neural integrator. Neurology. 1993; 43(9):1741–1749

[24] Leigh RJ, Zee DS. The Neurology of Eye Movements. 3rd ed. New York: Oxford University Press; 1999

[25] Campbell WW. The ocular motor nerves. In: DeJong's The Neurologic Examination. 7th ed. Philadelphia, PA: Lippincott Williams & Wilkins; 2013:179–226

[26] Avallone J, Bedell HE, Birch EE, et al. A Classification of Eye Movement Abnormalities and Strabismus (CEMAS). National Institutes of Health: Bethesda, MD. Retrieved from: https://nei.nih.gov/sites/default/files/nei-pdfs/cemas.pdf. Accessed February 24, 2018. Document based on February 9 and 10, 2001 symposium.

[27] Adeyemo B, Angelaki DE. Similar kinematic properties for ocular following and smooth pursuit eye movements. J Neurophysiol. 2005; 93(3):1710–1717

[28] Bertolini G, Tarnutzer AA, Olasagasti I, et al. Gaze holding in healthy subjects. PLoS One. 2013; 8(4):e61389

[29] Citek K, Elmont AD, Jons CL, et al. Sleep deprivation does not mimic alcohol intoxication on field sobriety testing. J Forensic Sci. 2011; 56(5): 1170–1179

[30] Dell'Osso LF. Biologically relevant models of infantile nystagmus syndrome: the requirement for behavioral ocular motor system models. Semin Ophthalmol. 2006; 21(2):71–77

[31] Kattah JC, Talkad AV, Wang DZ, Hsieh YH, Newman-Toker DE. HINTS to diagnose stroke in the acute vestibular syndrome: three-step bedside oculomotor examination more sensitive than early MRI diffusion-weighted imaging. Stroke. 2009; 40(11):3504–3510

[32] Gottlob I, Wizov SS, Reinecke RD. Spasmus nutans. A long-term follow-up. Invest Ophthalmol Vis Sci. 1995; 36(13):2768–2771

[33] Young TL, Weis JR, Summers CG, Egbert JE. The association of strabismus, amblyopia, and refractive errors in spasmus nutans. Ophthalmology. 1997; 104(1):112–117

[34] Massry GG, Bloom JN, Cruz OA. Convergence nystagmus associated with spasmus nutans. J Neuroophthalmol. 1996; 16(3):196–198

[35] Arnoldi KA, Tychsen L. Prevalence of intracranial lesions in children initially diagnosed with disconjugate nystagmus (spasmus nutans). J Pediatr Ophthalmol Strabismus. 1995; 32(5):296–301

[36] Gottlob I, Zubcov A, Catalano RA, et al. Signs distinguishing spasmus nutans (with and without central nervous system lesions) from infantile nystagmus. Ophthalmology. 1990; 97(9):1166–1175

[37] Newman SA, Hedges TR, Wall M, Sedwick LA. Spasmus nutans-or is it? Surv Ophthalmol. 1990; 34(6):453–456

[38] Gottlob I, Wizov SS, Reinecke RD. Quantitative eye and head movement recordings of retinal disease mimicking spasmus nutans. Am J Ophthalmol. 1995; 119(3):374–376

[39] Lambert SR, Newman NJ. Retinal disease masquerading as spasmus nutans. Neurology. 1993; 43(8):1607–1609

[40] Smith DE, Fitzgerald K, Stass-Isern M, Cibis GW. Electroretinography is necessary for spasmus nutans diagnosis. Pediatr Neurol. 2000; 23(1): 33–36

[41] Gottlob I, Helbling A. Nystagmus mimicking spasmus nutans as the presenting sign of Bardet-Biedl syndrome. Am J Ophthalmol. 1999; 128(6): 770–772

[42] Davey K, Kowal L, Friling R, Georgievski Z, Sandbach J. The Heimann-Bielschowsky phenomenon: dissociated vertical nystagmus. Aust N Z J Ophthalmol. 1998; 26(3):237–240

[43] Good WV, Koch TS, Jan JE. Monocular nystagmus caused by unilateral anterior visual-pathway disease. Dev Med Child Neurol. 1993; 35(12):1106–1110

[44] Stahl JS, Averbuch-Heller L, Leigh RJ. Acquired nystagmus. Arch Ophthalmol. 2000; 118(4):544–549

[45] Goldberg RT. Vertical pendular nystagmus in chronic myositis of medial and lateral rectus. Ann Ophthalmol. 1978; 10(12):1697–1702

[46] Oishi M, Mochizuki Y. Ipsilateral oculomotor nerve palsy and contralateral downbeat nystagmus: a syndrome caused by unilateral paramedian thalamopeduncular infarction. J Neurol. 1997; 244(2):132–133

[47] Matsuzono K, Manabe Y, Takahashi Y, Narai H, Omori N, Abe K. Combined ipsilateral oculomotor nerve palsy and contralateral downbeat nystagmus in a case of cerebral infarction. Case Rep Neurol. 2014; 6(1):134–138

[48] Jacome DE, FitzGerald R. Monocular ictal nystagmus. Arch Neurol. 1982; 39(10):653–656

[49] Burde RM, Savino PJ, Trobe JD. Clinical Decisions in Neuro-ophthalmology. 2nd ed. St Louis: Mosby Yearbook; 1991:289–320

[50] Komai K, Mimura O, Uyama J, et al. Neuro-ophthalmological evaluation of superior oblique myokymia. Neuro-ophthalmology. 1992; 12:135–140

[51] De , Haene I, Casselman J. Left superior oblique myokymia and right superior oblique paralysis due to a posterior fossa tumor. Neuro-ophthalmology. 1993; 13:13–16

[52] Morrow MJ, Sharpe JA, Ranalli PJ. Superior oblique myokymia associated with a posterior fossa tumor: oculographic correlation with an idiopathic case. Neurology. 1990; 40(2):367–370

[53] Brazis PW, Miller NR, Henderer JD, Lee AG. The natural history and results of treatment of superior oblique myokymia. Arch Ophthalmol. 1994; 112(8):1063–1067

[54] Hashimoto M, Ohtsuka K, Hoyt WF. Vascular compression as a cause of superior oblique myokymia disclosed by thin-slice magnetic resonance imaging. Am J Ophthalmol. 2001; 131(5):676–677

[55] Yousry I, Dieterich M, Naidich TP, Schmid UD, Yousry TA. Superior oblique myokymia: magnetic resonance imaging support for the neurovascular compression hypothesis. Ann Neurol. 2002; 51(3):361–368

[56] Geis TC, Newman NJ, Dawson RC. Superior oblique myokymia associated with a dural arteriovenous fistula. J Neuroophthalmol. 1996; 16(1):41–43

[57] Neetens A, Martin JJ. Superior oblique myokymia in a case of adrenoleukodystrophy and in a case of lead intoxication. Neuroophthalmology. 1983; 3:103–107

[58] Rosenberg ML, Glaser JS. Superior oblique myokymia. Ann Neurol. 1983; 13(6):667–669

[59] Tyler TD, Ruiz RS. Propranolol in the treatment of superior oblique myokymia. Arch Ophthalmol. 1990; 108(2):175–176

[60] de Sa LC, Good WV, Hoyt CS. Surgical management of myokymia of the superior oblique muscle. Am J Ophthalmol. 1992; 114(6):693–696

[61] Hayakawa Y, Takagi M, Hasebe H, et al. A case of superior oblique myokymia observed by an image-analysis system. J Neuroophthalmol. 2000; 20(3):163–165

[62] Kosmorsky GS, Ellis BD, Fogt N, Leigh RJ. The treatment of superior oblique myokymia utilizing the Harada-Ito procedure. J Neuroophthalmol. 1995; 15(3):142–146

[63] Samii M, Rosahl SK, Carvalho GA, Krzizok T. Microvascular decompression for superior oblique myokymia: first experience. Case report. J Neurosurg. 1998; 89(6):1020–1024

[64] May EF, Truxal AR. Loss of vision alone may result in seesaw nystagmus. J Neuroophthalmol. 1997; 17(2):84–85

[65] Halmagyi GM, Aw ST, Dehaene I, Curthoys IS, Todd MJ. Jerk-waveform seesaw nystagmus due to unilateral meso-diencephalic lesion. Brain. 1994; 117(Pt 4):789–803

[66] Halmagyi GM, Hoyt WF. See-saw nystagmus due to unilateral mesodiencephalic lesion. J Clin Neuroophthalmol. 1991; 11(2):79–84

[67] Barton JJS. Blink- and saccade-induced seesaw nystagmus. Neurology. 1995; 45(4):831–833

[68] Samkoff LM, Smith CR. See-saw nystagmus in a patient with clinically definite MS. Eur Neurol. 1994; 34(4):228–229

[69] Bennett JL, Galetta SL, Frohman LP, et al. Neuro-ophthalmologic manifestations of a paraneoplastic syndrome and testicular carcinoma. Neurology. 1999; 52(4):864–867

[70] Epstein JA, Moster ML, Spiritos M. Seesaw nystagmus following whole brain irradiation and intrathecal methotrexate. J Neuroophthalmol. 2001; 21(4):264–265

[71] Prakash S, Dumoulin SO, Fischbein N, Wandell BA, Liao YJ. Congenital achiasma and see-saw nystagmus in VACTERL syndrome. J Neuroophthalmol. 2010; 30(1):45–48

[72] Rambold H, Helmchen C, Straube A, Büttner U. Seesaw nystagmus associated with involuntary torsional head oscillations. Neurology. 1998; 51(3):831–837

[73] Pieh C, Gottlob I. Arnold-Chiari malformation and nystagmus of skew. J Neurol Neurosurg Psychiatry. 2000; 69(1):124–126

[74] Cochin JP, Hannequin D, Do Marcolino C, Didier T, Augustin P. Intermittent sea-saw nystagmus successfully treated with clonazepam [in French]. Rev Neurol (Paris). 1995; 151(1):60–62

[75] Pullicino P, Lincoff N, Truax BT. Abnormal vergence with upper brainstem infarcts: pseudoabducens palsy. Neurology. 2000; 55(3):352–358

[76] Rambold H, Kömpf D, Helmchen C. Convergence retraction nystagmus: a disorder of vergence? Ann Neurol. 2001; 50(5):677–681

[77] Mossman SS, Bronstein AM, Gresty MA, Kendall B, Rudge P. Convergence nystagmus associated with Arnold-Chiari malformation. Arch Neurol. 1990; 47(3):357–359

[78] Schnyder H, Bassetti C. Bilateral convergence nystagmus in unilateral dorsal midbrain stroke due to occlusion of the superior cerebellar artery. Neuro-ophthalmology. 1996; 16:59–63

[79] Selhorst JB. (1987). Pendular vergence oscillations. In: Ishikawa H, ed. Highlights in Neuro-ophthalmology. Proceedings of the Sixth Meeting of the International Neuro-Ophthalmology Society. Amsterdam, Aeolus, pp. 153–162

[80] Noda S, Ide K, Umezaki H, Itoh H, Yamamoto K. Repetitive divergence. Ann Neurol. 1987; 21(1):109–110

[81] Nelson KR, Brenner RP, Carlow TJ. Divergent-convergent eye movements and transient eyelid opening associated with an EEG burst-suppression pattern. J Clin Neuroophthalmol. 1986; 6(1):43–46

[82] Adler CH, Galetta SL. Oculo-facial-skeletal myorhythmia in Whipple disease: treatment with ceftriaxone. Ann Intern Med. 1990; 112(6):467–469

[83] Louis ED, Lynch T, Kaufmann P, Fahn S, Odel J. Diagnostic guidelines in central nervous system Whipple's disease. Ann Neurol. 1996; 40(4):561–568

[84] Tison F, Louvet-Giendaj C, Henry P, Lagueny A, Gaujard E. Permanent bruxism as a manifestation of the oculo-facial syndrome related to systemic Whipple's disease. Mov Disord. 1992; 7(1):82–85

[85] Lynch T, Odel J, Fredericks DN, et al. Polymerase chain reaction-based detection of Tropheryma whippelii in central nervous system Whipple's disease. Ann Neurol. 1997; 42(1):120–124

[86] von Herbay A, Ditton H-J, Schuhmacher F, Maiwald M. Whipple's disease: staging and monitoring by cytology and polymerase chain reaction analysis of cerebrospinal fluid. Gastroenterology. 1997; 113(2):434–441

[87] Gresty MA, Bronstein AM, Page NG, Rudge P. Congenital-type nystagmus emerging in later life. Neurology. 1991; 41(5):653–656

[88] Hertle RW, Dell'Osso LF. Clinical and ocular motor analysis of congenital nystagmus in infancy. J AAPOS. 1999; 3(2):70–79

[89] Kerrison JB, Vagefi MR, Barmada MM, Maumenee IH. Congenital motor nystagmus linked to Xq26-q27. Am J Hum Genet. 1999; 64(2):600–607

[90] Oetting WS, Armstrong CM, Holleschau AM, DeWan AT, Summers GC. Evidence for genetic heterogeneity in families with congenital motor nystagmus (CN). Ophthalmic Genet. 2000; 21(4):227–233

[91] Tarpey P, Thomas S, Sarvananthan N, et al. Mutations in FRMD7, a newly identified member of the FERM family, cause X-linked idiopathic congenital nystagmus. Nat Genet. 2006; 38(11):1242–1244

[92] Thomas MG, Crosier M, Lindsay S, et al. The clinical and molecular genetic features of idiopathic infantile periodic alternating nystagmus. Brain. 2011; 134(Pt 3):892–902

[93] Jacobson L, Ygge J, Flodmark O. Nystagmus in periventricular leucomalacia. Br J Ophthalmol. 1998; 82(9):1026–1032

[94] Shawkat FS, Kriss A, Thompson D, Russell-Eggitt I, Taylor D, Harris C. Vertical or asymmetric nystagmus need not imply neurological disease. Br J Ophthalmol. 2000; 84(2):175–180

[95] Hertle RW, FitzGibbon EJ, Avallone JM, Cheeseman E, Tsilou EK. Onset of oscillopsia after visual maturation in patients with congenital nystagmus. Ophthalmology. 2001; 108(12):2301–2307, discussion 2307–2308

[96] Cibis GW, Fitzgerald KM. Electroretinography in congenital idiopathic nystagmus. Pediatr Neurol. 1993; 9(5):369–371

[97] Leigh RJ, Averbuch-Heller L, Tomsak RL, Remler BF, Yaniglos SS, Dell'Osso LF. Treatment of abnormal eye movements that impair vision: strategies based on current concepts of physiology and pharmacology. Ann Neurol. 1994; 36(2):129–141

[98] Yaniglos SS, Leigh RJ. Refinement of an optical device that stabilizes vision in patients with nystagmus. Optom Vis Sci. 1992; 69(6):447–450

[99] Carruthers J. The treatment of congenital nystagmus with Botox. J Pediatr Ophthalmol Strabismus. 1995; 32(5):306–308

[100] Atilla H, Erkam N, Işikçelik Y. Surgical treatment in nystagmus. Eye (Lond). 1999; 13(Pt 1):11–15

[101] Bilska C, Pociej-Zero M, Krzystkowa KM. Surgical treatment of congenital nystagmus in 463 children [in Polish]. Klin Oczna. 1995; 97(5):140–141

[102] Helveston EM, Ellis FD, Plager DA. Large recession of the horizontal recti for treatment of nystagmus. Ophthalmology. 1991; 98(8):1302–1305

[103] von Noorden GK, Sprunger DT. Large rectus muscle recessions for the treatment of congenital nystagmus. Arch Ophthalmol. 1991; 109(2):221–224

[104] Zubcov AA, Stärk N, Weber A, Wizov SS, Reinecke RD. Improvement of visual acuity after surgery for nystagmus. Ophthalmology. 1993; 100(10):1488–1497

[105] Lee IS, Lee JB, Kim HS, Lew H, Han SH. Modified Kestenbaum surgery for correction of abnormal head posture in infantile nystagmus: outcome in 63 patients with graded augmentation. Binocul Vis Strabismus Q. 2000; 15(1):53–58

[106] Evans BJ, Evans BV, Jordahl-Moroz J, Nabee M. Randomised double-masked placebo-controlled trial of a treatment for congenital nystagmus. Vision Res. 1998; 38(14):2193–2202

[107] Gresty MA, Metcalfe T, Timms C, Elston J, Lee J, Liu C. Neurology of latent nystagmus. Brain. 1992; 115(Pt 5):1303–1321

[108] Wagner RS, Caputo AR, Reynolds RD. Nystagmus in Down's syndrome. Ophthalmology. 1990; 97(11):1439–1444

[109] Zubcov AA, Reinecke RD, Gottlob I, Manley DR, Calhoun JH. Treatment of manifest latent nystagmus. Am J Ophthalmol. 1990; 110(2):160–167

[110] Tychsen L, Richards M, Wong A, Foeller P, Bradley D, Burkhalter A. The neural mechanism for Latent (fusion maldevelopment) nystagmus. J Neuroophthalmol. 2010; 30(3):276–283

[111] Kushner BJ. Infantile uniocular blindness with bilateral nystagmus. A syndrome. Arch Ophthalmol. 1995; 113(10):1298–1300

[112] Lee J, Gresty M. A case of "voluntary nystagmus" and head tremor. J Neurol Neurosurg Psychiatry. 1993; 56(12):1321–1322

[113] Sato M, Kurachi T, Arai M, Abel LA. Voluntary nystagmus associated with accommodation spasms. Jpn J Ophthalmol. 1999; 43(1):1–4

[114] Davis BJ. Voluntary nystagmus as a component of a nonepileptic seizure. Neurology. 2000; 55(12):1937

[115] Averbuch-Heller L, Zivotofsky AZ, Das VE, DiScenna AO, Leigh RJ. Investigations of the pathogenesis of acquired pendular nystagmus. Brain. 1995; 118(Pt 2):369–378

[116] Barton JJS, Cox TA. Acquired pendular nystagmus in multiple sclerosis: clinical observations and the role of optic neuropathy. J Neurol Neurosurg Psychiatry. 1993; 56(3):262–267

[117] Lopez LI, Bronstein AM, Gresty MA, Du Boulay EP, Rudge P. Clinical and MRI correlates in 27 patients with acquired pendular nystagmus. Brain. 1996; 119(Pt 2):465–472

[118] Barton JJS, Cox TA, Digre KB. Acquired convergence-evoked pendular nystagmus in multiple sclerosis. J Neuroophthalmol. 1999; 19(1):34–38

[119] Revol A, Vighetto A, Confavreux C, Trillet M, Aimard G. Oculo-palatal myoclonus and multiple sclerosis [in French]. Rev Neurol (Paris). 1990; 146(8–9):518–521

[120] Schon F, Hart PE, Hodgson TL, et al. Suppression of pendular nystagmus by smoking cannabis in a patient with multiple sclerosis. Neurology. 1999; 53(9):2209–2210

[121] Starck M, Albrecht H, Pöllmann W, Straube A, Dieterich M. Drug therapy for acquired pendular nystagmus in multiple sclerosis. J Neurol. 1997; 244(1):9–16

[122] Talks SJ, Elston JS. Oculopalatal myoclonus: eye movement studies, MRI findings and the difficulty of treatment. Eye (Lond). 1997; 11(Pt 1):19–24

[123] Strupp M, Thurtell MJ, Shaikh AG, Brandt T, Zee DS, Leigh RJ. Pharmacotherapy of vestibular and ocular motor disorders, including nystagmus. J Neurol. 2011; 258(7):1207–1222

[124] Shaikh AG, Hong S, Liao K, et al. Oculopalatal tremor explained by a model of inferior olivary hypertrophy and cerebellar plasticity. Brain. 2010; 133(Pt 3):923–940

[125] Kori AA, Robin NH, Jacobs JB, et al. Pendular nystagmus in patients with peroxisomal assembly disorder. Arch Neurol. 1998; 55(4):554–558

[126] Maas EF, Ashe J, Spiegel P, Zee DS, Leigh RJ. Acquired pendular nystagmus in toluene addiction. Neurology. 1991; 41(2 (Pt 1)):282–285

[127] Trobe JD, Sharpe JA, Hirsh DK, Gebarski SS. Nystagmus of Pelizaeus-Merzbacher disease. A magnetic search-coil study. Arch Neurol. 1991; 48(1):87–91

[128] Rambold H, Heide W, Sprenger A, Haendler G, Helmchen C. Perilymph fistula associated with pulse-synchronous eye oscillations. Neurology. 2001; 56(12):1769–1771

[129] Good WV, Brodsky MC, Hoyt CS, Ahn JC. Upbeating nystagmus in infants: a sign of anterior visual pathway disease. Binocular Vis Q. 1990; 5:13–18

[130] Bronstein AM, Gresty MA, Mossman SS. Pendular pseudonystagmus arising as a combination of head tremor and vestibular failure. Neurology. 1992; 42(8):1527–1531

[131] Verhagen WI, Huygen PL, Nicolasen MG. Pendular pseudonystagmus. Neurology. 1994; 44(6):1188–1189

[132] Yen MT, Herdman SJ, Tusa RJ. Oscillopsia and pseudonystagmus in kidney transplant patients. Am J Ophthalmol. 1999; 128(6):768–770

[133] Eggenberger E, Cornblath W, Stewart DH. Oculopalatal tremor with tardive ataxia. J Neuroophthalmol. 2001; 21(2):83–86

[134] Nakada T, Kwee IL. Oculopalatal myoclonus. Brain. 1986; 109(Pt 3):431–441

[135] Wolin MJ, Trent RG, Lavin PJM, Cornblath WT. Oculopalatal myoclonus after the one-and-a-half syndrome with facial nerve palsy. Ophthalmology. 1996; 103(1):177–180

[136] Barton JJS, Huaman AG, Sharpe JA. Muscarinic antagonists in the treatment of acquired pendular and downbeat nystagmus: a double-blind, randomized trial of three intravenous drugs. Ann Neurol. 1994; 35(3):319–325

[137] Leigh RJ, Burnstine TH, Ruff RL, Kasmer RJ. Effect of anticholinergic agents upon acquired nystagmus: a double-blind study of trihexyphenidyl and tridihexethyl chloride. Neurology. 1991; 41(11):1737–1741

[138] Jabbari B, Rosenberg M, Scherokman B, Gunderson CH, McBurney JW, McClintock W. Effectiveness of trihexyphenidyl against pendular nystagmus and palatal myoclonus: evidence of cholinergic dysfunction. Mov Disord. 1987; 2(2):93–98

[139] Traccis S, Rosati G, Monaco MF, Aiello I, Agnetti V. Successful treatment of acquired pendular elliptical nystagmus in multiple sclerosis with isoniazid and base-out prisms. Neurology. 1990; 40(3 Pt 1):492–494

[140] Stahl JS, Rottach KG, Averbuch-Heller L, von Maydell RD, Collins SD, Leigh RJ. A pilot study of gabapentin as treatment for acquired nystagmus. Neuroophthalmology. 1996; 16(2):107–113

[141] Averbuch-Heller L, Tusa RJ, Fuhry L, et al. A double-blind controlled study of gabapentin and baclofen as treatment for acquired nystagmus. Ann Neurol. 1997; 41(6):818–825

[142] Bandini F, Castello E, Mazzella L, Mancardi GL, Solaro C. Gabapentin but not vigabatrin is effective in the treatment of acquired nystagmus in multiple sclerosis: How valid is the GABAergic hypothesis? J Neurol Neurosurg Psychiatry. 2001; 71(1):107–110

[143] Leigh RJ, Tomsak RL, Grant MP, et al. Effectiveness of botulinum toxin administered to abolish acquired nystagmus. Ann Neurol. 1992; 32(5):633–642

[144] Repka MX, Savino PJ, Reinecke RD. Treatment of acquired nystagmus with botulinum neurotoxin A. Arch Ophthalmol. 1994; 112(10):1320–1324

[145] Ruben S, Dunlop IS, Elston J. Retrobulbar botulinum toxin for treatment of oscillopsia. Aust N Z J Ophthalmol. 1994; 22(1):65–67

[146] Ruben ST, Lee JP, O'Neil D, Dunlop I, Elston JS. The use of botulinum toxin for treatment of acquired nystagmus and oscillopsia. Ophthalmology. 1994; 101(4):783–787

[147] Tomsak RL, Remler BF, Averbuch-Heller L, Chandran M, Leigh RJ. Unsatisfactory treatment of acquired nystagmus with retrobulbar injection of botulinum toxin. Am J Ophthalmol. 1995; 119(4):489–496

[148] Herishanu Y, Louzoun Z. Trihexyphenidyl treatment of vertical pendular nystagmus. Neurology. 1986; 36(1):82–84

[149] Shallo-Hoffmann J, Faldon M, Tusa RJ. The incidence and waveform characteristics of periodic alternating nystagmus in congenital nystagmus. Invest Ophthalmol Vis Sci. 1999; 40(11):2546–2553

[150] Troost BT, Janton F, Weaver R. Periodic alternating oscillopsia: a symptom of alternating nystagmus abolished by baclofen. J Clin Neuroophthalmol. 1990; 10(4):273–277

[151] Furman JMR, Wall C, III, Pang DL. Vestibular function in periodic alternating nystagmus. Brain. 1990; 113(Pt 5):1425–1439

[152] Gradstein L, Reinecke RD, Wizov SS, Goldstein HP. Congenital periodic alternating nystagmus. Diagnosis and Management. Ophthalmology. 1997; 104(6):918–928, discussion 928–929

[153] Abadi RV, Pascal E. Periodic alternating nystagmus in humans with albinism. Invest Ophthalmol Vis Sci. 1994; 35(12):4080–4086

[154] Huygen PLM, Verhagen WIM, Cruysberg JRM, Koch PAM. Familial congenital periodic alternating nystagmus with presumably X-linked dominant inheritance. Neuroophthalmology. 1995; 15:149–155

[155] Ito K, Murofushi T, Mizuno M. Periodic alternating nystagmus and congenital nystagmus: similarities in possibly inherited cases. ORL J Otorhinolaryngol Relat Spec. 2000; 62(1):53–56

[156] Hertle RW, Yang D, Kelly K, Hill VM, Atkin J, Seward A. X-linked infantile periodic alternating nystagmus. Ophthalmic Genet. 2005; 26(2):77–84

[157] Furman JM, Crumrine PK, Reinmuth OM. Epileptic nystagmus. Ann Neurol. 1990; 27(6):686–688

[158] Whyte C, Kramer PD, Rudzinskiy P, Fouladvand M. Periodic alternating nystagmus in HIV-induced primary cerebellar degeneration. Neuro-ophthalmology. 2008; 32:67–68

[159] Grant MP, Cohen M, Petersen RB, et al. Abnormal eye movements in Creutzfeldt-Jakob disease. Ann Neurol. 1993; 34(2):192–197

[160] Yokota T, Tsuchiya K, Yamane M, Hayashi M, Tanabe H, Tsukagoshi H. Geotropic ocular deviation with skew and absence of saccade in Creutzfelt-Jakob disease. J Neurol Sci. 1991; 106(2):175–178

[161] Mackay DD, Zepeda Garcia R, Galetta SL, Prasad S. Periodic alternating gaze deviation and nystagmus in posterior reversible encephalopathy syndrome. Neurol Clin Pract. 2014; 4:482–485

[162] Jeong SH, Nam J, Kwon MJ, Kim JK, Kim JS. Nystagmus and ataxia associated with antiganglioside antibodies. J Neuroophthalmol. 2011; 31(4):326–330

[163] Tilikete C, Vighetto A, Trouillas P, Honnorat J. Anti-GAD antibodies and periodic alternating nystagmus. Arch Neurol. 2005; 62(8):1300–1303

[164] Tilikete C, Vighetto A, Trouillas P, Honnorat J. Potential role of anti-GAD antibodies in abnormal eye movements. Ann N Y Acad Sci. 2005; 1039:446–454

[165] Averbuch-Heller L, Meiner Z. Reversible periodic alternating gaze deviation in hepatic encephalopathy. Neurology. 1995; 45(1):191–192

[166] Matsumoto S, Ohyagi Y, Inoue I, et al. Periodic alternating nystagmus in a patient with MS. Neurology. 2001; 56(2):276–277

[167] Lee MS, Lessell S. Lithium-induced periodic alternating nystagmus. Neurology. 2003; 60(2):344

[168] Moster ML, Schnayder E. Epileptic periodic alternating nystagmus. J Neuroophthalmol. 1998; 18(4):292–293

[169] Porges Y, Blumen S, Fireman Z, Sternberg A, Zamir D. Cyclosporine-induced optic neuropathy, ophthalmoplegia, and nystagmus in a patient with Crohn disease. Am J Ophthalmol. 1998; 126(4):607–609

[170] Remler BF, Leigh RJ, Osorio I, Tomsak RL. The characteristics and mechanisms of visual disturbance associated with anticonvulsant therapy. Neurology. 1990; 40(5):791–796

[171] Harris CM, Boyd S, Chong K, Harkness W, Neville BG. Epileptic nystagmus in infancy. J Neurol Sci. 1997; 151(1):111–114

[172] Kaplan PW, Tusa RJ. Neurophysiologic and clinical correlations of epileptic nystagmus. Neurology. 1993; 43(12):2508–2514

[173] Stolz SE, Chatrian GE, Spence AM. Epileptic nystagmus. Epilepsia. 1991; 32(6):910–918

[174] Tusa RJ, Kaplan PW, Hain TC, Naidu S. Ipsiversive eye deviation and epileptic nystagmus. Neurology. 1990; 40(4):662–665

[175] Gire C, Somma-Mauvais H, Niçaise C, Roussel M, Garnier JM, Farnarier G. Epileptic nystagmus: electroclinical study of a case. Epileptic Disord. 2001; 3(1):33–37

[176] Dieterich M, Brandt T. Episodic vertigo related to migraine (90 cases): vestibular migraine? J Neurol. 1999; 246(10):883–892

[177] Lopez L, Bronstein AM, Gresty MA, Rudge P, du Boulay EP. Torsional nystagmus. A neuro-otological and MRI study of thirty-five cases. Brain. 1992; 115(Pt 4):1107–1124

[178] Stearns MQ, Sinoff SE, Rosenberg ML. Purely torsional nystagmus in a patient with stiff-man syndrome: a case report. Neurology. 1993; 43:220

[179] Helmchen C, Glasauer S, Bartl K, Büttner U. Contralesionally beating torsional nystagmus in a unilateral rostral midbrain lesion. Neurology. 1996; 47(2):482–486

[180] FitzGibbon EJ, Calvert PC, Dieterich M, Brandt T, Zee DS. Torsional nystagmus during vertical pursuit. J Neuroophthalmol. 1996; 16(2):79–90

[181] Rosenthal JG, Selhorst JB. Continuous non-rhythmic cycloversion: a possible paraneoplastic disorder. Neuroophthalmology. 1987; 7:291–295

[182] Buttner U, Helmchen C, Buttner-Ennever JA. The localizing value of nystagmus in brainstem disorders. Neuro-ophthalmology. 1995; 15(6):283–290

[183] Walker MF, Zee DS. The effect of hyperventilation on downbeat nystagmus in cerebellar disorders. Neurology. 1999; 53(7):1576–1579

[184] Minagar A, Sheremata WA, Tusa RJ. Perverted head-shaking nystagmus: a possible mechanism. Neurology. 2001; 57(5):887–889

[185] Wagner JN, Glaser M, Brandt T, Strupp M. Downbeat nystagmus: aetiology and comorbidity in 117 patients. J Neurol Neurosurg Psychiatry. 2008; 79(6):672–677

[186] Vale TC, Pedroso JL, Alquéres RA, Dutra LA, Barsottini OG. Spontaneous downbeat nystagmus as a clue for the diagnosis of ataxia associated with anti-GAD antibodies. J Neurol Sci. 2015; 359(1–2):21–23

[187] Schniepp R, Wuehr M, Huth S, et al. The gait disorder in downbeat nystagmus syndrome. PLoS One. 2014; 9(8):e105463

[188] Ances BM, Dalmau JO, Tsai J, Hasbani MJ, Galetta SL. Downbeating nystagmus and muscle spasms in a patient with glutamic-acid decarboxylase antibodies. Am J Ophthalmol. 2005; 140(1):142–144

[189] Chen Y, Morgan ML, Palau AE, Mudd JA, Lee AG, Barton JJ. Downbeat down south. Surv Ophthalmol. 2015; 60(2):177–181

[190] Bussière M, Al-Khotani A, Steckley JL, Nicolle M, Nicolle D. Paraneoplastic downbeat nystagmus. Can J Ophthalmol. 2008; 43(2):243–245

[191] Ogawa E, Sakakibara R, Kawashima K, et al. VGCC antibody-positive paraneoplastic cerebellar degeneration presenting with positioning vertigo. Neurol Sci. 2011; 32(6):1209–1212

[192] Russell GE, Wick B, Tang RA. Arnold-Chiari malformation. Optom Vis Sci. 1992; 69(3):242–247

[193] Harada H, Tamaoka A, Watanabe M, Ishikawa K, Shoji S. Downbeat nystagmus in two siblings with spinocerebellar ataxia type 6 (SCA 6). J Neurol Sci. 1998; 160(2):161–163

[194] Bour LJ, van Rootselaar AF, Koelman JH, Tijssen MA. Oculomotor abnormalities in myoclonic tremor: a comparison with spinocerebellar ataxia type 6. Brain. 2008; 131(Pt 9):2295–2303

[195] Zivotofsky AZ, Siman-Tov T, Gadoth N, Gordon CR. A rare saccade velocity profile in Stiff-Person Syndrome with cerebellar degeneration. Brain Res. 2006; 1093(1):135–140

[196] Cai CX, Siringo FS, Odel JG, et al. Downbeat nystagmus secondary to familial hemophagocytic lymphohistiocytosis. J Neuroophthalmol. 2014; 34(1):57–60

[197] Bertholon P, Bronstein AM, Davies RA, Rudge P, Thilo KV. Positional down beating nystagmus in 50 patients: cerebellar disorders and possible anterior semicircular canalithiasis. J Neurol Neurosurg Psychiatry. 2002; 72(3):366–372

[198] Chan T, Logan P, Eustace P. Intermittent downbeat nystagmus secondary to vermian arachnoid cyst with associated obstructive hydrocephalus. J Clin Neuroophthalmol. 1991; 11(4):293–296

[199] Olson JL, Jacobson DM. Comparison of clinical associations of patients with vasculopathic and idiopathic downbeat nystagmus. J Neuroophthalmol. 2001; 21(1):39–41

[200] Rousseaux M, Dupard T, Lesoin F, Barbaste P, Hache JC. Upbeat and downbeat nystagmus occurring successively in a patient with posterior medullary haemorrhage. J Neurol Neurosurg Psychiatry. 1991; 54(4):367–369

[201] Choi JH, Yang TI, Cha SY, Lee TH, Choi KD, Kim JS. Ictal downbeat nystagmus in cardiogenic vertigo. Neurology. 2010; 75(23):2129–2130

[202] Gans MS, Melmed CA. Downbeat nystagmus associated with dolichoectasia of the vertebrobasilar artery. Arch Neurol. 1990; 47(8):843

[203] Himi T, Kataura A, Tokuda S, Sumi Y, Kamiyama K, Shitamichi M. Downbeat nystagmus with compression of the medulla oblongata by the dolichoectatic vertebral arteries. Am J Otol. 1995; 16(3):377–381

[204] Krespi Y, Verstichel P, Masson C, Cambier J. Downbeat nystagmus and vertebrobasilar arterial dolichoectasia [in French]. Rev Neurol (Paris). 1995; 151(3):196–197

[205] Lee AG. Downbeat nystagmus associated with caudal brainstem compression by the vertebral artery. J Neuroophthalmol. 2001; 21(3):219–220

[206] Noh Y, Kwon OK, Kim HJ, Kim JS. Rotational vertebral artery syndrome due to compression of nondominant vertebral artery terminating in posterior inferior cerebellar artery. J Neurol. 2011; 258(10):1775–1780

[207] Choi KD, Shin HY, Kim JS, et al. Rotational vertebral artery syndrome: oculographic analysis of nystagmus. Neurology. 2005; 65(8):1287–1290

[208] Marti S, Hegemann S, von Büdingen HC, Baumgartner RW, Straumann D. Rotational vertebral artery syndrome: 3D kinematics of nystagmus suggest bilateral labyrinthine dysfunction. J Neurol. 2008; 255(5):663–667

[209] Rosengart A, Hedges TR, III, Teal PA, et al. Intermittent downbeat nystagmus due to vertebral artery compression. Neurology. 1993; 43(1):216–218

[210] Yoshimoto Y, Koyama S. A case of acquired nystagmus alternans associated with acute cerebellitis. Acta Otolaryngol Suppl. 1991; 481:371–373

[211] Van Stavern GP, Biousse V, Newman NJ, Leingang JC. Downbeat nystagmus from heat stroke. J Neurol Neurosurg Psychiatry. 2000; 69(3):403–404

[212] Orwitz JI, Galetta SL, Teener JW. Bilateral trochlear nerve palsy and downbeat nystagmus in a patient with cephalic tetanus. Neurology. 1997; 49(3):894–895

[213] Rowlands A, Sgouros S, Williams B. Ocular manifestations of hindbrain-related syringomyelia and outcome following craniovertebral decompression. Eye (Lond). 2000; 14(Pt 6):884–888

[214] Mulder AH, Raemaekers JM, Boerman RH, Mattijssen V. Downbeat nystagmus caused by thiamine deficiency: an unusual presentation of CNS localization of large cell anaplastic CD 30-positive non-Hodgkin's lymphoma. Ann Hematol. 1999; 78(2):105–107

[215] Merkin-Zaborsky H, Ifergane G, Frisher S, Valdman S, Herishanu Y, Wirguin I. Thiamine-responsive acute neurological disorders in nonalcoholic patients. Eur Neurol. 2001; 45(1):34–37

[216] Hammack J, Kotanides H, Rosenblum MK, Posner JB. Paraneoplastic cerebellar degeneration. II. Clinical and immunologic findings in 21 patients with Hodgkin's disease. Neurology. 1992; 42(10):1938–1943

[217] Peterson K, Rosenblum MK, Kotanides H, Posner JB. Paraneoplastic cerebellar degeneration. I. A clinical analysis of 55 anti-Yo antibody-positive patients. Neurology. 1992; 42(10):1931–1937

[218] Hage R, Jr, Merle H, Jeannin S, Cabre P. Ocular oscillations in the neuromyelitis optica spectrum. J Neuroophthalmol. 2011; 31(3):255–259

[219] Pelak VS, Galetta SL, Grossman RI, Townsend JJ, Volpe NJ. Evidence for preganglionic pupillary involvement in superficial siderosis. Neurology. 1999; 53(5):1130–1132

[220] Shinmei Y, Kase M, Suzuki Y, et al. Ocular motor disorders in mitochondrial encephalopathy with lactic acid and stroke-like episodes with the 3271 (T-C) point mutation in mitochondrial DNA. J Neuroophthalmol. 2007; 27(1): 22–28

[221] Du Pasquier R, Vingerhoets F, Safran AB, Landis T. Periodic downbeat nystagmus. Neurology. 1998; 51(5):1478–1480

[222] Henderson RD, Wijdicks EF. Downbeat nystagmus associated with intravenous patient-controlled administration of morphine. Anesth Analg. 2000; 91(3):691–692

[223] Hwang TL, Still CN, Jones JE. Reversible downbeat nystagmus and ataxia in felbamate intoxication. Neurology. 1995; 45(4):846

[224] Monteiro ML, Sampaio CM. Lithium-induced downbeat nystagmus in a patient with Arnold-Chiari malformation. Am J Ophthalmol. 1993; 116(5): 648–649

[225] Young YH, Huang TW. Role of clonazepam in the treatment of idiopathic downbeat nystagmus. Laryngoscope. 2001; 111(8):1490–1493

[226] Hirose G, Kawada J, Tsukada K, Yoshioka A, Sharpe JA. Upbeat nystagmus: clinicopathological and pathophysiological considerations. J Neurol Sci. 1991; 105(2):159–167

[227] Wray SH, Dalmau J, Chen A, King S, Leigh RJ. Paraneoplastic disorders of eye movements. Ann N Y Acad Sci. 2011; 1233:279–284

[228] Kanaya T, Nonaka S, Kamito M, Unno T, Sako K, Takei H. Primary position upbeat nystagmus localizing value. ORL J Otorhinolaryngol Relat Spec. 1994; 56(4):236–238

[229] Munro NAR, Gaymard B, Rivaud S, Majdalani A, Pierrot-Deseilligny C. Upbeat nystagmus in a patient with a small medullary infarct. J Neurol Neurosurg Psychiatry. 1993; 56(10):1126–1128

[230] Hirose G, Ogasawara T, Shirakawa T, et al. Primary position upbeat nystagmus due to unilateral medial medullary infarction. Ann Neurol. 1998; 43(3):403–406

[231] Janssen JC, Larner AJ, Morris H, Bronstein AM, Farmer SF. Upbeat nystagmus: clinicoanatomical correlation. J Neurol Neurosurg Psychiatry. 1998; 65(3): 380–381

[232] Ohkoshi N, Komatsu Y, Mizusawa H, Kanazawa I. Primary position upbeat nystagmus increased on downward gaze: clinicopathologic study of a patient with multiple sclerosis. Neurology. 1998; 50(2):551–553

[233] Mizuno M, Kudo Y, Yamane M. Upbeat nystagmus influenced by posture: report of two cases. Auris Nasus Larynx. 1990; 16(4):215–221

[234] Choi H, Kim CH, Lee KY, Lee YJ, Koh SH. A probable cavernoma in the medulla oblongata presenting only as upbeat nystagmus. J Clin Neurosci. 2011; 18(11):1567–1569

[235] Hirose G, Kawada J, Yoshioka A. Primary position upbeat nystagmus: clinicopathologic study in three patients. Neurology. 1990; 40 Suppl:312

[236] Choi KD, Jung DS, Park KP, Jo JW, Kim JS. Bowtie and upbeat nystagmus evolving into hemi-seesaw nystagmus in medial medullary infarction: possible anatomic mechanisms. Neurology. 2004; 62(4):663–665

[237] Bruce BB, Newman NJ, Biousse V. Ophthalmoparesis in idiopathic intracranial hypertension. Am J Ophthalmol. 2006; 142(5):878–880

[238] Hawthorne KM, Compton CJ, Vaphiades MS, Roberson GH, Kline LB. Ocular motor and imaging abnormalities of midbrain dysfunction in osmotic demyelination syndrome. J Neuroophthalmol. 2009; 29(4):296–299

[239] Alroughani R, Thussu A, Guindi RT. Yet another atypical presentation of anti-GQ1b antibody syndrome. Neurol Int. 2015; 7(2):5770

[240] Nakamagoe K, Fujizuka N, Koganezawa T, et al. Residual central nervous system damage due to organoarsenic poisoning. Neurotoxicol Teratol. 2013; 37:33–38

[241] Albera R, Luda E, Canale G, et al. Cyclosporine A as a possible cause of upbeating nystagmus. Neuro-ophthalmology. 1997; 17:163–168

[242] Garcia-Reitboeck P, Thompson G, Johns P, Al Wahab Y, Omer S, Griffin C. Upbeat nystagmus in anti-Ma2 encephalitis. Pract Neurol. 2014; 14(1):36–38

[243] Goldblum TA, Effron LA. Upbeat nystagmus associated with tonic downward deviation in healthy neonates. J Pediatr Ophthalmol Strabismus. 1994; 31 (5):334–335

[244] Dieterich M, Straube A, Brandt T, Paulus W, Büttner U. The effects of baclofen and cholinergic drugs on upbeat and downbeat nystagmus. J Neurol Neurosurg Psychiatry. 1991; 54(7):627–632

[245] Martidis A, Yee RD, Azzarelli B, Biller J. Neuro-ophthalmic, radiographic, and pathologic manifestations of adult-onset Alexander disease. Arch Ophthalmol. 1999; 117(2):265–267

[246] Baloh RW, Winder A. Acetazolamide-responsive vestibulocerebellar syndrome: clinical and oculographic features. Neurology. 1991; 41(3):429–433

[247] Baloh RW, Yue Q, Furman JM, Nelson SF. Familial episodic ataxia: clinical heterogeneity in four families linked to chromosome 19p. Ann Neurol. 1997; 41(1):8–16

[248] Brandt T, Strupp M. Episodic ataxia type 1 and 2 (familial periodic ataxia/vertigo). Audiol Neurootol. 1997; 2(6):373–383

[249] Lin CY, Young YH. Clinical significance of rebound nystagmus. Laryngoscope. 1999; 109(11):1803–1805

[250] Yee RD, Farlow MR, Suzuki DA, Betelak KF, Ghetti B. Abnormal eye movements in Gerstmann-Sträussler-Scheinker disease. Arch Ophthalmol. 1992; 110(1):68–74

[251] Oliva A, Rosenberg ML. Convergence-evoked nystagmus. Neurology. 1990; 40(1):161–162

[252] Baloh RW, Yue Q, Jacobson KM, Honrubia V. Persistent direction-changing positional nystagmus: another variant of benign positional nystagmus? Neurology. 1995; 45(7):1297–1301

[253] Brandt T. Positional and positioning vertigo and nystagmus. J Neurol Sci. 1990; 95(1):3–28

[254] Brandt T. Man in motion. Historical and clinical aspects of vestibular function. A review. Brain. 1991; 114(Pt 5):2159–2174

[255] Furman JM, Cass SP. Benign paroxysmal positional vertigo. N Engl J Med. 1999; 341(21):1590–1596

[256] Lawden MC, Bronstein AM, Kennard C. Repetitive paroxysmal nystagmus and vertigo. Neurology. 1995; 45(2):276–280

[257] Weider DJ, Ryder CJ, Stram JR. Benign paroxysmal positional vertigo: analysis of 44 cases treated by the canalith repositioning procedure of Epley. Am J Otol. 1994; 15(3):321–326

[258] Baloh RW, Jacobson K, Honrubia V. Horizontal semicircular canal variant of benign positional vertigo. Neurology. 1993; 43(12):2542–2549

[259] De la Meilleure G, Dehaene I, Depondt M, Damman W, Crevits L, Vanhooren G. Benign paroxysmal positional vertigo of the horizontal canal. J Neurol Neurosurg Psychiatry. 1996; 60(1):68–71

[260] Arbusow V, Strupp M, Brandt T. Amiodarone-induced severe prolonged head-positional vertigo and vomiting. Neurology. 1998; 51(3):917

[261] Sakata E, Ohtsu K, Itoh Y. Positional nystagmus of benign paroxysmal type (BPPN) due to cerebellar vermis lesions. Pseudo-BPPN. Acta Otolaryngol Suppl. 1991; 481:254–257

[262] Minor LB, Haslwanter T, Straumann D, Zee DS. Hyperventilation-induced nystagmus in patients with vestibular schwannoma. Neurology. 1999; 53 (9):2158–2168

[263] Ehrhardt D, Eggenberger E. Medical treatment of acquired nystagmus. Curr Opin Ophthalmol. 2012; 23(6):510–516

[264] Etzion Y, Grossman Y. Highly 4-aminopyridine sensitive delayed rectifier current modulates the excitability of guinea pig cerebellar Purkinje cells. Exp Brain Res. 2001; 139(4):419–425

[265] Alviña K, Khodakhah K. The therapeutic mode of action of 4-aminopyridine in cerebellar ataxia. J Neurosci. 2010; 30(21):7258–7268

[266] Strupp M, Schüler O, Krafczyk S, et al. Treatment of downbeat nystagmus with 3,4-diaminopyridine: a placebo-controlled study. Neurology. 2003; 61 (2):165–170

[267] Shallo-Hoffmann J, Sendler B, Mühlendyck H. Normal square wave jerks in differing age groups. Invest Ophthalmol Vis Sci. 1990; 31(8):1649–1652

[268] Friedman DI, Jankovic J, McCrary JA, III. Neuro-ophthalmic findings in progressive supranuclear palsy. J Clin Neuroophthalmol. 1992; 12(2):104–109

[269] Rascol O, Sabatini U, Simonetta-Moreau M, Montastruc JL, Rascol A, Clanet M. Square wave jerks in parkinsonian syndromes. J Neurol Neurosurg Psychiatry. 1991; 54(7):599–602

[270] Stark KL, Gibson JB, Hertle RW, Brodsky MC. Ocular motor signs in an infant with carbohydrate-deficient glycoprotein syndrome type Ia. Am J Ophthalmol. 2000; 130(4):533–535

[271] Averbuch-Heller L, Stahl JS, Hlavin ML, Leigh RJ. Square-wave jerks induced by pallidotomy in parkinsonian patients. Neurology. 1999; 52(1):185–188

[272] Averbuch-Heller L, Kori AA, Rottach KG, Dell'Osso LF, Remler BF, Leigh RJ. Dysfunction of pontine omnipause neurons causes impaired fixation: macrosaccadic oscillations with a unilateral pontine lesion. Neuroophthalmology. 1996; 16(2):99–106

[273] Komiyama A, Toda H, Johkura K. Edrophonium-induced macrosaccadic oscillations in myasthenia gravis. Ann Neurol. 1999; 45(4):522–525

[274] Traccis S, Marras MA, Puliga MV, et al. Square-wave jerks and square wave oscillations: treatment with valproic acid. Neuroophthalmology. 1997; 18(2):51–58

[275] Ashe J, Hain TC, Zee DS, Schatz NJ. Microsaccadic flutter. Brain. 1991; 114 Pt 1B:461–472

[276] Foroozan R, Brodsky MC. Microsaccadic opsoclonus: an idiopathic cause of oscillopsia and episodic blurred vision. Am J Ophthalmol. 2004; 138(6):1053–1054

[277] Hattori T, Takaya Y, Tsuboi Y, Hirayama K. Opsoclonus showing only during eye closure in hereditary cerebellar ataxia. J Neurol Neurosurg Psychiatry. 1993; 56(9):1037–1038

[278] Gizzi M, Rudolph S, Perakis A. Ocular flutter in vidarabine toxicity. Am J Ophthalmol. 1990; 109(1):105

[279] Kaminski HJ, Zee DS, Leigh RJ, et al. Ocular flutter and ataxia associated with AIDS-related complex. Neuro-ophthalmology. 1991; 11(3):163–167

[280] Skeie GO, Eldøen G, Skeie BS, Midgard R, Kristoffersen EK, Bindoff LA. Opsoclonus myoclonus syndrome in two cases with neuroborreliosis. Eur J Neurol. 2007; 14(12):e1–e2

[281] van Erp WS, Bakker NA, Aries MJ, Vroomen PC. Opsoclonus and multiple cranial neuropathy as a manifestation of neuroborreliosis. Neurology. 2011; 77(10):1013–1014

[282] Vukelic D, Bozinovic D, Morovic M, et al. Opsoclonus-myoclonus syndrome in a child with neuroborreliosis. J Infect. 2000; 40(2):189–191

[283] Connolly AM, Pestronk A, Mehta S, Pranzatelli MR, III, Noetzel MJ. Serum autoantibodies in childhood opsoclonus-myoclonus syndrome: an analysis of antigenic targets in neural tissues. J Pediatr. 1997; 130(6):878–884

[284] Sheth RD, Horwitz SJ, Aronoff S, Gingold M, Bodensteiner JB. Opsoclonus myoclonus syndrome secondary to Epstein-Barr virus infection. J Child Neurol. 1995; 10(4):297–299

[285] Tabarki B, Palmer P, Lebon P, Sébire G. Spontaneous recovery of opsoclonus-myoclonus syndrome caused by enterovirus infection. J Neurol Neurosurg Psychiatry. 1998; 64(3):406–407

[286] Versino M, Mascolo A, Piccolo G, Alloni R, Cosi V. Opsoclonus in a patient with cerebellar dysfunction. J Neuroophthalmol. 1999; 19(4):229–231

[287] Wiest G, Safoschnik G, Schnaberth G, Mueller C. Ocular flutter and truncal ataxia may be associated with enterovirus infection. J Neurol. 1997; 244(5):288–292

[288] Wong A. An update on opsoclonus. Curr Opin Neurol. 2007; 20(1):25–31

[289] Gyllenborg J, Milea D. Ocular flutter as the first manifestation of Lyme disease. Neurology. 2009; 72(3):291

[290] Peter L, Jung J, Tilikete C, Ryvlin P, Mauguiere F. Opsoclonus-myoclonus as a manifestation of Lyme disease. J Neurol Neurosurg Psychiatry. 2006; 77(9):1090–1091

[291] Kruer MC, Hoeftberger R, Lim KY, et al. Aggressive course in encephalitis with opsoclonus, ataxia, chorea, and seizures: the first pediatric case of γ-aminobutyric acid type B receptor autoimmunity. JAMA Neurol. 2014; 71(5):620–623

[292] DeFelipe-Mimbrera A, Masjuan J, Corral Í, Villar LM, Graus F, García-Barragán N. Opsoclonus-myoclonus syndrome and limbic encephalitis associated with GABAB receptor antibodies in CSF. J Neuroimmunol. 2014; 272(1–2):91–93

[293] Player B, Harmelink M, Bordini B, Weisgerber M, Girolami M, Croix M. Pediatric opsoclonus-myoclonus-ataxia syndrome associated with anti-N-methyl-D-aspartate receptor encephalitis. Pediatr Neurol. 2015; 53(5):456–458

[294] Fisher PG, Wechsler DS, Singer HS. Anti-Hu antibody in a neuroblastoma-associated paraneoplastic syndrome. Pediatr Neurol. 1994; 10(4):309–312

[295] Mitchell WG, Snodgrass SR. Opsoclonus-ataxia due to childhood neural crest tumors: a chronic neurologic syndrome. J Child Neurol. 1990; 5(2):153–158

[296] Aggarwal A, Williams D. Opsoclonus as a paraneoplastic manifestation of pancreatic carcinoma. J Neurol Neurosurg Psychiatry. 1997; 63(5):687–688

[297] Bataller L, Graus F, Saiz A, Vilchez JJ, Spanish Opsoclonus-Myoclonus Study Group. Clinical outcome in adult onset idiopathic or paraneoplastic opsoclonus-myoclonus. Brain. 2001; 124(Pt 2):437–443

[298] Caviness JN, Forsyth PA, Layton DD, McPhee TJ. The movement disorder of adult opsoclonus. Mov Disord. 1995; 10(1):22–27

[299] Corcia P, De Toffol B, Hommet C, Saudeau D, Autret A. Paraneoplastic opsoclonus associated with cancer of the gall bladder. J Neurol Neurosurg Psychiatry. 1997; 62(3):293

[300] Honnorat J, Trillet M, Antoine JC, Aguera M, Dalmau J, Graus F. Paraneoplastic opsomyoclonus, cerebellar ataxia and encephalopathy associated with anti-Purkinje cell antibodies. J Neurol. 1997; 244(5):333–335

[301] Hormigo A, Dalmau J, Rosenblum MK, River ME, Posner JB. Immunological and pathological study of anti-Ri-associated encephalopathy. Ann Neurol. 1994; 36(6):896–902

[302] Koukoulis A, Cimas I, Gómara S. Paraneoplastic opsoclonus associated with papillary renal cell carcinoma. J Neurol Neurosurg Psychiatry. 1998; 64(1):137–138

[303] Luque FA, Furneaux HM, Ferziger R, et al. Anti-Ri: an antibody associated with paraneoplastic opsoclonus and breast cancer. Ann Neurol. 1991; 29(3):241–251

[304] Mitoma H, Orimo S, Sodeyama N, Tamaki M. Paraneoplastic opsoclonus-myoclonus syndrome and neurofibrosarcoma. Eur Neurol. 1996; 36(5):322

[305] Schwartz M, Sharf B, Zidan J. Opsoclonus as a presenting symptom in thymic carcinoma. J Neurol Neurosurg Psychiatry. 1990; 53(6):534

[306] Ploner CJ, Kupsch A. Ocular flutter in a patient with intracranial hypertension following cerebral venous thrombosis. Neurology. 2002; 59(6):959

[307] Shaikh AG, Wilmot G. Opsoclonus in a patient with increased titers of anti-GAD antibody provides proof for the conductance-based model of saccadic oscillations. J Neurol Sci. 2016; 362:169–173

[308] Galli JR, Clardy SL, Paz Soldán MM. Adult-onset opsoclonus-myoclonus syndrome associated with ganglionic acetylcholine receptor autoantibody. Neurologist. 2016; 21(6):99–100

[309] Blaes F, Jauss M, Kraus J, et al. Adult paraneoplastic opsoclonus-myoclonus syndrome associated with antimitochondrial autoantibodies. J Neurol Neurosurg Psychiatry. 2003; 74(11):1595–1596

[310] Boland T, Strause J, Hu M, et al. Posterior reversible encephalopathy syndrome presenting as opsoclonus-myoclonus. Neuroophthalmology. 2012; 36(4):149–152

[311] Schon F, Hodgson TL, Mort D, Kennard C. Ocular flutter associated with a localized lesion in the paramedian pontine reticular formation. Ann Neurol. 2001; 50(3):413–416

[312] Lubec D, Finsterer J, Müllbacher W, et al. Opsoclonus as a dominant sign in primary Sjögren's syndrome. Neuro-ophthalmology. 1999; 22(3):135–138

[313] Carstairs SD, Schneir AB. Images in clinical medicine. Opsoclonus due to diphenhydramine poisoning. N Engl J Med. 2010; 363(27):e40

[314] Irioka T, Yamanami A, Uchida N, Iwase M, Yasuhara H, Mizusawa H. Opsoclonus caused by diphenhydramine self-poisoning. J Neuroophthalmol. 2009; 29(1):72–73

[315] Apsner R, Schulenburg A, Steinhoff N, et al. Cyclosporin A-induced ocular flutter after marrow transplantation. Bone Marrow Transplant. 1997; 20(3):255–256

[316] Marchiori PE, Mies S, Scaff M. Cyclosporine A-induced ocular opsoclonus and reversible leukoencephalopathy after orthotopic liver transplantation: brief report. Clin Neuropharmacol. 2004; 27(4):195–197

[317] Fisher CM. Ocular flutter. J Clin Neuroophthalmol. 1990; 10(2):155–156

[318] Vigliani MC, Palmucci L, Polo P, et al. Paraneoplastic opsoclonus-myoclonus associated with renal cell carcinoma and responsive to tumour ablation. J Neurol Neurosurg Psychiatry. 2001; 70(6):814–815

[319] Pless M, Ronthal M. Treatment of opsoclonus-myoclonus with high-dose intravenous immunoglobulin. Neurology. 1996; 46(2):583–584

[320] Ishikawa H, Ishikawa S, Mukuno K. Short-cycle periodic alternating (ping-pong) gaze. Neurology. 1993; 43(6):1067–1070

[321] Crevits L, Decruyenaere J. "Ping-pong" gaze. Neuroophthalmology. 1992; 12: 121–123

[322] Johkura K, Komiyama A, Tobita M, Hasegawa O. Saccadic ping-pong gaze. J Neuroophthalmol. 1998; 18(1):43–46

[323] Simon RP, Aminoff MJ. Electrographic status epilepticus in fatal anoxic coma. Ann Neurol. 1986; 20(3):351–355

[324] Dehaene I, Lammens M, Marchau M. Paretic ocular bobbing. A clinico-pathological study of two cases. Neuro-ophthalmology. 1993; 13(3):143–146

[325] Gaymard B. Disconjugate ocular bobbing. Neurology. 1993; 43(10):2151

[326] Toshniwal P, Yadava R, Goldbarg H. Presentation of pinealoblastoma with ocular dipping and deafness. J Clin Neuroophthalmol. 1986; 6(2):128–136

[327] Shimazaki H, Morita M, Nakano I, Dalmau J. Inverse ocular bobbing in a patient with encephalitis associated with antibodies to the N-methyl-D-aspartate receptor. Arch Neurol. 2008; 65(9):1251

[328] Lennox G. Reverse ocular bobbing due to combined phenothiazine and benzodiazepine poisoning. J Neurol Neurosurg Psychiatry. 1993; 56(10): 1136–1137

[329] Keane JR. Pretectal pseudobobbing. Five patients with 'V'-pattern convergence nystagmus. Arch Neurol. 1985; 42(6):592–594

[330] Komiyama A, Toda H, Johkura K, Kataoka M, Yamamoto I. Pretectal pseudo-bobbing associated with an expanding posterior fossa cyst in tectocerebellar dysraphia: an electro-oculographic study. J Neurol. 1999; 246(3):221–223

[331] Keane JR. Acute vertical ocular myoclonus. Neurology. 1986; 36(1):86–89

18 Ptosis

Angeline Mariani Derham

Abstract

Ptosis is the abnormal drooping of one or both eyelids. It may be congenital or acquired, and isolated or associated with additional neurological features. This chapter discusses the clinical pathways in evaluating and diagnosing ptosis, by reviewing the literature in detail.

Keywords: ptosis, apraxia of eyelid opening, aponeurosis dehiscence, levator palpebrae superioris, pseudoptosis

18.1 Introduction

The causes of ptosis may be classified as mechanical, myogenic, neurogenic, neuromuscular junctional, or iatrogenic.[1,2] The first step in assessing an apparent ptosis is to determine whether the ptosis is real or pseudoptosis. Next, distinguishing between congenital or acquired and isolated or nonisolated forms of ptosis will guide evaluation and management. An approach to the evaluation of ptosis is outlined in ▶ Fig. 18.1.

18.2 What Is Pseudoptosis?

A number of conditions may cause downward displacement of the eyelid without true ptosis (pseudoptosis) including aberrant regeneration of the facial nerve, an anophthalmic socket, eyelid apraxia, downgaze paralysis, facial or eyelid spasms, hypertropia, hyperglobus, lash ptosis, contralateral lid retraction, microphthalmia, phthisis bulbi, and psychogenic pseudoptosis (Box 18.1).

Box 18.1 Causes of pseudoptosis

- Aberrant regeneration of the facial nerve.
- Anophthalmic socket.[3,4]
- Apraxia of lid opening.
- Downgaze paralysis and pseudoblepharoptosis.
- Blepharospasm or hemifacial spasm.
- Hypertropia or hyperglobus.
- Lash ptosis in floppy eyelid syndrome.[5,6]
- Lid retraction in the contralateral eye.[7,8]
- Microphthalmia or phthisis bulbi.
- Psychogenic pseudoptosis.[9]

Eye positioning or eye size alone may account for the pseudoptosis. Hypertropia or hyperglobus may result in an abnormal position of the eye under a normal eyelid. Fixation with the hypertropic eye may eliminate the pseudoptosis. In cases of reduced ocular surface area, such as microphthalmia or phthisis bulbi, the eyelid may appear to transverse more distance toward the center of the pupil. Anophthalmic sockets also produce a pseudoptosis due to the absence of ocular tissue and a decrease in levator function.[3,4]

Ptosis must be considered in the context of bilateral eyelid and globe symmetry and surrounding eye creases.[10] Eyelid retraction (e.g., thyroid eye disease) in one eye may produce an apparent ptosis (pseudoptosis) in the fellow (normal) eye.[7,8] Acquired ptosis can also cause mild retraction of the contralateral lid.[11] Acquisition of old imaging may be essential to determine the pathologic lid.[12] Manually lowering the retracted pathologic lid might allow the normal lid to elevate. Malfunction of the orbicularis oculi muscle may result in pseudoptosis. Involuntary lid closure, such as blepharospasm or hemifacial spasm, may produce a pseudoptosis due to the intermittent closure of the upper and lower eyelid(s) resulting from contraction of the orbicularis oculi muscles. The lid position during the periods without contraction of the orbicularis muscles is normal. A similar mechanism is true for aberrant regeneration of the facial nerve, where increased orbicularis tone may give rise to pseudoptosis. In this condition, ptosis will worsen during cheek puffing maneuvers.[13] Voluntary lid closure occurring in the context of a conversion-reaction may create pseudoptosis. In these cases, downward movement of the eyebrow is usually apparent.[9]

18.3 What Is Eyelid Apraxia?

Apraxia of eyelid opening is a supranuclear inability to open the eyelids voluntarily. Unilateral or bilateral hemispheric disease and extrapyramidal disease may produce apraxia of lid opening. The etiologies of apraxia of eye opening are listed in Box 18.2. Because spontaneous and reflex eyelid opening are normal, patients may manually open the lids or employ a head thrust as a compensatory movement.[14,15,16]

Box 18.2 Etiologies of apraxia of eyelid opening

- Extrapyramidal disease:
  - Parkinson disease.
  - MPTP(1-methyl-4-phenyl-1,2,3,6 tetrahydropyridine)-induced parkinsonism.
  - Progressive autosomal-dominant parkinsonism and dementia with pallido-ponto-nigral degeneration.[17]
  - Huntington's disease.
  - Multiple systems atrophy (e.g., Shy–Drager syndrome).
  - Progressive supranuclear palsy.
  - Wilson disease.
  - Neuroacanthocytosis.
  - Cortical-basal ganglionic degeneration.[18]
  - Pantothenate kinase-associated neurodegeneration.
  - Amyotrophic lateral sclerosis-parkinsonism-dementia complex.
- Unilateral (especially nondominant hemisphere) or bilateral hemispheric lesions.[19]
- Focal inferior and lateral frontal lobe cortical degeneration.[20]
- Motor neuron disease.[21,22]
- Postbilateral stereotactic subthalamotomy.[23]

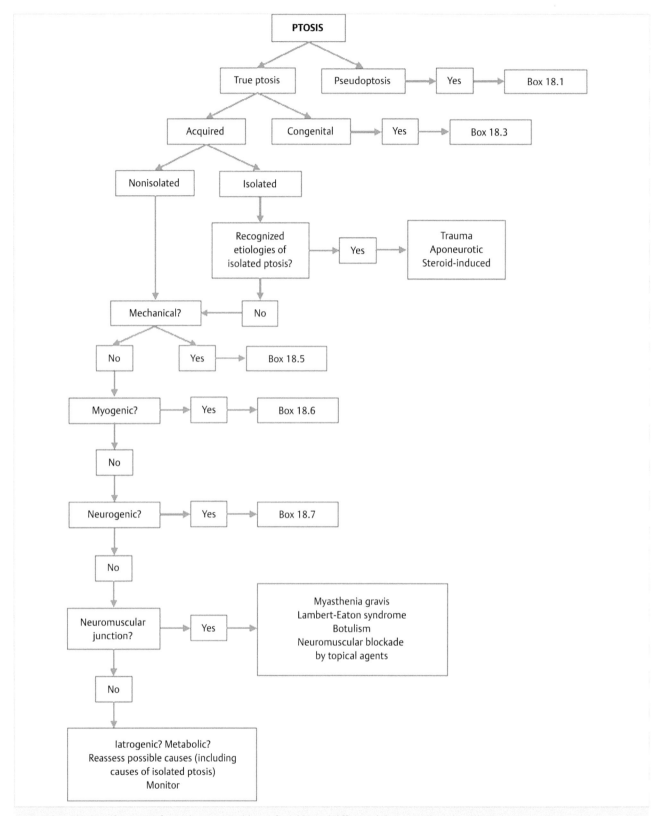

Fig. 18.1 Evaluation of ptosis. Refer to the associated boxes for additional differential diagnosis to guide evaluation.

- Postimplantation of bilateral subthalamic nucleus electrical stimulators.[24]
- Basal ganglia lesion:[25]
  - Unilateral putaminal hemorrhage.[26]
  - Unilateral lesions of the globus pallidus.
- Unilateral thalamic lesions.
- Anti-MA1/anti-MA2 antibody-associated encephalitis.
- Anti-Hu antibody encephalitis (paraneoplastic syndrome).[27]
- Acquired immune deficiency syndrome (AIDS).
- Benign unilateral apraxia of lid opening.[28]
- Isolated finding (may be levodopa responsive).[29]

Aramideh et al correlated the clinical findings of apraxia of eye opening with synchronous levator palpebrae (LP) and orbicularis oculi (OOc) electromyographic (EMG) recordings.[30] EMG was characterized by either intermittent LP inhibition (ILPI) or a continuation of OOc activity[31] following voluntary closure of the eyes (pretarsal motor persistence [PMP]). This study demonstrated the following:

1. In some patients, intermittent involuntary eye closure as a result of ILPI interferes with eye opening. When there is no ILPI, patients have no difficulty opening their eyes at will after voluntary closure.
2. In other patients, closure of the eyes due to ILPI may activate OOc. These patients have PMP in addition to ILPI and are unable to open their eyes at will following voluntary closure.
3. Patients who have PMP alone may be unable to open their eyes at will following voluntary closure but once open, eye opening can be sustained.

18.4 Is the Ptosis Congenital or Acquired?

Ptosis may occur on a congenital or acquired basis. Long-standing isolated and static congenital ptosis with no other signs of systemic neurogenic (e.g., third nerve palsy), myogenic (e.g., chronic progressive external ophthalmoplegia [CPEO]), or neuromuscular disease (e.g., myasthenia gravis) do not typically require additional evaluation. Other forms of congenital nonisolated ptosis necessitate the same evaluation as the patients with acquired nonisolated ptosis. Box 18.3 lists the various forms of congenital ptosis. Congenital ptosis may be associated with other ocular and nonocular defects.

Box 18.3 Congenital ptosis

- Isolated.
- Nonisolated or syndromic (e.g., Cornelia de Lange syndrome,[32] Jacobsen syndrome,[33] Noonan syndrome[34]).
- Associated ocular defects:
  - Congenital cataracts.
  - Blepharophimosis.[35]
  - Epicanthus inversus.
  - Punctal abnormalities.
  - Telecanthus.
  - Refractive error/anisometropia.
  - Strabismus and amblyopia.

- Associated nonocular defects (e.g., skeletal, central nervous system [CNS]):
  - Craniofacial anomalies.
  - Synkinetic ptosis (e.g., Marcus Gunn jaw-winking ptosis).
  - Myogenic (e.g., congenital fibrosis).
  - Neurogenic (e.g., third nerve palsy).
  - Neuromuscular junction (e.g., myasthenia gravis).
  - Combined valproate and hydantoin embryopathy with anomalous septum pellucidum.[36]
- X-linked congenital isolated ptosis.[37,38]

Although children with congenital ptosis in isolation do not usually require any further evaluation, they may need amblyopia treatment or surgical therapy to avoid amblyopia.[39,40,41,42,43] Intermittent lid retraction of a ptotic eyelid may occur during chewing, jaw movement, or sucking in a child due to aberrant innervation of the oculomotor (levator) and trigeminal nerves (synkinesis, the Marcus Gunn jaw-winking phenomenon). No additional evaluation is required in children with the jaw-winking phenomenon (class IV, level C). Patients with acquired forms of ptosis, including acquired synkinesis, should undergo further diagnostic evaluation (class III–IV, level B).

18.5 Is the Ptosis Isolated or Nonisolated?

A nonisolated acquired ptosis is defined as ptosis associated with other findings that may suggest a specific etiology, including mechanical, myogenic, neurogenic, or neuromuscular junction disease (Box 18.4). The causes of isolated ptosis include congenital ptosis, trauma (including surgery), steroid-induced ptosis, and aponeurotic ptosis. Intermittent isolated ptosis can rarely be associated with ophthalmoplegic migraine.[44] Ptosis may be the only sign/symptom of a more pervasive disease (e.g., myasthenia gravis).

Box 18.4 Etiologies of nonisolated ptosis

- Mechanical (e.g., lid mass, infection, or inflammation).
- Myogenic (e.g., external ophthalmoplegia).
- Neurogenic (e.g., ocular motor deficit and/or diplopia, other neurologic findings, Horner syndrome).
- Neuromuscular junction disease (e.g., signs of myasthenia gravis such as fatigue, enhancement, variability, Cogan lid twitch sign).

18.6 Is the Ptosis Due to Mechanical Causes?

Any mechanical disturbance of the upper eyelid may result in ptosis. Mechanical causes of ptosis are listed in Box 18.5. Traumatic injury may damage the skin, soft tissues, muscles, and levator complex creating a ptosis that is caused by either the initial insult or resultant scarring.[45] Patients with a mechanical ptosis that might be due to an underlying mass or infiltrative lesion should undergo imaging of the orbit (e.g., magnetic resonance imaging of the head and orbit with fat suppression and gadolinium contrast) (class IV, level C). An important sign suggesting malignancy infiltration of upper orbital tissue is a "hang-up" of the upper eyelid on downgaze.[46] Palpation of the lid is important in these cases.

Box 18.5 Mechanical causes of ptosis

- Redundant skin or fat on the upper eyelid (e.g., dermatochalasis).
- Tumors or cysts of the conjunctiva or eyelid.
- Infection (e.g., preseptal or orbital cellulitis; cysticercosis,[47,48] aspergillosis[49,50]).
- Cicatricial scarring (e.g., posttraumatic, postsurgical,[51] or postinflammatory).
- Inflammation and edema:
  - Graves disease.
  - Blepharochalasis.
  - Dermatomyositis.
  - Pachydermoperiostosis.[52,53]
  - Orbital inflammatory syndrome (orbital pseudotumor).
- Infiltration:
  - Amyloid.
  - Sarcoidosis.
  - Neoplastic (e.g., lymphoma, breast cancer[54]).
  - Waldenström macroglobulinemia.[55]
- Primary or metastatic tumors:
  - Neurofibroma.[56]
  - Schwannoma.
  - Hemangioma.
  - Dermoid.
  - Lymphoma.
- Contact lenses related:[1,57,58,59]
  - Foreign body reaction.
  - Blink-related microtrauma.[60]
  - Giant papillary conjunctivitis (GPC).
  - Contact lens migration.
  - Disinsertion of the levator from excessive eyelid manipulation.

---

fluid protein, other neurologic dysfunction (e.g., cerebellar, auditory, and vestibular dysfunction), cognitive dysfunction, short stature, and developmental delay. Muscle biopsy may show "ragged red fibers" or other changes in mitochondria.[61,62] Pathologic examination of the brain may demonstrate spongiform degeneration but is generally not required for the diagnosis.

Other systemic and ocular myopathies may cause ptosis but are usually associated with myopathic signs and symptoms due to involvement of extraocular and other muscles.[63] Detailed discussion of these myogenic forms of ptosis is beyond the scope of this text. Myopathies that may cause ptosis are listed in Box 18.6.

Box 18.6 Myopathies associated with ptosis

- CPEO.[64]
- Congenital fibrosis.[65,66,67]
- Myopathy:
  - Central core myopathy.
  - Centronuclear myopathy.
  - Multicore myopathy.
  - Nemaline myopathy.
  - Fiber-type disproportion.
  - Congenital muscular dystrophy.
  - Myotonia congenita and myotonic dystrophy.[68]
  - Oculopharyngeal muscular dystrophy.[69,70,71]
  - Inflammatory and infiltrative myopathies.
  - Hypothyroid myopathy.
  - Epidermolysis bullosa simplex associated with muscular dystrophy (EBS-MD).[72]
  - 3-Hydroxy-3-methyl-glutaryl coenzyme A reductase inhibitor-associated myopathy ("statin myopathy").
  - Rapidly progressive adolescent-onset oculopharyngeal somatic syndrome with rimmed vacuoles.[73]
- Diabetes (possibly due to hypoxia to levator).
- Familial periodic paralysis.
- Late-onset glycogenosis type II (acid maltase deficiency).[74]
- Lyme-associated orbital inflammation.[75]

18.7 Is the Ptosis Due to Myogenic Causes?

CPEO includes a spectrum of disorders that may result in a syndrome of painless, pupil-sparing, slowly progressive, and generally symmetric ophthalmoplegia often accompanied by ptosis. One subset of CPEO, the Kearns–Sayre syndrome, is characterized by the clinical triad of early-onset (usually before the age of 20 years) CPEO, pigmentary degeneration of the retina, and cardiac abnormalities (e.g., intraventricular conduction defects, bundle branch block, and complete heart block). Other features of Kearns–Sayre syndrome include elevation of cerebrospinal

18.8 Is the Ptosis Due to a Neurogenic Cause?

The neurogenic causes of ptosis are listed in Box 18.7. Denervation of the levator muscle due to a third nerve palsy may result in partial or complete ptosis. Levator excursion is decreased in all of these patients. As noted in Chapter 11, nuclear third nerve palsies result in bilateral ptosis or no ptosis because both levator muscles are innervated by a single central caudal nucleus. This type of ptosis is usually associated with other features of a third nerve palsy (e.g., pupil involvement, extraocular muscle dysfunction), but may rarely occur with other minimal third nerve signs.[76,77]

Box 18.7 Neurogenic conditions associated with ptosis

- Third nerve palsy:[78]
  - With or without partial or complete ophthalmoplegia.
  - With or without aberrant regeneration.
- Alternating ptosis in abetalipoproteinemia.
- Brainstem infarct.
- Horner syndrome.
- Miller Fisher syndrome.[79,80,81,82,83]
- Acute inflammatory polyradiculoneuropathy (Guillain–Barré syndrome).
- Chronic inflammatory polyradiculoneuropathy (CIDP).
- Cerebral ptosis.
- Cerebellar ptosis following craniovertebral decompression of Chiari I malformation.[84]
- Minor head trauma in patient with chronic hydrocephalus (supranuclear ptosis).[85]
- Midbrain lesion.[86,87,88]
- Hemispheric lesion.[89,90,91]
- Putaminal hemorrhage.[26]
- Paradoxic supranuclear inhibition of levator tonus.
- Seizure-induced.[92]
- Wernicke encephalopathy (thiamine deficiency).
- Recurrent isolated ptosis (lasting 6–10 weeks) in presumed ophthalmoplegic migraine of childhood.[93]
- Relapsing alternating ptosis (episodes lasting days).[94]

Sources: Zachariah.[91]

Ptosis and ipsilateral miosis may be due to a Horner syndrome. The associated features of the Horner syndrome are discussed in more detail in Chapter 20.

The Miller Fisher variant of Guillain–Barré syndrome of acute inflammatory demyelinating polyneuropathy may present with supranuclear ptosis, ophthalmoplegia, ataxia, and areflexia.[79,80,81,83]

Unilateral or bilateral hemispheric dysfunction (e.g., stroke, arteriovenous malformation, seizure) may produce supranuclear ptosis.[89,90,91,92] Midbrain lesions may result in ptosis with or without downgaze paralysis, fatigable ptosis,[95,96] or pseudoptosis.[86,97,98,99,100]

Primary headache disorders, such as cluster headaches, ophthalmic migraines, and hemicrania continua, can be associated with a transient ptosis but generally is a diagnosis of exclusion.[44]

18.9 Is the Ptosis Due to Neuromuscular Junction Disease?

Myasthenia gravis may result in a ptosis that is often variable and may worsen after sustained effort or fatigue. Fatigable ptosis, however, has also been reported in patients with intracranial etiologies (e.g., hematoma, metastasis).[95] As noted in Chapter 15, myasthenia gravis may result in ptosis with or without other extraocular muscle dysfunction. Other rare causes of neuromuscular junction ptosis include wound botulism, Lambert–Eaton syndrome, and topical neuromuscular

blockade (e.g., topical timolol).[101] We recommend that myasthenia gravis be considered in every case of unexplained, painless, unilateral, or bilateral ptosis with or without ophthalmoplegia (class IV, level C).

18.10 Is the Ptosis Iatrogenic?

Surgical trauma and/or myotoxicity from local anesthetic agents during dental, orbital, or ocular (including strabismus, retinal, corneal, cataract, glaucoma, and refractive) procedures may damage the eyelid structures and cause ptosis.[102,103,104,105,106] Kaplan et al performed a prospective analysis of ptosis and cataract surgery, and found that trauma to the superior rectus complex was the most critical factor.[107]

Even surgical manipulation as mild as lid speculum use can cause postoperative ptosis.[102,105] A patient with a narrower vertical palpebral aperture may be at increased risk for postoperative lid ptosis due to greater mechanical compression.[108]

Topical steroids have been implicated in some cases of ptosis.[109] Discontinuation of the steroids may reverse the ptosis in these cases. Sub-Tenon injection of steroids has been linked to ptosis due to orbital fat prolapse, dehiscence of the levator aponeurosis, and myopathy.[106,110,111,112]

Various types of cosmetic or therapeutic botulinum toxin treatments can also result in ptosis, usually temporarily but lasting months in some cases.[113,114,115,116,117,118] Apraclonidine eye drops may be used for symptomatic treatment of mild ptosis.[119] Botox-induced ptosis may be intentionally achieved to chemodenervate the levator muscle as corneal protection for conditions such as dry eye and corneal ulcers, and to achieve facial symmetry after Bell's palsy.[120,121]

18.11 Is Aponeurotic Ptosis Present?

Levator aponeurosis thinning and/or dehiscence may occur as a result of trauma, surgery, lid swelling, contact lens wear, patching, or, most commonly, as an age-related phenomenon.[122,123,124,125] Aponeurotic ptosis is acquired, often bilateral, with maintained levator function despite thinning of the eyelid above the tarsus and an elevated or absent lid crease (Box 18.8).

Box 18.8 Clinical features of aponeurotic ptosis

- Acquired.
- Good to excellent levator function (>12 mm).
- Elevated or absent lid crease.
- Thinning of the eyelid above the tarsus.
- Bilateral but may be unilateral or asymmetric.
- Elderly population.

Patients with aponeurotic ptosis may have significant ptosis in downgaze more than primary position.[126,127] The levator function is typically normal or near normal, the lid crease may be high and indistinct, and there may be a deep superior sulcus in age-related levator dehiscence. In the absence of findings to suggest mechanical, neurogenic, myogenic, or neuromuscular etiologies for ptosis, no further evaluation is necessary. Superior visual field loss may occur due to ptosis and may be an indication for surgical correction. The surgical treatment of aponeurotic ptosis is well described in the literature and is not reviewed here.[122,123,125] Aponeurotic ptosis does not require any neuroimaging (class III–IV, level B).

18.12 Is Ptosis Due to an Underlying Metabolic Disturbance?

Acute onset ptosis in an adult may result from various metabolic disturbances. Ptosis may also accompany transient physiologic states such as pregnancy or manifest as a response to metabolic stress such as in anorexia nervosa.[128,129,130] The high activity of metabolic activity in the extraocular muscles and eyelids can explain why ptosis may be striking in glycogen storage and mitochondrial diseases.[131] In these disease states, ptosis is often an early symptom, which is why they can be misdiagnosed as juvenile myasthenia gravis.[132]

References

[1] Kersten RC, de Conciliis C, Kulwin DR. Acquired ptosis in the young and middle-aged adult population. Ophthalmology. 1995; 102(6):924–928

[2] Oosterhuis HJ. Acquired blepharoptosis. Clin Neurol Neurosurg. 1996; 98(1):1–7

[3] Kaltreider SA, Shields MD, Hippeard SC, Patrie J. Anophthalmic ptosis: investigation of the mechanisms and statistical analysis. Ophthal Plast Reconstr Surg. 2003; 19(6):421–428

[4] Kim NJ, Khwarg SI. Decrease in levator function in the anophthalmic orbit. Ophthalmologica. 2008; 222(5):351–356

[5] Ezra DG, Beaconsfield M, Sira M, Bunce C, Wormald R, Collin R. The associations of floppy eyelid syndrome: a case control study. Ophthalmology. 2010; 117(4):831–838

[6] Sredkova MI. Lash ptosis as a characteristic sign of floppy eyelid syndrome. Folia Med. 2014; 56:170–174

[7] Kratky V, Harvey JT. Tests for contralateral pseudoretraction in blepharoptosis. Ophthal Plast Reconstr Surg. 1992; 8(1):22–25

[8] Lyon DB, Gonnering RS, Dortzbach RK, Lemke BN. Unilateral ptosis and eye dominance. Ophthal Plast Reconstr Surg. 1993; 9(4):237–240

[9] Hop JW, Frijns CJ, van Gijn J. Psychogenic pseudoptosis. J Neurol. 1997; 244 (10):623–624

[10] Ting SL, Koay AC, Yew YH, Chua CN. Challenges in diagnosis and management of pseudoptosis secondary to asymmetrical skin creases. Med J Malaysia. 2011; 66(2):121–123

[11] Meyer DR, Wobig JL. Detection of contralateral eyelid retraction associated with blepharoptosis. Ophthalmology. 1992; 99(3):366–375

[12] Mittal MK, Sloan JA, Rabinstein AA. Facebook: can it be a diagnostic tool for neurologists? BMJ Case Rep. 2012; 2012:bcr2012006426

[13] Chen C, Malhotra R, Muecke J, Davis G, Selva D. Aberrant facial nerve regeneration (AFR): an under-recognized cause of ptosis. Eye (Lond). 2004; 18(2):159–162

[14] Boghen D. Apraxia of lid opening: a review. Neurology. 1997; 48(6):1491–1494

[15] Jancovic J. Apraxia of lid opening. Mov Disord. 1995; 10:5

[16] Krack P, Marion MH. "Apraxia of lid opening," a focal eyelid dystonia: clinical study of 32 patients. Mov Disord. 1994; 9(6):610–615

[17] Wszolek ZK, Pfeiffer RF, Bhatt MH, et al. Rapidly progressive autosomal dominant parkinsonism and dementia with pallido-ponto-nigral degeneration. Ann Neurol. 1992; 32(3):312–320

[18] Riley DE, Lang AE, Lewis A, et al. Cortical-basal ganglionic degeneration. Neurology. 1990; 40(8):1203–1212

[19] Nazarian SM, Amiri M. Apraxia of eyelid opening in right hemisphere stroke. Neuroophthalmology. 1998; 20:25

[20] Adair JC, Williamson DJG, Heilman KM. Eyelid opening apraxia in focal cortical degeneration. J Neurol Neurosurg Psychiatry. 1995; 58(4):508–509

[21] Abe K, Fujimura H, Tatsumi C, Toyooka K, Yorifuji S, Yanagihara T. Eyelid "apraxia" in patients with motor neuron disease. J Neurol Neurosurg Psychiatry. 1995; 59(6):629–632

[22] Averbuch-Heller L, Helmchen C, Horn AKE, Leigh RJ, Büttner-Ennerver JA. Slow vertical saccades in motor neuron disease: correlation of structure and function. Ann Neurol. 1998; 44(4):641–648

[23] Klostermann W, Vieregge P, Kömpf D. Apraxia of eyelid opening after bilateral stereotaxic subthalamotomy. J Neuroophthalmol. 1997; 17(2):122–123

[24] Limousin P, Krack P, Pollak P, et al. Electrical stimulation of the subthalamic nucleus in advanced Parkinson's disease. N Engl J Med. 1998; 339(16):1105–1111

[25] Hirose M, Mochizuki H, Honma M, Kobayashi T, Nishizawa M, Ugawa Y. Apraxia of lid opening due to a small lesion in basal ganglia: two case reports. J Neurol Neurosurg Psychiatry. 2010; 81(12):1406–1407

[26] Verghese J, Milling C, Rosenbaum DM. Ptosis, blepharospasm, and apraxia of eyelid opening secondary to putaminal hemorrhage. Neurology. 1999; 53(3):652

[27] Choe CH, Gausas RE. Blepharospasm and apraxia of eyelid opening associated with anti-Hu paraneoplastic antibodies: a case report. Ophthalmology. 2012; 119(4):865–868

[28] Cherian V, Foroozan R. Benign unilateral apraxia of eyelid opening. Ophthalmology. 2010; 117(6):1265–1268

[29] Dewey RB, Jr, Maraganore DM. Isolated eyelid-opening apraxia: report of a new levodopa-responsive syndrome. Neurology. 1994; 44(9):1752–1754

[30] Aramideh M, Ongerboer de Visser BW, Koelman JH, Speelman JD. Motor persistence of orbicularis oculi muscle in eyelid-opening disorders. Neurology. 1995; 45(5):897–902

[31] Tozlovanu V, Forget R, Iancu A, Boghen D. Prolonged orbicularis oculi activity: a major factor in apraxia of lid opening. Neurology. 2001; 57(6):1013–1018

[32] Wygnanski-Jaffe T, Shin J, Perruzza E, Abdolell M, Jackson LG, Levin AV. Ophthalmologic findings in the Cornelia de Lange Syndrome. J AAPOS. 2005; 9(5):407–415

[33] Lee WB, O'Halloran HS, Grossfeld PD, Scher C, Jockin YM, Jones C. Ocular findings in Jacobsen syndrome. J AAPOS. 2004; 8(2):141–145

[34] van der Burgt I. Noonan syndrome. Orphanet J Rare Dis. 2007; 2:4

[35] Allen CE, Rubin PA. Blepharophimosis-ptosis-epicanthus inversus syndrome (BPES): clinical manifestation and treatment. Int Ophthalmol Clin. 2008; 48(2):15–23

[36] Gigantelli JW, Braddock SR, Johnson LN. Blepharoptosis and central nervous system abnormalities in combined valproate and hydantoin embryopathy. Ophthal Plast Reconstr Surg. 2000; 16(1):52–54

[37] McMullan TF, Collins AR, Tyers AG, Robinson DO. A novel X-linked dominant condition: X-linked congenital isolated ptosis. Am J Hum Genet. 2000; 66(4):1455–1460

[38] McMullan TF, Tyers AG. X linked dominant congenital isolated bilateral ptosis: the definition and characterisation of a new condition. Br J Ophthalmol. 2001; 85(1):70–73

[39] Cibis GW, Fitzgerald KM. Amblyopia in unilateral congenital ptosis: early detection by sweep visual evoked potential. Graefes Arch Clin Exp Ophthalmol. 1995; 233(10):605–609

[40] Gusek-Schneider GC, Martus P. Stimulus deprivation amblyopia in human congenital ptosis: a study of 100 patients. Strabismus. 2000; 8(4):261–270

[41] Hornblass A, Kass LG, Ziffer AJ. Amblyopia in congenital ptosis. Ophthalmic Surg. 1995; 26(4):334–337

[42] McCulloch DL, Wright KW. Unilateral congenital ptosis: compensatory head posturing and amblyopia. Ophthal Plast Reconstr Surg. 1993; 9(3):196–200

[43] Steel DH, Harrad RA. Unilateral congenital ptosis with ipsilateral superior rectus muscle overaction. Am J Ophthalmol. 1996; 122(4):550–556

[44] Gulkilik G, Cagatay HH, Oba EM, Uslu C. Ophthalmoplegic migraine associated with recurrent isolated ptosis. Ann Ophthalmol (Skokie). 2009; 41(3–4):206–207

[45] Keane JR. Ptosis and levator paralysis caused by orbital roof fractures. Three cases with subfrontal epidural hematomas. J Clin Neuroophthalmol. 1993; 13(4):225–228

[46] Uddin JM, Rose GE. Downgaze "hang-up" of the upper eyelid in patients with adult-onset ptosis: an important sign of possible orbital malignancy. Ophthalmology. 2003; 110(7):1433–1436

[47] Basu S, Muthusami S, Kumar A. Ocular cysticercosis: an unusual cause of ptosis. Singapore Med J. 2009; 50(8):e309–e311

[48] Labh RK, Sharma AK. Ptosis: a rare presentation of ocular cysticercosis. Nepal J Ophthalmol. 2013; 5(1):133–135

[49] Kim JW, Rha MS, Kim JH, Kang JW. Orbital apex syndrome caused by invasive aspergillosis. J Craniofac Surg. 2014; 25(2):e191–e193

[50] Wipfler P, Pilz G, Golaszewski S, et al. Invasive aspergillosis presenting with a painless complete ophthalmoplegia. Clin Neurol Neurosurg. 2010; 112(1):85–87

[51] Singh SK, Sekhar GC, Gupta S. Etiology of ptosis after cataract surgery. J Cataract Refract Surg. 1997; 23(9):1409–1413

[52] Ding J, Li B, Chen T, Hao L, Li D. Eyelid thickening and ptosis associated with pachydermoperiostosis: a case report and review of literature. Aesthetic Plast Surg. 2013; 37(2):464–467

[53] Neufeld KR, Price K, Woodward JA. Massive eyelid thickening in pachydermoperiostosis with myelofibrosis. Ophthal Plast Reconstr Surg. 2009; 25(4):316–318

[54] Po SM, Custer PL, Smith ME. Bilateral lagophthalmos. An unusual presentation of metastatic breast carcinoma. Arch Ophthalmol. 1996; 114(9):1139–1141

[55] Klapper SR, Jordan DR, Pelletier C, Brownstein S, Punja K. Ptosis in Waldenström's macroglobulinemia. Am J Ophthalmol. 1998; 126(2):315–317

[56] Avisar R, Leshem Y, Savir H. Unilateral congenital ptosis due to plexiform neurofibroma, causing refraction error and secondary amblyopia. Metab Pediatr Syst Ophthalmol (1985). 1991; 14(3–4):62–63

[57] Levy B, Stamper RL. Acute ptosis secondary to contact lens wear. Optom Vis Sci. 1992; 69(7):565–566

[58] Patel NP, Savino PJ, Weinberg DA. Unilateral eyelid ptosis and a red eye. Surv Ophthalmol. 1998; 43(2):182–187

[59] van den Bosch WA, Lemij HG. Blepharoptosis induced by prolonged hard contact lens wear. Ophthalmology. 1992; 99(12):1759–1765

[60] Cher I. Blink-related microtrauma: when the ocular surface harms itself. Clin Experiment Ophthalmol. 2003; 31(3):183–190

[61] Gross-Jendroska M, Schatz H, McDonald HR, Johnson RN. Kearns-Sayre syndrome: a case report and review. Eur J Ophthalmol. 1992; 2(1):15–20 (review)

[62] Simonsz HJ, Bärlocher K, Rötig A. Kearns-Sayre's syndrome developing in a boy who survived Pearson's syndrome caused by mitochondrial DNA deletion. Doc Ophthalmol. 1992; 82(1–2):73–79

[63] Parmeggiani A, Posar A, Leonardi M, Rossi PG. Neurological impairment in congenital bilateral ptosis with ophthalmoplegia. Brain Dev. 1992; 14(2):107–109

[64] Ohtaki E, Yamaguchi Y, Yamashita Y, et al. Complete external ophthalmoplegia in a patient with congenital myopathy without specific features (minimal change myopathy). Brain Dev. 1990; 12(4):427–430

[65] Engle EC, Marondel I, Houtman WA, et al. Congenital fibrosis of the extraocular muscles (autosomal dominant congenital external ophthalmoplegia): genetic homogeneity, linkage refinement, and physical mapping on chromosome 12. Am J Hum Genet. 1995; 57(5):1086–1094

[66] Gillies WE, Harris AJ, Brooks AM, Rivers MR, Wolfe RJ. Congenital fibrosis of the vertically acting extraocular muscles. A new group of dominantly inherited ocular fibrosis with radiologic findings. Ophthalmology. 1995; 102(4):607–612

[67] Tandon RK, Burke JP, Strachan IM. Unilateral congenital fibrosis syndrome presenting with hypertropia. Acta Ophthalmol (Copenh). 1993; 71(6):860–862

[68] Ashizawa T, Hejtmancik JF, Liu J, Perryman MB, Epstein HF, Koch DD. Diagnostic value of ophthalmologic findings in myotonic dystrophy: comparison with risks calculated by haplotype analysis of closely linked restriction fragment length polymorphisms. Am J Med Genet. 1992; 42(1):55–60

[69] Blumen SC, Nisipeanu P, Sadeh M, Asherov A, Tomé FM, Korczyn AD. Clinical features of oculopharyngeal muscular dystrophy among Bukhara Jews. Neuromuscul Disord. 1993; 3(5–6):575–577

[70] Lacomis D, Kupsky WJ, Kuban KK, Specht LA. Childhood onset oculopharyngeal muscular dystrophy. Pediatr Neurol. 1991; 7(5):382–384

[71] Rowland LP, Hirano M, DiMauro S, Schon EA. Oculopharyngeal muscular dystrophy, other ocular myopathies, and progressive external ophthalmoplegia. Neuromuscul Disord. 1997; 7 Suppl 1:S15–S21

[72] Auringer DE, Simon JW, Meyer DR, Malone A. Ptosis and ophthalmoplegia associated with epidermolysis bullosa simplex-muscular dystrophy. Ophthal Plast Reconstr Surg. 2010; 26(6):488–489

[73] Rose MR, Landon DN, Papadimitriou A, Morgan-Hughes JA. A rapidly progressive adolescent-onset oculopharyngeal somatic syndrome with rimmed vacuoles in two siblings. Ann Neurol. 1997; 41(1):25–31

[74] Groen WB, Leen WG, Vos AM, Cruysberg JR, van Doorn PA, van Engelen BG. Ptosis as a feature of late-onset glycogenosis type II. Neurology. 2006; 67(12):2261–2262

[75] Xu L, Winn BJ, Odel JG. Lyme-associated orbital inflammation presenting as painless subacute unilateral ptosis. J Neuroophthalmol. 2012; 32(3):246–248

[76] Good EF. Ptosis as the sole manifestation of compression of the oculomotor nerve by an aneurysm of the posterior communicating artery. J Clin Neuroophthalmol. 1990; 10(1):59–61

[77] Martin TJ, Corbett JJ, Babikian PV, Crawford SC, Currier RD. Bilateral ptosis due to mesencephalic lesions with relative preservation of ocular motility. J Neuroophthalmol. 1996; 16(4):258–263

[78] Tummala RP, Harrison A, Madison MT, Nussbaum ES. Pseudomyasthenia resulting from a posterior carotid artery wall aneurysm: a novel presentation: case report. Neurosurgery. 2001; 49(6):1466–1468, discussion 1468–1469

[79] al-Din SN, Anderson M, Eeg-Olofsson O, Trontelj JV. Neuro-ophthalmic manifestations of the syndrome of ophthalmoplegia, ataxia and areflexia: a review. Acta Neurol Scand. 1994; 89(3):157–163

[80] Berlit P, Rakicky J. The Miller Fisher syndrome. Review of the literature. J Clin Neuroophthalmol. 1992; 12(1):57–63

[81] Ishikawa H, Wakakura M, Ishikawa S. Enhanced ptosis in Fisher's syndrome after Epstein-Barr virus infection. J Clin Neuroophthalmol. 1990; 10(3):197–200

[82] Mori M, Kuwabara S, Fukutake T, Yuki N, Hattori T. Clinical features and prognosis of Miller Fisher syndrome. Neurology. 2001; 56(8):1104–1106

[83] Yip PK. Bilateral ptosis, ataxia and areflexia–a variant of Fisher's syndrome. (letter). J Neurol Neurosurg Psychiatry. 1991; 54(12):1121

[84] Holly LT, Batzdorf U. Management of cerebellar ptosis following craniovertebral decompression for Chiari I malformation. J Neurosurg. 2001; 94(1):21–26

[85] Suzuki H, Matsubara T, Kanamaru K, Kojima T. Chronic hydrocephalus presenting with bilateral ptosis after minor head injury: case report. Neurosurgery. 2000; 47(4):977–979, discussion 979–980

[86] Barton JJ, Kardon RH, Slagel D, Thompson HS. Bilateral central ptosis in acquired immunodeficiency syndrome. (review). Can J Neurol Sci. 1995; 22(1):52–55

[87] Mihaescu M, Brillman J, Rothfus W. Midbrain ptosis caused by periaqueductal infarct following cardiac catheterization: early detection with diffusion-weighted imaging. J Neuroimaging. 2000; 10(3):187–189

[88] Saeki N, Yamaura A, Sunami K. Bilateral ptosis with pupil sparing because of a discrete midbrain lesion: magnetic resonance imaging evidence of topographic arrangement within the oculomotor nerve. J Neuroophthalmol. 2000; 20(2):130–134

[89] Averbuch-Heller L, Leigh RJ, Mermelstein V, Zagalsky L, Streifler JY. Ptosis in patients with hemispheric strokes. Neurology. 2002; 58(4):620–624

[90] Averbuch-Heller L, Stahl JS, Remler BF, Leigh RJ. Bilateral ptosis and upgaze palsy with right hemispheric lesions. Ann Neurol. 1996; 40(3):465–468

[91] Zachariah SB, Wilson MC, Zachariah B. Bilateral lid ptosis on a supranuclear basis in the elderly. J Am Geriatr Soc. 1994; 42(2):215–217

[92] Afifi AK, Corbett JJ, Thompson HS, Wells KK. Seizure-induced miosis and ptosis: association with temporal lobe magnetic resonance imaging abnormalities. J Child Neurol. 1990; 5(2):142–146

[93] Stidham DB, Butler IJ. Recurrent isolated ptosis in presumed ophthalmoplegic migraine of childhood. Ophthalmology. 2000; 107(8):1476–1478

[94] Sieb JP, Hartmann A. Relapsing alternating ptosis in two siblings. J Neurol Neurosurg Psychiatry. 2000; 69(2):282–283

[95] Kao Y-F, Lan M-Y, Chou M-S, Chen W-H. Intracranial fatigable ptosis. J Neuroophthalmol. 1999; 19(4):257–259

[96] Ragge NK, Hoyt WF. Midbrain myasthenia: fatigable ptosis, 'lid twitch' sign, and ophthalmoparesis from a dorsal midbrain glioma. Neurology. 1992; 42(4):917–919

[97] Galetta SL, Gray LG, Raps EC, Grossman RI, Schatz NJ. Unilateral ptosis and contralateral eyelid retraction from a thalamic-midbrain infarction. Magnetic resonance imaging correlation. J Clin Neuroophthalmol. 1993; 13(4):221–224

[98] Johnson LN, Castro O. Monocular elevation paresis and incomplete ptosis due to midbrain infarction involving the fascicular segment of the oculomotor nerve. (letter). J Clin Neuroophthalmol. 1992; 12(1):73

[99] Lagreze WD, Warner JE, Zamani AA, Gouras GK, Koralnik IJ, Bienfang DC. Mesencephalic clefts with associated eye movement disorders. Arch Ophthalmol. 1996; 114(4):429–432

[100] Tomecek FJ, Morgan JK. Ophthalmoplegia with bilateral ptosis secondary to midbrain hemorrhage. A case with clinical and radiologic correlation. Surg Neurol. 1994; 41(2):131–136

[101] Brazis PW. Enhanced ptosis in Lambert-Eaton myasthenic syndrome. J Neuroophthalmol. 1997; 17(3):202–203

[102] Feibel RM, Custer PL, Gordon MO. Postcataract ptosis. A randomized, double-masked comparison of peribulbar and retrobulbar anesthesia. Ophthalmology. 1993; 100(5):660–665

[103] Liu D, Bachynski BN. Complete ptosis as a result of removal of epibulbar lipodermoid. Ophthal Plast Reconstr Surg. 1992; 8(2):134–136

[104] Loeffler M, Solomon LD, Renaud M. Postcataract extraction ptosis: effect of the bridle suture. J Cataract Refract Surg. 1990; 16(4):501–504

[105] Ropo A, Ruusuvaara P, Nikki P. Ptosis following periocular or general anaesthesia in cataract surgery. Acta Ophthalmol (Copenh). 1992; 70(2):262–265

[106] von Arx T, Lozanoff S, Zinkernagel M. Ophthalmologic complications after intraoral local anesthesia. Swiss Dent J. 2014; 124(7–8):784–806

[107] Kaplan LJ, Jaffe NS, Clayman HM. Ptosis and cataract surgery. A multivariant computer analysis of a prospective study. Ophthalmology. 1985; 92(2):237–242

[108] Crosby NJ, Shepherd D, Murray A. Mechanical testing of lid speculae and relationship to postoperative ptosis. Eye (Lond). 2013; 27(9):1098–1101

[109] McGhee CN, Dean S, Danesh-Meyer H. Locally administered ocular corticosteroids: benefits and risks. Drug Saf. 2002; 25(1):33–55

[110] Dal Canto AJ, Downs-Kelly E, Perry JD. Ptosis and orbital fat prolapse after posterior sub-Tenon's capsule triamcinolone injection. Ophthalmology. 2005; 112(6):1092–1097

[111] Ideta S, Noda M, Kawamura R, et al. Dehiscence of levator aponeurosis in ptosis after sub-Tenon injection of triamcinolone acetonide. Can J Ophthalmol. 2009; 44(6):668–672

[112] Morley AMS, Tumuluri K, Meligonis G, Collin JRO. Myopathic ptosis following posterior sub-Tenon's triamcinolone acetonide injection. Eye (Lond). 2009; 23(3):741–742

[113] Ababneh OH, Cetinkaya A, Kulwin DR. Long-term efficacy and safety of botulinum toxin A injections to treat blepharospasm and hemifacial spasm. Clin Experiment Ophthalmol. 2014; 42(3):254–261

[114] Brin MF, Boodhoo TI, Pogoda JM, et al. Safety and tolerability of onabotulinumtoxinA in the treatment of facial lines: a meta-analysis of individual patient data from global clinical registration studies in 1678 participants. J Am Acad Dermatol. 2009; 61(6):961–70.e1, 11

[115] Cavallini M, Cirillo P, Fundarò SP, et al. Safety of botulinum toxin A in aesthetic treatments: a systematic review of clinical studies. Dermatol Surg. 2014; 40(5):525–536

[116] Kowal L, Wong E, Yahalom C. Botulinum toxin in the treatment of strabismus. A review of its use and effects. Disabil Rehabil. 2007; 29(23):1823–1831

[117] Murthy R, Dawson E, Khan S, Adams GG, Lee J. Botulinum toxin in the management of internuclear ophthalmoplegia. J AAPOS. 2007; 11(5):456–459

[118] Steinsapir KD, Groth MJ, Boxrud CA. Persistence of upper blepharoptosis after cosmetic botulinum toxin type A. Dermatol Surg. 2015; 41(7):833–840

[119] Scheinfeld N. The use of apraclonidine eyedrops to treat ptosis after the administration of botulinum toxin to the upper face. Dermatol Online J. 2005; 11(1):9

[120] Naik MN, Gangopadhyay N, Fernandes M, Murthy R, Honavar SG. Anterior chemodenervation of levator palpebrae superioris with botulinum toxin type-A (Botox) to induce temporary ptosis for corneal protection. Eye (Lond). 2008; 22(9):1132–1136

[121] Reddy UP, Woodward JA. Abobotulinum toxin A (Dysport) and botulinum toxin type A (Botox) for purposeful induction of eyelid ptosis. Ophthal Plast Reconstr Surg. 2010; 26(6):489–491

[122] Frueh BR, Musch DC. Evaluation of levator muscle integrity in ptosis with levator force measurement. Ophthalmology. 1996; 103(2):244–250

[123] Liu D. Ptosis repair by single suture aponeurotic tuck. Surgical technique and long-term results. Ophthalmology. 1993; 100(2):251–259

[124] Martin JJ, Jr, Tenzel RR. Acquired ptosis: dehiscences and disinsertions. Are they real or iatrogenic? Ophthal Plast Reconstr Surg. 1992; 8(2):130–132, discussion 133

[125] Older JJ. Ptosis repair and blepharoplasty in the adult (review). Ophthalmic Surg. 1995; 26(4):304–308

[126] Dryden RM, Kahanic DA. Worsening of blepharoptosis in downgaze. Ophthal Plast Reconstr Surg. 1992; 8(2):126–129

[127] Wojno TH. Downgaze ptosis. Ophthal Plast Reconstr Surg. 1993; 9(2):83–88, discussion 88–89

[128] Garg P, Aggarwal P. Ocular changes in pregnancy. Nepal J Ophthalmol. 2012; 4(1):150–161

[129] Gaudiani JL, Braverman JM, Mascolo M, Mehler PS. Ophthalmic changes in severe anorexia nervosa: a case series. Int J Eat Disord. 2012; 45(5):719–721

[130] Omoti AE, Waziri-Erameh JM, Okeigbemen VW. A review of the changes in the ophthalmic and visual system in pregnancy. Afr J Reprod Health. 2008; 12(3):185–196

[131] Biousse V, Newman NJ. Neuro-ophthalmology of mitochondrial diseases. Curr Opin Neurol. 2003; 16(1):35–43

[132] Han J, Lee YM, Kim SM, Han SY, Lee JB, Han SH. Ophthalmological manifestations in patients with Leigh syndrome. Br J Ophthalmol. 2015; 99(4):528–535

19 Lid Retraction and Lid Lag

Benjamin A. Dake

Abstract

Lid retraction is the abnormal and excessive elevation of the upper eyelid or depression of the lower eyelid. Lid lag is the delayed lowering of the upper eyelid with the eyes in downward gaze. Disorders of lid movement can occur due to a variety of underlying etiologies. This chapter discusses the clinical pathways in evaluating and diagnosing lid retraction and lid lag, by reviewing the literature in detail.

Keywords: lid retraction, lid lag, lid nystagmus, sympathetic overactivity, thyroid eye disease

19.1 What Is the Anatomy of the Eyelids and What Brainstem Structures Control Lid Elevation?

In normal adults, the upper lid just covers the superior cornea (1–2 mm) and the lower lid lies slightly below the inferior corneal margin. Eyelid elevation occurs with contraction of the levator palpebrae superioris (LPS) muscle innervated by the oculomotor nerve. Accessory muscles include superior tarsal muscle (sympathetic innervation), which is embedded in the LPS and inserts mainly on the tarsal plate, and the frontalis muscle (innervated by the temporal branch of the facial nerve), which helps to retract the lid in extreme upgaze.[1] Tone in the LPS normally parallels that of the superior rectus muscle, and in extreme downgaze both muscles are completely inhibited. However, there is an inverse relationship between the LPS and the superior rectus during forced lid closure where the eye elevates (Bell's phenomenon). The motor neurons for both levator muscles are in the unpaired central caudal nucleus (CCN), located at the dorsal caudal pole of the oculomotor complex adjacent to the medial rectus and superior rectus subdivisions. Within the CCN, motor neurons of both LPS muscles are intermixed. The region of the nuclear complex of the posterior commissure (NPC) is involved in lid–eye movement coordination.[1]

The upper lid position is abnormal if it exposes a white band of sclera between the lid margin and the upper corneal limbus. This may be due to lid retraction (related to overactivity of the LPS, contracture of the LPS, or hyperactivity of superior tarsal muscle), or lid lag, which is noted on attempted downgaze. Bartley divided lid retraction into four categories: neurogenic, myogenic (including disease processes affecting the neuromuscular junction), mechanical, and miscellaneous.[2] This chapter adopts this classification, discusses the etiologies of lid lag and lid retraction, and suggests a diagnostic approach.

19.2 What Are the Neurogenic Causes of Lid Retraction and Lid Lag?

Neurogenic eyelid retraction and lid lag may be due to supranuclear, nuclear, or infranuclear lesions affecting the LPS or

conditions that produce hyperactivity of the sympathetically innervated superior tarsal muscle.[3] Preterm infants may have a benign transient conjugate downward gaze deviation with eyelid retraction thought to be due to immature myelination of vertical eye movement control pathways.[3,4] Approximately 80% of normal infants of 14 to 18 weeks of age may demonstrate bilateral transient lid retraction ("eye-popping reflex") when ambient light levels are suddenly reduced. Both of these phenomena are usually benign and typically require no evaluation if transient and in isolation (class IV, level C).

Dorsal mesencephalic supranuclear lesions may result in eyelid retraction, which is noted when the eyes are in the primary position of gaze or on looking upward (Collier sign or posterior fossa stare). Unlike the retraction from thyroid orbitopathy (see below), with midbrain lid retraction there is typically no retraction in downgaze. Patients with dorsal mesencephalic lesions often have associated vertical gaze palsies and other dorsal midbrain findings. The etiologies of the dorsal midbrain syndrome and the workup of these patients are discussed in Chapter 14. Spells of lid retraction lasting 20 to 30 seconds that may be seen with impending tentorial brain herniation may be due to a dorsal mesencephalic mechanism.[3]

Lesions of the medial and/or principal portion of the NPC are involved in lid–eye coordination and provide inhibitory modulation of levator motor neuronal activity.[1] Clinical and experimental evidence suggests an inhibitory premotor network in the periaqueductal gray (the supraoculomotor area or supra III) that is dorsal to the third cranial nerve nucleus and projects from the NPC to the central caudal subnucleus.[1,5,6,7] Lesions in the region of NPC may produce excessive innervation to the lids with lid retraction in primary position. Bilateral eyelid retraction and eyelid lag with minimal impairment of vertical gaze has been described with a circumscribed unilateral lesion immediately rostral and dorsal to the red nucleus involving the lateral periaqueductal gray area in the region of the NPC.[5,6,7] Eyelid lag without retraction has also been described in pretectal disease, implying that these lid signs may have separate neural mechanisms.[7] Vertical gaze paralysis without eyelid retraction may occur. In these cases, the fibers and nucleus of the posterior commissure are spared and the lesions involve the rostral interstitial nucleus of the medial longitudinal fasciculus (MLF), the interstitial nucleus of Cajal, and the periaqueductal gray area.[1] Ipsilateral ptosis and contralateral superior eyelid retraction may be due to a nuclear oculomotor nerve syndrome (plus-minus lid syndrome).[6,8,9] The plus-minus syndrome results from a unilateral lesion of the third nerve fascicle with extension rostrally and dorsally to involve the nucleus of the posterior commissure or its connections. The plus-minus syndrome has been described with mesencephalic infarct and glioma.[8,9] However, it must be differentiated from a pseudo plus-minus syndrome that can occur with myasthenia gravis and/or thyroid disease.[10] In a true plus-minus syndrome, elevation of the ptotic lid will not result in facilitated ptosis of the retracted lid. In pseudo plus-minus syndrome, raising the ptotic lid manually will result in decreased neural input to both levator muscles based on the Hering's law of equal innervation, and result in reduction of the lid retraction in the contralateral eye.[11] Also, a patient has been described with a nuclear third nerve palsy, sparing the caudal central nucleus and its efferent fibers, who had no ipsilateral ptosis but had contralateral lid retraction.[12] The contralateral eyelid retraction was thought to be due to damage to fibers from the NPC, most probably in the region of the supraoculomotor area, and it is inferred from this case that inhibitory connections between the NPC and the CCN are unilateral and crossed. A similar crossed pattern may also exist for excitatory afferents to the CCN as hemispheric lesions result in contralateral ptosis.

Paroxysmal superior rectus with LPS spasm is a rare and unique disorder described in a single patient with multiple sclerosis.[13] Paroxysms of vertical diplopia and lid retraction in this patient lasted 3 to 4 seconds, and examination revealed intermittent right hypertropia, lid retraction, and restriction of downgaze. Magnetic resonance imaging (MRI) revealed multiple lesions consistent with multiple sclerosis, including a lesion in the midbrain in the region of the third nerve fascicle. Carbamazepine stopped all the symptoms that were thought due to spontaneous spasm of the superior rectus/levator complex.

Bilateral episodic retraction of the eyelids may occur as a manifestation of epileptic discharges associated with petit mal or myoclonic seizures or due to "levator spasms" during an oculogyric crisis.[3] Lid lag may occur on a supranuclear basis in progressive supranuclear palsy, likely due to defective inhibition of the levator nuclei during downward gaze.[3,14] Lid lag may occur in the acute phases of Guillain–Barré syndrome,[15] and lid retraction may also occur with parkinsonism.[3,15] Lid retraction has also been described with Miller Fisher syndrome[16] and POEMS (peripheral neuropathy, organomegaly, endocrinopathy, M-protein, and skin changes) syndrome.[17]

Rhythmic upward jerking of the lids (eyelid nystagmus) refers to eyelid twitches that are synchronous with the fast phase of horizontal nystagmus on lateral gaze. It has been ascribed to lateral medullary disease where it may be inhibited by near effort. Lid nystagmus may also be provoked by convergence (Pick sign) in cerebellar or medullary pathology. There is a slow down drift of the lid corrected by an upward flick. Rhythmic upward jerking of the eyelids may also be associated with vertical nystagmus, palatal myoclonus, or convergence–retraction nystagmus (see Chapters 14 and 17).[3]

Eyelid retraction may also occur from paradoxic levator excitation that may be congenital or acquired supranuclear, nuclear, or infranuclear lesions.[3] Paradoxical lid retraction may occur with jaw movement or swallowing (the Marcus Gunn jaw-winking phenomenon). This trigemino-oculomotor synkinesis occurs on a congenital basis. Levator contraction with contraction of the external pterygoid muscle is the most common form of trigemino-oculomotor synkinesis.[3] The involved eyelid is usually ptotic, but may be normal or even retracted while the jaw muscles are inactive. Elevation of the lid occurs when the mandible is moved to the opposite side, the mandible is projected forward, the tongue protruded, or on wide opening of the mouth. These patients commonly have other associated ocular abnormalities including strabismus (e.g., double elevator palsy or superior rectus palsy), amblyopia, and anisometropia.[3] Another rare form of trigemino-oculomotor synkinesis is levator contraction with contraction of the internal pterygoid muscle (i.e., eyelid elevation with closure of the mouth or

clenching of the teeth). Treatment of cases of Marcus Gunn jaw-winking phenomenon includes occlusion therapy for amblyopia, strabismus surgery, and surgery to correct the ptosis or retraction.[3] Paradoxical eyelid retraction may also occur ipsilaterally in congenital or acquired horizontal gaze or abducens palsies.[3]

Eyelid retraction may also occur with aberrant regeneration of the third nerve. The lid may elevate when the eye adducts, elevates, or depresses (see Chapter 11).[18] Partial paresis of the superior rectus muscle[19] or orbital floor "blowout" fractures with globe hypotropia may produce an appearance of lid retraction. Secondary eyelid retraction (pseudoretraction) may also occur if there is ptosis of the opposite eyelid (especially when the ptosis is due to disease at or distal to the neuromuscular junction) when fixating with the eye with the unilateral ptosis (due to Hering's law). Compensatory unilateral orbicularis oculi contraction may mask lid retraction; therefore, if the orbicularis oculi muscle is also weakened as in myasthenia gravis, contralateral lid retraction becomes more evident. Occlusion of the eye on the side of the ptosis restores the retracted eyelid to a normal position.

Sympathetic overactivity may cause lid retraction by contraction of superior tarsal muscle. Intermittent oculosympathetic irritation may cause cyclic sympathetic spasm. The pupil dilates for 40 to 60 seconds and may be associated with lid retraction, facial hyperhidrosis, and headache (Pourfour du Petit syndrome).[20] Sympathetic overactivity may also play a role in the lid retraction rarely noted in ipsilateral orbital blowout fractures. Sympathomimetic drops used in routine dilation of the pupils for ophthalmoscopy (e.g., phenylephrine) may also cause lid retraction. Finally, volitional bilateral lid retraction may occur in anxious or psychotic patients.[20]

19.3 What Are the Neuromuscular and Myopathic Causes of Lid Retraction and Lid Lag?

Congenital maldevelopment or fibrosis of the LPS muscle or tendon may cause eyelid retraction or entropion at birth.[18,21,22] This eyelid retraction may be unilateral or bilateral and may be associated with congenital abnormalities.[3] Other causes of congenital eyelid retraction include maternal hyperthyroidism (transient), congenital myotonia, and myotonic dystrophy.

Dysthyroid disease (Graves ophthalmopathy) with involvement of the LPS is the most common cause of acquired unilateral or bilateral sustained eyelid retraction.[3,20] Patients may show retraction of the upper eyelid associated with infrequent or incomplete blinking (Stellwag sign) and abnormal widening of the palpebral fissure (Dalrymple sign). When the patient looks downward, there is often lid lag; the upper eyelid pauses and then incompletely follows the eye down (Graefe sign). The retracted upper eyelid remains elevated in downgaze in dysthyroid disease; this differentiates dysthyroid eyelid retraction from dorsal midbrain eyelid retraction (Collier sign), where the eyelids are also retracted in primary position but are typically normal in downgaze.[20]

Eyelid retraction in patients with thyroid ophthalmopathy may result from excessive sympathetic activity, superior tarsal muscle fibrosis, LPS fibrosis, local adhesions of the LPS to fixed orbital tissues, or contracture of the inferior rectus muscle.[23,24] The lid retraction may be controlled by botulinum toxin injection into the LPS.[25,26] Additionally, fornix and subconjunctival triamcinolone injections may effectively treat upper lid retraction.[27,28,29] Long-acting octreotide may have similar efficacy as full-thickness blepharotomy in treating patients with significant lid retraction.[30] Surgical procedures are available to improve eyelid retraction with options including lateral tarsorrhaphy, superior tarsal muscle and LPS muscle lengthening, lower eyelid elevation, and blepharoplasty with orbital fat excision.[31] Orbital decompression may improve lid retraction that is due to distortion from a proptotic globe. Strabismus surgery may relieve the compensatory component of lid retraction related to restrictive extraocular muscles, but recessions of the inferior rectus muscle often worsen the eyelid retraction. Therefore, the order of surgery for patients with thyroid ophthalmopathy who require different surgical procedures should in general be first orbital decompression followed by strabismus surgery and then lid surgery (class IV, level C).

In the pediatric population, the ophthalmic findings of Graves disease are typically mild and do not require surgery. Most pediatric patients require only lubricating eye drops. Surgery is indicated in a small proportion of patients for cosmesis and corneal exposure.[32,33]

Myasthenia gravis may also be associated with three types of eyelid retraction: (1) unilateral ptosis and contralateral eyelid retraction due to innervation to elevate the ptotic lid; (2) ptosis and brief eyelid retraction lasting only seconds following a saccade from downgaze to primary position (Cogan lid twitch sign); and (3) transient eyelid retraction lasting seconds or minutes after staring straight ahead or looking upward for several seconds (possibly due to posttetanic facilitation of the levator muscle).[3]

Other myopathic causes of lid retraction include hypokalemic or hyperkalemic periodic paralysis, myotonic muscular dystrophy, after botulinum toxin injections of the eyelids, and after eye surgery, including superior rectus recession, ptosis repair, and enucleation.[2,3,34] Fluctuating eyelid retraction caused by hypertrophied cranial nerves associated with chronic inflammatory demyelinating polyradiculoneuropathy (CIDP) has been described.[35]

19.4 What Are the Mechanical and Miscellaneous Etiologies of Lid Lag and Lid Retraction?

The eyelid retraction noted with mechanical causes often responds to correction of the underlying abnormality.[2] Prominence of the globe, such as may occur with severe myopia, buphthalmos, proptosis, cherubism, craniosynostosis, or Paget disease, may cause apparent lid retraction.[2,18,19,34] Cicatricial scarring of the eyelid and LPS fibrosis from eyelid tumors, hemangioma of the orbit, herpes zoster ophthalmicus, atopic dermatitis, scleroderma, or thermal or chemical burns may also mechanically retract or distort the eyelids.[2,18,20] Lid lag and retraction secondary to breast carcinoma metastasis to extraocular muscles and potentially the levator muscles has been

described.[36,37] Bilateral metastatic melanoma to the extraocular muscles causing lid retraction also has been described.[38] Pediatric cases of orbital myocysticercosis causing ptosis with lid lag have been described.[39] Blowout fractures of the orbital floor may cause upper eyelid retraction on either a neurogenic or mechanistic basis; hypotropia of the globe can stimulate increased innervation of the superior rectus, and LPS or traction on the connective sheath of the LPS can elevate the upper eyelid mechanically.[2] Contact lens wear may also cause upper eyelid retraction, presumably by mechanical irritation of the palpebral conjunctiva.[2] Lid retraction due to a lost hard contact lens becoming embedded in the upper eyelid has also been described.[40]

Eyelid retraction, often associated with enophthalmos and hypoglobus, may occur with chronic maxillary sinusitis, maxillary sinus hypoplasia, and orbital floor resorption (silent sinus syndrome).[41,42] Radiation or trauma to the orbit or sinus may also be associated with eyelid retraction.[43] A retracted eyelid may also be a complication of surgical procedures, including trabeculectomy for glaucoma, scleral buckle, frontal sinusotomy, blepharoplasty, orbicularis myectomy, orbital floor repair, and cataract extraction.[2,3,19,44]

Other miscellaneous entities that have been reported to be associated with eyelid retraction include optic nerve hypoplasia, microphthalmos, Down syndrome, hypertension, meningitis, sphenoid wing meningioma, Hutchinson–Gilford progeria syndrome, chronic hydrocephalus, and superior cul-de-sac lymphoma.[2,18,45,46] Bilateral upper and lower lid retraction may occur with hepatic cirrhosis (Summerskill's sign). The existence of this sign has been questioned, as many of the original patients described may well have had Graves ophthalmopathy in addition to liver disease, but rare cases without thyroid disease have been documented.[2,3,47,48] Etiologies of upper lid retraction and lid lag are listed in Box 19.1.

Box 19.1 Etiologies of upper lid retraction and lid lag

- Neurogenic:
  - Benign transient lid retraction in preterm infants ("eye-popping reflex" in infants).
  - Dorsal midbrain syndrome.
  - Paroxysmal superior rectus and levator spasm in multiple sclerosis.
  - Seizures (petit mal or myoclonic).
  - Oculogyric crisis.
  - Progressive supranuclear palsy.
  - Autosomal dominant cerebellar ataxias.
  - Parkinson disease.
  - Guillain–Barré syndrome (including Miller Fisher syndrome).
  - POEMS (polyneuropathy, organomegaly, endocrinopathy, M-protein, skin changes) syndrome.
  - Lid nystagmus.
  - Paradoxic levator excitation.
  - Marcus Gunn jaw-winking phenomenon.
  - Abducens nerve palsy.
  - Aberrant regeneration of the third nerve.
  - Partial superior rectus paresis.
  - Orbital floor fracture.
  - Pseudoretraction.

- Sympathetic overactivity:
  - Claude–Bernard syndrome.
  - Sympathomimetic drops.
- Volitional lid retraction.
- Neuromuscular and myopathic:
  - Congenital:
    - Congenital maldevelopment or fibrosis of the levator.
    - Maternal hyperthyroidism.
    - Congenital myotonia.
    - Myotonic dystrophy.
  - Graves ophthalmopathy.
  - Hypokalemic periodic paralysis.
  - Hyperkalemic periodic paralysis.
  - Chronic inflammatory demyelinating polyradiculoneuropathy.[35]
  - Myotonic muscular dystrophy.
  - Botulinum injection into lids.
- Mechanical:
  - Prominence of the globe:
    - Myopia.
    - Buphthalmos.
    - Proptosis.
    - Cherubism.
    - Craniosynostosis.
    - Paget disease.
  - Cicatricial scarring and fibrosis:
    - Eyelid tumors.
    - Metastatic breast carcinoma.[36,37]
    - Metastatic melanoma.[38]
    - Hemangioma of the orbit.
    - Herpes zoster ophthalmicus.
    - Atopic dermatitis.
    - Scleroderma.
    - Thermal or chemical burns.
    - Orbital myocysticercosis[39]
  - Blowout fracture of the orbital floor.
  - Contact lens wear.
  - Contact lens embedded in upper lid.
  - Enophthalmos and hypoglobus.
  - Silent sinus syndrome.[49,50]
  - Radiation therapy.
  - Trauma.
  - Surgical procedures:
    - Trabeculectomy.
    - Scleral buckle.
    - Frontal sinus surgery.
    - Blepharoplasty.
    - Orbicularis myectomy.
    - Orbital floor repair.[44]
    - Superior rectus recession.
    - Ptosis repair.
    - Enucleation.
- Miscellaneous:
  - Optic nerve hypoplasia.

- Microphthalmos.
- Down syndrome.
- Hypertension.
- Meningitis.
- Sphenoid wing meningioma.
- Superior cul-de-sac lymphoma.
- Hepatic cirrhosis.
- Hutchinson–Gilford progeria syndrome.[45]
- Chronic hydrocephalus.[46]

Source: Reprinted from Bartley GB. The differential diagnosis and classification of eyelid retraction. Ophthalmology. 1996; 103(1):168–176, with permission.

An approach to the diagnosis of unilateral or bilateral upper eyelid retraction is outlined in ▶ Fig. 19.1. An adequate history, ophthalmologic examination, and neurologic examination should be able to distinguish the major causes of lid retraction (class IV, level C).

19.5 What Are the Etiologies of Lower Eyelid Retraction?

Like upper eyelid retraction, retraction of the lower eyelid may be due to neurogenic, myogenic, and mechanical causes.[51] Congenital paradoxical lower eyelid retraction on upgaze and unilateral congenital lower eyelid retraction, due to the lid being tethered to the orbital margin, have been described. Lower eyelid retraction may be the earliest clinical lid sign of a lesion of the facial nerve, and facial nerve lesions are the most common cause of lower lid retraction.[51] Flaccidity of the lower lid may be an early manifestation of facial muscle paresis in myasthenia and myopathies. Lower lid retraction may occur with the following:

- Dysthyroid orbitopathy (with or without proptosis).
- Proptosis.
- Blepharochalasis.[52]
- Senile entropion or ectropion.
- Enophthalmos.
- After eye muscle (e.g., inferior rectus recession) or orbital surgery (e.g., orbital floor "blowout" fracture repair, orbitotomy, or maxillectomy).
- After scarring and contraction of lid tissue (e.g., from burns, tumors, trauma, granulomas of the orbital septum, dermatoses, or surgery).[2]

With a hypertropia, the ipsilateral lid may appear to be retracted, whereas with a hypotropia there may be an illusion of contralateral lid retraction. Pseudo lid retraction also may be due to elevation of the contralateral lower eyelid with facial contracture following Bell's palsy, spastic-paretic facial contracture with myokymia, hemifacial spasm, enophthalmos, or Horner syndrome "upside-down" ptosis.

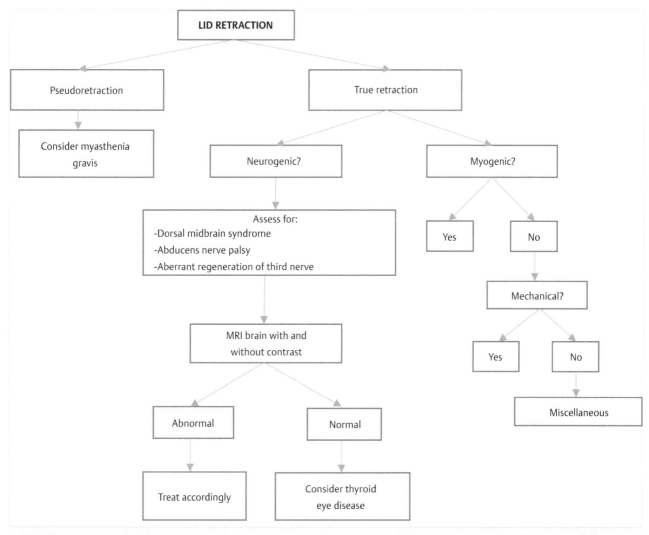

Fig. 19.1 Evaluation of lid retraction.

The etiologies of lower eyelid retraction are outlined in Box 19.2.

- Neurogenic:
  - Congenital paradoxical lower eyelid retraction on upgaze.
  - Unilateral congenital lower eyelid retraction due to the lid being tethered to the orbital margin.
  - Lesion of the facial nerve.
- Neuromuscular and myogenic:
  - Myasthenia gravis.
  - Myopathies.
  - Dysthyroid orbitopathy.
- Mechanical:
  - Proptosis.
  - Senile entropion or ectropion.
  - Enophthalmos.
  - Surgical procedures:
    - Inferior rectus recession.
    - Orbital floor blowout fracture repair.
    - Orbitotomy.
    - Maxillectomy.
  - Scarring and contraction of lid tissue (e.g., burns, tumors, granulomas of the orbital septum, dermatoses, or surgery).
- Miscellaneous:
  - Apparent lid retraction:
    - Ipsilateral with hypertropia.
    - Contralateral with hypotropia.
  - Pseudoretraction due to elevation of the contralateral lower eyelid from
    - Facial contracture following Bell's palsy.[53]
    - Spastic-paretic facial contracture with myokymia.
    - Hemifacial spasm.
    - Enophthalmos.
    - Horner syndrome ("upside-down" ptosis).

References

[1] Schmidtke K, Büttner-Ennever JA. Nervous control of eyelid function. A review of clinical, experimental and pathological data. Brain. 1992; 115(Pt 1): 227–247

[2] Bartley GB. The differential diagnosis and classification of eyelid retraction. Ophthalmology. 1996; 103(1):168–176

[3] Miller NR. Anatomy and physiology of normal and abnormal eyelid position and movement. In: Miller NR, ed. Walsh and Hoyt's Clinical Neuro-ophthalmology. 4th ed. Baltimore, Williams & Wilkins; 1985:932–995

[4] Kleiman MD, DiMario FJ, Jr, Leconche DA, Zalneraitis EL. Benign transient downward gaze in preterm infants. Pediatr Neurol. 1994; 10(4):313–316

[5] Galetta SL, Gray LG, Raps EC, Schatz NJ. Pretectal eyelid retraction and lag. Ann Neurol. 1993a; 33(5):554–557

[6] Galetta SL, Gray LG, Raps EC, Grossman RI, Schatz NJ. Unilateral ptosis and contralateral eyelid retraction from a thalamic-midbrain infarction. Magnetic resonance imaging correlation. J Clin Neuroophthalmol. 1993b; 13(4): 221–224

[7] Galetta SL, Raps EC, Liu GT, Saito NG, Kline LB. Eyelid lag without eyelid retraction in pretectal disease. J Neuroophthalmol. 1996; 16(2):96–98

[8] Gaymard B, Lafitte C, Gelot A, de Toffol B. Plus-minus lid syndrome. J Neurol Neurosurg Psychiatry. 1992; 55(9):846–848

[9] Vetrugno R, Mascalchi M, Marulli D, et al. Plus minus lid syndrome due to cerebral glioma: a case report. Neuroophthalmology. 1997; 18(3):149–151

[10] Bandini F. Pseudo plus-minus lid syndrome. Arch Neurol. 2009; 66(5): 668–669

[11] Gay AJ, Salmon ML, Windsor CE. Hering's law, the levators, and their relationship in disease states. Arch Ophthalmol. 1967; 77(2):157–160

[12] Gaymard B, Huynh C, Laffont I. Unilateral eyelid retraction. J Neurol Neurosurg Psychiatry. 2000; 68(3):390–392

[13] Ezra E, Plant GT. Paroxysmal superior rectus and levator palpebrae spasm: a unique presentation of multiple sclerosis. Br J Ophthalmol. 1996; 80(2): 187–188

[14] Friedman DI, Jankovic J, McCrary JA, III. Neuro-ophthalmic findings in progressive supranuclear palsy. J Clin Neuroophthalmol. 1992; 12(2):104–109

[15] Tan E, Kansu T, Kirkali P, Zileli T. Lid lag and the Guillain-Barré syndrome. J Clin Neuroophthalmol. 1990; 10(2):121–123

[16] al-Din SN, Anderson M, Eeg-Olofsson O, Trontelj JV. Neuro-ophthalmic manifestations of the syndrome of ophthalmoplegia, ataxia and areflexia: a review. Acta Neurol Scand. 1994; 89(3):157–163

[17] Gherardi RK, Chouaïb S, Malapert D, Bélec L, Intrator L, Degos JD. Early weight loss and high serum tumor necrosis factor-alpha levels in polyneuropathy, organomegaly, endocrinopathy, M protein, skin changes syndrome. Ann Neurol. 1994; 35(4):501–505

[18] Stout AU, Borchert M. Etiology of eyelid retraction in children: a retrospective study. J Pediatr Ophthalmol Strabismus. 1993; 30(2):96–99

[19] Mauriello JA, Jr, Palydowycz SB. Upper eyelid retraction after retinal detachment repair. Ophthalmic Surg. 1993; 24(10):694–697

[20] Burde RM, Savino PJ, Trobe JD. Clinical Decisions in Neuro-ophthalmology. 2nd ed. St. Louis: Mosby; 1992:362–364

[21] Collin JR, Allen L, Castronuovo S. Congenital eyelid retraction. Br J Ophthalmol. 1990; 74(9):542–544

[22] Gillies WE, Harris AJ, Brooks AM, Rivers MR, Wolfe RJ. Congenital fibrosis of the vertically acting extraocular muscles. A new group of dominantly inherited ocular fibrosis with radiologic findings. Ophthalmology. 1995; 102(4):607–612

[23] Feldon SE, Levin L. Graves' ophthalmopathy: V. Aetiology of upper eyelid retraction in Graves' ophthalmopathy. Br J Ophthalmol. 1990; 74(8):484–485

[24] Shih MJ, Liao SL, Kuo KT, Smith TJ, Chuang LM. Molecular pathology of Muller's muscle in Graves' ophthalmopathy. J Clin Endocrinol Metab. 2006; 91(3):1159–1167

[25] Biglan AW. Control of eyelid retraction associated with Graves' disease with botulinum A toxin. Ophthalmic Surg. 1994; 25(3):186–188

[26] Ebner R. Botulinum toxin type A in upper lid retraction of Graves' ophthalmopathy. J Clin Neuroophthalmol. 1993; 13(4):258–261

[27] Hamed-Azzam S, Mukari A, Feldman I, Saliba W, Jabaly-Habib H, Briscoe D. Fornix triamcinolone injection for thyroid orbitopathy. Graefes Arch Clin Exp Ophthalmol. 2015; 253(5):811–816

[28] Lee JM, Lee H, Park M, Baek S. Subconjunctival injection of triamcinolone for the treatment of upper lid retraction associated with thyroid eye disease. J Craniofac Surg. 2012; 23(6):1755–1758

[29] Chee E, Chee SP. Subconjunctival injection of triamcinolone in the treatment of lid retraction of patients with thyroid eye disease: a case series. Eye (Lond). 2008; 22(2):311–315

[30] Stan MN, Garrity JA, Bradley EA, et al. Randomized, double-blind, placebo-controlled trial of long-acting release octreotide for treatment of Graves' ophthalmopathy. J Clin Endocrinol Metab. 2006; 91(12):4817–4824

[31] Ceisler EJ, Bilyk JR, Rubin PA, Burks WR, Shore JW. Results of Müllerotomy and levator aponeurosis transposition for the correction of upper eyelid retraction in Graves' disease. Ophthalmology. 1995; 102(3):483–492

[32] Goldstein SM, Katowitz WR, Moshang T, Katowitz JA. Pediatric thyroid-associated orbitopathy: the Children's Hospital of Philadelphia experience and literature review. Thyroid. 2008; 18(9):997–999

[33] Chan W, Wong GW, Fan DS, Cheng AC, Lam DS, Ng JS. Ophthalmopathy in childhood Graves' disease. Br J Ophthalmol. 2002; 86(7):740–742

[34] Leatherbarrow B, Kwartz J, Sunderland S, Brammar R, Nichol E. The 'baseball' orbital implant: a prospective study. Eye (Lond). 1994; 8(Pt 5):569–576

[35] Alwan AA, Mejico LJ. Ophthalmoplegia, proptosis, and lid retraction caused by cranial nerve hypertrophy in chronic inflammatory demyelinating polyradiculoneuropathy. J Neuroophthalmol. 2007; 27(2):99–103

[36] Spitzer SG, Bersani TA, Mejico LJ. Multiple bilateral extraocular muscle metastases as the initial manifestation of breast cancer. J Neuroophthalmol. 2005; 25(1):37–39

[37] Luneau K, Falardeau J, Hardy I, Boulos PR, Boghen D. Ophthalmoplegia and lid retraction with normal initial orbit CT imaging in extraocular muscle metastases as the presenting sign of breast carcinoma. J Neuroophthalmol. 2007; 27(2):144–146

[38] Almeida AC, Fung A, Guedes ME, Costa JM. (2012). Bilateral metastatic melanoma to the extraocular-muscles simulating thyroid eye disease. BMJ Case Rep. http://www.ncbi.nlm.nih.gov/pmc/articles/PMC4543875/. Accessed February 15, 2016

[39] Sharma V, Saxena R, Betharia SM, Sharma P. Myocysticercosis: a cause of acquired ptosis in children simulating congenital ptosis with lid lag (report of two cases). J AAPOS. 2004; 8(4):390–392

[40] Weinstein GS, Myers BB. Eyelid retraction as a complication of an embedded hard contact lens. Am J Ophthalmol. 1993; 116(1):102–103

[41] Rubin PAD, Bilyk JR, Shore JW. Orbital reconstruction using porous polyethylene sheets. Ophthalmology. 1994; 101(10):1697–1708

[42] Soparkar CN, Patrinely JR, Cuaycong MJ, et al. The silent sinus syndrome. A cause of spontaneous enophthalmos. Ophthalmology. 1994; 101(4):772–778

[43] Smitt MC, Donaldson SS. Radiotherapy is successful treatment for orbital lymphoma. Int J Radiat Oncol Biol Phys. 1993; 26(1):59–66

[44] Kersey TL, Ng SG, Rosser P, Sloan B, Hart R. Orbital adherence with titanium mesh floor implants: a review of 10 cases. Orbit. 2013; 32(1):8–11

[45] Chandravanshi SL, Rawat AK, Dwivedi PC, Choudhary P. Ocular manifestations in the Hutchinson-Gilford progeria syndrome. Indian J Ophthalmol. 2011; 59(6):509–512

[46] Sanghvi CA, Richardson P, Leatherbarrow B. Unilateral lid retraction due to orbital fat entrapment in the anterior cranial fossa. Eye (Lond). 2005; 19(6): 695–697

[47] Bartley GB, Gorman CA. Hepatic cirrhosis as a doubtful cause of eyelid retraction. Am J Ophthalmol. 1991; 111(1):109–110

[48] Miller NR. Hepatic cirrhosis as a cause of eyelid retraction. Am J Ophthalmol. 1991; 112(1):94–95

[49] Kubis KC, Danesh-Meyer H, Bilyk JR. Unilateral lid retraction during pregnancy. Surv Ophthalmol. 2000; 45(1):69–76

[50] Wan MK, Francis IC, Carter PR, Griffits R, van Rooijen ML, Coroneo MT. The spectrum of presentation of silent sinus syndrome. J Neuroophthalmol. 2000; 20(3):207–212

[51] Brazis PW, Vogler JB, Shaw KE. The "numb cheek-limp lower lid" syndrome. Neurology. 1991; 41(2)(,)(Pt 1):327–328

[52] Koursh DM, Modjtahedi SP, Selva D, Leibovitch I. The blepharochalasis syndrome. Surv Ophthalmol. 2009; 54(2):235–244

[53] Meadows A, Hall N, Shah-Desai S, Low JL, Manners R. The House-Brackmann system and assessment of corneal risk in facial nerve palsy. Eye (Lond). 2000; 14 Pt 3A:353–357

20 Anisocoria and Pupillary Abnormalities

Noreen Shaikh

Abstract

Anisocoria is the asymmetry of pupil size. Evaluation of the pupils in the light and dark, as well as following instillation of specific topical pharmacological agents, can differentiate different pupil abnormalities and suggest the underlying etiology of the lesion. This chapter discusses the clinical pathways in evaluating and diagnosing anisocoria and other pupil abnormalities, by reviewing the literature in detail.

Keywords: anisocoria, Horner syndrome, Adie tonic pupil, Mydriasis, miosis

20.1 Introduction

Careful examination of pupillary reaction to light and near stimuli, the difference in anisocoria in light and dark, and attention to distinctive associated signs and symptoms facilitate differentiating the abnormalities in pupil size and response to stimuli. Old photographs may be helpful in defining the duration of anisocoria. Generally, the history and examination help distinguish the major entities causing an abnormal large pupil (e.g., third nerve palsy, tonic pupil, iris damage, pharmacologic dilation, or sympathetic irritation) or small pupil (e.g., Horner syndrome [HS], simple anisocoria, pharmacologic miosis). Pharmacologic testing confirms the diagnosis and facilitates topographic localization in many cases. Our algorithm cannot account for patients with multiple causes for anisocoria. For example, Slavin reported a case of physiologic anisocoria with HS and equal-sized pupils.[1]

20.2 Is the Anisocoria More Apparent in the Light or in the Dark?

If the anisocoria is greater in dim light (stimulates dilation of the pupils), then the defect is in the sympathetic innervation of the pupil. If the anisocoria is greater in bright light (stimulates constriction of the pupil), then the lesion is in the parasympathetic innervation of the pupil. If a large pupil poorly reactive to light and the visual afferent system is normal, then a defect in the efferent parasympathetic innervation to this pupil is likely.[2] If the light reaction is difficult to compare to the fellow eye, then a measurement of the anisocoria in light and dark may help determine the pupillary abnormality.

20.3 Is Light-Near Dissociation Present?

If the light reaction is poor but the near reaction is intact, the patient has light-near dissociation of the pupils. This can occur in one or both eyes depending on the underlying etiology. Box 20.1 lists the causes of light-near dissociation.

Box 20.1 Etiologies of light-near dissociation

- Systemic disease:
  - Diabetes (autonomic neuropathy).
  - Familial amyloidosis.
  - Spinocerebellar ataxia type 1 (SCA-1).[3]
- Midbrain lesions:
  - Dorsal midbrain syndrome (Parinaud syndrome).
  - Encephalitis/meningitis.
  - Wernicke encephalopathy and alcoholism.
  - Demyelination.
  - Pineal tumors.
  - Vascular disease.
- Ocular:
  - Argyll Robertson pupil.
  - Tonic pupils (e.g., local orbital, neuropathic, Adie pupil, ocular, or central nervous system [CNS] siderosis[4]).
  - Aberrant third nerve regeneration (not sparing of near but "restoring" of near).
  - Bilateral afferent disease (i.e., bilateral retinopathy or bilateral anterior visual pathway lesion (optic nerve, chiasm, tract).
- Other:
  - Syringomyelia (rare).

The quality of the near reaction may help differentiate the cause of the light-near dissociation. In a tonic pupil, the near reaction produces tonic constriction that then slowly relaxes. This is in contrast to the Argyll Robertson pupil (see below), where the near reaction is brisk.

20.4 Is There Other Evidence for a Third Nerve Palsy?

Patients with anisocoria and a poorly reactive pupil should be evaluated for an ipsilateral third nerve palsy. Sunderland suggested that an extra-axial lesion compressing the third nerve (e.g., unruptured intracranial aneurysm) may cause a dilated pupil in isolation or with minimal ocular motor nerve paresis. Anisocoria or a dilated pupil in the absence of an extraocular motility deficit and/or ptosis, however, is rarely due to a third nerve palsy.[5] Dhume and Paul described diabetic ischemic third nerve palsy-related mydriasis in 25% of the study subjects. Patients demonstrated 1 to 2 mm of anisocoria, with preserved minimal reactivity to light. These patients frequently had concurrent evidence of ophthalmoplegia that was more readily reversible than pupillary changes.[6] Intracranial aneurysms (e.g., posterior communicating artery-internal carotid artery junction) often produce a fixed and dilated pupil (pupil-involved third nerve palsy), but this is almost always associated with other signs of a third nerve palsy.[7] Walsh and Hoyt reported a patient with headache and a unilateral dilated pupil who was found to have an aneurysm at the junction of the superior cerebellar artery and basilar artery.[8] One week later, however, the patient developed other signs of a third nerve palsy. Payne and Adamkiewicz reported a case of unilateral internal ophthalmoplegia with a posterior communicating aneurysm, but this patient also had an intermittent exotropia and variable ptosis.[9] Crompton and Moore reported two cases of isolated pupil dilation due to aneurysm, but these patients developed severe headache and eventual signs of a third nerve palsy.[10] Fujiwara et al reviewed 26 patients with an oculomotor palsy due to cerebral aneurysm and reported three with only ptosis and anisocoria.[11]

Basilar aneurysms theoretically can produce isolated internal ophthalmoplegia, but this finding is rare and usually the patient rapidly develops signs of external ophthalmoplegia due to third nerve dysfunction. Gale and Crockard observed transient unilateral mydriasis in a patient with a basilar aneurysm.[12] Miller reported an isolated internal ophthalmoplegia in a patient with a basilar aneurysm.[7] Wilhelm et al described an oculomotor nerve paresis that began as an isolated internal ophthalmoplegia in 1979 and then developed into a more typical third nerve palsy in 1993 due to a neurinoma of the third nerve.[13] Kaye-Wilson et al also described a patient who initially had only minimal pupil signs due to a neurinoma of the third nerve.[14] A mydriatic pupil was the presenting sign of a common carotid artery dissection with the pupil dilation preceding other signs and symptoms of a third nerve palsy and cerebral ischemia.[15] These cases are uncommon presentations, and in general an isolated dilated pupil is more likely to be due to local iris abnormalities, the tonic pupil syndrome, or pharmacologic dilation than third nerve palsy (class IV, level C).

Other rare cases of interpeduncular cyst, mesencephalic hemorrhage, presumed ocular motor nerve inflammation due to meningitis (e.g., bacterial, cryptococcal or tuberculous basal meningitis), and direct head trauma to the third nerve at the posterior petroclinoid ligament have been described as presenting with an isolated, unilateral, fixed, and dilated pupil. Brookes et al describe unilateral mydriasis after maxillary osteotomy secondary to mechanical factors, including direct traction or local edema, or pharmacologics.[16] Other neurologic signs of a third nerve palsy, however, were present or appeared over time in almost all these patients. Unilateral pupillary involvement from probable preganglionic oculomotor nerve dysfunction (normal ductions but pupil minimally reactive to light; however, reactive to near stimuli) has also been described with superficial siderosis of the CNS with selective involvement of the superficially located pupillary fibers.[4] In a patient with an isolated dilated pupil in the presence of normal extraocular motility, a third nerve palsy can be safely excluded in almost every circumstance simply with close follow-up (class IV, level C).

In indeterminate cases, topical pilocarpine 1% can be used as a simple test for third nerve palsy versus pharmacologic blockade (see below). A pupil dilated from a third nerve palsy will constrict to pilocarpine 1%, but one with a parasympathetic pharmacologic blockade will not. Pupil reaction to topical pilocarpine 1 or 0.1%, however, does not differentiate between third nerve palsy and Adie tonic pupil. Please refer to Chapter 11 for a more detailed discussion of third nerve palsies.

20.5 Is There Evidence for Pharmacologic (or Toxic) Mydriasis or Miosis?

A careful history is usually all that is required for patients with inadvertent or intentional (e.g., glaucoma medication, treatment with topical cycloplegics for uveitis) exposure to agents that may affect pupil size (e.g., mydriatics or miotics). ▶ Table 20.1 and ▶ Table 20.2 list some medications and environmental agents that may result in mydriasis or miosis, respectively. Pharmacologically induced pupil abnormalities may produce a large pupil due to increased sympathetic tone with dilator stimulation (e.g., ocular decongestants, adrenergic

Table 20.1 Medications and environmental agents associated with mydriasis

Topical parasympatholytics	Topical sympathomimetics
• Atropine, drops or aerosolized[17]	• Apraclonidine (α-adrenergic agonist)[27]
• Cyclopentolate (Cyclogyl)	• Dexamethasone
• Eucatropine	• Epinephrine, dipivalyl epinephrine (Propine)
• Homatropine	• Phenylephrine (NeoSynephrine)
• Oxyphenonium	• Cocaine (e.g., topical nasal travels into conjunctival sac)
• Scopolamine	• Ocular decongestants (tetrahydrozoline hydrochloride, pheniramine maleate, chlorpheniramine maleate, naphazoline)[28,29]
• Tropicamide (Mydriacyl)	
• Gentamicin	
• Glycopyrrolate[18,19,20]	
• Lidocaine gel introduced to the eye[21]	
• Aerosolized ipratropium bromide given by loosely fitting mask[22,23,24,25,26]	

Local and systemic agents	Other
• Anesthetic agents for the airway (phenylephrine/lidocaine spray)[30]	• Siderosis bulbi/iron mydriasis—occult intraocular iron foreign body[39,40,41]
• Amphetamines	• Hypromellose viscoelastic in cataract surgery[42]
• Atropine (systemic)	• Alkaloids (belladonna alkaloids) (anticholinergic effect):
• Benztropine	• Jimson weed (Datura stramonium)
• Barracuda meat	• Blue nightshade or European bittersweet (Solanum dulcamara)
• Calcium	• Deadly nightshade (Atropa belladonna)
• Cocaine[31]	• Henbane (Hyoscyamus niger)
• Diphenhydramine	• Moonflower (Datura wrightii or D. meteloides)[43]
• Epinephrine[32]	• Other Datura species (D. suaveolans [angel's trumpet], aurea, candida, sanguinea, stramonium, wrightii)[44,45,46,47,48]
• Fenfluramine/norfenfluramine	• Brugmansia arborea (also known as angel's trumpet)[49]
• Glutethimide	
• Ipratropium (systemic)[33]	
• Levodopa	
• Lidocaine (e.g., orbital injection, anterior chamber injection)	
• Lysergic acid diethylamide	
• Magnesium	
• Nalorphine	
• Propantheline bromide (Pro-Banthine)	
• Scopolamine methylbromide,[34] transdermal scopolamine patches[35]	
• Selective serotonin reuptake inhibitors (SSRIs)[36,37,38]	
• Thiopental	
• Tricyclic antidepressants	

Table 20.2 Medications and environmental agents associated with miosis

Topical parasympathomimetics	Topical sympatholytics
• Aceclidine	• Thymoxamine hydrochloride
• Carbachol	• Dapiprazole ("RevEyes")
• Methacholine (Mecholyl)	• Dibenzyline (hemoxybenzamine)
• Organophosphate esters	• Phentolamine (Regitine)
• Pilocarpine	• Tolazoline (Priscoline)
• Physostigmine (eserine)	• Guanethidine
	• Timolol with epinephrine

Local and systemic agents	Other
• Chlorpromazine	• Flea collar (anticholinesterase)[50]
• Heroin	• Pyrethrins and piperonyl butoxide insecticides (anticholinesterase)
• Lidocaine (extradural anesthesia)	
• Marijuana	
• Methadone	
• Morphine and other narcotics	
• Phenothiazines	

inhalants in the intensive care unit, etc.) or decreased parasympathetic tone with sphincter block (e.g., belladonna alkaloids, scopolamine patch, anticholinergic inhalants, topical gentamicin, lidocaine injection in orbit, etc.). Small pupils might indicate decreased sympathetic tone or increased parasympathetic stimulation (e.g., pilocarpine glaucoma drops, anticholinesterases such as flea collar or insecticides, etc.).

Nurses, physicians, and other health care workers are particularly prone to inadvertent or intentional exposure to pharmacologic mydriatics. The pupil size of patients with pharmacologic sphincter blockade is often quite large (8–12 mm in diameter). This large, dilated pupil is much greater than the mydriasis usually seen in typical third nerve palsy or tonic pupil syndromes. The pupils are evenly affected for 360 degrees, unlike the irregular pupil seen in the tonic pupil or iris trauma. Topical pilocarpine 1% can be used as a simple test for pharmacologic blockade. A pupil dilated from a third nerve palsy will constrict to pilocarpine 1%, but a pupil with a parasympathetic pharmacologic blockade will constrict poorly or not at all to topical miotics. An acute tonic pupil may be unreactive to either light or near stimuli and may be difficult to distinguish from a pharmacologically dilated pupil or acute traumatic iridoplegia.

Adrenergic pharmacologic mydriasis (e.g., phenylephrine) typically produces blanched conjunctival vessels, retains residual light reaction, and produces a retracted upper lid due to sympathetic stimulation of the upper lid retractor muscle. Most "eye-whitening" over-the-counter eyedrops (e.g., oxymetazoline, phenylephrine) contain sympathomimetics too weak to dilate the pupil unless the corneal epithelium is breached (e.g., contact lens wear). Exposure to anticholinesterases can result in a miotic pupil.[51,52] There are reported cases of transient anisocoria under general anesthesia following administration of multiple agents, possibly due to altered autonomic tone. Acute causes of anisocoria should be considered before attributing the finding to an asymmetric reaction to systemic medications. In addition, in such settings, it is difficult to exclude direct topical exposure to a pharmacologic agent.[53,54,55,56,57,58] For cases of presumed isolated dilated or constricted pupils due to pharmacologic exposure, we recommend close follow-up to ensure that the pupil returns to normal size. Confirmatory pharmacologic

testing could be considered in atypical or persistent cases (class IV, level C).

20.6 Are Intermittent or Transient Pupillary Phenomena Present?

Transient mydriasis or miosis has been reported in the following conditions: migraine headaches,[59] trigeminal autonomic cephalalgias,[60] migraine aura without headache,[61] astrocytoma,[62] encephalopathy,[63] HS after carotid puncture, during or after seizure activity,[64] after reduction of bilateral orbital floor fractures,[65] and in normal individuals. Episodic miosis with ptosis accompanied by ipsilateral nasal stuffiness may occur without headache (cluster sine headache).[66] Tadpole-shaped pupils due to segmental spasm of the pupil sphincter may also be related to a partial postganglionic HS or migraine phenomenon (occurs between rather than with headache attacks). Tourney phenomenon describes anisocoria on lateral gaze with the adducting eye appearing smaller than the abducting eye in up to 10% of normal subjects. Though commonly reported to be of no clinical significant and considered by some to be a possible optical distortion,[67] if the phenomenon occurs in conjunction with oculomotor deficits, aberrant regeneration of the third nerve should be considered.[68] Some of these phenomena represent true sympathetic irritation or excess, but the mechanism remains controversial. If the transient or intermittent nature of the mydriasis can be firmly established, then these patients should not undergo arteriography or other testing and should simply be followed for 24 to 48 hours, at which point improvement would indicate the benign nature of the mydriasis.

Jacobson reported 24 patients with benign episodic unilateral mydriasis. Twenty of the 24 eyes were exclusively unilaterally affected. In two cases, either eye was affected independently and two cases did not specify laterally.[69] The median age of the patients was 31 (range, 14–50) and the median duration of events was 12 hours (range, 10 minutes–7 days). Associated symptoms included visual blur, headache, orbital pain, monocular photophobia, monocular red eye, monocular diplopia, and monocular positional transient obscurations. Some cases were thought due to parasympathetic insufficiency of the iris sphincter. These patients had associated impaired near vision, impaired accommodative function, and the anisocoria increased with added ambient light. Other patients had sympathetic hyperactivity of the iris dilator associated with normal near vision and normal reaction of the pupil during the attack. No associated neurologic disorders were found in these patients. Martín-Santana et al also describe seven individuals with benign episodic mydriasis. All seven patients were female, their mean age was 33 ± 10, and 4 of 10 patients endorsed history of migraine with prior migraine attacks with associated pupil changes. Six of seven patients presented with unilateral mydriasis and the duration ranged from < 5 minutes to 48 hours.[70] We do not recommend any further evaluation for isolated transient unilateral mydriasis (class IV, level C). If additional neurological symptoms are present, consider additional work-up as indicated by the overall clinical syndrome. In a case report presented by Clerici et al, a 56-year-old male presented with anisocoria during an episode of hypertensive crisis with vomiting, headache, retropulsion, postural instability, dysarthria, and incoordination. In the setting of these concurrent symptoms, imaging revealed a persistent left primitive hypoglossal artery with bilateral vertebral artery hypoplasia and slight aneurysmal dilation of the anterior communicating artery. With blood pressure control and IV antiplatelet therapy, the patient's neurological symptoms resolved within 12 hours. The persistent primitive hypoglossal artery was thought to contribute to a transient ischemic attack (TIA) in the setting of vascular compromise during the hypertensive crisis responsible for the pupillary and vertebra-basilar neurologic findings.[71]

20.7 Is a Structural Iris Abnormality Present?

Careful slit-lamp biomicroscopy of the iris should be performed in all patients with anisocoria to exclude structural iris abnormalities or damage. In many cases, the pupil is irregular and the structural abnormality can easily be identified. The clinical features of structural iris abnormality include irregular pupil, disruption of pupillary margin from iris sphincter tears, irregular contraction in light, poor response to parasympathomimetics, and the eventual development of iris atrophy. Notably, structural abnormalities are not associated with ocular motility disturbances or ptosis. Etiologies of iris structural damage are listed in Box 20.2.

Box 20.2 Etiologies of structural damage to the iris

- Congenital aplasia of the iris sphincter and dilator muscles.[72]
- Increased intraocular pressure due to acute angle closure glaucoma (sphincter paresis due to iris ischemia).
- Intraocular inflammation (e.g., iritis).
- Ischemia (e.g., ocular ischemic syndrome, iris ischemia after anterior chamber air/gas injection after deep lamellar keratoplasty for keratoconus).[73]
- Mechanical (e.g., iris tumor, intraocular lens).
- Surgical (e.g., iridectomy, iridotomy, iris damage).
- Trauma:
  - Blunt trauma (traumatic iridoplegia).
  - Sphincter tears at the pupillary margin.
- Atonic pupil after cataract extraction.[74]

Abnormalities of the iris are a common cause of anisocoria. False-positive pharmacologic testing may result in patients with structural abnormalities of the iris that prevent dilation or constriction to pharmacologic agents. In these cases, it may be necessary to test the integrity of the pupil dilation or constriction capacity by applying a topical direct sympathomimetic or parasympathomimetic (class IV, level C).

20.8 Is a Tonic Pupil Present?

The typical presentation of the tonic pupil is isolated anisocoria that is greater in light. Patients often present with acute awareness of the dilated pupil. The clinical features of a tonic pupil are listed in Box 20.3.

Box 20.3 Clinical features of a tonic pupil

- Poor pupillary light reaction.
- Segmental palsy of the sphincter.
- Tonic pupillary near response with light-near dissociation (near response not "spared" but "restored" due to aberrant regeneration).
- Cholinergic supersensitivity of the denervated muscles.
- Accommodation paresis (that tends to recover).
- Induced astigmatism at near.
- Tonicity of accommodation.
- Occasional ciliary cramp with near work.
- Occasionally regional corneal anesthesia (trigeminal ophthalmic division fibers in ciliary ganglion damaged).

Pharmacologic testing with low-dose pilocarpine (0.1%) may demonstrate cholinergic supersensitivity in the tonic pupil (a more miotic response than the fellow eye). Leavitt et al suggested a solution of 0.0625% pilocarpine to avoid false positives in a normal eye.[75] Unfortunately, cholinergic supersensitivity is not uniformly present in tonic pupils (80% with topical pilocarpine testing) and is not specific for postganglionic parasympathetic denervation. Supersensitivity has been reported after oculomotor nerve palsy.[68,76,77] In addition, larger-sized pupils normally constrict more than smaller pupils to the same dose of topical cholinergics. Jacobson recommends evaluating cholinergic supersensitivity responses in darkness to minimize the mechanical resistance factors of large and small pupil size.[76,77] A larger pupil that becomes the smaller pupil in darkness after topical cholinergics is more likely a supersensitive response.[76,77] Clinicians should use other clinical features (e.g., ptosis or motility deficit) to differentiate third nerve palsy anisocoria from the tonic pupil.

20.9 Is the Tonic Pupil Isolated?

The history and examination should be able to differentiate the various associations of secondary pupils from idiopathic Adie tonic pupil syndrome. ▶ Table 20.3 lists the causes of a tonic pupil.

Table 20.3 Etiologies of a tonic pupil

Infection[78]	Medication/Toxic
• Campylobacter jejuni enteritis[79]	• Local anesthesia[32] (i.e., inferior dental block or injection of retrobulbar alcohol)
• Cytomegalovirus[80]	• Quinine
• Cellulitis	• Trichloroethylene
• Choroiditis	• Siderosis from intraocular foreign body[86]
• Diphtheria	
• Herpes simplex virus	**Paraneoplastic**
• Herpes zoster virus[81]	• Eaton-Lambert syndrome[87]
• Human herpes Virus 6[82]	• Carcinomatous neuropathy
• HTLV-II[83]	• Congenital neuroblastoma with Hirschsprung's disease and central hypoventilation syndrome[88]
• Influenza	
• Measles (and postvaccination)[84]	
• Parvovirus B19[85]	• Unilateral or bilateral tonic pupil with anti-Hu antibodies[89,90,91]
• Pertussis	
• Sinusitis	• Reversible tonic pupil with non-Hodgkin lymphoma[92]
• Scarlet fever	
• Viral hepatitis	
• Syphilis	

Table 20.3 continued

Ischemia	Inflammation
• Orbital vasculitis • Lymphomatoid granulomatosis[93] • Giant cell arteritis[94] • Migraine[95] • Orbital or choroidal tumor[93] • Polyarteritis nodosa[96]	• Iritis/uveitis damage to ciliary ganglion; Heerfordt syndrome (uveoparotid fever)[97] • Rheumatoid arthritis • Vogt–Koyanagi–Harada syndrome[98,99] • Sarcoidosis • Post-operative edema[16]

Trauma (surgical and nonsurgical)	Neuropathic

• Surgery[100,101,102,103] ±:
  ○ Cataract surgery[103,104]
  ○ Cryotherapy
  ○ Diathermy
  ○ Penetrating keratoplasty
  ○ Retinal surgery
  ○ Strabismus surgery
  ○ Orbital surgery[100]
  ○ Laser therapy
• Blunt trauma to ciliary plexus
• Orbital floor fracture
• Retrobulbar hemorrhage[105]
• Damage to short ciliary nerves
	• Peripheral or autonomic neuropathies:
	  ○ Amyloidosis[106]
	  ○ Diabetes
	  ○ Alcohol-related
	• Familial dysautonomia
	• Hereditary neuropathy (e.g., Charcot–Marie–Tooth disease)
	• Guillain–Barré syndrome
	• Miller Fisher syndrome (including isolated bilateral internal ophthalmoplegia with IgG anti-GQ1b antibodies)[107, 108,109,110,111,112,113,114]
	• Chronic inflammatory demyelinating polyradiculoneuropathy[115]
	• Acute sensorimotor polyneuropathy with tonic pupils and abduction deficit with polyarteritis nodosa[96]
	• Pandysautonomia
	• Progressive autonomic failure
	• Shy–Drager syndrome
	• Ross syndrome (tonic pupil, hyporeflexia segmental anhidrosis)[80,116,117,118]

Other
• Sjögren syndrome[119,120] • Following oculomotor nerve palsy[68] • Adie tonic pupil syndrome • Endometriosis[121]

20.10 Is This Adie Tonic Pupil Syndrome?

The clinical features of Adie tonic pupil syndrome, based on Thompson's extensive review[122,123] and the literature, are reported in ▶ Table 20.4. With the tonic pupil, the iris sphincter and ciliary muscles become supersensitive to acetylcholine, and thus when they are stimulated their response is strong and tonic and their relaxation is slow and sustained. Initially, there is an isolated internal ophthalmoplegia, and in the acute stage there is no reaction to light or near stimuli at all. The diagnosis of a tonic pupil can usually be made on clinical grounds alone (class IV, level B).

Table 20.4 Clinical features of Adie syndrome

Prevalence	2 cases per 1,000 population
Mean age	32 years
Female-to-male ratio	2.6:1
Unilateral	80%
Reduced deep tendon reflexes	89%
Sector palsy	100%[a]
Accommodative paresis	66%
Bilateral	4% per year
Cholinergic supersensitivity	80%
Decreased regional corneal sensation	90%
Prognosis	Accommodative paresis resolves over months Pupil light reaction usually does not recover Pupil smaller with time ("little old Adie") Most symptoms resolve spontaneously

*In patients with some degree of light reaction.

20.10.1 What Causes the Adie Tonic Pupil Syndrome?

The pathophysiology of Adie tonic pupil is believed to be due to damage to the ciliary ganglion.[124,125,126] More than 90% of the ciliary ganglion cells normally serve the ciliary body and only 3% serve the iris sphincter. After damage to the ciliary ganglion, aberrant regeneration of fibers originally destined for the ciliary body now innervate the iris sphincter. The initially mydriatic pupil may become smaller over time ("little old Adie pupil") and indeed Adie tonic pupil may present as a miotic pupil (acute awareness rather than acute onset of anisocoria). Although most Adie tonic pupils present unilaterally, bilateral involvement may develop at a rate of 4% per year.[122] Thompson reviewed 220 cases from the literature and reported that 20% were bilateral.[122] Rarely, Adie syndrome may be associated with a chronic cough likely related to vagal involvement.[127] When associated with diminished deep tendon reflexes, it is referred to as Holmes–Adie pupillary syndrome.[128]

20.10.2 Should Neuroimaging Studies Be Performed in Adie Syndrome?

Once the diagnosis of the Adie tonic pupil is confirmed clinically and/or pharmacologically, no neuroimaging studies are required (class III–IV, level C).

20.10.3 What Treatment Is Recommended for Adie Syndrome?

Patients with Adie syndrome often complain of difficulty in reading due to accommodative paresis. The treatment of Adie tonic pupil is usually reassurance alone. Unequal bifocal reading aids or a unilateral frosted bifocal segment may be needed for patients with accommodative paresis. The use of topical low-dose pilocarpine or eserine has been suggested by some authors for Adie syndrome, but may precipitate ciliary spasm, induce myopia, cause browache, or worsen anisocoria due to miosis.[122,123] We do not generally recommend treatment for Adie tonic pupil (class IV, level C).

20.11 When Does One Perform Syphilis Serology in Bilateral, Tonic, or Miotic, Irregular Pupils with Light-Near Dissociation?

Thompson recommends that all patients with bilateral tonic pupils have serologic testing for syphilis.[122] Fletcher and Sharpe reported that 5 of 60 consecutive patients with tonic pupils had positive serology for syphilis.[129] Of these patients, all were bilateral tonic pupils and none presented with acute mydriasis or cycloplegia. We recommend syphilis serology for unexplained bilateral tonic pupils (class IV, level C).

Argyll Robertson pupils are small, irregular, and are characterized by light-near dissociation, variable iris atrophy, and normal afferent visual function. They are classically described with neurosyphilis, and the lesion is within the rostral midbrain and pretectal oculomotor light reflex fibers on the dorsal side of the Edinger–Westphal nucleus. There is sparing of the near fibers that approach this nucleus more ventrally. The pupils are small because supranuclear adrenergic inhibitory fibers to the Edinger–Westphal nucleus are blocked. The pupil abnormality is usually bilateral in neurosyphilis, but may be unilateral in some patients.[130]

Although classically described with neurosyphilis, other entities may produce a similar clinical syndrome. Patients with diabetes may also have small, poorly reactive pupils with light-near dissociation that may appear similar to the Argyll Robertson pupil. Other etiologies include chronic alcoholism, encephalitis, multiple sclerosis, degenerative diseases of the CNS (e.g., Charcot–Marie–Tooth), rare midbrain tumors, herpes zoster, neurosarcoidosis, and lymphocytic meningoradiculitis.

20.12 Is the Pupillary Light Reaction Normal?

If the pupillary light reaction is normal in both eyes, then physiologic (simple) anisocoria,[131] a Horner syndrome, sympathetic irritation, or pharmacologic mydriasis should be considered.

20.13 Is the Anisocoria Isolated?

If the patient has an isolated anisocoria (e.g., no ptosis or dilation lag, no evidence of iris injury or drugs, and not related to Adie tonic pupil or other innervational defects), then simple (physiologic or central) anisocoria is likely to be present.[131] Simple anisocoria may have a prevalence of up to 21% (range, 1–90% in various studies), and most of these patients have an anisocoria of less than 0.4 mm that is usually only intermittently present.[131]

The anisocoria tends to be equal in light or dark. Topical cocaine will dilate both pupils equally (see the "What Is Pharmacologic Localization of HS," section below). In newborns, anisocoria is also reported to occur at a prevalence of 21% with a difference less than 1.0 mm.[132] It is assumed that in these patients' inhibition of the sphincter nuclei in the midbrain is not "balanced" with any precision that is necessary for clear binocular vision. When associated with poor visual acuity, amaurotic mydriasis should be considered. Lepore describes mydriasis in eyes with pregeniculate vision loss.[133]

20.14 Is Horner Syndrome Present?

Interruption of the ocular sympathetic pathway is known as an HS. HS is characterized clinically by the signs listed in Box 20.4.

Box 20.4 Clinical signs of Horner syndrome

- Ipsilateral mild (usually < 2 mm) ptosis (due to denervation of the superior tarsal muscle of the upper eyelid).
- "Upside-down ptosis" (from sympathetic denervation to the lower eyelid retractors).
- Apparent enophthalmos.
- Anisocoria due to ipsilateral miosis.
- Dilation lag (slow dilation of the pupil after the lights are dimmed).
- Increased accommodative amplitude or accommodative paresis.[7]
- Transient (acute phase) ocular hypotony and conjunctival hyperemia.
- Variable ipsilateral facial anhidrosis.
- Ipsilateral straight hair in congenital cases.
- Heterochromia of the iris (usually congenital but rarely acquired).[7,134]
- Rarely, neurotrophic corneal endothelial failure with pain and stromal edema.[135]

HS may result from a lesion anywhere along a three-neuron pathway that arises as a first-order (central) neuron from the posterolateral hypothalamus, descends in the brainstem and lateral column of the spinal cord to synapse at the cervical (C8), and thoracic (T1-T2) levels (ciliospinal center of Budge) of the spinal cord as a second-order neuron. This second-order (intermediate) preganglionic neuron exits the ventral root and arches over the apex of the lung to ascend in the cervical sympathetic chain. The second-order neurons synapse in the superior cervical ganglion and exit as a third-order neuron. The neural fibers for sweating of the face travel with the external carotid artery. The third-order postganglionic neuron travels with the carotid artery into the cavernous sinus. Within the cavernous sinus, the sympathetic fibers join the abducens nerve for a short course and then travel with the ophthalmic division of the trigeminal nerve and join the nasociliary branch of the trigeminal nerve. The fibers pass through the ciliary ganglion and to the eye as the long and short ciliary nerves.[2,7] Depending on the location of the lesion, all features of the HS triad may not be present. Anhidrosis may be variable due to relatively early branching of these efferent nerves. Furthermore, confounding factors may mask symptoms as discussed by Pemberton et al in a patient with ptosis whose anisocoria was not evident with a carotid artery dissection due to naphazoline use.[29]

The evaluation of HS includes two stages[2,7]: (1) recognition of the clinical syndrome, and (2) confirmation and localization by pharmacologic testing.

20.14.1 Is the Horner Syndrome Isolated?

Nonisolated HS should undergo imaging with attention to the topographic localization of the clinical findings.

20.14.2 Is a Central Horner Syndrome Present?

Patients with a central HS can usually be identified by the presence of associated hypothalamic or brainstem signs or symptoms (e.g., contralateral fourth nerve palsy, diabetes insipidus, disturbed temperature or sleep regulation, meningeal signs, vertigo, sensory deficits, anhidrosis of the body, etc.). The etiologies of central HS are listed in ▶ Table 20.5.

Table 20.5 Etiologies of Horner syndrome

	Central	Preganglionic	Postganglionic
Vascular	Hemorrhage,[136] ischemia/infarction (i.e., midbrain,[137] hypothalamic,[138,139] thalamic[140]) Wallenberg syndrome,[141] Giant cell arteritis (unilateral internuclear ophthalmoplegia with ipsilateral Horner syndrome),[142] anterior spinal artery thrombosis[143]	Internal jugular vein thrombosis in polycythemia vera,[144] thoracic aneurysms[145]	Intracavernous aneurysm, ophthalmic artery aneurysm,[146] orbital vascular lesion (e.g., hemangioma),[147] vascular abnormalities of the internal carotid artery, carotid artery aneurysms or dissection,[148,149,150,151,152,153] arteriosclerosis or thrombosis of the internal carotid artery,[154] fibromuscular dysplasia, giant cell arteritis,[155] granulomatosis with polyangitis[156]
Infection	Syphilis, poliomyelitis, meningitis, herpes zoster meningitis[157]		Herpes zoster,[158] severe purulent otitis media (caroticotympanic plexus), herpetic geniculate neuralgia, meningitis, sinusitis, mononeuritis multiplex due to cytomegalovirus in an AIDS patient[159]
Neoplasm	Hypothalamic/pituitary, third ventricle, brainstem, spinal cord neoplasms	Neck and brachial plexus tumors, glomus tumors, breast cancer, sarcomas, Pancoast tumors, lymphoreticular neoplasms,[160] neurofibroma, neuroblastoma,[161,162] thyroid adenoma,[163] vagus nerve schwannoma,[164] sympathetic paraganglioma,[165] cervical sympathetic chain schwannoma or neurilemmomas,[166,167] cervical node metastasis	Orbital tumors, cavernous sinus tumors, nasopharyngeal tumors,[164] metastases
Inflammatory	Sarcoidosis	Mediastinal or neck lymphadenopathy (i.e., pachymeningitis, herpes zoster in T3-T4[168])	Sarcoidosis, Tolosa–Hunt syndrome, otitis media (caroticotympanic plexus), petrositis, sphenoid sinus mucocele, cervical lymphadenopathy [a,162,169,170,171]
Degenerative		Hypertrophic spinal arthritis, foraminal osteophyte, ruptured intervertebral disc	Amyloidosis[106,143]
Intoxication		Continuous thoracic epidural analgesia[172,173,174]	
Congenital		Cervicothoracic abnormalities, cervical rib	Congenital agenesis of internal carotid artery[175]
Neurologic	Demyelinating disease		Miller Fisher syndrome, Ross syndrome,[116] pure autonomic failure,[143] familial dysautonomia,[143] autonomic neuropathy (HSAN) type III,[143] Dopamine β-hydroxylase deficiency,[143] multiple system atrophy (Shy–Drager syndrome),[143] headache syndromes (e.g., cluster or migraine)[176,177,178]
Endocrine		Thoracic endometriosis[164] Thyroiditis (mass effect)[179]	Diabetes[a,143,180]

Table 20.5 continued

	Central	Preganglionic	Postganglionic
Mechanical/Trauma	Trauma,[181] Brown–Sequard Syndrome[182]	Syringomyelia,[183] neck or brachial plexus trauma or surgery,[184] birth trauma (Klumpke's paralysis), surgical or procedural trauma,[185] superior cervical ganglion injury,[186] upper cervical sympathectomies,[143] anterior C3–C6 fusion, radical thyroid surgery, chest trauma,[187] implantation of vagus nerve stimulator,[188] migration of foreign body from pharynx to soft tissues of neck,[189] first rib fracture,[190] pulmonary surgery (resection of ruptured pulmonary hydatid cyst)[191]	Cavernous sinus lesions,[7] basilar skull fracture, orbital fracture, radical middle ear surgery, injection or surgery of the Gasserian ganglion, intraoral trauma to internal carotid sympathetic plexus, intraoral anesthesia injection,[164] tonsillectomy, prolonged abnormal posture during coma,[192] head trauma with intracranial carotid artery injury,[193] carotid endarterectomy,[194] intracavernous carotid artery aneurysm repair[195]

[a]Exact localization of the lesion as pre- or postganglionic may vary by individual patient.
Additional Sources: Refs.[2,7,138,139,196,197].

20.14.3 Is a Preganglionic (Intermediate) Horner Syndrome Present?

The preganglionic (intermediate) HS occurs due to a lesion of the second-order neuron traveling in the sympathetic chain from the ciliospinal center of Budge to the superior cervical ganglion. The patient may have neck or arm pain, anhidrosis involving the face and neck, brachial plexopathy, vocal cord paralysis, or phrenic nerve palsy.[2] Ptosis and anisocoria may fluctuate.[162] The etiologies of preganglionic intermediate HS are listed in ▶ Table 20.5.

20.14.4 Is a Postganglionic Horner Syndrome Present?

The postganglionic HS occurs due to a lesion of the third-order neuron traveling from the superior cervical ganglion to the orbit. The patient may have ipsilateral pain and other symptoms suggestive of cluster or migraine headaches (e.g., tearing, facial flushing, rhinorrhea).[176,178] Anhidrosis in postganglionic HS is often absent.[123] Sweat glands of the forehead are supplied by the terminal branches of sympathetics to the internal carotid, and involvement of these fibers after they have separated from the remaining facial sweat fibers may explain the occurrence of anhidrosis of the forehead with sparing of the rest of the face in these patients. Postganglionic HS due to cavernous sinus lesions (e.g., thrombosis, infection, neoplasm) usually is associated with other localizing signs such as ipsilateral third, fourth, or sixth nerve palsy or trigeminal nerve dysfunction.[7]

Dissection of the internal carotid artery (e.g., traumatic, spontaneous) may result in HS. Biousse et al, for example, studied 146 patients with internal carotid artery dissections and found that 28% (41 of 146) had a painful HS that was isolated in half of the cases (32 of 65).[198] Kerty noted HS in 23 of 28 patients with internal carotid artery dissection.[199] A third-order HS and orbital and/or ipsilateral head pain or neck pain of acute onset is diagnostic of internal carotid artery dissection unless proven otherwise.[198] Box 20.5 lists the associated signs and symptoms of a possible carotid artery dissection.

Box 20.5 Associated signs and symptoms of carotid artery dissection

- Ipsilateral orbital, facial, or neck pain (present in 90% of cases; ipsilateral to involved vessel in 80%).
- Diplopia (transient or persistent):
  - May be due to cavernous carotid involvement.
  - More likely due to transient or permanent impairment of blood supply through inferolateral trunk supplying third, fourth, and sixth cranial nerves.
  - Also possible due to orbital (extraocular muscle) ischemia or ophthalmic artery occlusion.
  - May have third, fourth, and/or sixth cranial nerve palsies.
- Transient carotid distribution ischemic attacks (e.g., amaurosis fugax), sometimes evoked by changes in posture.
- Transient monocular "scintillations" or "flashing lights," often related to postural changes or exposure to bright lights (possible choroidal ischemia).
- Visual loss:
  - Anterior (AION) or posterior (PION) ischemic optic neuropathy.
  - Central retinal artery occlusion (CRAO), branch retinal artery occlusion (BRAO).
  - Ophthalmic artery occlusion (often associated with head or neck pain).
  - Ocular ischemic syndrome.
  - Homonymous hemianopia (due to ischemic stroke).
  - Cortical vision loss or disturbance due to posterior reversible encephalopathy syndrome.
- Horner syndrome (third order, often painful).
- Transient unilateral mydriasis (rare).[200]
- Neck bruit or swelling.

- Other neurologic deficits:
  - Dysgeusia.
  - Tinnitus (often pulsatile).
  - Syncope.
  - Unilateral speech, motor, and/or sensory deficits (due to ischemic stroke or transient ischemic attacks).
  - Other cranial neuropathy (VI, IX, X, XI, XII).
- Connective tissue abnormalities in overlying skin usually without other clinical manifestations of a connective tissue disease.

Source: Refs. [2,149,198,199,201,202,203,204,205,206,207,208,209,210,211].

Patients with these signs should undergo imaging of the head and neck. We recommend imaging of the head and neck in cases of HS due to suspected carotid dissection (class III–IV, level B). Initially, screening typically consists of computed tomography (CT) or magnetic resonance imaging (MRI) of the head and neck combined with angiography (CT angiography, CTA, or MR angiography, MRA). The gold standard test for definitive diagnosis remains catheter angiography. Chapter 11 discusses vascular imaging in detail. Other etiologies of a post-ganglionic HS are listed in ▶ Table 20.5.

Although facial sweating abnormalities may be helpful in localizing a HS, the performance of clinical testing with starch and iodine (e.g., thermoregulatory sweat test) as described by some authors is somewhat time consuming, messy, and may be difficult to perform in the outpatient setting. Other tests of facial sweating may not add to the clinical or pharmacologic localization of HS.

20.15 What Is Alternating Horner Syndrome?

HS that alternates from one eye to the other (usually over days to weeks) is an uncommon finding but has been reported in multiple system atrophy (MSA) and in cervical spinal cord lesions. Tan et al reported a case and reviewed 25 cases from the literature (1 vertebral luxation, 14 cervical cord injuries, 8 MSA, 1 syringomyelia, 1 unknown, and 1 radiation myelopathy).[212] Generalized peripheral or autonomic neuropathies (e.g., diabetes, Miller Fisher syndrome, Shy–Drager syndrome) may also result in HS.[7]

20.16 Is the Horner Syndrome Related to Trauma?

Patients with a clear temporal association of the onset of HS with surgical or nonsurgical trauma to the sympathetic chain in the neck or chest do not require additional evaluation. The trauma may be direct or indirect.[184] Pharmacologic testing may aid in localization and confirmation of the diagnosis (class IV, level C). The etiologies of traumatic HS are listed in Box 20.6.

- Medical procedures:
  - Chest tube above the third posterior rib.[2,7,213,214]
  - Anesthesia administration (extradural, lumbar epidural,[215,216,217,218] thoracic epidural,[173] intraoral[164,219]).
  - Internal jugular vein catheterization.[135,220,221,222,223,224,225,226,227]
  - Carotid artery damage (e.g., carotid angiography,[228] carotid endarterectomy[194]).
  - Implantation of vagus nerve stimulator.[188]
  - Interscalene brachial plexus block.
- Surgery:[2,7,167,184,185,213,214]
  - Cardiac surgery.[229]
  - Neck or brachial plexus trauma surgery.[184]
  - Median sternotomy.
  - Superior cervical ganglion injury during tonsillectomy.[186]
  - Intentional surgical damage (e.g., sympathectomy).[143]
  - Intracavernous carotid artery aneurysm repair.[195]
  - Thoracic esophageal surgery.[230]
  - Anterior cervical spine surgery.[231]
  - Pulmonary surgery.[227]
  - Cervical sympathetic chain schwannoma resection.[232]
  - Injection or surgery of the Gasserian ganglion.
  - Radical middle ear surgery.
  - Stereotactic thalamotomy.
- Other:
  - Patient malpositioning[192] or prolonged abnormal posture during coma.[192]
  - Trauma to the head,[193] neck,[210,233] or chest.[187,190]
  - Brown–Sequard syndrome.[182]
  - Birth trauma (Klumpke's paralysis).
  - Syringomyelia.[183]
  - Injection into the carotid artery of heroin.
  - Migration of foreign body from pharynx to soft tissues of neck.[189]

20.17 What Is Pharmacologic Evaluation of Horner Syndrome?

Patients with HS that cannot be localized by clinical examination alone should undergo pharmacologic studies to confirm the diagnosis of HS and localize it to the preganglionic or postganglionic levels (class III–IV, level B). Although the clinical features of HS are classic, they are not pathognomonic. Ipsilateral ptosis and miosis may occur in patients without HS (e.g., levator dehiscence and physiologic anisocoria). Pharmacologic confirmation is relatively easy to perform and is more specific and sensitive than clinical diagnosis alone.

Cocaine inhibits the reuptake of norepinephrine at the neuromuscular junction. Therefore, topical 5 to 10% cocaine dilates a normal pupil (the mydriatic effect is small and usually about 1 mm) but does not dilate a pupil with HS (regardless of the location of the affected sympathetic neuron) as well as it dilates a normal pupil. Therefore, there is an increase in the degree of anisocoria after the cocaine test in a patient with HS. Minimal dilation of the pupil may occur in patients with only partial disruption of the oculosympathetic pathway or first-order neuron involvement.[2,7] Minimal or no dilation of the pupil after topical cocaine confirms that HS exists, but does not localize the responsible process to a preganglionic or postganglionic location. The advantage of cocaine is that it will test positive even in acute cases of HS, as the mechanism does not require denervation hypersensitivity.[234] Friedman et al reported the response to topical cocaine of 10% in 24 normal volunteers and suggested that 0.5 mm or more of anisocoria was necessary for the diagnosis of HS.[235] Van der Wiel and Van Gijn compared 12 patients with HS and 20 normal patients and found that an anisocoria of 1.0 mm after topical 5% cocaine was sufficient to diagnose HS.[236] Kardon et al administered the cocaine test to 50 normal patients and 119 patients with HS.[237] A postcocaine test anisocoria value of 1.0 mm gave a mean odds ratio using logistic regression analysis of about 5990:1 that HS was present (lower 95% confidence limit 37:1). These authors stated that simply measuring the postcocaine test anisocoria (versus measuring the net change in anisocoria) was the best predictor of HS.[237] Friedman et al noted that the pupils of black patients (with heavily pigmented irides) dilated poorly with cocaine, and therefore the test should be interpreted with more caution in black patients.[235,237] Patients undergoing topical pharmacologic testing should be informed that urine drug screening tests (for occupational hiring reasons) remain positive for 24 to 48 hours following topical testing.[238] Due to the controlled substance status of cocaine, this test is not readily available in all settings.

Apraclonidine, an alpha-2-agonist with weak alpha-1 effect is also used as a pharmacologic test for HS, and may be used in settings where cocaine testing is not available. Physiologically, apraclonidine normally acts on the alpha-2 receptors to cause in a slight miosis of the pupil. In a subacute or chronic case of HS where denervation hypersensitivity has developed, the alpha-1 action of apraclonidine will predominate in the effected eye, resulting in a dilation of the pupil. Diagnosis is thus made by reversal of the anisocoria.[234] In 22 eyes with oculosympathetic paresis, apraclonidine caused a mean dilation of 2.04 mm in the effected eye and a mean elevation of 1.75 mm of the upper eyelid, with a reported sensitivity and specificity similar to cocaine.[239] Denervation hypersensitivity may take time (days) to develop, but there are reports of positive tests at 3 hours for carotid dissection and 36 hours for dorsolateral pontomedullary infarct.[240,241] Systemic use of sympathomimetic and/or sympatholytic medications could potentially impact the results of the apraclonidine test, but this has not been studied clinically.[29,242] In addition, brimonidine also acts as an alpha-2 agonist with a weaker alpha-1 that could mask HS. Indeed, some physicians report cosmetic use of topical brimonidine for HS-associated anisocoria (class IV, level C).[243]

Hydroxyamphetamine releases stored norepinephrine from the postganglionic adrenergic nerve endings at the dilator muscle of the pupil. Therefore, a preganglionic HS (with intact postganglionic third-order neuron) dilates after the administration of topical hydroxyamphetamine 1%, whereas a postganglionic HS pupil does not dilate (no norepinephrine stores due to nerve damage).[238] It should be noted that a false-negative hydroxyamphetamine test may occur with postganglionic HS during the first week after injury.[244] A positive test result is noted if the anisocoria increases after the test versus a negative result if the anisocoria is diminished or unchanged (this measurement accounts for any preexisting anisocoria and psychosensory transient dilation effects).[245,246]

In intermediate and central preganglionic lesions, the affected pupil usually dilates more in response to hydroxyamphetamine possibly because of enhanced receptor sensitivity at the dilator muscle.[245,246] There is no effective pharmacologic test to differentiate central from intermediate preganglionic HS. The hydroxyamphetamine test should be deferred for 24 to 48 hours following the cocaine test because cocaine will block the effects of the hydroxyamphetamine.[245,246] Similarly, apraclonidine and hydroxyamphetamine testing should not occur on the same day. If one is confident in the diagnosis of HS and localization is the most critical objective, some authors favor going directly to hydroxyamphetamine testing (class IV, level U).

Topical pharmacologic testing should be performed in both eyes (the fellow eye serves as a control) and iatrogenic disruption of the corneal epithelium (e.g., applanation tonometry or corneal sensitivity testing) should be avoided prior to testing. Patients with congenital HS may fail to dilate after topical hydroxyamphetamine due to orthograde transsynaptic dysgenesis of the postganglionic neuron and may in reality have a preganglionic lesion.

Maloney et al reviewed the clinical accuracy of the pharmacologic localization of HS in 267 patients.[228] The hydroxyamphetamine test correctly localized peripheral postganglionic HS in 75 (84%) of 89 patients. The reported sensitivity for identification of a postganglionic HS by hydroxyamphetamine was 96%.[228] Van der Wiel and Van Gijn reported a sensitivity of only 40%,[247] but their study had a relatively smaller number of patients and excluded patients with cluster headache. Cremer et al described the results of hydroxyamphetamine testing in 54 patients with HS and reported a sensitivity of 93% and specificity of 83%.[245,246] Patients with an isolated postganglionic HS usually have a benign HS, whereas patients with a preganglionic HS are at risk for harboring an underlying malignancy. Grimson and Thompson described 67 patients with HS.[248] The incidence of malignant neoplasm in the preganglionic HS was almost 50% versus 2% in postganglionic HS. Some authors have recommended a screening chest radiograph for all cases of HS of undetermined etiology due to the small risk of misdiagnosis of a preganglionic HS by the hydroxyamphetamine test.[213] Wilhelm et al reviewed 90 cases of HS and reported a specificity of 90% for postganglionic HS and 88% for preganglionic HS.[249]

Grimson and Thompson reported 120 patients with HS.[250] Of these 120 patients, 41% were preganglionic, and one half of these were due to underlying neoplasm.[250] Maloney et al reported an etiology in 270 (60%) of 450 cases of HS.[228] Of the 180 cases without a defined etiology, 65 (36%) were reexamined (6 months to 28 years later) without a definite etiology, and the authors thus felt this indicated a benign and stable origin of the HS. The etiology of the remaining 270 cases was as follows: 60 (22%) tumors (23 benign lesions and 37 malignant lesions); 54 (20%) cluster headaches; 45 (16%) iatrogenic cases (e.g., neck surgery and carotid angiography); 18 (7%) Raeder syndromes; 18 (7%) trauma; 13 (5%) cervical disc protrusions; 13 (5%) congenital cases; 13 (5%) vascular occlusions; 9 (3%) vascular anomalies; and 27 (10%) miscellaneous (e.g., pneumothorax, herpes zoster, cervical rib, and mediastinal lymphadenopathy) cases. Of these

270 cases, 34 (13%) were central preganglionic HS, 120 (44%) were intermediate preganglionic HS, and 116 (43%) were peripheral postganglionic HS. Of particular interest, 13 patients in this series had undetected malignancy, and 10 were due to primary or metastatic tumor involving the pulmonary apex. Nine of these 10 (90%) patients had arm pain (due to presumed involvement of the adjacent sympathetic chain and C8-T2 nerves).

Giles and Henderson reported a 35.6% incidence (77 cases) of HS due to underlying neoplasm.[251] Of these 77 cases, 58 were malignant (mostly bronchogenic carcinoma and metastatic disease) and 19 were benign (e.g., neurofibroma and thyroid adenoma).[251]

20.18 What Are the Indications for Imaging Based on Clinical and Pharmacologic Localization?

Digre et al prospectively performed MRI studies in 33 patients with HS.[252] Of these 33 patients, 13 were preganglionic HS and 20 were postganglionic HS. Patients with preganglionic HS without brainstem signs or symptoms underwent T1-weighted sagittal imaging of the entire neck, offset to the ipsilateral side; coronal imaging of the posterior spinal cord through anterior neck; and axial T1- and T2-weighted imaging from cervical level 2 (C2) to thoracic level 6 (T6). Preganglionic HS patients with brainstem signs or symptoms underwent extensive imaging of the sympathetic axis including (1) sagittal imaging of the entire brain; (2) axial T1- and T2-weighted sagittal brain and upper cervical spine; (3) imaging offset to the side of interest; (4) coronal T2-weighted imaging of the carotid and cavernous sinuses; and (5) axial T1- and T2-weighted images from the optic chiasm to C4. Four patients had a lateral medullary infarct out of six patients with central preganglionic HS; two patients had spinal cord/root compression secondary to disc disease, one had apical Pancoast lung tumor, and one had paravertebral metastatic mass out of seven patients with preganglionic HS. There were 3 carotid dissections out of 20 postganglionic HS. Though Sergott and colleagues recommend against imaging of the cavernous sinus or orbits as processes localized to those anatomic structures are unlikely to cause an isolated HS,[234] most neuro-ophthalmologists prefer extensive imaging (e.g., MRI with MRA with and without contrast) of the entire sympathetic pathway extending to the T2 level to rule out life-threatening and other causative factors of HS.[253]

20.19 When Can You Forgo Imaging with Horner Syndrome?

Long-standing isolated postganglionic HS does not necessarily require any evaluation (class IV, level C).[2] A number of headache syndromes may be associated with a postganglionic HS, including cluster headache, migraine,[59] and Raeder syndrome.[254] Cluster headache is typically characterized by the following ipsilateral clinical manifestations in addition to headache: conjunctival injection, lacrimation, miosis, ptosis, eyelid edema, nasal stuffiness, rhinorrhea, facial hyperhidrosis, or flushing. These cluster accompaniments are related to a combination of

sympathetic hypofunction (e.g., ptosis and myosis) and parasympathetic hyperfunction (e.g., lacrimation and rhinorrhea).[255] Cremer et al reported that 19 of 39 (49%) postganglionic HS were due to cluster headache.[245,246] The headache and facial pain of Raeder syndrome can be mimicked by internal carotid artery dissection however,[256] and patients suspected of harboring a dissection should undergo appropriate imaging of the carotid artery (class IV, level C). Thus, given the difficulty in proving the chronicity of HS, most of these patients will undergo evaluation and imaging to rule out occult dissection, which can often mimic more benign etiologies. Davagnanam et al described a comprehensive algorithm for the clinical, pharmacological, and imaging evaluation of HS.[257] We outline our approach to the evaluation of anisocoria, including HS, in ▶ Fig. 20.1.

20.20 Is the Evaluation of Horner Syndrome Different in Children?

Giles and Henderson reported birth trauma to be the most common etiology of HS in children.[251] In children, cervical or thoracic tumors (e.g., cervical neuroblastoma,[258] thoracic neuroblastoma,[259] neurilemmoma, and other congenital or acquired tumors) may cause HS. We recommend a complete evaluation including imaging (e.g., CT scan) of the cervicothoracic region in all children with unexplained HS (e.g., no history of birth trauma to the brachial plexus or other iatrogenic etiology).[2,7,260] Musarella et al reviewed 405 children with neuroblastoma and 14 had HS; 9 of these 14 patients presented with HS.[261] Woodruff et al reported that 2 out of 10 children with HS had neuroblastoma.[262] In a retrospective chart review over 12 years, Mahoney et al describe 56 children with HS. Half of the children had no previously identified a cause warranting further work-up. Six of the 18 children who received urine catecholamine metabolite studies and imaging studies of the brain, neck, and chest, had responsible mass lesions identified: neuroblastoma (4), Ewing sarcoma (1), and juvenile xanthogranuloma (1). Of note, urine studies were negative on all patients.[263] Sauer and Levingohn described seven patients (younger than 11 years old) with HS due to spinal cord tumor, traumatic brachial plexus palsy, intrathoracic aneurysm, embryonal cell carcinoma, neuroblastoma, rhabdomyosarcoma, and thrombosis of the internal carotid artery.[264] Gangaputra et al describes a patient with HS due to cervical lymphadenopathy secondary to rhabdomyosarcoma rather than the tumor itself.[170] Iris coloration is not established until several months of age, and therefore iris heterochromia is not a helpful differential feature of HS in these patients after the perinatal period.[2] According to a population-based study, ptosis may be absent in about 20% of pediatric patients with HS.[234] Patients with a substantial history of perinatal head trauma, such as forceps delivery or with evidence of brachial plexus injury (Klumpke's paralysis), and pharmacologic evidence of a postganglionic HS do not require additional evaluation. Childhood HS without a history of clear trauma (including surgical and birth trauma) to the sympathetic chain often have a preganglionic (intermediate) lesion, and therefore should undergo evaluation for an underlying neoplasm such as neuroblastoma.[2,7,262,264] Other etiologies of congenital HS include viral infections (e.g., cytomegalovirus or

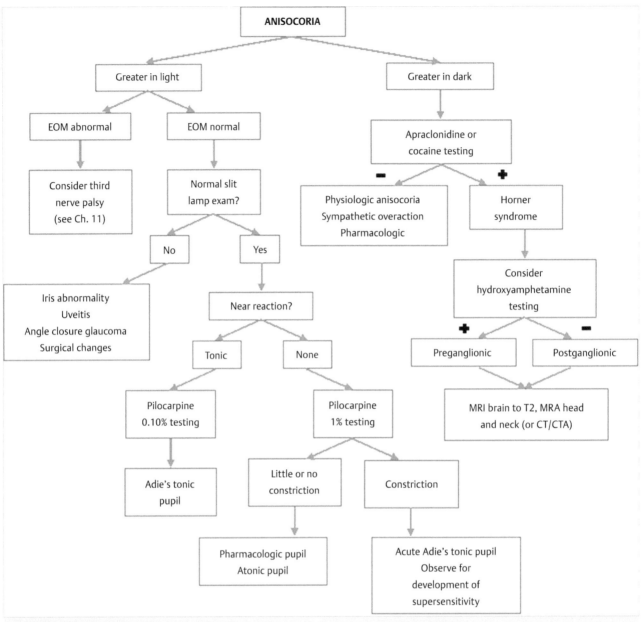

Fig. 20.1 Evaluation of anisocoria.

varicella), fibromuscular dysplasia of the internal carotid artery (possibly posttraumatic), and HS in association with other congenital anomalies (e.g., facial hemiatrophy, enterogenous cyst, and cervical vertebral anomaly).[7]

20.21 What Is Congenital HS?

Weinstein et al reported 11 patients with congenital HS and divided them into three groups based on clinical and pharmacologic testing[265]:
1. Obstetric perinatal forceps (high forceps and rotation for fetal malposition) trauma to the carotid sympathetic plexus.
2. Presumed superior cervical ganglion lesions (postganglionic lesions with facial anhidrosis).

3. Surgical (thoracic) or obstetric trauma (brachial plexus) to the preganglionic pathway.

Congenital HS[266] may result in heterochromia irides as the sympathetic innervation of the iris determines iris pigmentation. Acquired HS, however, has also been rarely reported to cause iris heterochromia.[7,134]

20.22 What Pupillary Signs May Be Observed in a Critically Ill Patient?

Box 20.7 reviews pupillary signs of importance in the intensive care unit (ICU) setting.

Box 20.7 Pupillary signs in the ICU

- Unilateral large, poorly reactive pupil:
  - Third nerve palsy (more commonly from increased intracranial pressure, but can also be seen in downward herniation due to intracranial hypotension).[267]
  - Brainstem bleed.[268]
  - Contusion of eye.
  - Accidental exposure to aerosolized anticholinergics or spilling of atropine droplets during preparation of the syringe.
  - Transient (ipsilateral or contralateral) during focal seizure or as part of an absence seizure.
- Oval unilateral nonreactive pupil:
  - Transitory appearance in brain death.
- Bilateral mydriasis with normal reaction to light:
  - Anxiety, delirium, pain.
  - Ictal state (during seizure activity).
  - Botulism.
  - Drugs: systemic atropine, aerosolized albuterol, amyl nitrate, magnesium sulfate, norepinephrine, dopamine, aminoglycoside, polypeptide, tetracycline overdose.
- Bilateral midposition and fixed to light*:
  - Brain death.
  - Midbrain lesion.
- Unilateral small, reactive:
  - Horner syndrome:
    - Traumatic carotid dissection.
    - Brachial plexopathy.
    - Internal jugular vein catheterization.
    - Extensive thoracic surgery.
  - Spastic miosis in acute corneal penetration injury.
- Bilateral miosis (reaction present but may be difficult to see):
  - Narcotic agents (e.g., morphine).
  - Any metabolic encephalopathy.
  - Respiratory distress with hypercapnia and tachypnea.
- Bilateral pinpoint, reactive*:
  - Acute pontine lesion (e.g., hemorrhage or basilar artery stroke).
  - Nonketotic hyperglycemia.

*Rarely, lesions involving both the midbrain and pons (e.g., infarcts from basilar artery thrombosis) may cause a combined syndrome with one pupil midposition and fixed and the other pinpoint and reactive.[269]

References

[1] Slavin ML. Horner syndrome with equal-sized pupils in a case with underlying physiologic anisocoria. J Neuroophthalmol. 2000; 20(1):1–2

[2] Burde RM, Savino PJ, Trobe JD. Clinical Decisions in Neuro-ophthalmology. St. Louis: Mosby Year Book; 1992:326–327, 330–332

[3] Mabuchi K, Yoshikawa H, Takamori M, Yokoji H, Takahira M. Pseudo-Argyll Robertson pupil of patients with spinocerebellar ataxia type 1 (SCA1). J Neurol Neurosurg Psychiatry. 1998; 65(4):612–613

[4] Pelak VS, Galetta SL, Grossman RI, Townsend JJ, Volpe NJ. Evidence for preganglionic pupillary involvement in superficial siderosis. Neurology. 1999; 53(5):1130–1132

[5] Sunderland S. Mechanism responsible for changes in the pupil unaccompanied by disturbances of extra-ocular muscle function. Br J Ophthalmol. 1952; 36(11):638–644

[6] Dhume KU, Paul KE. Incidence of pupillary involvement, course of anisocoria and ophthalmoplegia in diabetic oculomotor nerve palsy. Indian J Ophthalmol. 2013; 61(1):13–17

[7] Miller NR. Walsh and Hoyt's Clinical Neuro-ophthalmology. 4th ed. Baltimore: Williams and Wilkins; 1985:425–428, 500–511, 703–705, 1012–1015

[8] Walsh FB, Hoyt WF. Walsh and Hoyt's Clinical Neuro-Ophthalmology. Baltimore: Williams and Wilkins; 1969

[9] Payne JW, Adamkiewicz J, Jr. Unilateral internal ophthalmoplegia with intracranial aneurysm. Am J Ophthalmol. 1969; 68(2):349–352

[10] Crompton JL, Moore CE. Painful third nerve palsy: how not to miss an intracranial aneurysm. Aust J Ophthalmol. 1981; 9(2):113–115

[11] Fujiwara S, Fujii K, Nishio S, Matsushima T, Fukui M. Oculomotor nerve palsy in patients with cerebral aneurysms. Neurosurg Rev. 1989; 12(2):123–132

[12] Gale A, Crockard HA. Transient unilateral mydriasis with basilar aneurysm. J Neurol Neurosurg Psychiatry. 1982; 45(6):565–566

[13] Wilhelm H, Klier R, Toth B, Wilhelm B. Oculomotor nerve paresis starting as isolated internal ophthalmoplegia. Neuroophthalmology. 1995; 15:211–215

[14] Kaye-Wilson LG, Gibson R, Bell JE, Steers AJW, Cullen JF. Oculomotor nerve neurinoma, early detection by magnetic resonance imaging. Neuroophthalmology. 1994; 14:37–41

[15] Koennecke H, Seyfert S. Mydriatic pupil as the presenting sign of common carotid artery dissection. Stroke. 1998; 29(12):2653–2655

[16] Brookes CD, Golden BA, Lawrence SD, Turvey TA. Unilateral mydriasis after maxillary osteotomy: a case series and review of the literature. J Oral Maxillofac Surg. 2015; 73(6):1159–1168

[17] Nakagawa TA, Guerra L, Storgion SA. Aerosolized atropine as an unusual cause of anisocoria in a child with asthma. Pediatr Emerg Care. 1993; 9(3):153–154

[18] Coleman MJ, Tomsak RL. A 15-year-old girl with variable anisocoria. Digit J Ophthalmol. 2014; 20(1):13–14

[19] Ng J, Li Yim J. Accidental unilateral mydriasis from hyoscine patch in a care provider. Semin Ophthalmol. 2015; 30(5–6):462–463

[20] Pieris N, Baldwin AD, DeSilva P, Wong M. Unequal pupils following removal of hyoscine patch. Arch Dis Child. 2014; 99(3):196

[21] Gala PK, Henretig FM, Alpern ER, Sampayo EM. An interesting case of a unilaterally dilated pupil. Pediatr Emerg Care. 2013; 29(5):648–649

[22] Goldstein JB, Biousse V, Newman NJ. Unilateral pharmacologic mydriasis in a patient with respiratory compromise. Arch Ophthalmol. 1997; 115(6):806

[23] Ferreira-González L, Trigás-Ferrín M, Marcos PJ. Beware of nebulized bronchodilators. Arch Bronconeumol. 2015; 51(3):151

[24] Wehbe E, Antoun SA, Moussa J, Nassif I. Transient anisocoria caused by aerosolized ipratropium bromide exposure from an ill-fitting face mask. J Neuroophthalmol. 2008; 28(3):236–237

[25] Iosson N. Images in clinical medicine. Nebulizer-associated anisocoria. N Engl J Med. 2006; 354(9):e8

[26] Bisquerra RA, Botz GH, Nates JL. Ipratropium-bromide-induced acute anisocoria in the intensive care setting due to ill-fitting face masks. Respir Care. 2005; 50(12):1662–1664

[27] Morales J, Brown SM, Abdul-Rahim AS, Crosson CE. Ocular effects of apraclonidine in Horner syndrome. Arch Ophthalmol. 2000; 118(7):951–954

[28] Gelmi C, Ceccuzzi R. Mydriatic effect of ocular decongestants studied by pupillography. Ophthalmologica. 1994; 208(5):243–246

[29] Pemberton JD, MacIntosh PW, Zeglam A, Fay A. Naphazoline as a confounder in the diagnosis of carotid artery dissection. Ophthal Plast Reconstr Surg. 2015; 31(2):e33–e35

[30] Prielipp RC. Unilateral mydriasis after induction of anaesthesia. Can J Anaesth. 1994; 41(2):140–143

[31] Stewart D, Simpson GT, Nader ND. Postoperative anisocoria in a patient undergoing endoscopic sinus surgery. Reg Anesth Pain Med. 1999; 24(5):467–469

[32] Perlman JP, Conn H. Transient internal ophthalmoplegia during blepharoplasty. A report of three cases. Ophthal Plast Reconstr Surg. 1991; 7(2):141–143

[33] Alotaibi MA, Wali SO. Anisocoria with high dose ipratropium bromide inhaler. Saudi Med J. 2014; 35(5):508–509

[34] Nussdorf JD, Berman EL. Anisocoria associated with the medical treatment of irritable bowel syndrome. J Neuroophthalmol. 2000; 20(2):100–101

[35] Lee DT, Jenkins NL, Anastasopulos AJ, Volpe AG, Lee BT, Lalikos JF. Transdermal scopolamine and perioperative anisocoria in craniofacial surgery: a report of 3 patients. J Craniofac Surg. 2013; 24(2):470–472

[36] Yucel A, Yucel N, Ibis A, Ozcan H. Anisocoria associated with escitalopram. J Clin Psychopharmacol. 2015; 35(4):483–484

[37] Falavigna A, Kleber FD, Teles AR, Molossi C. Sertraline-related anisocoria. J Clin Psychopharmacol. 2010; 30(5):646–647

[38] Barrett J. Anisocoria associated with selective serotonin reuptake inhibitors. BMJ. 1994; 309(6969):1620

[39] Monteiro ML, Coppeto JR, Milani JA. Iron mydriasis. Pupillary paresis from occult intraocular foreign body. J Clin Neuroophthalmol. 1993; 13(4):254–257

[40] Scotcher SM, Canning CR, Dorrell D. Siderosis bulbi: an unusual cause of a unilaterally dilated pupil. Br J Hosp Med. 1995; 54(2–3):110–111

[41] Koutsonas A, Plange N, Roessler GF, Walter P, Mazinani BA. A case of siderosis bulbi without a radiologically detectable foreign body. Can J Ophthalmol. 2013; 48(1):e9–e11

[42] Tan AK, Humphry RC. The fixed dilated pupil after cataract surgery–is it related to intraocular use of hypromellose? Br J Ophthalmol. 1993; 77(10):639–641

[43] Meng K, Graetz DK. Moonflower-induced anisocoria. Ann Emerg Med. 2004; 44(6):665–666

[44] Wilhelm H. Pupil examination and evaluation of pupillary disorders. Neuroophthalmology. 1994; 14:283–295

[45] Macchiaiolo M, Vignati E, Gonfiantini MV, et al. An unusual case of anisocoria by vegetal intoxication: a case report. Ital J Pediatr. 2010; 36:50

[46] Andreola B, Piovan A, Da Dalt L, Filippini R, Cappelletti E. Unilateral mydriasis due to Angel's trumpet. Clin Toxicol (Phila). 2008; 46(4):329–331

[47] Firestone D, Sloane C. Not your everyday anisocoria: angel's trumpet ocular toxicity. J Emerg Med. 2007; 33(1):21–24

[48] Havelius U, Asman P. Accidental mydriasis from exposure to Angel's trumpet (Datura suaveolens). Acta Ophthalmol Scand. 2002; 80(3):332–335

[49] Van der Donck I, Mulliez E, Blanckaert J. Angel's trumpet (Brugmansia arborea) and mydriasis in a child–a case report. Bull Soc Belge Ophtalmol. 2004; 2004(292):53–56 Abstract

[50] Upshaw J, MacLean B, Losek JD. Anisocoria and topical carbamate exposure: illustrative case report. Clin Pediatr (Phila). 2010; 49(5):502–505

[51] Apt L. Flea collar anisocoria. Arch Ophthalmol. 1995; 113(4):403–404

[52] Ellenberg DJ, Spector LD, Lee A. Flea collar pupil. (letter). Ann Emerg Med. 1992; 21(9):1170

[53] Inchingolo F, Tatullo M, Abenavoli FM, et al. Severe anisocoria after oral surgery under general anesthesia. Int J Med Sci. 2010; 7(5):314–318

[54] Aceto P, Perilli V, Vitale E, Sollazzi L. Effect of anesthesia in a patient with pre-existing anisocoria. Eur Rev Med Pharmacol Sci. 2011; 15(2):211–213

[55] Orii R, Sugawara Y, Makuuchi M, Kokudo N, Yamada Y. Anisocoria in liver recipients during the perioperative period: two case reports. Biosci Trends. 2010; 4(3):148–150

[56] Jarmoc M, Shastri K, Davis F. Anisocoria after open reduction and internal fixation of a mandible fracture under general anesthesia: a case report. J Oral Maxillofac Surg. 2010; 68(4):898–901

[57] Gokcinar D, Karabeyoglu I, Ucar H, Gogus N. Post-operative nystagmus and anisocoria due to serotonin toxicity? Acta Anaesthesiol Scand. 2009; 53(5):694–695

[58] Kobayashi M, Takenami T, Kimotsuki H, Mukuno K, Hoka S. Adie syndrome associated with general anesthesia. Can J Anaesth. 2008; 55(2):130–131

[59] Drummond PD. Cervical sympathetic deficit in unilateral migraine headache. Headache. 1991; 31(10):669–672

[60] Antonaci F, Sances G, Loi M, Sandrini G, Dumitrache C, Cuzzoni MG. SUNCT syndrome with paroxysmal mydriasis: Clinical and pupillometric findings. Cephalalgia. 2010; 30(8):987–990

[61] Soriani S, Scarpa P, Arnaldi C, De Carlo L, Pausini L, Montagna P. Migraine aura without headache and ictal fast EEG activity in an 11-year-old boy. Eur J Pediatr. 1996; 155(2):126–129

[62] Berreen JP, Vrabec MP, Penar PL. Intermittent pupillary dilatation associated with astrocytoma. (letter). Am J Ophthalmol. 1990; 109(2):237–239

[63] Johkura K, Hasegawa O, Kuroiwa Y. Episodic encephalopathy with dilated pupils. Neurology. 2001; 56(8):1115–1116

[64] Masjuan J, García-Segovia J, Barón M, Alvarez-Cermeño JC. Ipsilateral mydriasis in focal occipitotemporal seizures. J Neurol Neurosurg Psychiatry. 1997; 63(6):810–811

[65] Stromberg BV, Knibbe M. Anisocoria following reduction of bilateral orbital floor fractures. Ann Plast Surg. 1988; 21(5):486–488

[66] Salvesen R. Cluster headache sine headache: case report. Neurology. 2000; 55(3):451

[67] Robert MP, Plant GT. Tournay's description of anisocoria on lateral gaze: reaction, myth, or phenomenon? Neurology. 2014; 82(5):452–456

[68] Cox TA, Goldberg RA, Rootman J. Tonic pupil and Czarnecki's sign following third nerve palsy. J Clin Neuroophthalmol. 1991; 11(1):55–56, discussion 57

[69] Jacobson DM. Benign episodic unilateral mydriasis. Clinical characteristics. Ophthalmology. 1995; 102(11):1623–1627

[70] Martín-Santana I, González-Hernández A, Tandón-Cárdenes L, López-Méndez P. Benign episodic mydriasis. Experience in a specialist neuro-ophthalmology clinic of a tertiary hospital. Neurologia. 2015; 30(5):290–294

[71] Clerici AM, Craparo G, Cafasso G, Micieli C, Bono G. De-novo headache with transient vertebro-basilar symptoms: role of embryonic hypoglossal artery. J Headache Pain. 2011; 12(6):639–643

[72] Buys Y, Buncic JR, Enzenauer RW, Mednick E, O'Keefe M. Congenital aplasia of the iris sphincter and dilator muscles. Can J Ophthalmol. 1993; 28(2):72–75

[73] Maurino V, Allan BDS, Stevens JD, Tuft SJ. Fixed dilated pupil (Urrets-Zavalia syndrome) after air/gas injection after deep lamellar keratoplasty for keratoconus. Am J Ophthalmol. 2002; 133(2):266–268

[74] Behndig A. Small incision single-suture-loop pupilloplasty for postoperative atonic pupil. J Cataract Refract Surg. 1998; 24(11):1429–1431

[75] Leavitt JA, Wayman LL, Hodge DO, Brubaker RF. Pupillary response to four concentrations of pilocarpine in normal subjects: application to testing for Adie tonic pupil. Am J Ophthalmol. 2002; 133(3):333–336

[76] Jacobson DM. Pupillary responses to dilute pilocarpine in preganglionic 3rd nerve disorders. Neurology. 1990; 40(5):804–808

[77] Jacobson DM. A prospective evaluation of cholinergic supersensitivity of the iris sphincter in patients with oculomotor nerve palsies. Am J Ophthalmol. 1994; 118(3):377–383

[78] Caputo AR, Mickey KJ, Guo S. A varicella-induced pupil abnormality. (letter). Pediatrics. 1992; 89(4 Pt 1):685–686

[79] Roberts BN, Mills PV, Hawksworth NJ. Bilateral ptosis, tonic pupils and abducens palsies following Campylobacter jejuni enteritis. Eye (Lond). 1995; 9(Pt 5):657–658

[80] Nagane Y, Utsugisawa K. Ross syndrome associated with cytomegalovirus infection. Muscle Nerve. 2008; 38(1):924–926

[81] Hodgkins PR, Luff AJ, Absolon MJ. Internal ophthalmoplegia–a complication of ocular varicella. Aust N Z J Ophthalmol. 1993; 21(1):53–54

[82] Oberacher-Velten IM, Jonas JB, Jünemann A, Schmidt B. Bilateral optic neuropathy and unilateral tonic pupil associated with acute human herpesvirus 6 infection: a case report. Graefes Arch Clin Exp Ophthalmol. 2005; 243(2):175–177

[83] Hjelle B, Appenzeller O, Mills R, et al. Chronic neurodegenerative disease associated with HTLV-II infection. Lancet. 1992; 339(8794):645–646

[84] Aydin K, Elmas S, Guzes EA. Reversible posterior leukoencephalopathy and Adie's pupil after measles vaccination. J Child Neurol. 2006; 21(6):525–527

[85] Corridan PG, Laws DE, Morrell AJ, Murray PI. Tonic pupils and human parvovirus (B19) infection. J Clin Neuroophthalmol. 1991; 11(2):109–110

[86] Weiss MJ, Hofeldt AJ, Behrens M, Fisher K. Ocular siderosis. Diagnosis and management. Retina. 1997; 17(2):105–108

[87] Wirtz PW, de Keizer RJW, de Visser M, Wintzen AR, Verschuuren JJ. Tonic pupils in Lambert-Eaton myasthenic syndrome. Muscle Nerve. 2001; 24(3):444–445

[88] Lambert SR, Yang LLH, Stone C. Tonic pupil associated with congenital neuroblastoma, Hirschsprung disease, and central hypoventilation syndrome. Am J Ophthalmol. 2000; 130(2):238–240

[89] Bruno MK, Winterkorn JM, Edgar MA, Kamal A, Stübgen JP. Unilateral Adie pupil as sole ophthalmic sign of anti-Hu paraneoplastic syndrome. J Neuroophthalmol. 2000; 20(4):248–249

[90] Wabbels BK, Elflein H, Lorenz B, Kolling G. Bilateral tonic pupils with evidence of anti-hu antibodies as a paraneoplastic manifestation of small cell lung cancer. Ophthalmologica. 2004; 218(2):141–143

[91] Müller NG, Prass K, Zschenderlein R. Anti-Hu antibodies, sensory neuropathy, and Holmes-Adie syndrome in a patient with seminoma. Neurology. 2005; 64(1):164–165

[92] Hulsman CA, Langerhorst CT. Reversible tonic pupils. J Neuroophthalmol. 2007; 27(4):308–309

[93] Haider S. Tonic pupil in lymphomatoid granulomatosis. J Clin Neuroophthalmol. 1993; 13(1):38–39

[94] Prasad S, Baccon J, Galetta SL. Mydriatic pupil in giant cell arteritis. J Neurol Sci. 2009; 284(1–2):196–197

[95] Purvin VA. Adie's tonic pupil secondary to migraine. J Neuroophthalmol. 1995; 15(1):43–44

[96] Bennett JL, Pelak VA, Mourelatos Z, Bird S, Galetta SL. Acute sensorimotor polyneuropathy with tonic pupils and an abduction deficit: an unusual

presentation of polyarteritis nodosa. Surv Ophthalmol. 1999; 43(4): 341–344

[97] Blair MP, Rizen M. Heerfordt syndrome with internal ophthalmoplegia. Arch Ophthalmol. 2005; 123(7):1017

[98] Kim JS, Yun CH, Moon CS. Bilateral tonic (Adie's) pupils in Vogt-Koyanagi-Harada syndrome. J Neuroophthalmol. 2001; 21(3):205–206

[99] Garza Leon M, Herrera-Jimenez IP, González-Madrigal PM. Complete Vogt-Koyanagi-Harada disease and Holmes-Adie syndrome: case report. Ocul Immunol Inflamm. 2014; 22(4):336–340

[100] Bodker FS, Cytryn AS, Putterman AM, Marschall MA. Postoperative mydriasis after repair of orbital floor fracture. Am J Ophthalmol. 1993; 115(3): 372–375

[101] Golnik KC, Hund PW, III, Apple DJ. Atonic pupil after cataract surgery. J Cataract Refract Surg. 1995; 21(2):170–175

[102] Halpern BL, Pavilack MA, Gallagher SP. The incidence of atonic pupil following cataract surgery. Arch Ophthalmol. 1995; 113(4):448–450

[103] Saiz A, Angulo S, Fernandez M. Atonic pupil: an unusual complication of cataract surgery. Ophthalmic Surg. 1991; 22(1):20–22

[104] Monson MC, Mamalis N, Olson RJ. Toxic anterior segment inflammation following cataract surgery. J Cataract Refract Surg. 1992; 18(2):184–189

[105] Miller D, Thomson J, Williams G, Olson S. Unilateral pupil dilation following head injury: thinking outside the (brain) box. QJM. 2011; 104(5):449

[106] Davies DR, Smith SE. Pupil abnormality in amyloidosis with autonomic neuropathy. J Neurol Neurosurg Psychiatry. 1999; 67(6):819–822

[107] Berlit P, Rakicky J. The Miller Fisher syndrome. Review of the literature. J Clin Neuroophthalmol. 1992; 12(1):57–63

[108] Caccavale A, Mignemi L. Acute onset of a bilateral areflexical mydriasis in Miller-Fisher syndrome: a rare neuro-ophthalmologic disease. J Neuroophthalmol. 2000; 20(1):61–62

[109] Cher LM, Merory JM. Miller Fisher syndrome mimicking stroke in immunosuppressed patient with rheumatoid arthritis responding to plasma exchange. J Clin Neuroophthalmol. 1993; 13(2):138–140

[110] Igarashi Y, Takeda M, Maekawa H, Ohguro H, Ohyachi H, Ogasawara K. Fisher's syndrome without total ophthalmoplegia. Ophthalmologica. 1992; 205(3):163–167

[111] Ishikawa H, Wakakura M, Ishikawa S. Enhanced ptosis in Fisher's syndrome after Epstein-Barr virus infection. J Clin Neuroophthalmol. 1990; 10(3): 197–200

[112] Mori M, Kuwabara S, Fukutake T, Yuki N, Hattori T. Clinical features and prognosis of Miller Fisher syndrome. Neurology. 2001; 56(8):1104–1106

[113] Radziwill AJ, Steck AJ, Borruat F-X, Bogousslavsky J. Isolated internal ophthalmoplegia associated with IgG anti-GQ1b antibody. Neurology. 1998; 50(1):307

[114] Sawada T, Kimura T, Kimura W, et al. Two cases of Fisher's syndrome with tectal pupil. Nippon Ganka Kiyo. 1990; 41:1833–1838

[115] Midroni G, Dyck PJ. Chronic inflammatory demyelinating polyradiculoneuropathy: unusual clinical features and therapeutic responses. Neurology. 1996; 46(5):1206–1212

[116] Shin RK, Galetta SL, Ting TY, Armstrong K, Bird SJ. Ross syndrome plus: beyond Horner, Holmes-Adie, and harlequin. Neurology. 2000; 55(12): 1841–1846

[117] Weller M, Wilhelm H, Sommer N, Dichgans J, Wiethölter H. Tonic pupil, areflexia, and segmental anhidrosis: two additional cases of Ross syndrome and review of the literature. J Neurol. 1992; 239(4):231–234

[118] Wolfe GI, Galetta SL, Teener JW, Katz JS, Bird SJ. Site of autonomic dysfunction in a patient with Ross' syndrome and postganglionic Horner's syndrome. Neurology. 1995; 45(11):2094–2096

[119] Bachmeyer C, Zuber M, Dupont S, Blanche P, Dhôte R, Mas JL. Adie syndrome as the initial sign of primary Sjögren syndrome. Am J Ophthalmol. 1997; 123(5):691–692

[120] Vetrugno R, Liguori R, Cevoli S, Salvi F, Montagna P. Adie's tonic pupil as a manifestation of Sjögren's syndrome. Ital J Neurol Sci. 1997; 18(5):293–295

[121] Morelli N, Gallerini S, Cafforio G, et al. Adie tonic pupil associated to endometriosis. Neurol Sci. 2006; 27(1):80–81

[122] Thompson HS. Adie's syndrome: some new observations. Trans Am Ophthalmol Soc. 1977; 75:587–626

[123] Thompson HS. Diagnosing Horner's syndrome. Trans Sect Ophthalmol Am Acad Ophthalmol Otolaryngol. 1977; 83(5):840–842

[124] Kardon RH, Corbett JJ, Thompson HS. Segmental denervation and reinnervation of the iris sphincter as shown by infrared videographic transillumination. Ophthalmology. 1998; 105(2):313–321

[125] Phillips PH, Newman NJ. Tonic pupil in a child. J Pediatr Ophthalmol Strabismus. 1996; 33(6):331–332

[126] Söylev MF, Saatci O, Kavukcu S, Ergin M. Adie's syndrome in childhood. Acta Paediatr Jpn. 1997; 39(3):395–396

[127] Kimber J, Mitchell D, Mathias CJ. Chronic cough in the Holmes-Adie syndrome: association in five cases with autonomic dysfunction. J Neurol Neurosurg Psychiatry. 1998; 65(4):583–586

[128] Moeller JJ, Maxner CE. The dilated pupil: an update. Curr Neurol Neurosci Rep. 2007; 7(5):417–422

[129] Fletcher WA, Sharpe JA. Tonic pupils in neurosyphilis. Neurology. 1986; 36(2):188–192

[130] Jivraj I, Johnson M. A rare presentation of neurosyphilis mimicking a unilateral Adie's tonic pupil. Semin Ophthalmol. 2014; 29(4):189–191

[131] Lam BL, Thompson HS, Walls RC. Effect of light on the prevalence of simple anisocoria. Ophthalmology. 1996; 103(5):790–793

[132] Roarty JD, Keltner JL. Normal pupil size and anisocoria in newborn infants. Arch Ophthalmol. 1990; 108(1):94–95

[133] Lepore FE. Amaurotic mydriasis. J Clin Neuroophthalmol. 1993; 13(3): 200–203

[134] Diesenhouse MC, Palay DA, Newman NJ, To K, Albert DM. Acquired heterochromia with horner syndrome in two adults. Ophthalmology. 1992; 99(12):1815–1817

[135] Zamir E, Chowers I, Banin E, Frucht-Pery J. Neurotrophic corneal endothelial failure complicating acute Horner syndrome. Ophthalmology. 1999; 106(9): 1692–1696

[136] Muri RM, Baumgartner RW. Horner's syndrome and contralateral trochlear nerve palsy. Neuroophthalmology. 1995; 15:161–163

[137] Bassetti C, Staikov IN. Hemiplegia vegetativa alterna (ipsilateral Horner's syndrome and contralateral hemihyperhidrosis) following proximal posterior cerebral artery occlusion. Stroke. 1995; 26(4):702–704

[138] Austin CP, Lessell S. Horner's syndrome from hypothalamic infarction. Arch Neurol. 1991; 48(3):332–334

[139] Mutschler V, Sellal F, Maillot C, et al. Horner's syndrome and thalamic lesions. Neuroophthalmology. 1994; 14:231–236

[140] Kauh CY, Bursztyn LL. Positive apraclonidine test in Horner syndrome caused by thalamic hemorrhage. J Neuroophthalmol. 2015; 35(3):287–288

[141] Kim JS, Lee JH, Suh DC, Lee MC. Spectrum of lateral medullary syndrome. Correlation between clinical findings and magnetic resonance imaging in 33 subjects. Stroke. 1994; 25(7):1405–1410

[142] Askari A, Jolobe OM, Shepherd DI. Internuclear ophthalmoplegia and Horner's syndrome due to presumed giant cell arteritis. J R Soc Med. 1993; 86(6):362

[143] Smith SA, Smith SE. Bilateral Horner's syndrome: detection and occurrence. J Neurol Neurosurg Psychiatry. 1999; 66(1):48–51

[144] Glemarec J, Berthelot JM, Chevalet P, Guillot P, Maugars Y, Prost A. Brachial plexopathy and Horner's syndrome as the first manifestations of internal jugular vein thrombosis inaugurating polycythemia vera. (English Version). Rev Rhum Engl Ed. 1998; 65(5):358–359

[145] Delabrousse E, Kastler B, Bernard Y, Couvreur M, Clair C. MR diagnosis of a congenital abnormality of the thoracic aorta with an aneurysm of the right subclavian artery presenting as a Horner's syndrome in an adult. Eur Radiol. 2000; 10(4):650–652

[146] Pritz MB. Ophthalmic artery aneurysm associated with Horner's syndrome. Acta Neurochir (Wien). 1999; 141(8):891–892

[147] Voide N, Borruat FX. Isolated Horner syndrome and orbital hemangioma. Klin Monatsbl Augenheilkd. 2013; 230(4):365–366

[148] Assaf M, Sweeney PJ, Kosmorsky G, Masaryk T. Horner's syndrome secondary to angiogram negative, subadventitial carotid artery dissection. Can J Neurol Sci. 1993; 20(1):62–64

[149] Cullom RD, Jr, Cullom ME, Kardon R, Digre K. Two neuro-ophthalmic episodes separated in time and space. Surv Ophthalmol. 1995; 40(3):217–224

[150] Foster RE, Kosmorsky GS, Sweeney PJ, Masaryk TJ. Horner's syndrome secondary to spontaneous carotid dissection with normal angiographic findings. (letter). Arch Ophthalmol. 1991; 109(11):1499–1500

[151] Mokri B, Schievink WI, Olsen KD, Piepgras DG. Spontaneous dissection of the cervical internal carotid artery. Presentation with lower cranial nerve palsies. Arch Otolaryngol Head Neck Surg. 1992; 118(4):431–435

[152] Vighetto A, Lisovoski F, Revol A, Trillet M, Aimard G. Internal carotid artery dissection and ipsilateral hypoglossal nerve palsy. (letter). J Neurol Neurosurg Psychiatry. 1990; 53(6):530–531

[153] Zander DR, Just N, Schipper HM. Aneurysm of the intrapetrous internal carotid artery presenting as isolated Horner's syndrome: case report. Can Assoc Radiol J. 1998; 49(1):46–48

[154] Koivunen P, Löppönen H. Internal carotid artery thrombosis and Horner's syndrome as complications of parapharyngeal abscess. Otolaryngol Head Neck Surg. 1999; 121(1):160–162

[155] Pascual-Sedano B, Roig C. Horner's syndrome due to giant cell arteritis. Neuroophthalmology. 1998; 20(2):75–77

[156] Nishino H, Rubino FA. Horner's syndrome in Wegener's granulomatosis: report of four cases. J Neurol Neurosurg Psychiatry. 1993; 56(8):897–899

[157] Cho BJ, Kim JS, Hwang JM. Horner's syndrome and contralateral abducens nerve palsy associated with zoster meningitis. Korean J Ophthalmol. 2013; 27(6):474–477

[158] Smith EF, Santamarina L, Wolintz AH. Herpes zoster ophthalmicus as a cause of Horner syndrome. J Clin Neuroophthalmol. 1993; 13(4):250–253

[159] Harada H, Tamaoka A, Yoshida H, et al. Horner's syndrome associated with mononeuritis multiplex due to cytomegalovirus as the initial manifestation in a patient with AIDS. J Neurol Sci. 1998; 154(1):91–93

[160] Emir S, Kutluk MT, Göğüş S, Büyükpamukçu M. Paraneoplastic cerebellar degeneration and Horner syndrome: association of two uncommon findings in a child with Hodgkin disease. J Pediatr Hematol Oncol. 2000; 22(2):158–161

[161] Simon T, Voth E, Berthold F. Asymmetric salivary gland 123I-meta-iodobenzylguanidine uptake in a patient with cervical neuroblastoma and Horner syndrome. Med Pediatr Oncol. 2001; 36(4):489–490

[162] Pollard ZF, Greenberg MF, Bordenca M, Lange J. Atypical acquired pediatric Horner syndrome. Arch Ophthalmol. 2010; 128(7):937–940

[163] Freeman JL, van den Brekel MW, Brown D. Carcinoma of the thyroid presenting as Horner's syndrome. J Otolaryngol. 1997; 26(6):387–388

[164] Martin TJ. Horner's syndrome, Pseudo-Horner's syndrome, and simple anisocoria. Curr Neurol Neurosci Rep. 2007; 7(5):397–406

[165] Birchler MT, Landau K, Went PT, Stoeckli SJ. Paraganglioma of the cervical sympathetic trunk. Ann Otol Rhinol Laryngol. 2002; 111(12 Pt 1): 1087–1091

[166] Ganesan S, Harar RP, Owen RA, Dawkins RS, Prior AJ. Horner's syndrome: a rare presentation of cervical sympathetic chain schwannoma. J Laryngol Otol. 1997; 111(5):493–495

[167] Hamza A, Fagan JJ, Weissman JL, Myers EN. Neurilemomas of the para-pharyngeal space. Arch Otolaryngol Head Neck Surg. 1997; 123(6):622–626

[168] Poole TR, Acheson JF, Smith SE, Steiger MJ. Horner's syndrome due to herpes zoster in the T3-T4 dermatome. J R Soc Med. 1997; 90(7):395–396

[169] Bollen AE, Krikke AP, de Jager AEJ. Painful Horner syndrome due to arteritis of the internal carotid artery. Neurology. 1998; 51(5):1471–1472

[170] Gangaputra S, Babiuch A, Bradfield YS. Cervical lymphadenopathy secondary to rhabdomyosarcoma presenting as Horner syndrome in an infant. J AAPOS. 2015; 19(2):194–196

[171] Cahill JA, Ross J. Eye on children: acute work-up for pediatric Horner's syndrome. Case presentation and review of the literature. J Emerg Med. 2015; 48(1):58–62

[172] Aronson LA, Parker GC, Valley R, Norfleet EA. Acute Horner syndrome due to thoracic epidural analgesia in a paediatric patient. Paediatr Anaesth. 2000; 10(1):89–91

[173] Liu M, Kim PS, Chen CK, Smythe WR. Delayed Horner's syndrome as a complication of continuous thoracic epidural analgesia. J Cardiothorac Vasc Anesth. 1998; 12(2):195–196

[174] Menendez C, MacMillan DT, Britt LD. Transient Horner's syndrome in a trauma patient with thoracic epidural analgesia: a case report. Am Surg. 2000; 66(8):756–758

[175] Ryan FH, Kline LB, Gomez C. Congenital Horner's syndrome resulting from agenesis of the internal carotid artery. Ophthalmology. 2000; 107(1):185–188

[176] De Marinis M. Pupillary abnormalities due to sympathetic dysfunction in different forms of idiopathic headache. Clin Auton Res. 1994; 4(6):331–338

[177] De Marinis M, Assenza S, Carletto F. Oculosympathetic alterations in migraine patients. Cephalalgia. 1998; 18(2):77–84

[178] Manzoni GC, Micieli G, Zanferrari C, Sandrini G, Bizzi P, Nappi G. Cluster headache. Recent developments in clinical characterization and pathogenesis. Acta Neurol (Napoli). 1991; 13(6):506–513

[179] Okamoto T, Kase M, Yokoi M, Suzuki Y. Reversible Horner's syndrome and dysthyroid ocular myopathy associated with Hashimoto's disease. Jpn J Ophthalmol. 2003; 47(6):587–590

[180] Pishdad GR, Pishdad P, Pishdad R. Pupillary autonomic neuropathy simulating partial Horner syndrome in diabetes mellitus and its reversal with control of blood glucose. J Neuroophthalmol. 2008; 28(3):241–242

[181] Worthington JP, Snape L. Horner's syndrome secondary to a basilar skull fracture after maxillofacial trauma. J Oral Maxillofac Surg. 1998; 56(8):996–1000

[182] Johnson S, Jones M, Zumsteg J. Brown-Séquard syndrome without vascular injury associated with Horner's syndrome after a stab injury to the neck. J Spinal Cord Med. 2016; 39(1):111–114

[183] Kerrison JB, Biousse V, Newman NJ. Isolated Horner's syndrome and syringomyelia. J Neurol Neurosurg Psychiatry. 2000; 69(1):131–132

[184] Oono S, Saito I, Inukai G, Morisawa K. Traumatic Horner syndrome without anhidrosis. J Neuroophthalmol. 1999; 19(2):148–151

[185] Naimer SA, Weinstein O, Rosenthal G. Congenital horner syndrome: a rare though significant complication of subclavian flap aortoplasty. J Thorac Cardiovasc Surg. 2000; 120(2):419–421

[186] Giannikas C, Pomeranz HD, Smith LP, Fefer Z. Horner syndrome after tonsillectomy: an anatomic perspective. Pediatr Neurol. 2014; 51(3): 417–420

[187] Hassan AN, Ballester J, Slater N. Bilateral first rib fractures associated with Horner's syndrome. Injury. 2000; 31(4):273–274

[188] Kim W, Clancy RR, Liu GT. Horner syndrome associated with implantation of a vagus nerve stimulator. Am J Ophthalmol. 2001; 131(3):383–384

[189] Scaglione M, Pinto F, Grassi R, Laporta A, Di Lorenzo G, Di Salle F. Migration of a foreign body from the pharynx to the soft tissues of the neck: delayed presentation with Horner's syndrome. AJR Am J Roentgenol. 1999; 172(4): 1131–1132

[190] Ozel SK, Kazez A. Horner syndrome due to first rib fracture after major thoracic trauma. J Pediatr Surg. 2005; 40(10):e17–e19

[191] Bayhan Gİ, Karaca M, Yazici Ü, Tanir G. A case of Horner's syndrome after the surgical treatment of pulmonary hydatid cyst. Turkiye Parazitol Derg. 2010; 34(4):196–199

[192] Thompson CG. Horner's syndrome resulting from a prolonged abnormal posture during a coma. Aust N Z J Ophthalmol. 1998; 26(2):165–167

[193] Fujisawa H, Marukawa K, Kida S, Hasegawa M, Yamashita J, Matsui O. Abducens nerve palsy and ipsilateral Horner syndrome: a predicting sign of intracranial carotid injury in a head trauma patient. J Trauma. 2001; 50(3): 554–556

[194] Perry C, James D, Wixon C, Mills J, Ericksen C. Horner's syndrome after carotid endarterectomy–a case report. Vasc Surg. 2001; 35(4):325–327

[195] Castillo BV, Jr, Khan AM, Gieser R, Shownkeen H. Purtscher-like retinopathy and Horner's syndrome following coil embolization of an intracavernous carotid artery aneurysm. Graefes Arch Clin Exp Ophthalmol. 2005; 243(1): 60–62

[196] Attar S, Krasna MJ, Sonett JR, et al. Superior sulcus (Pancoast) tumor: experience with 105 patients. Ann Thorac Surg. 1998; 66(1):193–198

[197] Everett CM, Gutowski NJ. Prostatic carcinoma presenting as brain stem dysfunction. J Neurol Neurosurg Psychiatry. 1999; 66(4):546

[198] Biousse V, Touboul P-J, D'Anglejan-Chatillon J, Lévy C, Schaison M, Bousser MG. Ophthalmologic manifestations of internal carotid artery dissection. Am J Ophthalmol. 1998; 126(4):565–577

[199] Kerty E. The ophthalmology of internal carotid artery dissection. Acta Ophthalmol Scand. 1999; 77(4):418–421

[200] Inzelberg R, Nisipeanu P, Blumen SC, Kovach I, Groisman GM, Carasso RL. Transient unilateral mydriasis as the presenting sign of aortic and carotid dissection. Neurology. 2000; 55(12):1934–1935

[201] Baumgartner RW, Arnold M, Baumgartner I, et al. Carotid dissection with and without ischemic events: local symptoms and cerebral artery findings. Neurology. 2001; 57(5):827–832

[202] Bilbao R, Amoros S, Murube J. Horner syndrome as an isolated manifestation of an intrapetrous internal carotid artery dissection. Am J Ophthalmol. 1997; 123(4):562–564

[203] Brandt T, Orberk E, Weber R, et al. Pathogenesis of cervical artery dissections: association with connective tissue abnormalities. Neurology. 2001; 57(1):24–30

[204] Brown J, Jr, Danielson R, Donahue SP, Thompson HS. Horner's syndrome in subadventitial carotid artery dissection and the role of magnetic resonance angiography. Am J Ophthalmol. 1995; 119(6):811–813

[205] Cintron R, Kattah J. Oculosympathetic paresis and hemicrania in spontaneous dissection of the internal carotid artery: Four cases and review of the literature. Neuroophthalmology. 1995; 15(5):241–248

[206] Grau AJ, Brandt T, Forsting M, Winter R, Hacke W. Infection-associated cervical artery dissection. Three cases. Stroke. 1997; 28(2):453–455

[207] Leira EC, Bendixen BH, Kardon RH, Adams HP, Jr. Brief, transient Horner's syndrome can be the hallmark of a carotid artery dissection. Neurology. 1998; 50(1):289–290

[208] Mokhtari F, Massin P, Paques M, et al. Central retinal artery occlusion associated with head or neck pain revealing spontaneous internal carotid artery dissection. Am J Ophthalmol. 2000; 129(1):108–109

[209] Purvin V, Wall M, Slavin M. Unilateral headache and ptosis in a 30-year-old woman. Surv Ophthalmol. 1997; 42(2):163–168

[210] Schievink WI, Atkinson JL, Bartleson JD, Whisnant JP. Traumatic internal carotid artery dissections caused by blunt softball injuries. Am J Emerg Med. 1998; 16(2):179–182

[211] Venketasubramanian N, Singh J, Hui F, Lim MK. Carotid artery dissection presenting as a painless Horner's syndrome in a pilot: fit to fly? Aviat Space Environ Med. 1998; 69(3):307–310

[212] Tan E, Kansu T, Saygi S, Zileli T. Alternating Horner's syndrome. A case report and review of the literature. Neuroophthalmology. 1990; 10:19–22

[213] Gasch AT. Horner's syndrome secondary to chest tube placement. Ann Ophthalmol. 1996; 28:235–239

[214] Resnick DK. Delayed pulmonary perforation. A rare complication of tube thoracostomy. Chest. 1993; 103(1):311–313

[215] Biousse V, Guevara RA, Newman NJ. Transient Horner's syndrome after lumbar epidural anesthesia. Neurology. 1998; 51(5):1473–1475

[216] Hered RW, Cummings RJ, Helffrich R. Persistent Horner's syndrome after spinal fusion and epidural analgesia. A case report. Spine. 1998; 23(3): 387–390

[217] Jeret JS, Mazurek AA. Acute postpartum Horner's syndrome due to epidural anesthesia. Arch Ophthalmol. 1995; 113(5):560

[218] Paw HG. Horner's syndrome following low-dose epidural infusion for labour: a cautionary tale. Eur J Anaesthesiol. 1998; 15(1):110–111

[219] Peñarrocha-Diago M, Sanchis-Bielsa JM. Ophthalmologic complications after intraoral local anesthesia with articaine. Oral Surg Oral Med Oral Pathol Oral Radiol Endod. 2000; 90(1):21–24

[220] Moreno E, Gómez SR, Gonzalez J, et al. Neurologic complications in liver transplantation. Acta Neurol Scand. 1993; 87(1):25–31

[221] Guccione P, Gagliardi MG, Bevilacqua M, Parisi F, Marino B. Cardiac catheterization through the internal jugular vein in pediatric patients. An alternative to the usual femoral vein access. Chest. 1992; 101(6):1512–1514

[222] Peake ST, Bollen B. Unilateral fixed dilated pupil after aortic valve replacement: an unusual combination of causes. J Cardiothorac Anesth. 1990; 4(6):737–739

[223] Reddy G, Coombes A, Hubbard AD. Horner's syndrome following internal jugular vein cannulation. Intensive Care Med. 1998; 24(2):194–196

[224] Vaswani S, Garvin L, Matuschak GM. Postganglionic Horner's syndrome after insertion of a pulmonary artery catheter through the internal jugular vein. Crit Care Med. 1991; 19(9):1215–1216

[225] Zeligowsky A, Szold A, Seror D, Vromen A, Pfeffermann R. Horner syndrome: a rare complication of internal jugular vein cannulation. JPEN J Parenter Enteral Nutr. 1991; 15(2):199

[226] Ford S, Lauder G. Case report of Horner's syndrome complicating internal jugular venous cannulation in a child. Paediatr Anaesth. 2007; 17(4): 396–398

[227] Butty Z, Gopwani J, Mehta S, Margolin E. Horner's syndrome in patients admitted to the intensive care unit that have undergone central venous catheterization: a prospective study. Eye (Lond). 2016; 30(1):31–33

[228] Maloney WF, Younge BR, Moyer NJ. Evaluation of the causes and accuracy of pharmacologic localization in Horner's syndrome. Am J Ophthalmol. 1980; 90(3):394–402

[229] Barbut D, Gold JP, Heinemann MH, Hinton RB, Trifiletti RR. Horner's syndrome after coronary artery bypass surgery. Neurology. 1996; 46(1): 181–184

[230] Szawłowski AW, Falkowski S, Morysiński T, et al. Preoperative concurrent chemotherapy and radiotherapy for local-regional and advanced squamous cell carcinoma of the thoracic oesophagus: preliminary results of a pilot study. Eur J Surg Oncol. 1991; 17(6):575–580

[231] Ebraheim NA, Lu J, Yang H, Heck BE, Yeasting RA. Vulnerability of the sympathetic trunk during the anterior approach to the lower cervical spine. Spine. 2000; 25(13):1603–1606

[232] Hood RJ, Reibel JF, Jensen ME, Levine PA. Schwannoma of the cervical sympathetic chain. The Virginia experience. Ann Otol Rhinol Laryngol. 2000; 109(1):48–51

[233] Crönlein M, Sandmann GH, Beirer M, Wunderlich S, Biberthaler P, Huber-Wagner S. Traumatic bilateral carotid artery dissection following severe blunt trauma: a case report on the difficulties in diagnosis and therapy of an often overlooked life-threatening injury. Eur J Med Res. 2015; 20:62

[234] Peterson JD, Bilyk JR, Sergott RC. But it's not all there. Surv Ophthalmol. 2013; 58(5):492–499

[235] Friedman JR, Whiting DW, Kosmorsky GS, Burde RM. The cocaine test in normal patients. Am J Ophthalmol. 1984; 98(6):808–810

[236] Van der Wiel HL, Van Gijn J. The diagnosis of Horner's syndrome. Use and limitations of the cocaine test. J Neurol Sci. 1986; 73(3):311–316

[237] Kardon RH, Denison CE, Brown CK, Thompson HS. Critical evaluation of the cocaine test in the diagnosis of Horner's syndrome. Arch Ophthalmol. 1990; 108(3):384–387

[238] Burde RM, Thompson HS. Hydroxyamphetamine. A good drug lost? (editorial). Am J Ophthalmol. 1991; 111(1):100–102

[239] Koc F, Kavuncu S, Kansu T, Acaroglu G, Firat E. The sensitivity and specificity of 0.5% apraclonidine in the diagnosis of oculosympathetic paresis. Br J Ophthalmol. 2005; 89(11):1442–1444

[240] Lebas M, Seror J, Debroucker T. Positive apraclonidine test 36 hours after acute onset of Horner syndrome in dorsolateral pontomedullary stroke. J Neuroophthalmol. 2010; 30(1):12–17

[241] Cooper-Knock J, Pepper I, Hodgson T, Sharrack B. Early diagnosis of Horner syndrome using topical apraclonidine. J Neuroophthalmol. 2011; 31(3): 214–216

[242] Martín-Moro JG, Botín DM, Muñoz-Negrete FJ. Possible effect of systemic sympatholytic drugs on apraclonidine test. Can J Ophthalmol. 2009; 44(4): 463–464

[243] deSousa JL, Malhotra R. Brimonidine for anisocoria. Ophthalmology. 2007; 114(7):1419

[244] Donahue SP, Lavin PJM, Digre K. False-negative hydroxyamphetamine (Paredrine) test in acute Horner's syndrome. Am J Ophthalmol. 1996; 122 (6):900–901

[245] Cremer SA, Thompson HS, Digre KB, Kardon RH. Hydroxyamphetamine mydriasis in normal subjects. Am J Ophthalmol. 1990; 110(1):66–70

[246] Cremer SA, Thompson HS, Digre KB, Kardon RH. Hydroxyamphetamine mydriasis in Horner's syndrome. Am J Ophthalmol. 1990; 110(1):71–76

[247] Van der Wiel HL, Van Gijn J. Localization of Horner's syndrome. Use and limitations of the hydroxyamphetamine test. J Neurol Sci. 1983; 59(2): 229–235

[248] Grimson BS, Thompson HS. Drug testing in Horner's syndrome. In: Glaser JS, et al, eds. Neuro-Ophthalmology Symposium of the University of Miami and the Bascom Palmer Eye Institute. Vol. 8. St. Louis: Mosby Year Book; 1975:265

[249] Wilhelm H, Ochsner H, Kopyciok E, Trauzettel-Klosinski S, Schiefer U, Zrenner E. Horner's syndrome: a retrospective analysis of 90 cases and recommendations for clinical handling. Ger J Ophthalmol. 1992; 1(2): 96–102

[250] Grimson BS, Thompson HS. Horner's syndrome: overall view of 120 cases. In. Thompson HS, ed. Topics in Neuro-ophthalmology. Baltimore: Williams and Wilkins; 1979:151–156

[251] Giles CL, Henderson JW. Horner's syndrome: an analysis of 216 cases. Am J Ophthalmol. 1958; 46(3 Pt 1):289–296

[252] Digre KB, Smoker WRK, Johnston P, et al. Selective MR imaging approach for evaluation of patients with Horner's syndrome. AJNR Am J Neuroradiol. 1992; 13(1):223–227

[253] Chen Y, Morgan ML, Barros Palau AE, Yalamanchili S, Lee AG. Evaluation and neuroimaging of the Horner syndrome. Can J Ophthalmol. 2015; 50(2): 107–111

[254] Pimentel J, Martins IP. Raeder's syndrome. A case with an unusual localization. Cephalalgia. 1993; 13(2):135

[255] Matharu MS, Goadsby PJ. Trigeminal autonomic cephalgias. J Neurol Neurosurg Psychiatry. 2002; 72 Suppl 2:ii19–ii26

[256] Dihné M, Block F, Thron A, Küker W. Raeder's syndrome: a rare presentation of internal carotid artery dissection. Cerebrovasc Dis. 2000; 10(2):159–160

[257] Davagnanam I, Fraser CL, Miszkiel K, Daniel CS, Plant GT. Adult Horner's syndrome: a combined clinical, pharmacological, and imaging algorithm. Eye (Lond). 2013; 27(3):291–298

[258] Abramson SJ, Berdon WE, Ruzal-Shapiro C, Stolar C, Garvin J. Cervical neuroblastoma in eleven infants–a tumor with favorable prognosis. Clinical and radiologic (US, CT, MRI) findings. Pediatr Radiol. 1993; 23(4):253–257

[259] Pelton JJ, Ratner IA. Neuroblastoma of the thoracic inlet. J Pediatr Surg. 1990; 25(5):547–549

[260] Gibbs J, Appleton RE, Martin J, Findlay G. Congenital Horner syndrome associated with non-cervical neuroblastoma. Dev Med Child Neurol. 1992; 34(7):642–644

[261] Musarella MA, Chan HS, DeBoer G, Gallie BL. Ocular involvement in neuroblastoma: prognostic implications. Ophthalmology. 1984; 91(8): 936–940

[262] Woodruff G, Buncic JR, Morin JD. Horner's syndrome in children. J Pediatr Ophthalmol Strabismus. 1988; 25(1):40–44

[263] Mahoney NR, Liu GT, Menacker SJ, Wilson MC, Hogarty MD, Maris JM. Pediatric Horner syndrome: etiologies and roles of imaging and urine

studies to detect neuroblastoma and other responsible mass lesions. Am J Ophthalmol. 2006; 142(4):651–659

[264] Sauer C, Levingohn MW. Horner's syndrome in childhood. Neurology. 1976; 26(3):216–220

[265] Weinstein JM, Zweifel TJ, Thompson HS. Congenital Horner's syndrome. Arch Ophthalmol. 1980; 98(6):1074–1078

[266] Weissberg D. Congenital Horner syndrome. J Thorac Cardiovasc Surg. 2001; 121(4):819–820

[267] Bonow RH, Bales JW, Morton RP, Levitt MR, Zhang F. Reversible coma and Duret hemorrhage after intracranial hypotension from remote lumbar spine surgery: case report. J Neurosurg Spine. 2016; 24(3):389–393

[268] Fugate JE, Mallory GW, Wijdicks EF. Ultra-early aneurysmal rebleeding and brainstem destruction. Neurocrit Care. 2012; 17(3):439–440

[269] Burns JD, Schiefer TK, Wijdicks EF. Large and small: a telltale sign of acute pontomesencephalic injury. Neurology. 2009; 72(19):1707

Index

Note: Page numbers set **bold** or *italic* indicate headings or figures, respectively.